a LANGE medical book

SYMPTOM TO DIAGNOSIS

An Evidence-Based Guide

Scott D. C. Stern, MD
Associate Professor of Medicine
Co-Director, Junior Clerkship in Medicine
Clinical Director of Clinical Pathophysiology and Therapeutics
University of Chicago
Pritzker School of Medicine
Chicago, Illinois

Adam S. Cifu, MD
Associate Professor of Medicine
Co-Director, Junior Clerkship in Medicine
University of Chicago
Pritzker School of Medicine
Chicago, Illinois

Diane Altkorn, MD
Associate Professor of Medicine
Director, Senior Student Clerkships in Medicine
University of Chicago
Pritzker School of Medicine
Chicago, Illinois

Lange Medical Books/McGraw-Hill
Medical Publishing Division

New York   St. Louis   San Francisco   Auckland   Bogota   Caracas   Lisbon   London
Madrid   Mexico City   Milan   Montreal   New Delhi   San Juan
Singapore   Sydney   Tokyo   Toronto

Symptom to Diagnosis: An Evidence-Based Guide

567890 DOC/DOC 0987

ISBN 0-07-146389-5

ISSN 1556-2719

Notice

Medicine is an ever-changing science. As new research and clinical experience broaden our knowledge, changes in treatment and drug therapy are required. The authors and the publisher of this work have checked with sources believed to be reliable in their efforts to provide information that is complete and generally in accord with the standards accepted at the time of publication. However, in view of the possibility of human error or changes in medical sciences, neither the authors nor the publisher nor any other party who has been involved in the preparation or publication of this work warrants that the information contained herein is in every respect accurate or complete, and they disclaim all responsibility for any errors or omissions or for the results obtained from use of the information contained in this work. Readers are encourage to confirm the information contained herein with other sources. For example and in particular, readers are advised to check the product information sheet included in the package of each drug they plan to administer to be certain that the information contained in this work is accurate and that changes have not been made in the recommended dose or in the contraindications for administration. This recommendation is of particular importance in connection with new or infrequently used drugs.

This book was set in Adobe Garamond by Rainbow Graphics.
The editors were Janet Foltin, Harriet Lebowitz, and Karen Davis.
The production supervisor was Sherri Souffrance.
The text designer was Eve Siegel.
The illustrator was Keyword House.
The cover designer was Aimée Nordin.
The index was prepared by Andover Publishing Services.
R.R. Donnelley and Sons, Inc. was printer and binder.

This book is printed on acid-free paper

In memory of Kim Michele Stern
Scott Stern

To Sarah for your support and confidence,
and to Amelia and Ben for your
attempts at distraction
Adam Cifu

To Bob, Danny, and Emily
Diane Altkorn

Contents

Preface

Our goal in creating *Symptom to Diagnosis* was to develop an interesting, practical, and informative approach to learning the diagnostic process in internal medicine. Interesting, because real patient cases are integrated within each chapter, complementing what can otherwise be dry and soporific. Informative, because *Symptom to Diagnosis* articulates the most difficult process in becoming a physician; namely, making an accurate diagnosis. Many other textbooks describe *diseases*, but fail to characterize the process that leads from patient presentation to diagnosis. Although students can, and often do, learn this process through intuition and experience without adequate instruction, we feel that diagnostic reasoning is a teachable skill. Furthermore, in many books the description of the disease is oversimplified, and the available evidence on the predictive value of symptoms, signs, and diagnostic test results is not included. Teaching based on the classic presentation often fails to help less experienced physicians recognize the common, but atypical presentation. This oversight, combined with a lack of knowledge of test characteristics, often leads to prematurely dismissing diagnoses.

Symptom to Diagnosis aims to help students and residents learn internal medicine and focuses on the challenging task of diagnosis. Using the framework and terminology presented in Chapter 1, each chapter addresses one common complaint, such as chest pain. The chapter begins with a case and an explanation of a way to frame, or organize, the differential diagnosis. As the case progresses, clinical reasoning is clearly articulated. The differential diagnosis for that particular case is summarized in tables that delineate the clinical clues and important tests for the leading diagnostic hypothesis and important alternative diagnostic hypotheses. As the chapter progresses, the pertinent diseases are reviewed. Just as in real life, the case unfolds in a stepwise fashion as tests are performed and diagnoses are confirmed or refuted. Readers are continually engaged by a series of questions that direct the evaluation. Each chapter contains several cases and most conclude with a diagnostic algorithm.

Symptom to Diagnosis can be used in three ways. First it is designed to be read in its entirety to guide the reader through a third-year medicine clerkship. We are confident that the text does an excellent job of teaching the basics of internal medicine. Second, it is perfect for learning about a particular problem by studying an individual chapter. Focusing on one chapter will provide the reader with a comprehensive approach to the problem being addressed: a framework for the differential diagnosis, an opportunity to work through several interesting cases, and a review of pertinent diseases. Third, *Symptom to Diagnosis* is well suited to for reviewing specific diseases through the use of the index to identify information on a particular disorder of immediate interest.

Our approach to the discussion of a particular disease is different than most other texts. Not only is the information bulleted to make it concise and readable, but the discussion of each disease is divided into 4 sections. The *Textbook Presentation*, which serves as a concise statement of the common, or classic, presentation of that particular disease, is the first part. The next section, *Disease Highlights*, reviews the most pertinent epidemiologic and pathophysiologic information. The third part, *Evidence-Based Diagnosis*, reviews the *accuracy* of the history, physical exam, and laboratory and radiologic tests for that specific disease. Whenever possible, we have listed the sensitivities, specificities, and likelihood ratios for these findings and test results. This section allows us to point out the findings that help to "rule in" or "rule out" the various diseases. We often suggest a test of choice. It is this part of the book in particular that separates this text from many others. In the final section, *Treatment,* we review the basics of therapy for the disease being considered. Recognizing that treatment evolves at an rapid pace, we have chosen to limit our discussion to the fundamentals of therapy rather than details that would become quickly out of date.

The recommendations of the Core Medicine Clerkship Guide of the Society of General Internal Medicine/Clerkship Directors in Internal Medicine was used to guide our choices of the most important presenting symptoms and diseases to be included, so that the book could serve as a textbook for students during their internal medicine rotation. To be comprehensive, the book has a companion Web site—www.symptomtodiagnosis.com—that presents the following 5 additional chapters

1. AIDS
2. Diabetes
3. Hypertension
4. Rashes
5. Screening and Health Maintenance

For generations the approach to diagnosis has been learned through apprenticeship and intuition. Diseases have been described in detail, but the approach to diagnosis has not been formalized. In *Symptom to Diagnosis* we feel we have succeeded in articulating this science and art and, at the same time, making it interesting to read.

ACKNOWLEDGMENTS

We would like to thank Sarah Stein, MD, and John Luc Benoit, MD, for their co-authorship of two chapters, Rashes and AIDS, respectively. These chapters appear on the companion Web site www.symptomtodiagnosis.com. We would also like to thank Harriet Lebowitz and Janet Foltin at McGraw Hill, who have helped us throughout this process and believed in our vision. Thanks to Jennifer Bernstein for her meticulous copyediting. Finally, our patients deserve special praise, for sharing their lives with us, trusting us, and forgiving us when our limited faculties err, as they inevitably do. It is for them that we practice our art.

Scott Stern: I would like to thank a few of the many people who have contributed to this project either directly or indirectly. First I would like to thank my wife Laura, whose untiring support throughout the last 28 years of our lives and during this project, made this work possible. Other members of my family have also been very supportive including my children, Michael, David, and Elena; my parents, Suzanne Black and Robert Stern; and grandmother, Elsie Clamage. Two mentors deserve special mention. David Sischy shared his tremendous clinical wisdom and insights with me over 10 wonderful years that we worked together. David is the best diagnostician I have met and taught me more about clinical medicine than any one else in my career. I remain in his debt. I would also like to note my appreciation to my late advisor, Dr. John Ultmann. Dr. Ultmann demonstrated the art of compassion in his dealings with patients on a day-to-day basis on a busy hematology–oncology service in 1983. Other wonderful teachers have included Dr. Gotoff, who introduced me to problem-oriented medical diagnosis, Eric Lombard, Nathan Sugarman, Bertram Kohler, and Mr. Gulla. I would like to thank Larry Wood for teaching me as a student and supporting this project as Faculty Dean, Harvey Golomb for his support as chairman, and Alex Lickerman and Halinka Brukner who encouraged me at the conception of this project.

Adam Cifu: I have always wondered: can someone be your mentor if you never informed him that he was your mentor? I thought I would take this opportunity to acknowledge my formerly unrecognized mentors and thus make the above quandary irrelevant. Each has mentored in a very different way. My parents have given me every opportunity imaginable. Claude Wintner taught me the importance of organization, dedication, and focus and gave me a model of a gifted educator. Olaf Andersen nurtured my interest in science and guided my entry into medicine. Carol Bates showed me what it means to be a specialist in general medicine and a clinician educator. Thank you.

Diane Altkorn: I want to thank the students and house officers at the University of Chicago for helping me to continually examine and refine my thinking about clinical medicine and how to practice and teach it. I have been fortunate to have many wonderful mentors and teachers. I particularly want to mention Dr. Steven MacBride, who first taught me clinical reasoning and influenced me to become a general internist and clinician educator. As a resident and junior faculty member, I had the privilege of being part of Dr. Arthur Rubenstein's Department of Medicine at the University of Chicago. Dr. Rubenstein's commitment to excellence in all aspects of medicine is a standard to which I will always aspire. His kind encouragement and helpful advice have been invaluable in my professional development. Finally, I want to thank my family. My parents have provided lifelong support and encouragement. My husband, Bob, is eternally patient and supportive of everything I do. And without my son, Danny, and my daughter, Emily, my life would be incomplete.

Scott D. C. Stern, MD
Adam S. Cifu, MD
Diane Altkorn, MD

1

I have a patient with a problem.
How do I figure out the possible causes?

THE DIAGNOSTIC PROCESS

Constructing a differential diagnosis, choosing diagnostic tests, and interpreting the results are key skills for all physicians and are some of the primary new skills medical students begin to learn during their third year. The process is similar to that used in trying to answer any scientific question and can be thought of as "bringing the scientific method to the bedside."

A. Using the information from the history and physical exam, analyze preliminary data and then pose a hypothesis regarding the most likely cause of the patient's problem. In other words, using the information from the history and physical exam, decide which diagnosis has the highest probability of being the true cause of the patient's problem.

B. Design an experiment that will obtain more data to either support or refute your hypothesis; in other words, decide which test will rule in or rule out your diagnosis.

C. Analyze the results of your experiment and decide whether you need further data, or if you need to re-formulate your hypothesis.

1. Did the test rule in the disease? If so, you can treat.

2. Did the test support the diagnosis, but left you still uncertain? If so, you need another test.

3. Did the test rule out the diagnosis? If so, you need to consider alternative diagnoses.

This chapter will take you through the steps an experienced clinician uses to construct a differential diagnosis, decide which tests to order, and interpret and apply the test results.

CONSTRUCTING A DIFFERENTIAL DIAGNOSIS

I have a patient with a problem. How do I figure out the possible causes?

PATIENT ▽1

Mrs. S is a 58-year-old woman who comes to an urgent care clinic complaining of painful swelling of her left calf that has lasted for 2 days. She feels slightly feverish but has no other symptoms such as chest pain, shortness of breath, or abdominal pain. She has been completely healthy except for mild osteoarthritis of her knees, with no history of other medical problems, surgeries, or fractures. She takes no medications and had a normal pelvic exam and Pap smear 1 month ago. Physical exam shows that the circumference of her left calf is 3.5 cm greater than her right calf, and there is 1+ pitting edema. The left calf is uniformly red and very tender, and there is slight tenderness along the popliteal vein and medial left thigh. There is a healing cut on her left foot. Her temperature is 37.7 °C. The rest of her exam is normal.

 How would you construct a differential diagnosis for Mrs. S's problem, unilateral leg swelling with erythema?

Although the "scientific method" framework forms the basis of diagnostic reasoning, in reality it is more complicated. The physician must integrate sometimes conflicting or unreliable data from the history and physical, and then sort through an often long list of possible diagnoses ranging from common to quite rare diseases. It is helpful to divide the process of constructing a differential into 2 steps.

Step 1: Develop a List of Possible Causes

There are several ways to develop a list of possible causes.

A. Memorize long lists from textbooks, which is *not* a useful approach.

B. Use an **anatomic** framework.

   1. Works well for problems such as chest pain

   2. Example list for chest pain: chest wall, pleura, lung parenchyma, heart (blood supply, valves, muscle), esophagus

C. Use an **organ/system** framework.

   1. This works well for symptoms with very broad differential diagnoses, such as fatigue.

   2. Start with broad categories, and then construct a list for each category.

   3. Example list for fatigue: endocrine (hypothyroidism, adrenal insufficiency), psychiatric (depression, anxiety), cardiovascular (ischemia, congestive heart failure), pulmonary, GI, infectious disease, etc.

D. Use a **pathophysiologic** framework.

E. Use **mnemonics.**

F. Be flexible and **combine frameworks** to fit the problem.

An anatomic framework works well for Mrs. S's unilateral swollen and red leg:

A. Skin: Stasis dermatitis

B. Soft tissue: Cellulitis

C. Calf veins: Distal deep venous thrombosis (DVT)

D. Knee: Ruptured Baker cyst

E. Thigh veins: Proximal DVT

F. Pelvis: Mass causing lymphatic obstruction

Step 2: Prioritize the List

There are 4 approaches to organizing and prioritizing the differential diagnosis for a given problem.

A. **Possibilistic approach:** Consider all known causes equally likely and simultaneously test for all of them. This is not a useful approach.

B. **Probabilistic approach:** Consider first those disorders that are more likely; that is, those with the highest **pretest probability.** (Pretest probability is the probability that a disease is present before further testing is done.)

C. **Prognostic approach:** Consider the most serious diagnoses first.

D. **Pragmatic approach:** Consider the diagnoses most responsive to treatment first.

Experienced physicians often simultaneously integrate probabilistic, prognostic, and pragmatic approaches when constructing a differential diagnosis and deciding how to choose tests (Table 1–1).

If both the leading hypothesis and active alternatives are disproved, it is extremely important to continue the diagnostic process, prioritizing and testing for other hypotheses. Sometimes the correct diagnosis seems unlikely initially.

Table 1–1. Prioritizing the differential diagnosis.

Diagnostic Hypotheses	Description	Implications for Choosing Tests
Leading hypothesis ("working diagnosis")	Single best overall explanation	Choose tests to confirm this disease (those with high specificity and high LR+)
Active alternatives ("rule outs")	Not as likely as the leading hypothesis, but serious, treatable, or likely enough to be actively sought in the patient (**"most common"** and **"must not miss"** diagnoses)	Choose tests to exclude these diseases (those with high sensitivity and very low LR–)
Other hypotheses	Not excluded, but not serious, treatable, or likely enough to be tested for initially	Test for these only if the leading hypothesis and active alternatives are disproved
Excluded hypotheses	Disproved causes	No further tests necessary

Source: Adapted from Richardson WS et al. How to use an article about disease probability for differential diagnosis. *JAMA.* 1999;281: 1214–1219.

Mrs. S has a constellation of symptoms and signs supporting the diagnosis of cellulitis as the leading hypothesis: fever; an entry site for infection on her foot; and a red, tender, swollen leg. Even without risk factors for DVT, either proximal or calf vein DVT are the active alternatives, being both common and "must not miss" diagnoses. Ruptured Baker cyst and a pelvic mass would be other hypotheses, to be looked for if cellulitis and DVT are not present. Finally, stasis dermatitis is excluded in a patient without a history of chronic leg swelling.

How certain are you that Mrs. S has cellulitis? Should you treat her with antibiotics? How certain are you that she does not have DVT? Should you test for DVT?

THE ROLE OF DIAGNOSTIC TESTING

I have a leading hypothesis and an active alternative—how do I know if I need to do a test, or if I should start treatment?

Once you have generated a leading hypothesis, with or without active alternatives, you need to decide whether you need further information before proceeding to treatment or before excluding the diagnosis. One way to think about this is in terms of certainty: how certain are you that your hypothesis is correct, and how much more certain do you need to be before starting treatment? Another way to think about this is in terms of **probability:** is **your pretest probability** of disease high enough or low enough that you do not need any further information from a test?

Step 1: Determine the Pretest Probability

There are 3 ways to determine the pretest probability of your leading diagnosis and your most important (usually most serious) active alternatives: use a validated scoring model, use information about the prevalence of certain symptoms in a given disease, and use your overall clinical impression.

A. Use a validated scoring model

1. History and physical exam findings are assigned point values, and different point totals correspond to different pretest probabilities (see Box, Validated Clinical Model for Determining Pretest Probability of DVT).

VALIDATED CLINICAL MODEL FOR DETERMINING PRETEST PROBABILITY OF DVT

Symptoms or Finding	Score
Active cancer	+1
Paralysis, paresis, or recent casting of lower extremity	+1
Recently bedridden > 3 days, major surgery within weeks	+1
Localized tenderness along deep venous system	+1
Swelling of entire leg	+1
Calf swelling > 3 cm compared with asymptomatic leg	+1
Pitting edema greater in symptomatic leg	+1
Nonvaricose collateral superficial veins	+1
Alternative diagnosis as likely or greater than DVT	−2

Key:
Score 3 or more = high probability = prevalence 75%.
Score 1 or 2 = moderate probability = prevalence 17%.
Score 0 or less = low probability = prevalence 3%.

Mrs. S has the likely alternative diagnosis of cellulitis (−2), asymmetric calf swelling (+1) and edema (+1), and slight tenderness along the deep venous system (+1), for a total score of 1, suggesting her pretest probability is 17%.

---

2. Validated scoring models are rarely available but are the most precise way of estimating pretest probability.

3. If you can find a validated scoring model, you can come up with an exact number (or a small range of numbers) for your pretest probability.

B. Use information about the prevalence of certain symptoms in a given disease.

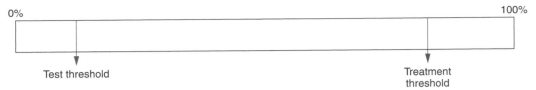

Figure 1–1. The threshold model.

1. For example, 73% of patients with pulmonary embolism (PE) have dyspnea.
2. However, this does not tell you how many patients with dyspnea have PE.
3. There is often a lot of information available about symptom prevalence.

C. Use your overall clinical impression.
   1. This is a combination of what you know about symptom prevalence and disease prevalence, mixed with your clinical experience, and the ever elusive attribute, "clinical judgment."
   2. This is just as imprecise as it sounds, and it has been shown that physicians are disproportionately influenced by their most recent clinical experience.
   3. Nevertheless, it has also been shown that the overall clinical impression of experienced clinicians has significant predictive value.
   4. Clinicians generally categorize pretest probability as low, moderate, or high.
      a. This rather vague categorization is still helpful.
      b. Do not get distracted thinking a number is necessary.

Step 2: Consider the Potential Harms

Consider the potential harms of both the disease and the treatment.

A. It is very harmful to miss certain diagnoses, such as myocardial infarction (MI) or PE, while it is not so harmful to miss others, such as mild carpal tunnel syndrome. You need to be very certain that harmful diagnoses are not present (that is, have a very low pretest probability), before excluding them without testing.

B. Some treatments, such as thrombolytics, are more harmful than others, such as oral antibiotics; you need to be very certain that harmful treatments are needed (that is the pretest probability is very high) before prescribing them without testing.

THE THRESHOLD MODEL: CONCEPTUALIZING PROBABILITIES

The ends of the bar in the threshold model represent 0% and 100% pretest probability. The **treatment threshold** is the probability above which the diagnosis is so likely you would treat the patient without further testing. The **test threshold** is the probability below which the diagnosis is so unlikely it is excluded without further testing (Figure 1–1).

For example, consider Ms. A, a 19-year-old woman, who complains of 30 seconds of sharp right-sided chest pain after lifting a heavy box. The pretest probability of cardiac ischemia is so low that no further testing is necessary (Figure 1–2).

Now consider Mr. B, a 60-year-old man who smokes and has diabetes, hypertension, and 15 minutes of crushing substernal chest pain accompanied by nausea and diaphoresis, with an ECG showing ST-segment elevations in the anterior leads. The pretest probability of

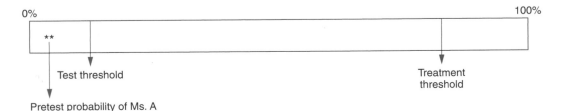

Figure 1–2. Ms. A's threshold model.

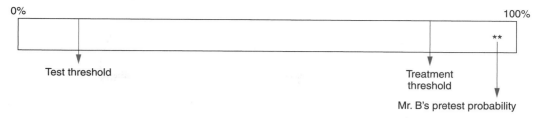

0%   **100%**

Test threshold

Treatment
threshold

Mr. B's pretest probability

Figure 1–3. Mr. B's threshold model.

an acute MI is so high you would treat without further testing, such as cardiac enzymes (Figure 1–3).

Diagnostic tests are necessary when the pretest probability of disease is in the middle, above the test threshold and below the treatment threshold. A really useful test shifts the probability of disease so much that the **posttest probability** (the probability of disease after the test is done) crosses one of the thresholds (Figure 1–4).

You are unable to find much information about estimating the pretest probability of cellulitis. You consider the potential risk of starting antibiotics to be low, and your overall clinical impression is that the pretest probability of cellulitis is high enough to cross the treatment threshold, so you start antibiotics.

You consider the pretest probability of DVT to be low, but not so low you can exclude it without testing. You are able to find a clinical scoring model that helps you quantify the pretest probability, and calculate that her pretest probability is 17% (see Box, Validated Clinical Model for Determining Pretest Probability of DVT).

You have read that duplex ultrasonography is the best noninvasive test for DVT. How good is it? Will a negative test rule out DVT?

UNDERSTANDING TEST RESULTS

How do I know whether a test is really useful—whether it will really shift the probability of disease across a threshold?

A perfect diagnostic test would always be positive in patients with the disease and would always be negative in patients without the disease (Figure 1–5). Since there are no perfect diagnostic tests, some patients with the disease have negative tests (false-negatives {FN}), and some without the disease have positive tests (false-positives {FP}) (Figure 1–6).

The **test characteristics** help you to know how often false results occur. They are determined by performing the test in patients known to have or not have the disease, and recording the distribution of results (Table 1–2).

Table 1–3 shows the test characteristics of duplex ultrasonography for the diagnosis of proximal DVT, based on a hypothetical group of 200 patients, 90 of whom have DVT.

The **sensitivity** is the percentage of patients with DVT who have a true-positive (TP) test result:

$$\text{Sensitivity} = \text{TP/total number of patients with DVT}$$
$$= 86/90 = 0.96 = 96\%$$

Since tests with very high sensitivity have a very low percentage of false-negative results (in Table 1–3, 4/90 = 0.04 = 4%), they tend to rule out disease. In other words, if you get a negative result, it is very unlikely to be a false-negative, and it is very likely the patient really does not have the disease.

The **specificity** is the percentage of patients without DVT who have a true-negative (TN) test result:

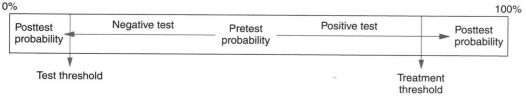

0%   **100%**

| Posttest probability | Negative test | Pretest probability | Positive test | Posttest probability |

Test threshold

Treatment threshold

Figure 1–4. The role of diagnostic testing.

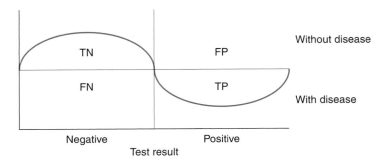

Figure 1–5. A perfect diagnostic test.

Specificity = TN/total number of patients without DVT
= 108/110 = 0.98 = 98%

Since tests with very high specificity have a low percentage of false-positive results (in Table 1–3, 2/110 = 0.02 = 2%), they tend to rule in disease. In other words, if you get a positive result, it is very unlikely to be a false-positive, and it is very likely the patient actually has the disease.

The sensitivity and specificity are important attributes of a test, but they do not tell you whether the test result will change your pretest probability enough to move beyond the test or treatment thresholds. The like-lihood ratio (**LR**), the likelihood that a given test result would be expected in a patient with the disease compared with the likelihood that the same result would not be expected in a patient without the disease, tells you how much the probability will shift.

Table 1–2. Test characteristics.

	Disease Present	**Disease Absent**
Test positive	True-positives	False-positives
Test negative	False-negatives	True-negatives

Table 1–3. Results for calculating the test characteristics of duplex ultrasonography.

	Proximal DVT Present	**Proximal DVT Absent**
Abnormal duplex US	TP = 86 patients	FP = 2 patients
Normal duplex US	FN = 4 patients	TN = 108 patients
	Total number of patients with DVT = 90	Total number of patients without DVT = 110

US, ultrasound; TP, true-positive; FP, false-positive; FN, false-negative; TN, true-negative.

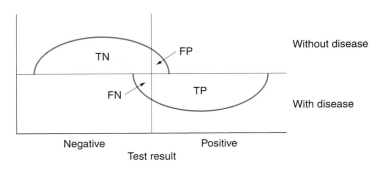

Figure 1–6. A pictorial representation of test characteristics.

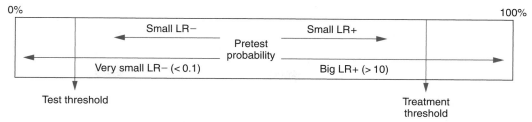

Figure 1–7. Incorporating likelihood ratios (LRs) into the threshold model.

The LR+ tells you how likely it is that a result is a true-positive (TP), rather than a false-positive (FP):

$$\text{LR+} = \frac{\text{TP/total with DVT}}{\text{FP/total without DVT}} = \frac{\%\text{TP}}{\%\text{FP}} = \frac{\textbf{sensitivity}}{\textbf{1-specificity}} = \frac{0.96}{0.02} = 48$$

LR+ should be significantly above 1, indicating that a true-positive is much more likely than a false-positive, pushing you across the treatment threshold. In general, an LR+ should be greater than 10, although a test with an LR+ between 5 and 10 is somewhat useful.

The negative likelihood ratio (**LR−**) tells you how likely it is that a result is a false-negative (FN), rather than a true-negative (TN):

$$\text{LR−} = \frac{\text{FN/total with DVT}}{\text{TN/total without DVT}} = \frac{\%\text{FN}}{\%\text{TN}} = \frac{\textbf{1-sensitivity}}{\textbf{specificity}} = \frac{0.04}{0.98} = 0.04$$

LR− should be significantly less than 1, indicating that a false-negative is much less likely than a true-negative, pushing you below the test threshold. In general, an LR− should be less than 0.1; a test with an LR− between 0.1 and 0.5 is somewhat helpful. The following threshold model incorporates LRs and illustrates how tests can change disease probability (Figure 1–7).

The closer the LR is to 1, the less useful the test; tests with an LR = 1 do not change probability at all and are useless.

When you have a specific pretest probability, you can use the LR to calculate an exact posttest probability (see Box, Calculating an Exact Posttest Probability). Table 1–4 shows some examples of how much LRs of different magnitudes change the pretest probability.

If you are using descriptive pretest probability terms such as low, moderate, and high, you can use LRs as follows:

A. A test with an LR− of 0.1 or less will rule out a disease of low or moderate pretest probability.

B. A test with an LR+ of 10 or greater will rule in a disease of moderate or high probability.

CALCULATING AN EXACT POSTTEST PROBABILITY

For mathematical reasons, it is not possible to just multiply the pretest probability by the LR to calculate the posttest probability. Instead, it is necessary to convert to odds and then back to probability.

A. **Step 1**
  1. Convert pretest probability to pretest odds.
  2. Pretest odds = pretest probability/ (1 − pretest probability).

B. **Step 2**
  1. Multiply pretest odds by the LR to get the posttest odds.
  2. Posttest odds = pretest odds × LR.

C. **Step 3**
  1. Convert posttest odds to posttest probability.
  2. Posttest probability = posttest odds/(1 + posttest odds).

For Mrs. S, the pretest probability of DVT was 17%, and the LR− for duplex ultrasound was 0.04.

A. Step 1: pretest odds = pretest probability/(1 − pretest probability) = 0.17/(1 − 0.17) = 0.17/0.83 = 0.2

B. Step 2: posttest odds = pretest odds × LR = 0.2 × 0.04 = 0.008

C. Step 3: posttest probability = posttest odds/(1 + posttest odds) = 0.008/(1 + 0.008) = 0.008/ 1.008 = 0.008

So Mrs. S's posttest probability of proximal DVT is 0.8%.

Table 1–4. Calculating posttest probabilities using likelihood ratios (LRs) and pretest probabilities.

	Pretest Probability = 5%	Pretest Probability = 10%	Pretest Probability = 20%	Pretest Probability = 30%	Pretest Probability = 50%	Pretest Probability = 70%
LR = 10	34%	53%	71%	81%	91%	96%
LR = 3	14%	25%	43%	56%	75%	88%
LR = 1	5%	10%	20%	30%	50%	70%
LR = 0.3	1.5%	3.2%	7%	11%	23%	41%
LR = 0.1	0.5%	1%	2.5%	4%	9%	19%

C. **Beware if the test result is the opposite of what you expected!**

1. If your pretest probability is high, a negative test rarely rules out the disease, no matter what the LR– is.

2. If you pretest probability is low, a positive test rarely rules in the disease, no matter what the LR+ is.

3. *In these situations, you need to perform another test.*

Mrs. S has a normal duplex ultrasound scan. Since your pretest probability was moderate and the LR– is < 0.1, proximal DVT has been ruled out. Since the test is less sensitive for calf DVT, you tentatively plan to repeat the ultrasound in 1 week. When she returns for reexamination after 2 days, her leg looks much better, with minimal erythema, no edema, and no tenderness. The clinical response confirms your diagnosis of cellulitis, and you cancel the repeat ultrasound.

I have a patient with abdominal pain. How do I determine the cause?

CHIEF COMPLAINT

PATIENT 1

Mr. C is a 22-year-old man who complains of diffuse abdominal pain.

 What is the differential diagnosis of abdominal pain? How would you frame the differential?

CONSTRUCTING A DIFFERENTIAL DIAGNOSIS

Abdominal pain is the most common cause for hospital admission in the United States. Diagnoses range from benign entities (eg, irritable bowel syndrome [IBS]) to life-threatening diseases (eg, ruptured abdominal aortic aneurysms [AAAs]). The first step in diagnosing abdominal pain is to identify the **location** of the pain. The differential diagnosis can then be narrowed to a subset of conditions that cause pain in that particular quadrant of the abdomen (Figure 2–1 and Summary table of abdominal pain by location at the end of the chapter). The **character** and **acuity** of the pain are also critical in ranking the differential diagnosis.

Other important historical points include factors that make the pain better or worse (eg, eating), radiation of the pain, duration of the pain, and associated symptoms (nausea, vomiting, anorexia, inability to pass stool and flatus, melena, hematochezia, fever, chills, weight loss, altered bowel habits, orthostatic symptoms, or urinary symptoms). Pulmonary symptoms or a cardiac history can be clues to pneumonia or myocardial infarction (MI) presenting as abdominal pain. In women, sexual and menstrual histories are important. The patient should be asked about alcohol consumption.

A few points about the physical exam are worth emphasizing. First, vital signs are just that, vital. Hypoten-

sion, fever, tachypnea, and tachycardia are important clinical clues that must not be overlooked. The HEENT exam should look for pallor or icterus. Careful heart and lung exams can reveal pneumonia or other extra-abdominal causes of abdominal pain. Of course, the abdominal exam is key. Inspection assesses for distention (often associated with obstruction or ascites). Auscultation evaluates whether bowel sounds are present. Absent bowel sounds may suggest an intra-abdominal catastrophe; high-pitched tinkling sounds and rushes suggest an intestinal obstruction. Palpation should be done last. *It is useful to slightly distract the patient by continuing to talk with him or her during abdominal palpation.* This allows the examiner to get a better appreciation of the location and severity of maximal tenderness. The clinician should palpate the area of pain last. The rectal exam should be performed, and the stool tested for occult blood. Finally, the pelvic exam should be performed in adult women and the testicular exam in men.

1

Mr. C felt well until the onset of pain several hours ago. He reports that the pain is a pressure-like sensation in the mid-abdomen, which is not particularly severe. He reports no fever, nausea, or vomiting. His appetite is diminished, and he has been unable to have a bowel movement since the onset of pain. He reports no history of urinary symptoms such as frequency, dysuria, or hematuria. His past medical history is unremarkable. On physical exam, his vital signs are stable, and he is afebrile. His cardiac and pulmonary exams are normal. Abdominal exam reveals a flat abdomen with hypoactive but positive bowel sounds. He has no rebound or guarding; although he has some mild diffuse

(continued)

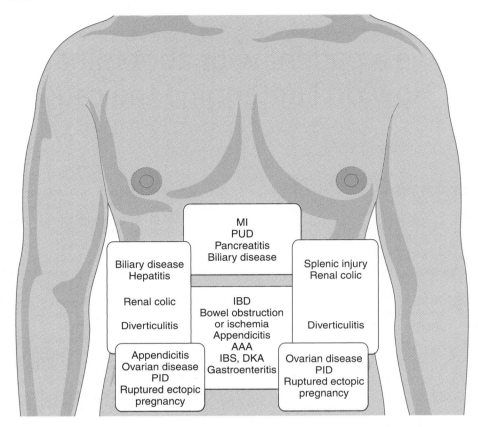

MI
PUD
Pancreatitis
Biliary disease

Biliary disease
Hepatitis

Splenic injury
Renal colic

Renal colic

IBD
Bowel obstruction
or ischemia
Appendicitis
AAA
IBS, DKA
Gastroenteritis

Diverticulitis

Diverticulitis

Appendicitis
Ovarian disease
PID
Ruptured ectopic
pregnancy

Ovarian disease
PID
Ruptured ectopic
pregnancy

PUD, peptic ulcer disease; MI, myocardial infarction; IBD, inflammatory bowel disease;
AAA, abdominal aortic aneurysm; IBS, irritable bowel syndrome; DKA, diabetic ketoacidosis;
PID, pelvic inflammatory disease.

Figure 2–1. The differential diagnosis of abdominal pain by location.

tenderness, he has no focal or marked tenderness. There is no hepatosplenomegaly. Rectal exam is nontender and stool is guaiac negative.

 At this point, what is the leading hypothesis, and what are the active alternatives? What other tests should be ordered?

ORGANIZING THE DIFFERENTIAL DIAGNOSIS

The patient's history is not particularly suggestive of any diagnosis. Focus your attention on diseases associated with mid-abdominal pain. Appendicitis should always

be considered in young, otherwise healthy patients with unexplained abdominal pain. Peptic ulcer disease (PUD) and pancreatitis may also present with epigastric or mid-abdominal pain. Table 2–1 lists the differential diagnosis.

 Mr. C reports no history of NSAID, aspirin, or alcohol ingestion. He has no known gallstones and no prior history of abdominal surgery. He reports that he is passing flatus and denies vomiting.

 Is the clinical information sufficient to make a diagnosis? If not, what other information do you need?

Table 2–1. Diagnostic hypotheses for Mr. C.

Diagnostic Hypotheses	Clinical Clues	Important Tests
Leading Hypothesis		
Appendicitis	Migration of pain from periumbilical region to right lower quadrant	Clinical exam CT scan
Active Alternatives—Most Common		
PUD	NSAID use *Helicobacter pylori* infection Melena Pain relieved by eating	EGD *H pylori* serology
Pancreatitis	Alcohol abuse Gallstones	Serum lipase
Active Alternatives—Must Not Miss		
Early bowel obstruction	Inability to pass stool or flatus Nausea, vomiting Prior abdominal surgery	Abdominal x-rays CT scan Small bowel study Barium enema

Leading Hypothesis: Appendicitis

Textbook Presentation

The classic presentation of appendicitis is abdominal pain that is initially diffuse and then migrates toward the RLQ to McBurney point (1.5–2 inches from the anterior superior iliac crest toward umbilicus). Patients often complain of bloating and anorexia. With time, parietal peritoneal inflammation results in localization of the pain, increased intensity of the pain, and guarding and rebound.

Disease Highlights

A. Appendicitis, one of most common causes of acute abdomen, is secondary to obstruction of appendiceal orifice, with subsequent swelling, ischemia, necrosis, and perforation.

B. The risk of perforation increases steadily with age (ages 10–40, 10%; age 60, 30%; and age > 75, 50%).

Evidence-Based Diagnosis

A. History is particularly important in women. Consider pelvic inflammatory disease (PID), ruptured ectopic pregnancy, and ruptured ovarian cyst, which can mimic appendicitis. The most useful clinical clues that suggest PID include the following:

1. History of PID

2. Vaginal discharge

3. Cervical motion tenderness on pelvic exam

 Rule out ectopic pregnancy in women of child-bearing age who complain of abdominal pain by testing urine for β-HCG.

B. Fever (temperature > 38.1 °C) is neither sensitive nor specific for appendicitis.

1. Sensitivity, 15–67%; specificity, 85%

2. LR+, 1; LR−, 1

3. Even among patients with perforated appendices, the sensitivity of fever is only 40%.

C. Abdominal exam evaluates tenderness, guarding, and rebound.

1. Tenderness over McBurney point is present in only 50% of patients with appendicitis

2. Guarding (moderate to severe)

   a. Sensitivity, 46%; specificity, 92%

   b. LR+, 5.5; LR−, 0.59

   c. Guarding was completely absent in 22% of patients with appendicitis.

3. Rebound (moderate to severe)

   a. Sensitivity, 61%; specificity, 82%

   b. LR+, 3.45; LR−, 0.47

   c. Rebound was completely absent in 16%.

 Fever, severe tenderness, guarding, and rebound may be absent in patients with appendicitis.

D. WBC

1. Only *very low* WBC in patients without severe rebound or guarding makes appendicitis unlikely.

   a. WBC < 7000/mcL: sensitivity, 98%; LR−, 0.1

   b. A low WBC does not exclude appendicitis in

patients who have severe rebound or guarding; 80% of such patients had appendicitis even when WBC < 8000/mcL.

2. Elevated WBCs (> 17,000) increase the LR of appendicitis: Sensitivity, 15%; specificity, 98%; LR+, 7.5

3. WBCs closer to normal are not diagnostic.

    a. WBC > 11,000: Sensitivity, 76%; specificity, 74%

    b. LR+, 3.1; LR–, 0.3

 The WBC is not reliably elevated in patients with acute appendicitis.

E. Urine β-HCG test should be done to rule out ectopic pregnancy.

F. Plain radiography is useful only to detect free air or signs of another process (ie, small bowel obstruction [SBO]).

G. CT scanning is an accurate imaging method and is cost effective when clinical suspicion is high.

    1. 96–98% sensitive, 98% specific; LR+, 49; LR–, 0.05–0.08

    2. Recent study results show only 3% of patients who had a CT scan performed preoperatively underwent unnecessary appendectomy versus 6–13% of patients who did not have a CT scan performed.

    3. Although ultrasonography is inferior to CT scanning, it should be substituted for CT scanning in pregnant patients.

MAKING A DIAGNOSIS

Mr. C's symptoms are consistent with—but certainly not diagnostic of—appendicitis. None of the historical features (ie, no alcohol use, NSAID ingestion, or prior abdominal surgery) suggest any of the alternative diagnoses of pancreatitis, PUD, or bowel obstruction. Diagnostic options include obtaining a CBC (clearly of limited value), continued observation and reexamination, surgical consultation, and obtaining a CT scan. Given the lack of evidence for any of the less concerning possibilities you remain somewhat concerned that the patient may have early appendicitis. You elect to observe the patient, obtain a CBC and lipase, and ask for a surgical consult.

 Frequent clinical observations are exceptionally useful when evaluating a patient with possible appendicitis.

 The CBC reveals a WBC of 8.7% (86% neutrophils, 0% basophils) and a Hct of 44%. The lipase is normal. The surgical resident evaluates the patient who complains that the pain is now more severe in the RLQ. On exam, the patient's abdomen is moderately tender but still without rebound or guarding. The surgical resident agrees that the normal CBC and absence of fever do not exclude appendicitis and recommends an abdominal CT scan.

The migration of pain to the RLQ is suggestive of appendicitis as well as diverticulitis, Crohn disease, and colon cancer (unlikely in this age group). If our patient were a woman, PID and ovarian pathology (ruptured ectopic pregnancy, ovarian torsion, or ruptured ovarian cyst) would also need to be considered. The patient's age argues against diverticulitis or colon cancer.

 Diffuse abdominal pain that subsequently localizes and becomes more constant, suggests parietal peritoneal inflammation.

 The CT scan reveals a hypodense fluid collection on the right side inferior to the cecum. An appendolith is seen. The interpretation is possible appendiceal perforation versus Crohn disease.

CASE RESOLUTION

The patient's symptom complex, particularly the migration, localization, and intensification of pain are highly suggestive of appendicitis. CT findings make this diagnosis likely. At this point, surgical exploration is appropriate.

 The patient undergoes surgery and purulent material is found in the peritoneal cavity. A necrotic appendix is removed, and the peritoneal cavity is irrigated. The patient is treated with broad-spectrum antibiotics and does well postoperatively.

Treatment of Appendicitis

A. Observation is critical

B. Monitor urinary output, vital signs

C. IV fluid resuscitation

D. Broad-spectrum antibiotics

E. Urgent appendectomy

CHIEF COMPLAINT

PATIENT ⑂2

Ms. R is a 50-year-old woman who comes to the office complaining of abdominal pain. The patient reports that she has been having "episodes" or "attacks" of abdominal pain over the last several months. She reports that the attacks of pain are in the epigastrium, last up to 4 hours, and often awaken her at night. The pain is described as a severe cramping-like sensation that is very intense and steady for hours. Occasionally, the pain radiates to the right back. The pain is associated with emesis. She may get several attacks in a week or go weeks or months without them. She reports that the color of her urine and stool are normal. On physical exam, her vital signs are stable. She is afebrile. On HEENT exam, she is anicteric. Her lungs are clear, and cardiac exam is unremarkable. Abdominal exam is soft with only mild epigastric discomfort to deep palpation. Murphy sign (tenderness in the right upper quadrant [RUQ] with palpation during inspiration) is negative. Rectal exam reveals guaiac-negative stool.

 At this point, what is the leading hypothesis, and what are the active alternatives? What tests should be ordered?

ORGANIZING THE DIFFERENTIAL DIAGNOSIS

The key features of Ms. R's abdominal pain are its epigastric location, episodic nature, and its severe intensity. Epigastric pain is commonly caused by PUD, biliary colic, and pancreatitis. Episodic abdominal pain is often caused by IBS, biliary colic, mesenteric ischemia, and renal colic. Severe, intense, crampy pain suggests obstruction of a hollow visceral (ie, biliary colic, bowel obstruction, or ureteral obstruction from stone). Given the epigastric location, recurring episodic nature, and intensity of the pain, biliary colic is most likely. Table 2–2 lists the differential diagnosis.

 Biliary colic, renal colic, mesenteric ischemia, and IBS can all present with recurring well-defined discrete *"episodes"* of pain.

 Ms. R has no prior history of abdominal pain, nor are the episodes relieved by defecation. There is no history of alcohol bingeing, NSAID use, known PUD, or abdominal surgery. The pain does not improve with food or antacids. She denies any history of flank pain or hematuria. She denies inability to pass stool or flatus. There is no history of atrial fibrillation, MI, congestive heart failure, coronary artery disease, or peripheral vascular disease.

 Is the clinical information sufficient to make a diagnosis? If not, what other information do you need?

Leading Hypothesis: Biliary Colic

Textbook Presentation

Gallstone disease may present as asymptomatic cholelithiasis, biliary colic, cholecystitis, cholangitis, or pancreatitis. The pattern depends on the location of the stone and its chronicity. Patients with biliary colic typically present with intense abdominal pain that begins 1 or more hours after eating. The pain is usually located in the RUQ, although epigastric pain is also common. The pain may radiate to the back and may be associated with nausea and vomiting. The pain usually lasts for more than 30 minutes and may last for hours.

Table 2–2. Diagnostic hypotheses for Ms. R.

Diagnostic Hypotheses	Clinical Clues	Important Tests
Leading Hypothesis		
Biliary colic	Episodic and crampy pain may radiate to back	Ultrasonography
Active Alternatives—Most Common		
IBS	Long history (years) of intermittent pain relieved by defecation or associated with diarrhea	Absence of alarm symptoms (eg, anemia, fever, weight loss, positive fecal occult blood test) Exclusion of other diagnoses
PUD	NSAID use *Helicobacter pylori* infection Melena Pain relieved by eating or by antacids	EGD *H pylori* serology
Pancreatitis	Alcohol abuse Gallstones	Serum lipase
Renal colic	Hematuria Radiation to flank, groin, genitals	Urinalysis Renal CT scan
Active Alternatives—Must Not Miss		
Early bowel obstruction	Inability to pass stool or flatus Nausea, vomiting Prior surgery	Abdominal x-rays CT scan Small bowel study Barium enema
Mesenteric ischemia	Postprandial pain Associated weight loss Atrial fibrillation, MI, CHF, CAD, peripheral vascular disease	Mesenteric Doppler, angiography

Disease Highlights

A. Asymptomatic cholelithiasis

  1. Predisposing factors

    a. Increasing age is the predominant risk factor. The prevalence is 8% in patients older than 40 years and 20% in those older than 60 years (Figure 2–2).

    b. Obesity

    c. High fat diets

    d. Gender: more women are affected than men (risk increased during pregnancy)

    e. Prolonged fasting

    f. Malabsorption of bile salts (Crohn disease)

    g. Hemolytic anemias can lead to increased bilirubin excretion and bilirubin stones (ie, thalassemia, sickle cell disease)

  2. Annual risk of developing biliary colic in patients with asymptomatic gallstones is 1–4%.

  3. Cholecystectomy not advised for patients with asymptomatic cholelithiasis.

 Make sure the gallstones are causing the pain before advising cholecystectomy.

B. Biliary colic

  1. Occurs when gallstone becomes lodged in cystic duct and the gallbladder contracts against the obstruction

  2. Presents as one of the classic visceral obstructive syndromes with severe, constant, and crampy waves of pain that incapacitate the patient

  3. The pain usually lasts < 2–4 hours. Longer episodes suggest cholecystitis.

  4. Characterized by episodes of pain with pain free intervals of weeks to years.

  5. Pain begins 1–4 hours after eating or may awaken the patient during the night. May be precipitated by fatty meals.

  6. The pain is usually associated with nausea and vomiting.

  7. Resolution occurs if the stone comes out of the gallbladder neck. The intense pain improves fairly rapidly, although mild discomfort may persist for 1 to 2 days.

  8. Biliary colic recurs in 50% of symptomatic patients.

  9. Complications (eg, pancreatitis, acute cholecystitis, or ascending cholangitis) occur in 1–2% of patients with biliary colic per year.

  10. Colic occasionally develops in patients without stones secondary to sphincter of Oddi dysfunction or scarring leading to obstruction.

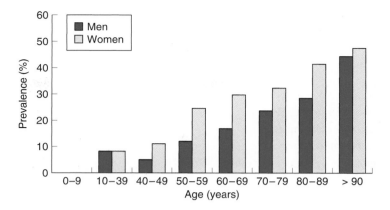

Figure 2–2. Prevalence of asymptomatic gallstones by age. (Reproduced, with permission, from the BMJ Publishing Group, Bateson MC. Gallbladder disease. *BMJ*. 1999;318:1745–1748.)

Evidence-Based Diagnosis

A. Pain is located in RUQ in 54% of cases and in the epigastrium in 34% of cases. It may occur as a band across the entire upper abdomen, or rarely in the mid-abdomen. Pain may radiate to back, right flank, or chest.

B. Ultrasonography is the test of choice; it is 89% sensitive, 97% specific, and has an LR+ of 30. (CT scan is only 79% sensitive.)

MAKING A DIAGNOSIS

Ms. R's history suggests biliary colic. You order an ultrasound of the RUQ.

A RUQ ultrasound reveals multiple small gallstones within the gallbladder. The common bile duct (CBD) is normal and no other abnormalities are seen. A serum lipase is normal and serology for *Helicobacter pylori* is negative.

Have you crossed a diagnostic threshold for the leading hypothesis, biliary colic? Have you ruled out the active alternatives? Do other tests need to be done to exclude the alternative diagnoses?

Alternative Diagnosis: IBS

Textbook Presentation

Patients often complain of intermittent diarrhea or constipation or both of *years* duration. The diarrhea is often associated with cramps that are relieved by defecation. Pain cannot be explained by structural or biochemical abnormalities. Weight loss or anemia should alert the clinician to other possibilities.

New persistent *changes* in bowel habits (either diarrhea or constipation) should be thoroughly evaluated to exclude colon cancer, IBD, or other process. An assumption of IBS in such patients is inappropriate.

Disease Highlights

A. Affects 20% of adults, women 3 times more than men

B. Etiology is a combination of altered motility, visceral hypersensitivity, and psychological factors.

Evidence-Based Diagnosis

A. History: Manning criteria (≥ 2 of the following)
   1. Abdominal distention
   2. Pain relief with bowel movement
   3. Pain associated with more frequent stools
   4. Pain associated with loose stools
   5. Sensitivity, 91%; specificity 70%
   6. LR+, 3.0; LR–, 0.13

B. Alarm symptoms (suggest alternative diagnosis and necessitate evaluation)

1. Positive fecal occult blood test or rectal bleeding

2. Anemia

3. Weight loss

4. Fever

5. Persistent diarrhea causing dehydration

6. Severe constipation or fecal impaction

7. Family history of colorectal cancer

8. Onset of symptoms at age 50 years or older

C. Laboratory studies

1. No known biochemical or structural markers for IBS.

2. Diagnostic studies performed to exclude other disorders.

3. Common recommendations include a CBC, liver function tests, TSH, basic metabolic panel (electrolytes, BUN, and creatinine) and flexible sigmoidoscopy for patients under 50; perform colonoscopy for those over 50 and obtain a biopsy to rule out microscopic colitis.

4. There is no evidence that routine flexible sigmoidoscopy or colonoscopy is necessary in young patients without alarm symptoms.

Treatment

A. Nonspecific management

1. Certain foods may worsen symptoms in some patients.

2. Common offenders include milk products, caffeine, alcohol, fatty foods, gas-producing vegetables, sorbitol products (sugarless gum and diet candy).

3. A food diary can help identify triggers.

B. Specific therapy based on predominant syndrome.

1. When abdominal pain is the predominant symptom

a. Modify diet when applicable

b. Medications include anticholinergics (dicyclomine, hyoscyamine), nitrates, tricyclics (amitriptyline or nortriptyline) or smooth muscle relaxants (effective but not available in United States).

2. When diarrhea is the predominant symptom

a. Change diet when applicable

b. Medications include loperamide, diphenoxylate, and cholestyramine.

3. When constipation is the predominant symptom

a. Change in diet (fiber, psyllium)

b. Osmotic laxative: Lactulose, polyethylene glycol, or other

c. Tegaserod, a visceral serotonin receptor agonist, has been approved for women with IBS in whom constipation is the dominant symptom.

(1) Adverse effects include diarrhea.

(2) Avoided in patients with gallbladder disease.

C. Treat underlying lactose intolerance. Such treatment in lactase deficient individuals with IBS markedly reduces outpatient visits.

Alternative Diagnosis: PUD

See Chapter 22, Unintentional Weight Loss.

Alternative Diagnosis: Ischemic Bowel

Three distinct clinical subtypes of ischemic bowel include chronic mesenteric ischemia (chronic small bowel ischemia), acute mesenteric ischemia (acute ischemia of small bowel) and ischemic colitis (ischemia of the large bowel).

1. Chronic Mesenteric Ischemia

Textbook Presentation

Chronic mesenteric ischemia typically occurs in patients with vascular disease. Presenting manifestations include chronic postprandial abdominal pain (often in the first hour and diminishing 1–2 hours later), food fear, and weight loss.

Disease Highlights

A. Secondary to near obstructive atherosclerotic disease of the superior mesenteric artery (SMA) or celiac artery

B. Although asymptomatic stenosis and occlusions of the SMA and celiac artery are common, symptomatic chronic mesenteric ischemia is rare (2/100,000).

C. 74% of cases occur in women

Evidence-Based Diagnosis

A. Exclude more common disorders (ie, PUD and gallstone disease).

B. Vascular screening with Doppler ultrasonography, followed by magnetic resonance angiography or angiography for patients with abnormal results.

C. The finding of stenosis does not prove that symptoms are secondary to ischemia.

Treatment

Surgical repair or angioplasty (with stent) is the only treatment.

2. Acute Mesenteric Ischemia

Textbook Presentation

Acute mesenteric ischemia occurs in patients with risk factors for systemic embolization (ie, recent MI, atrial fibrillation). Patients have acute severe abdominal pain that is typically out of proportion to their relatively benign physical exam.

Disease Highlights

A. Secondary to acute embolization or thrombosis of an artery supplying the small bowel (75%); SMA affected more often than celiac artery.

B. In 25% of cases, acute mesenteric ischemia is secondary to low flow and nonocclusive mesenteric ischemia (NOMI).

C. Patients have acute abdominal pain that is often out of proportion to their abdominal exam. If left untreated, bowel infarction will develop.

D. Incidence: 0.1–0.3% of hospital admissions

E. Atrial fibrillation, MI, congestive heart failure, and angiography of abdominal aorta as well as NOMI may cause acute mesenteric ischemia.

F. Mortality is 65%.

Evidence-Based Diagnosis

A. Some cases are diagnosed intraoperatively due to acute presentation.

B. Doppler ultrasonography is insensitive due to distended bowel.

C. Sensitivity of CT is poor (64%).

D. Angiography is gold standard.

Treatment

A. Surgery or angiographic thrombolytic therapy or both

B. Broad-spectrum antibiotics

C. Volume resuscitation

D. For patients with NOMI, improved perfusion is paramount.

3. Ischemic Colitis

Textbook Presentation

Ischemic colitis typically presents with rectal bleeding, and patients may have mild to moderate left-sided abdominal pain.

Disease Highlights

Disease is secondary to inadequate blood supply to the watershed areas of the colon, most commonly the splenic flexure, descending colon, and rectosigmoid junction. Vascular occlusion is *uncommon* and the precipitating event is often unclear.

Evidence-Based Diagnosis

A. Colonoscopy is the preferred test to evaluate ischemic colitis.

B. Vascular studies are usually normal and not indicated.

Treatment

Therapy is primarily supportive with bowel rest, hydration, and broad-spectrum antibiotics. Colonic infarction occurs in a small percentage of patients (15%) and requires segmental resection.

CASE RESOLUTION

Ms. R discussed her case with her primary care physician and surgeon. Both agree that her symptom complex and ultrasound suggest biliary colic. Furthermore, there was no evidence of any of the alternative diagnoses. The normal lipase effectively rules out pancreatitis, and the combination of no NSAIDs and a negative H pylori serology makes PUD very unlikely. She also lacked any risk factors for mesenteric ischemia. They recommend surgery, which she schedules for the end of the summer.

Treatment of Biliary Colic

A. Patients with biliary colic should be offered cholecystectomy.

B. Lithotripsy is not advised.

C. Dissolution therapies are slow and reserved for non-surgical candidates.

FOLLOW-UP

Ms. R returns 3 weeks later (and prior to her scheduled surgery) in acute distress. She

(continued)

reports that her pain began last evening, is in the same location as her previous bouts of pain, but unlike her previous episodes, the pain has persisted. She is very uncomfortable. She reports that her urine has changed color and is now quite dark "like tea." In addition, she complains of "teeth chattering" chills. On physical exam, Ms. R is febrile (38.5 °C). Her other vital signs are stable. Sclera are anicteric and cardiac and pulmonary exams are all completely normal. Abdominal exam reveals moderate tenderness in the epigastrium and RUQ. Murphy sign is positive.

At this point, what is the leading hypothesis and what are the active alternatives? What other tests should be ordered?

ORGANIZING THE DIFFERENTIAL DIAGNOSIS

The persistence of Ms. R's prior abdominal pain raises several possibilities. The first consideration should be that the current symptom complex is in some way related to her known biliary colic.

Although the persistent pain may suggest cholecystitis (due to a stone lodged in the cystic duct), the dark urine is an important clinical clue. Dark urine suggests bile in the urine (bilirubinuria).

Dark urine suggests bilirubinuria and may precede icterus.

Bilirubinuria only occurs in patients with conjugated hyperbilirubinemia. Bilirubinuria or conjugated hyperbilirubinemia occur in patients with either CBD obstruction or hepatitis. In our patient, the preexistent biliary colic and RUQ pain makes the most likely etiology CBD obstruction due to migration of a stone into the CBD (choledocholithiasis.) Isolated cystic duct obstruction (ie, cholecystitis) does not cause hyperbilirubinemia or significant increases in ALT (SGPT) or AST (SGOT). Finally, Ms. R's fever suggests that the CBD obstruction has been complicated by ascending infection (ascending cholangitis), a life-threatening condition.

Rigors (defined as visibly shaking or teeth chattering chills) suggests bacteremia and should increase the suspicion of a life-threatening bacterial infection.

Other considerations include pancreatitis, which may be caused by CBD obstruction and hepatitis. While hepatitis can cause RUQ pain, bilirubinuria, and hyperbilirubinemia, it would also require giving Ms. R. another unrelated diagnosis and is therefore less likely. Table 2–3 lists the differential diagnosis.

Laboratory results include WBC 17,000/mcL (84% neutrophils, 10% bands). Hct is 38%, lipase 17 units/L, alkaline phosphatase 467 units/L (nl 30–120), bilirubin 4.2 mg/dL (nl 3.0 mg/dL conjugated), GGT 246 units/L (nl 8–35), ALT, 100 units/L (nl 15–59). Ultrasound shows sludge and stones within the gallbladder. No CBD dilatation or CBD stone is seen. Blood cultures are ordered and you initiate broad-spectrum IV antibiotics (ie, ampicillin, gentamicin, and metronidazole).

Is the clinical information sufficient to make a diagnosis of ascending cholangitis? If not, what other information do you need?

Table 2–3. Diagnostic hypotheses for Ms. R on follow-up.

Diagnostic Hypotheses	Clinical Clues	Important Tests
Leading Hypothesis		
Ascending cholangitis	Right upper quadrant or epigastric pain Dark urine Fever Rigors	Ultrasound ERCP CBC Blood cultures
Active Alternatives—Most Common		
Acute cholecystitis	Right upper quadrant pain Fever	Ultrasound
Pancreatitis	Alcohol abuse, gallstones	Serum lipase
Hepatitis	Right upper quadrant pain Nausea Dark urine	Elevated ALT and AST Viral serologies

Leading Hypothesis: Choledocholithiasis and Ascending Cholangitis

Textbook Presentation

Patients typically have some form of CBD obstruction (most often from gallstones); RUQ pain, fever, and jaundice are presenting symptoms.

Disease Highlights

A. 10–15% of patients with symptomatic gallstones have stones within the CBD.

B. 55% of patients with retained stones in the CBD become symptomatic.

C. Ascending infection may follow obstruction (ascending cholangitis) and should be suspected in patients with fever and leukocytosis.

D. Complications: Pancreatitis 5%, severe pancreatitis 0.7%, death 0.2%

Evidence-Based Diagnosis

A. Ultrasound is *not* sensitive for choledocholithiasis. Dilated CBD is seen in only 25%.

B. CT scanning is only 75% sensitive for choledocholithiasis.

C. ERCP
1. Invasive endoscopy that allows for direct cannulation of CBD, extraction of CBD stones, and sphincterotomy
2. > 90% sensitive, 99% specific for diagnosis
3. Any of the following suggests choledocholithiasis and should prompt preoperative ERCP or intraoperative cholangiogram (Table 2–4):
   a. Cholangitis, jaundice, dilated CBD on ultrasound, elevated alkaline phosphatase, pancreatitis.
   b. CBD stones are present in 5–8% of patients without any of the aforementioned risk factors.

D. Magnetic resonance cholangiopancreatography (MRCP)
1. Noninvasive scan visualizes CBD and adjacent structures
2. For obstruction: 97% sensitive, 98% specific; LR+ is 49, LR– is 0.03
3. For stone detection: 92% sensitive, 97% specific; LR+ is 31, LR– is 0.08
4. Less sensitive for malignancy (88%)

Table 2–4. Test characteristics for choledocholithiasis.

Finding	Sensitivity	Specificity	LR+	LR–
Cholangitis	11%	99%	18.3	0.93
Preoperative jaundice	36%	97%	10.1	0.69
Dilated CBD on ultrasound	42%	96%	6.9	0.77
Elevated alkaline phosphatase	57%	86%	2.6	0.65
Elevated amylase	11%	95%	1.5	0.99

CBD, common bile duct.

Modified with permission from Springer. Paul, A. Diagnosis and treatment of common bile duct stones. *Surg Endosc.* 1998; 12:856–864.

5. Probably most useful in patients for whom index of suspicion of CBD obstruction is low (and unlikely to need sphincterotomy or stone extraction.)

MAKING A DIAGNOSIS

Neither dilation of the CBD nor CBD stone can be seen on ultrasound (but is only 25% sensitive). You still suspect choledocholithiasis because of the jaundice and increased transaminases.

Twenty-four hours later, blood cultures are positive for *E coli* (consistent with ascending cholangitis).

Have you crossed a diagnostic threshold for the leading hypothesis, ascending cholangitis? Have you ruled out the active alternatives? Do other tests need to be done to exclude the alternative diagnoses?

Alternative Diagnosis: Acute Hepatitis

See Abnormal liver tests in Chapter 18, Jaundice.

Alternative Diagnosis: Acute Cholecystitis

Textbook Presentation

Persistent RUQ or epigastric pain, fever, nausea, and vomiting are typical presenting symptoms.

Disease Highlights

A. Secondary to prolonged cystic duct obstruction (> 12 hours).

B. Persistent obstruction results in increasing gallbladder inflammation and pain.

C. Jaundice and marked elevation of liver enzymes are seen only if the stone migrates into the CBD and causes obstruction.

Evidence-Based Diagnosis

A. No clinical finding is sufficiently sensitive to rule out cholecystitis.

   1. Fever: present in 35% of patients

   2. Leukocytosis (> 10,000 mcL) present in 63% of patients.

   3. Murphy sign

      a. Sensitivity, 65%; specificity, 87%

      b. LR+ = 2.8, LR− = .05

B. Ultrasound findings that suggest acute cholecystitis include gallstones *with* gallbladder wall thickening, enlargement, or tenderness.

   1. Sensitivity, 88%; specificity, 80%

   2. LR+, 4.4, LR−, 0.15

C. Cholescintigraphy (HIDA) scans

   1. Radioisotope is excreted by the liver into the biliary system. In normal patients, the gallbladder concentrates the isotope and is visualized.

   2. Useful when the pretest probability is high and the ultrasound is surprisingly normal.

   3. Nonvisualization of the gallbladder suggests cystic duct obstruction and is highly specific for acute cholecystitis.

   4. Nonvisualization can also be seen in prolonged fasting, hepatitis, and alcohol abuse.

   5. Visualization of the gallbladder essentially excludes acute cholecystitis.

D. Ultrasound is the test of choice. If it is normal, consider HIDA.

Treatment

Antibiotics and cholecystectomy.

Alternative Diagnosis: Acute Pancreatitis

Textbook Presentation

Abdominal pain associated with acute pancreatitis is often described as constant and boring and of moderate to severe intensity that is localized to the epigastrium. It may radiate to the back (50%) and may be exacerbated in the supine position. Patients often have nausea and vomiting (75%) and low-grade fever (< 38.3 °C) (60%). Abdominal distention can be present due to concomitant ileus and ascites.

Disease Highlights

A. Etiology

   1. Alcohol abuse and choledocholithiasis or biliary microlithiasis cause 80% of acute pancreatitis cases.

   2. 10% of cases are idiopathic (67% of patients with idiopathic pancreatitis were found to have small gallstones at ERCP)

   3. ERCP (pancreatitis complicates 5% of ERCP procedures)

   4. Drugs commonly associated with pancreatitis include pentamidine, didanosine (DDI), estrogens, hydrochlorothiazide, and sulfonamides among others.

   5. Less common causes include trauma, hyperlipidemia, hypercalcemia, ischemia, pancreatic carcinoma, and organ transplantation.

B. Complications

   1. Necrotizing pancreatitis

   2. Pancreatic pseudocyst

   3. Shock

   4. Hypocalcemia

   5. Acute renal failure (ARF)

   6. Acute respiratory distress syndrome (ARDS)

   7. Disseminated intravascular coagulation (DIC)

   8. **Ranson's criteria** predict mortality (≤ 2 criteria, < 1% mortality; 3–4 criteria, 16% mortality; ≥ 5 criteria, 40% mortality)

      a. On admission:

         (1) Age > 55 years

         (2) WBC > 16,000/mcL

         (3) Glucose > 198 mg/dL

         (4) LDH > 350 international units/L

         (5) AST > 250 units/L

b. During initial 48 hours:

    (1) Hct decrease > 10%

    (2) BUN increase > 5 mg/dL

    (3) Calcium < 8 mg/dL

    (4) PaO_2 < 60 mm Hg

    (5) Base deficit > 4 mEq/L

    (6) Fluid sequestration > 6 L

Evidence-Based Diagnosis

A. History and physical

  1. Low-grade fevers are common.

  2. Rebound rare on presentation; guarding is common (50%).

  3. Periumbilical bruising (Cullen sign) is rare.

  4. Flank bruising (Grey-Turner's syndrome) is rare.

B. Laboratory studies

  1. Lipase

    a. 94% sensitive, 96% specific; LR+ = 23, LR− = .06

    b. Remains elevated longer than serum amylase

    c. Marked elevations suggest pancreatitis secondary to gallstones.

  2. Amylase

    a. Less sensitive and specific than lipase

    b. Should not be routinely ordered

  3. Alkaline phosphatase: Elevations in alkaline phosphatase and bilirubin suggest pancreatitis secondary to gallstone disease

  4. Plain radiography is useful to rule out free air or SBO

  5. Cross sectional imaging

    a. Ultrasound should be performed in *all* patients to look for gallstones or dilatation of CBD.

    b. CT scans should be performed in patients with severe pancreatitis to evaluate for pseudocysts or pancreatic necrosis, especially if symptoms fail to improve over the first 72 hours.

  6. ERCP

    a. ERCP can remove persistent stones in the CBD in patients with gallstone pancreatitis.

    b. Studies have documented that early ERCP is safe

    c. Most studies have demonstrated that ERCP leads to fewer complications (eg, biliary sepsis) and reduces length of stay in patients with severe gallstone pancreatitis.

    d. Early ERCP should be considered for patients with severe pancreatitis suspected to be of gallstone origin (ie, patients with dilated CBD, elevated alkaline phosphatase, aminotransferase, or bilirubin).

Treatment

A. Vital signs, orthostatic BPs, and urinary output critical to assess intravascular volume.

B. IV fluid to maintain appropriate BP and urinary output (> 0.5 mL/kg/h)

C. No oral intake

D. Parenteral pain medication

E. Nasogastric (NG) tube if recurrent vomiting

F. ICU admission for severe pancreatitis

G. Antibiotics are recommended in patients with severe pancreatitis.

H. If infection is suspected, evaluate with fine-needle aspiration and culture. If infection is confirmed, surgical debridement should be considered.

I. Elective cholecystectomy if secondary to gallstones

J. Alcohol abstinence

Alternative Diagnosis: Chronic Pancreatitis

See Chapter 22, Unintentional Weight Loss.

CASE RESOLUTION

An ERCP demonstrates multiple small stones within the CBD, which are extracted. Ms. R underwent cholecystectomy and recovered without incident.

Treatment of Ascending Cholangitis

A. IV broad-spectrum antibiotics

B. Emergent decompression of the biliary system (ERCP or transhepatic stent)

C. Cholecystectomy

CHIEF COMPLAINT

PATIENT 3

Mr. J is a 63-year-old man with severe abdominal pain for 48 hours. The pain is periumbilical with severe crampy exacerbations that last for several minutes and then subside. He notes loud intestinal noises (borborygmi) during the periods of increased pain. The pain is associated with nausea and vomiting. He reports decreased appetite with no oral intake in the last 48 hours.

At this point, what is the leading hypothesis, and what are the active alternatives? What other tests should be ordered?

ORGANIZING THE DIFFERENTIAL DIAGNOSIS

Mr. J's severe crampy abdominal pain suggests some type of visceral obstruction. The syndromes associated with pain of this quality include ureteral obstruction secondary to stones, biliary obstruction, or intestinal obstruction (large or small bowel). The associated nausea and vomiting can be seen with any of those diseases. However, the loud intestinal sounds associated with exacerbations of the pain suggest some form of intestinal obstruction. In addition, the periumbilical location is more suggestive of intestinal obstruction rather than renal or biliary colic. Table 2–5 lists the differential diagnosis.

3

Three weeks ago, Mr. J noted a small amount of blood on the stool. He reports no other change in bowel habits until 4 days ago. Since that time, he has been constipated and has not passed stool or flatus. He has no prior history of intra-abdominal surgeries, hernias, or diverticulitis. He reports no history of flank pain, groin pain, or hematuria. He has no history of gallstones and has not noticed any

Table 2–5. Diagnostic hypotheses for Mr. J.

Diagnostic Hypothesis	Clinical Clues	Important Tests
Leading Hypothesis		
Bowel obstruction	Inability to pass stool or flatus Nausea, vomiting Prior abdominal surgery or altered bowel habits, hematochezia Abdominal distention, hyperactive bowel sounds (with tinkling) or hypoactive bowel sounds	Abdominal x-rays CT scan
Active Alternatives—Most Common		
Biliary colic	Episodic, crampy pain Dark urine	Ultrasound
Renal colic	Flank or groin pain Hematuria	Urinalysis Renal CT scan

tea-colored urine. On physical exam, he is intermittently very uncomfortable with episodes of severe cramping pain. Vital signs reveal orthostatic hypotension: supine BP, 110/75 mm Hg; pulse, 90 bpm; upright BP, 85/50 mm Hg; pulse, 125 bpm; temperature, 37.0 °C; RR, 18 breaths per minute. He is anicteric. Cardiac and lung exams are unremarkable. Abdominal exam reveals prominent distention. Bowel sounds show intermittent rushes. He has mild diffuse tenderness to exam without rebound or guarding. Stool is brown and heme positive.

The constipation, absence of flatus, abdominal distention and rushing bowel sounds further increase the suspicion of bowel obstruction. Many small bowel obstructions (SBO) are due to adhesions from prior surgery. Mr. J's negative surgical history makes this unlikely. However, the hematochezia raises the possibility of some malignant obstruction. The orthostatic hypotension suggests significant dehydration.

Laboratory findings are WBC 10,000/mcL (70% neutrophils, 0% bands); Hct, 41%. Electrolytes: Na, 141; K, 3.0; HCO₃, 32; Cl, 99; BUN, 45; Creatinine 1.0 mg/dL. An abdominal upright x-ray is shown Figure 2–3.

 Is the clinical information sufficient to make a diagnosis? If not, what other information do you need?

Leading Hypothesis: Large Bowel Obstruction (LBO)

Textbook Presentation

Bowel obstructions present with severe crampy abdominal pain that is accentuated in waves, which the patient finds incapacitating. Vomiting is common. The pain is often diffuse and poorly localized. Initially, the patient may have several bowel movements as the bowel is emptied *distal* to the obstruction. Bowel sounds are hyperactive early in the course. Abdominal distention is often present. (Distention is less marked in proximal SBOs.) At first, the pain is intermittent; later, the pain often becomes more constant, bowel sounds may diminish and become absent, constipation progresses and the patient becomes unable to pass flatus. If bowel infarction occurs, peritoneal findings may be seen.

 In patients with abdominal pain, the inability to pass stool or flatus suggests bowel obstruction.

Disease Highlights

Etiology and related prevalence is as follows:

1. Cancer, 53%
2. Sigmoid or cecal volvulus, 17%
3. Diverticular disease, 12%
4. Extrinsic compression from metastatic cancer, 6%
5. Other, 12% (adhesions rarely cause LBO)

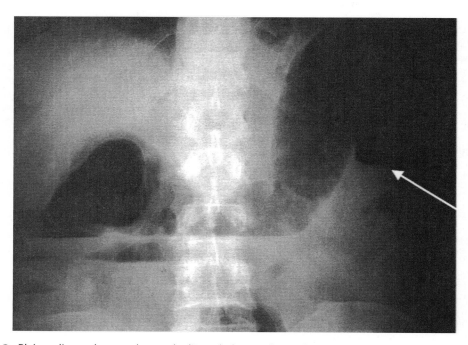

Figure 2–3. Plain radiography reveals grossly distended ascending colon, multiple air-fluid levels and an abrupt termination of air in the descending colon (arrow) suggestive of large bowel obstruction.

Evidence-Based Diagnosis

A. History and physical exam (Table 2–6)

   1. None of the expected clinical findings are very sensitive

      a. Vomiting, 75%

      b. Abdominal distention, 63%

   2. Certain findings are fairly specific

      a. Constipation, 95%; LR+, 8.8

      b. Prior abdominal surgery, 94%; LR+, 11.5

      c. Abdominal distention, 89%; LR+, 5.7

   3. Certain combinations are insensitive (27–48%) but highly specific.

      a. Distention associated with any of the following highly suggestive (LR+ ≈ 10): increased bowel sounds, vomiting, constipation, or prior surgery

      b. Increased bowel sounds with prior surgery or vomiting also very suggestive of obstruction (LR+ of 11 and 8, respectively)

B. A CBC and electrolytes should be obtained: Anion gap acidosis suggests bowel infarction or sepsis.

 Marked leukocytosis, left shift or anion gap acidosis in a patient with bowel obstruction is a *late* finding and suggests bowel infarction.

C. Plain radiography may show air-fluid levels and distention of large bowel (> 6 cm).

   1. 84% sensitive for presence of LBO (not etiology)

   2. Small bowel distention also occurs if ileocecal valve is incompetent.

D. Barium enema (water soluble) or colonoscopy

   1. Can determine etiology preoperatively (if patient stable)

   2. Can exclude acute colonic pseudo-obstruction (distention of the cecum and colon without mechanical obstruction)

   3. Colonoscopy can decompress pseudo-obstruction and prevent cecal perforation.

E. CT scan is more useful in patients with SBO than in those with LBO.

MAKING A DIAGNOSIS

 After reviewing the plain films, you order a barium enema.

 Have you crossed a diagnostic threshold for the leading hypothesis, large bowel obstruction? Have you ruled out the active alternatives? Do other tests need to be done to exclude the alternative diagnoses?

Alternative Diagnosis: SBO

Textbook Presentation

The presentation is similar to that for LBO with the exception that more patients have a history of prior abdominal surgery.

Disease Highlights

A. Bowel obstruction accounts for 4% of patients presenting with abdominal pain

B. SBO accounts for 80% of all bowel obstructions

C. Etiology

   1. Adhesions present in 70% of cases

      a. Usually postoperative

Table 2–6. Test characteristics for predicting bowel obstruction.

Finding	Sensitivity	Specificity	LR+	LR–
Visible peristalsis	6%	99.7%	20	0.94
Prior abdominal surgery	69%	94%	11.5	0.33
History of constipation	44%	95%	8.8	0.59
Distended abdomen	63%	89%	5.7	0.42
Increased bowel sounds	40%	89%	3.6	0.67
Reduced bowel sounds	23%	93%	3.3	0.83
Colicky pain	31%	89%	2.8	0.78
Vomiting	75%	65%	2.1	0.38

Modified with permission from Taylor & Francis Ltd. Böhmer H. *Simple Data from History and Physical Examination Help to Exclude Bowel Obstruction and to Avoid Radiographic Studies in Patients with Acute Abdominal Pain.* http://www.tandf.co.UK/journals.

   b. 93% of patients with prior abdominal surgery have adhesions

   c. 3–5% of patients with prior surgery require readmission for adhesions over the next 10 years

   d. Even in patients with prior malignancy, 39% of SBO cases are secondary to adhesion or benign cause.

2. Malignant tumor 10–20%; usually metastatic

3. Hernia 10%

   a. Ventral, inguinal, or internal

   b. More often complicated by strangulation than adhesions

4. Inflammatory bowel disease 5%

5. Radiation

D. SBOs may be partial or complete. Complete obstructions may strangulate and then infarct.

   1. Partial SBO

      a. Rarely progress to strangulation or infarction

      b. Characterized by continuing ability to pass stool or flatus (> 6–12 hours after symptom onset) or passage of contrast into cecum

      c. Resolves spontaneously (without surgery) in 60–85% of patients

      d. Enteroclysis (an air-contrast study of the small bowel) is test of choice.

      e. CT scan only 48% sensitive for partial SBO

      f. Therapy

         (1) Fluid resuscitation

         (2) Careful observation over several days

   2. Complete SBO

      a. 20–40% progress to strangulation and infarction

      b. Clinical signs do *not* allow for identification of strangulation prior to infarction: Fever, leukocytosis, and metabolic acidosis are late signs of strangulation and suggest infarction

Evidence-Based Diagnosis

A. See characteristics of history and physical under LBO.

B. WBC may be normal even in presence of ischemia.

C. Plain x-ray films may show air-fluid levels (> 2) or dilated loops of bowel proximal to obstruction (> 2.5 cm diameter of small bowel).

   1. Sensitivity 50–90%

   2. Rarely determines etiology

D. Ultrasound is seldom used for this indication.

E. CT scanning

   1. 80–93% sensitive for high-grade obstruction

   2. May delineate etiology of obstruction

   3. Perform *before* NG suction is initiated

F. Small bowel series

   1. Water-soluble contrast and barium have been used

   2. Barium is superior because it is not diluted by intraluminal water.

   3. Barium can become inspissated in colon. Contraindicated in LBO.

   4. 93% sensitive, 97% specific

Treatment

A. Fluid resuscitation (monitor urinary output carefully)

B. NG suction (controversy exists about efficacy of long tube vs NG)

C. Broad-spectrum antibiotics (59% of patients have bacterial translocation to mesenteric lymph nodes)

D. Careful, frequent surgical observation over first 12–24 hours

E. Frequent plain x-ray films and CBC

F. Indications for surgery include any of the following

   1. Signs of ischemia (increased pain, fever, tenderness, peritoneal findings, acidosis, or worsening leukocytosis)

   2. CT findings of infarction

   3. SBO secondary to hernia

   4. SBO clearly not secondary to adhesion (no prior surgery)

   5. Some clinicians recommend surgery when bowel obstruction fails to resolve in 24 hours. Others suggest a small bowel study.

CASE RESOLUTION

The barium enema reveals an obstructive apple core lesion in the sigmoid colon suggestive of carcinoma of the colon. Mr. J underwent surgical exploration, which confirmed an obstructing colonic mass. The mass was resected and a colostomy created. Pathologic evaluation revealed adenocarcinoma of the colon.

Treatment of LBO

A. Aggressive rehydration and monitoring of urinary output is vital.

B. Broad-spectrum antibiotics advised: 39% of patients have microorganisms in the mesenteric nodes

C. Surgery

   1. Emergent indications: perforation or ischemia

   2. Nonemergent indications: increasing distention, failure to resolve

CHIEF COMPLAINT

PATIENT 4

Mr. L is a 55-year-old man who arrives in the emergency department complaining of 1 hour of excruciating constant abdominal pain radiating to his flank. He has suffered 1 episode of vomiting and feels light headed. The emesis was yellow. He has moved his bowels once this morning. There is no change in his bowel habits, melena, or hematochezia. Nothing seems to make the pain better or worse. He was without any pain until this morning. His past medical history is remarkable for hypertension and tobacco use. On physical exam, he is diaphoretic and in obvious acute distress. Vital signs are BP, 110/65 mm Hg; pulse, 90 bpm; temperature, 37.0 °C; RR, 20 breaths per minute. HEENT, cardiac, and pulmonary exams are all within normal limits. Abdominal exam reveals moderate diffuse tenderness, without rebound or guarding. Bowel sounds are present and hypoactive. Stool is guaiac negative.

At this point, what is the leading hypothesis, and what are the active alternatives? What other tests should be ordered?

Table 2–7. Diagnostic hypotheses for Mr. L.

Diagnostic Hypotheses	Clinical Clues	Important Tests
Leading Hypothesis		
Renal colic	Flank pain Radiation to groin Hematuria	Urinalysis Renal CT
Active Alternatives—Most Common		
Biliary colic	Episodic, crampy pain Dark urine	Ultrasound
Diverticulitis	Left lower quadrant pain (usually) Diarrhea Fever	CT scan
Pancreatitis	Alcohol abuse Gallstones	Serum lipase
Active Alternatives—Must Not Miss		
AAA	Orthostatic hypotension Pulsatile abdominal mass Decreased lower extremity pulses	Abdominal CT scan

ORGANIZING THE DIFFERENTIAL DIAGNOSIS

Given Mr. L's extreme distress, life-threatening diagnoses must be considered carefully. The location of the pain is not terribly helpful in this case although the radiation of the pain to the flank raises the possibilities of renal colic, biliary colic, pancreatitis, or AAA. Clearly, AAA is a must not miss diagnosis. The acuity of the pain is consistent with renal colic, biliary colic, pancreatitis, AAA, or bowel obstruction (although the rapidity is somewhat unusual for bowel obstruction). Diverticular rupture can result in severe sudden onset of pain, although the pain is more often in the left lower quadrant (LLQ) than diffuse. PUD rarely causes such severe pain unless associated with perforation, and the abdominal exam does not suggest peritonitis. Table 2–7 lists the differential diagnosis.

Mr. L has no history of renal stones or hematuria, gallstones, dark urine, or light stools. He has never had this pain before. He does not drink alcohol. On reexamination, orthostatic maneuvers reveal profound orthostatic hypotension. Supine BP and pulse were 110/65 mm Hg and 90 bpm. Upon standing his BP falls to 65/40 mm Hg with a pulse of 140 bpm. He remains afebrile. Again, you find that he lacks rebound or guarding and is not particularly tender in the LLQ. He has moderate flank and back tenderness to percussion. His abdominal aorta cannot be palpated due to his abdominal girth. Lower extremity pulses are intact. Plain abdominal x-rays do not demonstrate free air.

 Is the clinical information sufficient to make a diagnosis? If not, what other information do you need?

The most dramatic and important physical finding is the presence of profound orthostatic hypotension. This suggests significant intravascular depletion and is a critical clinical clue. It is unlikely that dehydration is responsible for the profound orthostasis given the absence of significant emesis, diarrhea, or prolonged period of no oral intake. Therefore, the profound orthostasis suggests acute blood loss; either GI or intra-abdominal hemorrhage. GI hemorrhage almost always traverses the bowel quickly resulting in either melena or hematochezia and is rarely subtle. Therefore, you are more concerned about intra-abdominal hemorrhage. Massive intra-abdominal hemorrhage can occur in AAAs, splenic rupture, or ectopic pregnancy. The patient's history is most suggestive of AAA rupture. You revise your leading diagnosis to AAA rupture. You call for a stat vascular surgery consult.

 Orthostatic BPs should be considered the 5th vital sign. Orthostatic hypotension significantly alters the diagnostic and therapeutic management and may be marked despite a normal supine BP and pulse.

Leading Hypothesis: AAAs

Textbook Presentation

Typically, patients are men with a history of hypertension who have the triad of severe abdominal pain, a pulsatile abdominal mass, and hypotension.

Disease Highlights

A. 10,000 deaths per year in United States

B. Misdiagnosis (most commonly renal colic) occurs in 16% of cases.

C. Subtypes of AAA

1. Asymptomatic: rupture rates rise as aneurysm increases in size

   a. AAA 5.5–6.5 cm: 10%/y

   b. AAA 6.5–7.0 cm: 20%/y

   c. AAA > 7 cm: 30%/y

2. Ruptured

   a. Hypotension is a late finding, and palpable mass often not present.

   b. Mortality with rupture is 70–90%.

   c. Syncope may be present.

   d. Patient may live for days if rupture is contained.

   e. Rupture into the duodenum is a rare complication, is more common in patients with prior AAA graft, and may result in GI bleeding over weeks.

3. Symptomatic, contained

   a. Although rarely considered, some patients present nonemergently with symptomatic contained rupture of the abdominal aorta. Symptoms are primarily secondary to retroperitoneal hemorrhage and are occasionally present for weeks or even months.

   b. Manifestations include

      (1) Abdominal pain 83%

      (2) Flank or back pain 61%

      (3) Syncope 26%

      (4) Abdominal mass on careful exam 52% (only 18% had abdominal mass noted on routine abdominal exam)

      (5) Hypotension or orthostasis 48%

      (6) Leukocytosis (> 11,000/mcL) 70%

      (7) Anemia (unusual)

D. Risk factors

1. Smoking is the most significant risk factor.

2. Men are affected 4 to 5 times more often than women.

3. Family history

4. Increased age

5. Hypertension

Evidence-Based Diagnosis

A. Physical exam is *not* sufficiently sensitive to rule out AAA.

B. Bruits do not contribute to diagnosis.

C. Sensitivity of *focused* exam for *asymptomatic* AAA: (normal width < 2.5 cm, at level of umbilicus)

1. AAA 3.0–3.9 cm: 29–61%; LR+ 12, LR– 0.72
2. AAA 4.0–4.9 cm: 50–69%
3. AAA ≥ 5.0 cm: 76–82%
4. If aorta palpable, 82%
5. Waistline < 40 in: 91%
6. Waistline > 40 in: 52%

D. Sensitivity of abdominal exam *in symptomatic AAA*

1. Abdominal pain, distention, and rupture all limit sensitivity.
2. Distention was reported in 52–100% in different series.
3. Palpable mass was found 18%.

E. Laboratory and radiologic tests

1. Ultrasound is preferred screening method because its sensitivity is ≈ 100%.
2. Preoperative evaluation prior to repair of asymptomatic AAA includes CT scanning, helical CT, or aortography.

MAKING A DIAGNOSIS

Further evaluation at this point depends on the index of suspicion. If AAA is very likely and the patient unstable, many vascular surgeons proceed directly to the operating room without further studies in order to avoid the potential lethal delay of obtaining a CT scan. If AAA is less likely and the patient is stable, CT scanning is appropriate.

Have you crossed a diagnostic threshold for the leading hypothesis, AAA? Have you ruled out the active alternatives? Do other tests need to be done to exclude the alternative diagnoses?

Alternative Diagnosis: Nephrolithiasis

Textbook Presentation

Patients typically experience rapid onset of excruciating back and flank pain, which may radiate to the abdomen or groin. The intensity of the pain is often dramatic as patients writhe and move about constantly in an unsuccessful attempt to get comfortable. The pain may be associated with nausea and vomiting. Abdominal *tenderness* is unusual and should raise the possibility of other diagnoses.

Disease Highlights

A. Incidence: Symptomatic stones develop in 3–12% of people in the United States

1. 50% recurrence at 10 years
2. Men affected 2 to 3 times more often than women
3. Positive family history 2.6 relative risk

B. Etiology

1. CaOxalate stones 75%
2. Struvite (Mg NH4PO4) 10–20%
3. Calcium phosphate stones (CAPO4) 5%
4. Uric acid stones 5%
5. Other: Cystine and indinavir stones

C. Complications

1. Ureteral obstruction
2. Renal failure (bilateral obstruction or obstruction of solitary functioning kidney)
3. Pyelonephritis
4. Sepsis

Evidence-Based Diagnosis

A. Hematuria is present in 80% of patients, LR– is 0.57. The absence of hematuria does not rule out nephrolithiasis.

B. Radiographs (KUB) are not terribly sensitive for stones (29–68%).

C. Noncontrast helical renal CT is the test of choice: Sensitivity, 95%; Specificity, 98%; LR+, 48; LR–, 0.05

Treatment

A. Pain control

1. NSAIDS

   a. Treat pain and diminish spasm
   b. Create less dependence than narcotics
   c. To be avoided 3 days before lithotripsy due to antiplatelet effects

2. Narcotics

B. Hydration (oral if tolerated, otherwise IV)

C. Sepsis or renal failure

   1. Necessitate emergent drainage

      a. Percutaneous nephrostomy tube or

      b. Ureteral stent and stone extraction

   2. For sepsis, give broad-spectrum IV antibiotics to cover gram-negative organisms and enterococcus

D. Stone extraction

   1. Stones < 5 mm

      a. Depending on location in ureter, 38–74% of stones < 5 mm will pass within 1–2 weeks.

      b. Observation during this period is appropriate.

      c. Monitor for sepsis or renal decline.

   2. Stones > 5 mm

      a. Unlikely to pass spontaneously (< 25%)

      b. Lithotripsy recommended

Alternative Diagnosis: Diverticulitis

Textbook Presentation

Patients typically complain of a constant gradually increasing abdominal pain lasting hours to days. Diarrhea and fever are often present. Pain is usually localized to LLQ. Epigastric pain is less common. Guarding and rebound may be seen.

Disease Highlights

A. Diverticulosis is asymptomatic outpouchings in colonic wall without inflammation.

   1. Incidence: 5–10% of patients aged > 45 years, 50% in persons aged > 60 years, and 80% in those aged > 85 years

   2. Diverticulitis develops in 10–25%.

B. Diverticulitis

   1. Develops secondary to obstruction of diverticula

   2. 85% of diverticulitis occurs in sigmoid or descending colon

   3. Complications of diverticulitis

      a. Abscess

      b. Peritonitis

      c. Sepsis

      d. Obstruction

      e. Fistula formation (colovesicular fistula most common)

   4. Simultaneous diverticular hemorrhage and *diver-ticulitis* unusual; Diverticular hemorrhage is discussed in Chapter 14, GI Bleeding.

Evidence-Based Diagnosis (Diverticulitis)

A. CBC may demonstrate leukocytosis

B. Plain x-ray films may demonstrate free air or obstruction

C. CT scan is test of choice.

   1. May demonstrate diverticula, thickened bowel wall, pericolonic fat stranding, or abscess formation

   2. 79–99% sensitive

D. Carcinoma may be difficult to distinguish from inflammation.

E. Acute colonoscopy is not advised due to concern of perforation.

Treatment

A. Mild attack (pain manageable with oral analgesics, tolerating oral intake)

   1. Ciprofloxacin and metronidazole for 7–10 days

   2. Liquid diet

   3. High-fiber diet after attack resolved

   4. Follow-up colonoscopy to exclude cancer when stable

B. Moderate to severe attack (unable to tolerate oral intake, more severe pain)

   1. Broad-spectrum IV antibiotics

   2. No oral intake

   3. CT guided drainage for abscesses > 5 cm

   4. Surgery (sigmoid resection) for the following:

      a. Frank peritonitis

      b. Uncontrolled sepsis

      c. Clinical deterioration

      d. Frank fecal contamination of abscess

      e. Fistula formation

      f. Recurrent episodes (2 or more): Likelihood of third attack > 50%

      g. Immunocompromised

   5. High-fiber diet once the attack has resolved

   6. Follow-up colonoscopy is advised 4–6 weeks after resolution of symptoms to exclude carcinoma in patients without a recent colonoscopy. (Colon cancer is found in 17% of patients thought to have complicated diverticular disease.)

CASE RESOLUTION

The surgical resident evaluates the patient and agrees with your concern about an AAA. He orders a stat CT scan and contacts his attending. The attending immediately evaluates the patient and redirects the patient directly to the operating room bypassing the CT scan. Surgery reveals a leaking AAA that ruptures on the table. The aorta is cross clamped, repaired, and the patient is stabilized.

Treatment of AAA

A. For ruptured AAA, proceed directly to the operating room.

B. Asymptomatic AAA

　1. Most clinicians recommend elective repair if diameter > 5.5 cm.

　2. If diameter < 5.5 cm, monitor every 6 months with ultrasonography.

Summary table of abdominal pain by location.

Location	Differential Diagnosis	Quality and Frequency	Radiation and Associated Symptoms	Clinical Clues
RUQ	Biliary disease	Obstructive Episodic	Back, right shoulder; N & V	Postprandial or nocturnal pain Dark urine
	Pancreatitis	See below		
	Renal colic: Usually flank pain	Obstructive Episodic	Groin; N & V	Hematuria (usually microscopic) Writhing, unable to get comfortable
LUQ	Splenic infarct or rupture	Constant	Left shoulder pain	Endocarditis, trauma, orthostatic hypotension
Epigastrium	Peptic ulcer	Hunger like, intermittent, gradual changes	Back; early satiety	Melena, history of NSAIDs Food may increase or decrease pain
	Pancreatitis	Boring, constant	Back; N & V	Worse supine; history of alcohol abuse or gallstones
	Biliary disease	See above		
Diffuse peri-Umbilical	Appendicitis	Steady, worsening; migrates to RLQ	Groin; occasionally back; N & V, anorexia	Migration and progression No prior similar episodes
	Bowel obstruction	Obstructive	N & V, anorexia	Inability to pass stool or flatus, prior surgery
	Mesenteric ischemia	Severe	Weight loss	Out of proportion to exam, brought on by food, bruit
	AAA	Excruciating	Back	Low BP or abdominal mass
	Irritable bowel syndrome	Crampy, recurring	Intermittent diarrhea, constipation	Absence of weight loss or alarm symptoms, recurring nature of symptoms
RLQ	Appendicitis	See above		
	Diverticulitis	See below		
	Cecal volvulus	Similar to bowel obstruction; See above		
	Ovarian disease	Differential includes ovarian torsion, Mittelschmerz, ectopic pregnancy, and PID		
LLQ	Diverticulitis	Persistent, increasing	Back; fever, N & V	May have prior episodes, localized tenderness, diarrhea
	Ovarian disease	See above		
	Sigmoid volvulus	Similar to bowel obstruction		

RUQ, right upper quadrant; N & V, nausea and vomiting; LUQ, left upper quadrant; NSAIDs, nonsteroidal anti-inflammatory drugs; RLQ, right lower quadrant; AAA, abdominal aortic aneurysm; BP, blood pressure; PID, pelvic inflammatory disease; LLQ, left lower quadrant.

3

I have a patient with an acid-base abnormality. How do I determine the cause?

CHIEF COMPLAINT

PATIENT 1

Mr. L is a 42-year-old man who complains of weakness, anorexia, abdominal pain, and vomiting. Laboratory studies demonstrate a HCO_3^- of 6 mEq/L.

What is the differential diagnosis of acid-base disorders? How would you frame the differential?

CONSTRUCTING A DIFFERENTIAL DIAGNOSIS

Listed below are the steps to analyze an acid-base disorder.

Step 1: Generate Clinical Hypotheses

A. Each clinical scenario suggests a few possible acid-base disorders.

B. The first step considers those possibilities before analyzing the laboratory results.

Step 2: Check the pH

A. pHs < 7.4 indicates the *primary* disorder is an acidosis.

B. pHs > 7.4 indicates the *primary* disorder is an alkalosis.

Step 3: Determine Whether the Primary Disorder Is Due to a Metabolic or Respiratory Process

A. Check HCO_3^- and $PaCO_2$

B. $CO_2 + H_2O \leftrightarrow H_2CO_3 \leftrightarrow HCO_3^- + H^+$; therefore

C. HCO_3^- changes drive pH as follows:

1. Elevated HCO_3^- drives the reaction to left: This decreases H^+ which raises the pH resulting in a metabolic alkalosis.

2. Decreased HCO_3^-: An increase in H^+ production lowers pH and consumes HCO_3^-. Therefore, a decreased HCO_3^- is associated with a metabolic acidosis.

D. $PaCO_2$ changes drive pH as follows:

1. Increased $PaCO_2$ drives reaction to right: This increases H^+ which lowers pH resulting in a respiratory acidosis.

2. Decreased $PaCO_2$ drives reaction to left: This decreases H^+ which raises pH resulting in a respiratory alkalosis.

Step 4: Calculate Whether Compensation Is Appropriate

A. The acid-base system attempts to maintain homeostasis. Alterations in 1 system (respiratory or metabolic) trigger compensatory changes in the other system to minimize the impact on pH.

B. Formulas predict the expected degree of compensation (Table 3–1).

C. Compensation that is greater or less than expected suggests that an *additional* disease process is affecting the compensating system.

Step 5: Calculate the Anion Gap

A. Anion gap = $Na^+ - (HCO_3^- + Cl^-)$

B. An increased anion gap indicates that an anion gap metabolic acidosis is present (even when the HCO_3^- is elevated).

1. Optimal cutoff is 14 mEq/L.

2. Cutoff of 16 mEq/L is often used.

Table 3–1. Compensation in acid-base disorders.[a]

Primary Disorder	Duration	Expected Compensation
Metabolic acidosis	Acute/Chronic	$PaCO_2$ ↓ 1.2 mm Hg per 1 mEq/L ↓ HCO_3^- (To a minimum $PaCO_2$ of 10–15 mm Hg)
Metabolic alkalosis	Acute/Chronic	$PaCO_2$ ↑ 0.7 mm Hg per 1 mEq/L ↑ HCO_3^-
Respiratory acidosis	Acute	HCO_3^- ↑ 1 mEq/L per 10 mm Hg ↑ $PaCO_2$
	Chronic	HCO_3^- ↑ 3.5 mEq/L per 10 mm Hg ↑ $PaCO_2$
Respiratory alkalosis	Acute	HCO_3^- ↓ 2 mEq/L per 10 mm Hg ↓ $PaCO_2$
	Chronic	HCO_3^- ↓ 4 mEq/L per 10 mm Hg ↓ $PaCO_2$

[a]Metabolic compensation takes time and is more complete in chronic than in acute disorders.

Reproduced with permission from the McGraw-Hill Companies. Rose BD. *Clinical Physiology of Acid-Base and Electrolyte Disorders,* 2000.

 Always check the anion gap. An elevated gap always suggests an anion gap metabolic acidosis even when the HCO_3^- is above normal.

Step 6: Reach Final Diagnosis

Figure 3–1 outlines the stepwise approach to acid-base disorders.

Differential Diagnosis of Acid-Base Disorders

A. Metabolic acidosis
  1. **Anion gap metabolic acidosis** occurs when there is an abnormal accumulation of an un-measured anion (either ketones, lactate, sulfates and phosphates, or organic anions).
    a. Ketoacidosis
      (1) Diabetic ketoacidosis (DKA)
      (2) Starvation ketoacidosis
      (3) Alcoholic ketoacidosis
    b. Lactic acidosis
      (1) Secondary to any impairment of aerobic metabolism
      (2) The differential diagnosis of lactic acidosis can be remembered by considering the steps of oxygen transport from the environment to the mitochondria. Any disease that interrupts oxygen transport can cause lactic acidosis. Common causes include hypoxia or hypotension (due to cardiogenic shock, septic shock, or hypovolemic shock) (Table 3–2).

    c. Uremia (associated with sulfate and phosphate accumulation)
    d. Toxin, drugs, and miscellaneous
      (1) Salicylate toxicity
      (2) Methanol ingestion
      (3) Ethylene glycol ingestion
      (4) D-Lactic acidosis (secondary to production of D-lactic acid by intestinal bacteria in patients with jejunoileal bypass or short bowel)
  2. **Nonanion gap metabolic acidosis**
    a. Diarrhea
    b. Renal tubular acidosis (RTA) (type IV most common in adults)
    c. Carbonic anhydrase inhibitor
    d. Dilutional (large volume normal saline administration)
    e. Early renal failure
B. Metabolic alkalosis
  1. Vomiting or nasogastric drainage
  2. Dehydration
    a. Diuretics
    b. Vomiting
  3. Hypokalemia
  4. Hyperaldosteronism
C. Respiratory acidosis

 Any process that interferes with the normal ventilation (from brain to brainstem, spinal cord, nerve, neuromuscular junction, muscle, chest wall, or lung) can be deranged, causing ventilatory failure and respiratory acidosis.

Stepwise Approach to the Diagnosis of Acid-Base Disorders

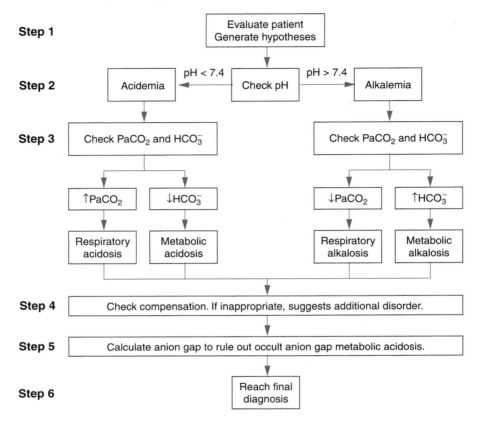

Figure 3–1.

1. Brain
   a. Stroke
   b. Drugs and intoxicants
   c. Hemorrhage
   d. Trauma
   e. Sleep apnea
2. Brainstem: Herniation
3. Spinal cord
   a. Trauma
   b. Amyotrophic lateral sclerosis
   c. Polio
4. Nerve: Guillain-Barré syndrome
5. Neuromuscular junction: Myasthenia gravis
6. Chest wall or muscle
   a. Flail chest
   b. Muscular dystrophy

7. Pleural disease
   a. Effusions
   b. Pneumothorax
8. Lung diseases are the most common etiology.
   a. Chronic obstructive pulmonary disease (COPD)
   b. Asthma
   c. Pulmonary edema
   d. Pneumonia
D. Respiratory alkalosis
   1. Hypoxemia
   2. Pulmonary disorders (via both hypoxic and vagal mechanisms)
      a. Pneumonia
      b. Asthma
      c. Pulmonary embolism

Table 3–2. Differential diagnosis of lactic acidosis.

Pathophysiology of Disorder	Examples
Low environmental oxygen	High altitude
Inadequate oxygen absorption resulting in hypoxemia	Lung disease (eg, pneumonia, congestive heart failure, and pulmonary embolism)
Inadequate Hgb saturation	Carbon monoxide poisoning (or hypoxemia)
Inadequate oxygen delivery to tissues (Demand > supply) Increase demand	Intense anaerobic activity, seizures
Decreased supply	Cardiogenic shock Hypovolemic shock Septic shock Obstruction to regional blood flow (eg, mesenteric ischemia)
Mitochondrial disorder	Cyanide poisoning

     d. Pulmonary edema

     e. Interstitial lung disease

     f. Mechanical ventilation

   3. Extrapulmonary disorders

     a. Anxiety

     b. Pain

     c. Fever

     d. Pregnancy

     e. CNS insult

     f. Drugs (salicylates, nicotine, catecholamines)

     g. Cirrhosis

   4. Compensatory respiratory alkalosis (ie, due to metabolic acidosis)

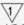

Mr. L reports that he has had diabetes since he was 10 years old. His diabetes has been complicated by peripheral vascular disease requiring a below the knee amputation and laser surgeries for retinopathy. Two days ago, he began experiencing nausea and some vomiting. He continued to take his insulin. Physical exam reveals supine

BP of 90/50 mm Hg and pulse of 100 bpm. Upon standing, his vital signs are BP, 60/30 mm Hg; pulse, 150 bpm; RR, 24 breaths per minute; and temperature, 37.0 °C. Retinal exam reveals dot-blot hemorrhages and multiple laser scars. Lungs are clear to percussion and auscultation. Cardiac exam reveals a regular rate and rhythm with a grade I/VI systolic murmur at the upper left sternal border. Abdominal exam is soft and nontender. Stool is guaiac-negative. Lab studies reveal Na^+, 138 mEq/L; K^+, 6.2 mEq/L; HCO_3^-, 6 mEq/L; Cl^-, 100 mEq/L; BUN, 40 mg/dL; creatinine, 1.8 mg/dL; glucose, 389 mg/dL; WBC, 10,500/mcL; Hct, 42%; ALT (SGPT), AST (SGOT), and lipase are normal.

At this point what is the leading hypothesis and what are the active alternatives? What other tests should be ordered?

ORGANIZING THE DIFFERENTIAL DIAGNOSIS

Although an arterial pH has not yet been obtained, the patient's very low HCO_3^- strongly suggests a metabolic acidosis.

Step 1: Generate Clinical Hypotheses

The history of childhood-onset diabetes mellitus strongly suggests insulin-dependent diabetes mellitus. This form of diabetes is associated with total or near total insulin deficiency placing patients at risk for DKA. This is the leading hypothesis (Table 3–3). In addition, patients with longstanding diabetes and renal insufficiency have a significant incidence of type IV RTA (a nonanion gap acidosis). Yet, another possibility is uremic acidosis from Mr. L's renal insufficiency. Finally, lactic acidosis from sepsis is a "must not miss diagnosis" that should always be considered in sick patients with metabolic acidosis.

Step 2: Check the pH

ABG: pH of 7.15, PaO_2 of 80 mm Hg, and $PaCO_2$ of 20 mm Hg. The low pH confirms that the primary disorder is an acidosis.

Table 3–3. Diagnostic hypotheses for Mr. L.

Diagnostic Hypothesis	Clinical Clues	Important Tests
Leading Hypothesis		
Diabetic ketoacidosis (DKA)	History of insulin-dependent diabetes Noncompliance with insulin Precipitating illness (eg, infection or stress)	Increased anion gap Increased serum or urine ketones Tests to identify precipitant (urinalysis, chest x-ray, ECG, lipase, abdominal imaging as indicated)
Active Alternatives—Most Common		
Uremic acidosis	Oliguria	Elevated BUN, creatinine, and anion gap Elevated FENa Renal ultrasound
Type IV renal tubular acidosis	Longstanding diabetes mellitus Nonanion gap acidosis Hyperkalemia	Basic metabolic panel
Active Alternatives—Must Not Miss		
Lactic acidosis from sepsis	Fever Rigors Urinary frequency Dysuria Cough Diarrhea Abdominal pain	Elevated WBC, anion gap, and serum lactate Urinalysis Chest x-ray (imaging as indicated) Blood cultures

Step 3: Determine Whether the Primary Disorder Is Due to a Metabolic or Respiratory Process

$HCO_3^- = 6$ mEq/L and $PaCO_2 = 20$ mm Hg.

A low HCO_3^- is associated with metabolic acidosis which drives the pH down whereas a low $PaCO_2$ drives the pH up (see above). Since the patient's pH is low (acidemic) the primary disorder must be a metabolic acidosis.

Step 4: Calculate Whether Compensation Is Appropriate

For metabolic acidosis, we can use the formula $PaCO_2$ drops by 1.2 mm Hg per 1 mEq/L fall in HCO_3^- (see Table 3–1). The patient's HCO_3^- is 6 mEq/L (normal is 24 mEq/L), which is a 18 mEq/L fall from normal. The $PaCO_2$ should fall by $1.2 \times 18 = 21.6$ mm Hg. Since the

normal $PaCO_2$ is approximately 40 mm Hg, we would expect the $PaCO_2$ to be approximately $40 - 21.6 \approx 18$. The actual $PaCO_2$ is close to the predicted value suggesting that respiratory compensation is indeed appropriate. Therefore, Mr. L is suffering from a metabolic acidosis with appropriate respiratory compensation.

Step 5: Calculate the Anion Gap

Anion gap $= 138 - (6 + 100) = 32$ (Normal $= 14$)

Clearly, Mr. L is suffering from an anion gap metabolic acidosis. This excludes RTA and focuses our attention on the remaining possibilities of DKA, lactic acidosis from sepsis, or uremia.

 Is the clinical information sufficient to make a diagnosis? If not, what other information do you need?

Leading Hypothesis: DKA

Textbook Presentation

DKA often begins with an acute illness (ie, urinary tract infection). Patients often complain of fever, nausea, vomiting, abdominal pain, and weakness. Patients are profoundly dehydrated and exhibit orthostatic changes or frank hypotension. Confusion, lethargy, and coma may occur secondary to dehydration, hyperglycemia, acidosis, or the underlying precipitating event.

Disease Highlights

A. Occurs primarily in patients with complete or near complete insulin deficiency

1. Type 1 autoimmune insulin-dependent diabetes mellitus

2. Diabetes mellitus secondary to severe chronic pancreatitis and near complete islet cell obliteration

3. DKA occasionally occurs in patients with type 2 diabetes mellitus

a. Type 2 diabetes mellitus accounts for 6–73% of DKA episodes in adults. Many such patients do not require lifelong insulin for management of their diabetes.

b. Precipitants include

(1) Severe stress

(2) Marked hyperglycemia (may transiently impair insulin secretion)

B. 4.6–8.0 cases/1000 person years in patients with diabetes

C. Precipitated by low insulin levels or a rise in insulin's counterregulatory hormones (cortisol, epinephrine, or glucagon).

1. Most common precipitants

a. New onset type 1 diabetes mellitus

b. Noncompliance with insulin

c. Infection (Urinary tract infections and pneumonia are most common.)

2. Other precipitants

a. Other infections

b. Myocardial infarction (MI)

c. Cerebrovascular accident

d. Acute pancreatitis

e. Pulmonary embolism

f. GI hemorrhage

g. Severe emotional stress

h. Drugs (eg, corticosteroids)

D. Pathogenesis: A *marked* decrease in insulin levels together with an increase in counterregulatory hormones lead to the following events:

1. Reduced glucose uptake by cells leads to hyperglycemia.

2. Increased hepatic gluconeogenesis augments hyperglycemia.

3. Glucosuria helps prevent extreme hyperglycemia (> 500–600 mg/dL)

4. More extreme hyperglycemia occurs if urinary output falls.

5. Hyperglycemia leads to an osmotic shift of water from the intracellular space to intravascular space, resulting in hyponatremia.

6. Marked insulin deficiency also causes increased lipase activity leading to increased FFA mobilization resulting in ketonemia (β hydroxybutyric acid and acetoacetic acid)

7. Ketonemia leads to anion gap metabolic acidosis.

8. Ketonemia and hyperglycemia result in osmotic diuresis.

9. Osmotic diuresis causes profound dehydration and significant potassium deficit.

a. Typical fluid loss is 5–7 L.

b. Typical potassium deficit is 3–5 mEq/kg body weight

10. Acidosis shifts potassium out of cells, producing *hyperkalemia* despite total body potassium deficit. Profound *hypokalemia* may develop when acidosis is corrected.

E. Mortality rate of DKA is 5–15%. Risk factors for death include:

1. Severe coexistent disease (adjusted OR 16.3)

2. pH < 7.0 at presentation (adjusted OR 8.7)

3. > 50 U insulin required in first 12 h (adjusted OR 7.9)

4. Glucose > 300 after 12 h (adjusted OR 8.3)

5. Depressed mental status after 24 hours (adjusted OR 8.6)

6. Fever (axillary temp $\geq$ 38.0 °C) after 24 hours (adjusted OR 5.8)

7. Increasing age

a. Mortality rate < 1.25% in persons younger than 55 years

b. Mortality rate of 11.8% in persons older than 55 years

Evidence-Based Diagnosis

A. Signs and symptoms

1. Polyuria and increased thirst are common.

2. Lethargy and obtundation may be seen with marked increased osmolality (> 320 mOsm/L)

   a. Osmolality can be calculated:

   (1) $(2 \times Na^+) + BUN/2.8 + Glucose/18$

   (2) ie, Na^+ of 140 mEq/L, BUN of 28 mg/dL, and glucose of 540 mg/dL = osmolality of 320 mOsm/L

   b. Consider neurologic insult if neurologic changes are present in patients without marked hyperosmolality or if neurologic abnormalities fail to resolve with therapy.

3. Abdominal pain

   a. May be secondary to DKA or another process precipitating DKA (ie, appendicitis, cholecystitis, abscess)

   b. Abdominal pain is increasingly common with increasing severity of DKA (Table 3–4).

   c. Likelihood that another process is causing abdominal pain increases if DKA is *mild.*

 Always consider an intra-abdominal cause of abdominal pain in patients with DKA, especially if the abdominal pain persists, occurs in patients with mild acidosis ($HCO_3^- > 10$), or in patients older than 40 years.

4. Nausea and vomiting are common and nonspecific.

B. Hyperglycemia

1. Glucose level is variable.

2. 15% of patients with DKA have glucose levels < 350 mg/dL (particularly in pregnancy or in patients with poor oral intake)

Table 3–4. Frequency and etiology of abdominal pain in patients with DKA.

Serum HCO_3^-	Frequency of Abdominal Pain	Patients with DKA as Etiology of Pain	Patients with Other Etiology of Pain
0–10 mEq/L	25–75%	70%	30%
> 10 mEq/L	12%	16%	84%

DKA, diabetic ketoacidosis.

C. Ketones

1. 3 ketones: β hydroxybutyrate, acetoacetate, acetone

2. Nitroprusside reaction detects acetoacetate but is insensitive for β hydroxybutyrate. In severe DKA, β hydroxybutyrate may be the prominent ketone causing a falsely negative ketone measurement.

   a. Anion gap still elevated

   b. In such cases, lactic acid should be measured to rule out lactic acidosis.

3. Urine ketones are an excellent screen for DKA.

   a. 99% sensitive, 69% specific

   b. LR+ 3.2; LR– 0.01

D. Anion gap

1. 90% sensitive for DKA (cutoff of 16 mEq/L)

2. 85% specific

E. Nonspecific findings

1. Amylase: Nonspecific elevations in amylase are common.

2. Leukocytosis

   a. Mild leukocytosis (10,000–15,000 cells/mcL) is common and may occur secondary to stress or infection.

   b. One study documented higher WBCs in patients with major infection than in patients without infection (17,900/mcL vs 13,700/mcL).

   c. Band counts were also higher in patients with infection (23% vs 6%).

MAKING A DIAGNOSIS

 Have you crossed a diagnostic threshold for the leading hypothesis, DKA? Have you ruled out the active alternatives or uremia or lactic acidosis (from sepsis)? Do other tests need to be done to exclude the alternative diagnoses?

Alternative Diagnosis: Uremic Acidosis

Textbook Presentation

Typically, patients with chronic renal failure have low HCO_3^- levels, high creatinine levels (often > 4–5 mg/dL) and elevated BUN and phosphate levels. Patients often complain of a variety of constitutional symptoms secondary to their renal failure including fatigue, nausea, vomiting, anorexia, and pruritus.

Disease Highlights

A. Pathophysiology: Each day, ingested nonvolatile acids neutralize HCO_3^-. Maintenance of acid-base equilibrium requires the kidneys to regenerate the HCO_3^-. Renal impairment results in failed HCO_3^- regeneration and metabolic acidosis.

B. Acidosis in patients with renal failure may be of the anion gap type or nonanion gap type.

   1. In early renal failure, ammonia-genesis is impaired resulting in reduced acid secretion and a nonanion gap metabolic acidosis.

   2. In more advanced chronic renal failure, the kidney is still unable to excrete the daily acid load and also becomes unable to excrete anions such as sulfates, phosphates, and urate. Therefore, an anion gap acidosis develops. HCO_3^- levels stabilize between 12 mEq/L and 20 mEq/L.

C. The acidosis has several adverse effects.

   1. Increased calcium loss from bone

   2. Increased skeletal muscle breakdown

Treatment

A. Some but not all clinicians recommend HCO_3^- replacement.

B. Hemodialysis

CASE RESOLUTION

Mr. L's serum ketones are large. Lactate level is 1 mEq/L (normal 0.5–1.5 mEq/L).

The high serum ketones confirm DKA. The normal lactate effectively rules out lactic acidosis, and uremic acidosis is very unlikely with mild renal insufficiency. Evaluation and treatment identifies the precipitant of DKA and treats the acidosis, hyperglycemia, and profound dehydration.

Mr. L confirms he has been taking his insulin. He reports no fever, rigors, dysuria, cough, shortness of breath, diarrhea, or abdominal pain. Uri-

nalysis, chest x-ray, and lipase were sent to search for the precipitating event. All of the results were normal. An ECG revealed T wave inversion in leads V1–V4, suggesting anterior myocardial ischemia. Troponin T levels were elevated consistent with acute MI (believed to be the precipitant of his DKA). He was given IV normal saline, and an insulin drip was initiated. He was transferred to the ICU for monitoring.

Always search for the precipitant of DKA (eg, infection, MI).

Treatment of DKA

A. Detect and treat underlying precipitant.

   1. Urinalysis, chest film, CBC with differential, blood cultures, lipase, ECG, troponin levels

   2. β-HCG should be measured in women of childbearing age.

B. Evaluate hydration status: Urinary output, BP, orthostatic BP and pulse, FENa

C. Check renal function, electrolytes, ABG

   1. Serum creatinine may be artificially elevated due to interference of assay by ketone bodies.

   2. Qualitative serum ketones should be measured to confirm ketoacidosis.

   3. Electrolytes should be measured frequently (every 1–2 hours) and the anion gap calculated.

D. Hydration

   1. IV normal saline 0.5–1.0 L bolus initially.

      a. Higher rates (1 L) are useful for patients with significant hypotension.

      b. Lower rates (500 mL/h) may allow for more rapid correction of acidosis in patients without marked volume depletion.

   2. Reevaluate after each liter checking BP, orthostatic BP and pulse, urinary output, and cardiac and pulmonary exams. Repeat boluses until hypotension and oliguria resolves.

   3. Normal saline should be switched to 0.45% normal saline when intravascular volume improves to restore free water deficit.

E. Insulin

   1. Most clinicians recommend regular insulin IV at 0.1 U/kg/h (some physicians start with a 0.1–0.2 U/kg bolus).

2. Administer in monitored setting.

3. Monitor glucose levels hourly: Target reduction 75–90 mg/dL/h and adjust insulin dose accordingly

4. Insulin should be continued until anion gap normalizes.

    a. Premature discontinuation of IV insulin before the anion gap normalizes may result in rebound ketoacidosis.

    b. If patient's glucose normalizes (< 250 mmol/d) before the anion gap returns to normal, the insulin dose may be reduced by 50% and glucose (D5W) added to the IV to prevent hypoglycemia.

In DKA, it is important to continue IV insulin until the anion gap returns to normal. Administer glucose as necessary to prevent hypoglycemia.

F. Potassium replacement

    1. Hypokalemia is a common complication of therapy.

    2. Potassium therapy should be initiated when urinary output resumes and potassium is < 4.0–5.0 mEq/L.

G. HCO_3^- therapy

    1. Use is controversial; if used, monitor patient for hypokalemia

    2. Does not improve outcomes in patients with serum pH > 7.0. May also paradoxically lower CNS pH.

    3. Reserve for patients with serum pH < 6.9–7.0 or when shock is present.

H. Observation: Hourly assessment of volume status (orthostatic BP and pulse, urinary output, lung and cardiac exam) and review of glucose and electrolytes is critical to ensure a good outcome.

Careful, frequent observation and evaluation of patients with DKA is critical to success.

Mr. L was stabilized in the ICU. He received fluid resuscitation, IV insulin, and potassium until his ketoacidosis resolved. His MI was treated with β-blockers and aspirin. Subsequent cardiac catheterization revealed triple vessel disease. After stabilization, he underwent coronary artery bypass grafting and did well.

CHIEF COMPLAINT

PATIENT 2

Ms. S is a 32-year-old woman who complains of nausea and vomiting. She reports that she felt well until 5 days ago when she noticed urinary frequency and burning on urination. She increased her intake of fluids and cranberry juice but noticed some increasing right back pain 2 days ago. Yesterday, she felt warm and noticed that she had a fever of 38.8 °C and teeth-chattering chills. Subsequently, she has been unable to keep down any food or liquids and has persistent nausea and vomiting. She feels weak and dizzy. Physical exam: supine BP, 95/62 mm Hg, pulse, 120 bpm; temperature, 38.9 °C; RR, 24 breaths per minute. On standing, her BP falls to 72/40 mm Hg with a pulse of 145 bpm. Cardiac and pulmonary exam are notable only for the tachycardia. She has 2+ right costovertebral angle tenderness. Abdominal exam is soft without rebound, guarding, or focal tenderness.

At this point, what is the leading hypothesis, and what are the active alternatives? What other tests should be ordered?

ORGANIZING THE DIFFERENTIAL DIAGNOSIS

Step 1: Generate Clinical Hypotheses

Ms. S's history of persistent vomiting combined with her dehydration (as evidenced by her orthostatic hypotension) may cause a metabolic alkalosis. On the other hand, the combination of fever, dysuria, and flank pain suggest urinary tract infection and pyelonephritis. Furthermore, her teeth-chattering chills suggest bacteremia, which combined with her hypotension suggests severe sepsis. Septic shock can cause lactic acid production and thereby generate an anion gap metabolic acidosis. This is the leading hypothesis and must not miss diagnosis (Table 3–5).

 Patients with either teeth-chattering or physically shaking chills (rigors) are at significant risk for bacteremia.

Step 2: Check the pH

An ABG reveals a pH of 7.29, $PaCO_2$ of 30 mm Hg, PaO_2 of 90 mm Hg.

The low pH on the ABG confirms the primary process is an acidosis.

Step 3: Determine Whether the Primary Disorder Is Due to a Metabolic or Respiratory Process

Other initial laboratory results include Na^+, 138 mEq/L; K^+, 5.4 mEq/L; HCO_3^-, 14 mEq/L; Cl^-, 94

Table 3–5. Diagnostic hypotheses for Ms. S.

Diagnostic Hypotheses	Clinical Clues	Important Tests
Leading Hypothesis		
Sepsis causing lactic acidosis	Fever Shaking chills Hypotension Localized symptoms and signs of infection (eg, skin redness, cough, dysuria)	Elevated anion gap and lactate Leukocytosis Left shift Blood cultures Urinalysis Chest x-ray
Active Alternatives—Most Common		
Metabolic alkalosis	Vomiting Dehydration Nasogastric tube drainage Diuretics	Elevated HCO_3^- Hypokalemia

mEq/L; BUN, 30 mg/dL; creatinine, 1.2 mg/dL. Glucose, 90 mg/dL; WBC, 18,500 cells/mcL with 62% granulocytes and 30% bands. Urinalysis reveals > 20 WBC/hpf.

Ms. S's HCO_3^- *and* $PaCO_2$ are both low. Only the low HCO_3^- would create an acidosis. (A low $PaCO_2$ would drive the pH up and cause an alkalosis.) Since her pH is low the primary process is a metabolic acidosis.

Step 4: Calculate Whether Compensation Is Appropriate

The expected compensation for a metabolic acidosis = $PaCO_2$ falls by 1.2 mm Hg per 1 mEq/L fall in HCO_3^- (see Table 3–1). The patient's HCO_3^- is 14 mEq/L (10 mEq/L below normal). The $PaCO_2$ should fall by 1.2 × 10 = 12. Since normal $PaCO_2$ is approximately 40 mm Hg, we would expect the $PaCO_2$ to be approximately 40 − 12 = 28 mm Hg. The actual $PaCO_2$ is 30 mm Hg, quite close to the prediction. This suggests that respiratory compensation is appropriate. Therefore, Ms. S is suffering from a metabolic acidosis with appropriate respiratory compensation.

Step 5: Calculate the Anion Gap

The next vital step in the differential diagnosis is to calculate the anion gap. Her anion gap = 138 − (94 + 14) = 30.

Clearly, Ms. S is suffering from an anion gap metabolic acidosis. This is alarming. It excludes the possibility of metabolic alkalosis and focuses our attention on the remaining possibility of lactic acidosis due to sepsis. (The clinical history and laboratory results suggest neither DKA nor uremic acidosis.)

 Is the clinical information sufficient to make a diagnosis? If not, what other information do you need?

Although the clinical picture strongly suggests lactic acidosis secondary to sepsis, it is instructive to review the other causes of lactic acidosis before focusing on sepsis.

General Principles of Lactic Acidosis

Textbook Presentation

The presentation of lactic acidosis depends on the underlying etiology. The most common clinical scenarios arise secondary to hypoxemia, septic shock, cardiogenic shock, or hypovolemic shock.

Disease Highlights

A. Lactic acidosis develops when oxygen delivery to the cells is inadequate. This results in anaerobic metabolism and the production of lactic acid. Therefore, the differential diagnosis can be remembered by tracing the pathway of oxygen from the environment through the blood to the cells and mitochondria. Any disease that interferes with oxygen delivery can cause lactic acidosis (Table 3–2).

1. Low oxygen carrying capacity
   a. Low Hgb oxygen saturation due to hypoxemia (from pulmonary or cardiac disease).
   b. Low Hgb oxygen saturation due to carbon monoxide poisoning.
2. Inadequate tissue perfusion (shock)
   a. Hypovolemic shock
   b. Cardiogenic shock
   c. Septic shock
3. Regional obstruction to blood flow (eg, ischemic bowel or gangrene)
4. Inadequate cellular utilization of oxygen (cyanide poisoning)
5. Occasionally, lactic acidosis develops secondary to unusually high demand exceeding oxygen supply (eg, intense exercise, seizures).

B. As noted above, a common cause of lactic acidosis is shock, defined as inadequate tissue perfusion. Manifestations of shock include hypotension, oliguria, and impaired mentation. Since hypotension almost always accompanies shock, the differential of shock can be deduced by considering the components of BP:

$$BP = cardiac\ output\ (CO) \times total\ peripheral\ resistance\ (TPR)$$

$$CO = stroke\ volume\ (SV) \times heart\ rate\ (HR)$$

$$Simple\ substitution:\ BP = SV \times HR \times TPR$$

$$SV = end\text{-}diastolic\ volume\ (EDV) - end\text{-}systolic\ volume\ (ESV)$$

$$Simple\ substitution:\ BP = (EDV - ESV) \times HR \times TPR$$

Evaluating each constituent in turn illustrates the differential diagnosis of hypotension and shock.

1. *Low EDV* causes decreased CO and if severe, results in *hypovolemic shock*. The low CO causes a compensatory increase in systemic vascular resistance (SVR) producing cold extremities and oliguria. Common causes include massive hemorrhage and dehydration. Less common causes include massive pulmonary embolism and cardiac tamponade.

2. *Elevated ESV* develops when CO is impaired. When severe, this defines *cardiogenic shock*. The decreased CO causes decreased BP and a compensatory increase in SVR. Patients are usually hypotensive, oliguric, and have cold extremities. The left ventricular filling volume is often elevated due to poor contractility and poor emptying. Etiologies include massive MI, severe congestive heart failure (CHF), and severe arrhythmias.

3. *Low TPR* is usually caused by *septic shock*. In this case, infection and the body's response to infection triggers excessive vasodilatation. Patients are often febrile and may complain of rigors or symptoms specific to their underlying infection. Urinary tract infection, pneumonia, and bacteremia from an indwelling catheter are some of the common causes of septic shock. Extremities are often warm (due to the vasodilatation). Less common causes of low TPR include adrenal crisis and anaphylaxis.

4. Hemodynamic features of shock are summarized in Table 3–6.

Evidence-Based Diagnosis for Lactic Acidosis

A. Serum lactate levels are more sensitive than the anion gap.

B. Anion gap is 44–67% sensitive and 83–91% specific.

C. An elevated anion gap may suggest a lactic acidosis, but a normal anion gap does not exclude a lactic acidosis.

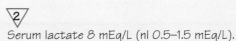

Serum lactate 8 mEq/L (nl 0.5–1.5 mEq/L).

The serum lactate levels confirm a significant lactic acidosis. However, there are several etiologies of lactic acidosis.

Leading Hypothesis: Lactic Acidosis Secondary to Sepsis

Textbook Presentation

Patients with septic shock typically have fever, tachypnea, tachycardia, and hypotension. Whereas patients with cardiogenic or hemorrhagic shock often have cold extremities, patients with septic shock often have warm extremities and bounding pulses after fluid resuscitation. (Pulses are bounding due to a widened pulse pres-

Table 3–6. The hemodynamic features of shock.[a,b]

Etiology	Clinical Clues	Mechanism	Cardiac Output	Systemic Vascular Resistance	Left Ventricular Filling Volume[c] (PcW)
Cardiogenic shock	Massive MI Severe CHF Cold extremities Arrhythmias	↑**ESV**	↓↓	↑↑	↑
Hypovolemic shock	Hematemesis Melena Vomiting Diarrhea Heatstroke Hematochezia Abdominal pain	↓**EDV**	↓↓	↑↑	↓↓
Septic shock	Fevers Rigors Dysuria Flank pain Cough Indwelling line	↓**TPR**	↑ then ↓	↓↓	↓ to normal

[a]Principal abnormality is bolded.
[b]BP = (EDV − ESV) × HR × TPR
[c]Left ventricular filling can be estimated by using an invasive catheter and measuring the pulmonary capillary wedge pressure (PcW). This estimates LV end-diastolic pressure and thereby LV filling.
EDV, end-diastolic volume; ESV, end-systolic volume; HR, heart rate; TPR, total peripheral resistance; MI, myocardial infarction; CHF, congestive heart failure.

sure.) Mentation may be impaired and urinary output decreased.

Disease Highlights

A. Pathophysiology

   1. Sepsis occurs when an infection (viral, bacterial, fungal, or mycobacterial) triggers a proinflammatory reaction that is poorly regulated and becomes systemic.

   2. In early stages of sepsis, hyperimmune responses may play a role in the organ dysfunction and cause multiple organ dysfunction syndrome (MODS), hypotension, disseminated intravascular coagulation, and death.

   3. In later stages of sepsis, patients may be hypoimmune. Hypoimmunity may also contribute to infection and death.

   4. Mechanisms of hypotension include

      a. Vasodilatation (decreased SVR) mediated by elevated nitrous oxide levels, increased prostacyclin levels, and low vasopressin levels.

      b. Leakage of fluid out of intravascular space leads to decreased venous return, which leads to decreased CO.

      c. Reduced myocardial function causes decreased CO. (Early in sepsis, CO may be elevated after fluid resuscitation due to the low SVR.)

      d. Typically, the *initial* hemodynamic response is decreased SVR and increased CO.

   5. MODS

      a. Lung involvement: Acute respiratory distress syndrome secondary to increased permeability

      b. Renal failure secondary to

         (1) Hypotension

         (2) Renal vasoconstriction

         (3) Increased tumor necrosis factor

      c. Disseminated intravascular coagulation: Multiple mediators are involved, including decreased protein C.

6. Lactic acidosis multifactorial

   a. Microcirculatory lesion impairs oxygen delivery.

      (1) Dysregulation of supply and demand

      (2) Microvascular occlusion

   b. Hypotension impairs oxygen delivery.

   c. Mitochondrial injury impairs oxygen utilization.

B. The definitions of sepsis, severe sepsis, and septic shock and their associated mortality rates are shown in Table 3–7.

C. There is an increased risk of septic shock in patients with bacteremia (21%), advanced age, abdominal infection, and markedly elevated WBC.

D. Predictors of mortality

   1. Age > 40 years

   2. Comorbidities: AIDS, hepatic failure, CHF, diabetes mellitus, cancer, or immunocompromise

   3. Temperature < 35.5 °C

   4. Leukopenia < 4000 cells/mcL

   5. Nosocomial infection

   6. *Candida* or *Pseudomonas* infection

   7. Inappropriate antibiotics: appropriate antibiotics associated with 50% decrease in mortality

   8. Multiple organ failure

E. Etiology: Most common sources of infection include urine, lung, and IV catheters. Commonly overlooked sources include sinusitis (associated with nasogastric tubes), acalculous cholecystitis and *Clostridium difficile* colitis

Evidence-Based Diagnosis

A. Skin findings: Certain life-threatening infections may produce characteristic rashes. Rapid recognition and treatment is vital.

B. Predictors of bacteremia (Table 3–8):

   1. WBC > 15,000/mcL is only 28% sensitive for bacteremia.

 A normal WBC does not rule out bacteremia.

   2. When present, history of injection drug use, acute abdomen, or WBC > 15,000/mcL are associated with an increased risk of bacteremia.

   3. Incidence of bacteremia is low (2%) in patients without *any* of the following risk factors: temperature > 38.3 °C, shaking chills, injection drug use, acute abdomen on exam, major comorbidity.

   4. Fever

      a. 18% of patients with gram-negative bacteremia are afebrile (temperature < 37.6 °C)

      b. 13% of patients with bacteremia were hypothermic (< 36.4 °C)

      c. 5% of patients with bacteremia were neither hypothermic nor febrile

      d. The absence of fever was associated with increased mortality among patients with bacteremia.

Table 3–7. Definitions of stages of sepsis.

Category	Definition	Mortality
Sepsis	Infection and ≥ 2 of following: Temperature > 38.0 °C or < 36.0 °C Pulse > 90 bpm RR > 20/min or PaCO₂ < 32 mm Hg WBC > 12,000/mcL or < 4000/mcL or > 10% bands	16%
Severe sepsis	Sepsis with hypotensionᵃ and evidence of inadequate tissue perfusion (altered mental status, oliguria, lactic acidosis)	20%
Septic shock	Severe sepsis despite fluid resuscitation	46%

ᵃHypotension defined systolic BP < 90 mm Hg or > 40 mm Hg fall from baseline value.

Table 3–8. Predictors of bacteremia.

Finding	Sensitivity	Specificity	LR+	LR−
Injection drug use	7%	98%	2.9	0.95
Acute abdomen	20%	91%	2.2	0.9
WBC > 15,000/mcL	28%	87%	2.2	0.8
WBC < 1000/mcL	14%	94%	2.3	0.9
Bandemia ≥ 1500/mcL	44%	69%	1.4	0.8
Shaking chills	65%	69%	2.1	0.5
Comorbidity	86%	37%	1.4	0.14

Providers should have a low threshold for ordering blood cultures.

MAKING A DIAGNOSIS

Blood cultures and urine cultures grew Escherichia coli.

The positive blood cultures confirm the overwhelming clinical impression of severe sepsis. (Cultures can be negative in 10% of patients with sepsis.) Other tests are not necessary to confirm the diagnosis.

CASE RESOLUTION

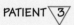
Ms. S was treated with broad-spectrum antibiotics and intensive IV fluids. After initial stabilization, hypotension recurred and urinary output dropped. She was transferred to the ICU. Four hours later her oxygenation deteriorated and a chest film revealed a diffuse infiltrate consistent with acute respiratory distress syndrome. She was intubated.

Treatment of Septic Shock

The treatment of septic shock is complex and recommendations evolve frequently. Readers are referred to specialized texts for details.

Ms. S received IV fluids, norepinephrine, antibiotics, mechanical ventilation, and activated protein C. Over the next 24 hours, her BP stabilized and her anion gap lactic acidosis resolved. Forty-eight hours later she was extubated. She eventually made a full recovery.

CHIEF COMPLAINT

PATIENT 3
Mr. R is a 55-year-old man with a history of COPD whose chief complaint is dyspnea. He reports that his symptoms began 5 days ago with a cough productive of green sputum. The cough worsened, and 4 days ago he had a low-grade fever of 37.2 °C. He noticed increasing shortness of breath 3 days ago. He reports that previously he was able to walk about 25 feet before becoming short of breath but now he is short of breath at rest. Last night his fever reached 38.8 °C, and today his dyspnea intensified. He is unable to complete a sentence without pausing to take a breath. On physical exam he appears older than his stated age. He is gaunt, sitting upright, breathing through pursed lips, and in obvious distress. Vital signs are temperature, 38.9 °C; RR, 28 breaths per minute; BP, 110/70 mm Hg; pulse, 110 bpm. His pulsus paradox is 20 mm Hg. Lung exam reveals significant use of accessory muscles and markedly decreased breath sounds. Cardiac exam is notable only for diminished heart sounds.

At this point, what is the leading hypothesis, and what are the active alternatives? What other tests should be ordered?

ORGANIZING THE DIFFERENTIAL DIAGNOSIS

Step 1: Generate Clinical Hypotheses

Mr. R's history of very poor exercise tolerance at *baseline* suggests severe COPD. Such severe COPD could result in chronic carbon dioxide retention and chronic respiratory acidosis. Another "must not miss" possibility is that his acute respiratory infection has precipitated *acute* respiratory failure (and acute respiratory acidosis). This is suggested by his worsening symptoms, respiratory distress, upright posture, pursed lip breathing, pulsus paradox, and decreased breath sounds. *It is critical to distinguish acute respiratory acidosis from chronic respiratory acidosis* because the former is more likely to progress rapidly to *complete* respiratory failure. Therefore, acute respiratory acidosis is both the leading hypothesis and the "must not miss" diagnosis. Another "must not miss" diagnosis is sepsis. His symptoms of fever and cough suggest the possibility of pneumonia, which can be complicated by sepsis resulting in an anion gap metabolic lactic acidosis. Finally, fever and lung disease may also result in *excessive* ventilation and a respiratory alkalosis. The differential diagnosis is listed in (Table 3–9).

Ask patients about a prior history of intubation or ICU admission. Such patients are at greater risk for respiratory failure.

Table 3–9. Diagnostic hypotheses for Mr. R.

Diagnostic Hypotheses	Clinical Clues	Important Tests
Leading Hypothesis		
Acute respiratory acidosis	Severe underlying lung disease Worsening symptoms Distress Pulsus paradox Decreased breath sounds Prior history of intubation, ICU admission	Decreased pH Elevated PCO₂ Near *normal* HCO₃⁻
Active Alternatives—Most Common		
Chronic respiratory acidosis	Severe underlying lung disease Decreased breath sounds	Decreased pH Elevated PaCO₂ *Elevated* HCO₃⁻
Respiratory alkalosis	Fever Pain Anxiety	Elevated pH Decreased PaCO₂ Normal HCO₃⁻
Active Alternatives—Must Not Miss		
Sepsis: anion gap metabolic acidosis	Fever Source of infection Shaking chills Oliguria Hypotension Altered mental status	Decreased pH, HCO₃⁻, and PaCO₂ Increased anion gap Positive blood cultures

Step 2: Check the pH

An ABG reveals a pH of 7.22, PaCO₂ of 70 mm Hg, and PaO₂ of 55 mm Hg.

The low pH on the ABG confirms the primary process is due to an acidosis.

Step 3: Determine Whether the Primary Disorder Is Due to a Metabolic or Respiratory Process

Na⁺, 138 mEq/L; K⁺, 5.1 mEq/L; HCO₃⁻, 27 mEq/L; Cl⁻, 102 mEq/L; BUN, 30 mg/dL; creatinine, 1.2 mg/dL.

The PaCO₂ and HCO₃⁻ are elevated. Since an elevated PaCO₂ would lower pH and cause an acidemia (whereas an elevated HCO₃⁻ would not), the primary process is a respiratory acidosis.

Step 4: Calculate Whether Compensation Is Appropriate

In this case, it is critical to determine whether the PaCO₂ is chronically elevated or whether this represents an acute decompensation. Acute respiratory acidosis can be distinguished from chronic respiratory acidosis by evaluating the degree of metabolic compensation. Metabolic compensation takes time since it requires renal generation of HCO₃⁻. Therefore, metabolic compensation is more complete in chronic respiratory acidosis. Formulas (see Table 3–1) allow us to calculate the HCO₃ levels we might expect in an acute versus chronic respiratory acidosis. In acute respiratory acidosis, the HCO₃ increases by only 1 mEq/L for every 10 mm Hg increase in PaCO₂. In Mr. R's case, the PaCO₂ is up by 30 mm Hg (from a normal of 40 mm Hg), so *if this were an acute respiratory acidosis* we would expect the HCO₃⁻ to increase by only 3 mEq/L (from a normal of 24 mEq/L to 27 mEq/L).

On the other hand, in chronic respiratory acidosis we expect an increase of 3.5 mEq/L of HCO₃⁻ per 10 mm Hg increase in PaCO₂. For a 30 mm Hg increase in PaCO₂, you would predict an increase in HCO₃ of 3 × 3.5 = 10.5 mEq *if this were a chronic respiratory acidosis.*

Mr. R's laboratory results reveal a HCO₃ of 27 mEq/L, an increase of only 3 mEq/L from a normal baseline of 24 mEq/L. Therefore, the tiny metabolic compensation suggests that Mr. R is suffering from an acute respiratory acidosis and is in imminent danger of complete respiratory failure.

Step 5: Calculate the Anion Gap

The anion gap = $138 - (102 + 27) = 9$.

Clearly, Mr. R has a normal anion gap, ruling out a co-existent hidden metabolic acidosis. His laboratory test results suggest an acute respiratory acidosis.

Other initial laboratory test results include WBC, 16,500/mcL with 62% granulocytes and 10% bands. Chest x-ray reveals hyperinflated lung fields and a left lower lobe infiltrate.

 Is the clinical information sufficient to make a diagnosis? If not, what other information do you need?

Leading Hypothesis: Respiratory Acidosis

Textbook Presentation

The presentation of respiratory acidosis depends primarily on the underlying cause. The most common causes are severe underlying lung or heart disease (ie, COPD or CHF). Such patients are typically in extreme respiratory distress.

Disease Highlights

A. Insufficient ventilation results in increasing levels of $PaCO_2$. This in turn lowers arterial pH. Compensation occurs over several days, with increased renal HCO_3^- regeneration.

B. Ventilation is assessed by measuring the arterial $PaCO_2$ and pH. Significant hypoventilation and acidosis may occur *without* significant hypoxia.

 Pulse oxymetry should never be used to assess adequate ventilation. An ABG is required in patients at risk for respiratory failure.

C. Etiology: Although most commonly due to lung or heart disease, respiratory acidosis may result from any disease affecting ventilation—from the brain to the alveoli.

D. Manifestations are primarily CNS.

   1. Severity depends on acuity. Patients with chronic hypercapnia have markedly fewer CNS effects than patients with acute hypercapnia.

   2. Anxiety, irritability, confusion, and lethargy

   3. Headache may be prominent in the morning due to the worsening hypoventilation that occurs with sleep.

   4. Stupor and coma may occur when the $PaCO_2$ > 70–100 mm Hg

   5. Tremor, asterixis, slurred speech, and papilledema may be seen.

Evidence-Based Diagnosis

A. Typically characterized by $PaCO_2$ > 43 mm Hg.

   1. Occasionally, a normal $PaCO_2$ suggests respiratory failure. For example, patients with a metabolic acidosis should hyperventilate to compensate and the expected $PaCO_2$ is actually below normal. In such states, a $PaCO_2$ of 40 mm Hg would be inappropriate and represent a respiratory acidosis.

   2. The alveolar-arterial oxygen gradient (PAO_2-PaO_2) can help distinguish hypercapnia associated with pulmonary disease from hypercapnia due to CNS disease (central hypoventilation). A normal A-a gradient (around 10 mm Hg) suggests central hypoventilation.

B. Pulsus paradox

   1. Defined as > 10 mm Hg drop in systolic BP with inspiration

   2. May be seen in patients using unusually strong inspiratory effort to breath

   3. Insensitive for severe asthma

   4. When increase is marked, there is a high LR of severe disease (Table 3–10).

CASE RESOLUTION

Mr. R is transferred to the ICU where he is placed on ventilatory support with biphasic positive airway pressure (BiPAP) and antibiotics. Over the next 5 days, his pneumonia improves. On day 8, BiPAP is discontinued and he is sent to the medical floors.

Table 3–10. Pulsus paradox in severe asthma.

	Sensitivity	Specificity	LR+	LR–
Pulsus > 10 mm Hg	53–68%	69–92%	2.7	0.5
Pulsus > 20 mm Hg	19–39%	92–100%	8.2	0.8
Pulsus > 25 mm Hg	16%	99%	22.6	0.8

Reprinted from McGee S. Evidence Based Physical Diagnosis, p. 143; Copyright © 2001 with permission from Elsevier.

Treatment of Respiratory Acidosis

A. Treat underlying disease process (ie, bronchodilators for asthma, naloxone for narcotic overdose).

B. Supplemental oxygen should be given as necessary to prevent hypoxemia.

 Supplemental oxygen occasionally worsens hypercapnia in some patients with severe COPD, asthma, and sleep apnea but should never be withheld from hypoxic patients.

C. Avoid hypokalemia and dehydration that may worsen metabolic alkalosis and inadvertently further suppress ventilation.

D. Mechanical ventilation with either intubation or BiPAP is lifesaving in some patients.

1. Mechanical ventilation is considered when pH < 7.1–7.25 or $PaCO_2$ > 80–90 mm Hg.

2. In general, patients with acute hypoventilation require mechanical ventilation with milder hypercarbia than patients with chronic hypoventilation.

REVIEW OF OTHER IMPORTANT DISEASES

Renal Tubular Acidosis (RTA)

Textbook Presentation

Although there are a variety of RTAs, the most common type in adults is hyperkalemic type IV or hyporenin hypoaldosterone RTA. Classically, patients have long-standing diabetes, mild renal insufficiency, and a mild nonanion gap metabolic acidosis. Patients have hyperkalemia secondary to hypoaldosteronism. Only the highlights of type IV RTA will be reviewed here.

Disease Highlights

A. Patients with RTAs have a nonanion gap acidosis due to the inability to excrete the daily acid load.

B. Defect is primarily secondary to impaired ammoniagenesis (and inability to buffer acid secretion).

C. Usually associated with hypoaldosteronism or pseudohypoaldosteronism. Hypoaldosteronism causes hyperkalemia.

D. Etiologies are numerous, but RTA is most commonly seen in diabetic patients with hyporeninism and mild renal impairment. Other causes include Addison disease, systemic lupus erythematosus, AIDS nephropathy, chronic interstitial renal disease, ACE inhibitors, cyclooxygenase inhibitors, potassium-sparing diuretics, β-blockers, α-blockers, and digitalis.

Treatment

Loop diuretics and fludrocortisone may be useful.

Starvation Ketosis

Typically, starvation ketosis occurs in patients with diminished carbohydrate intake. Ketosis is usually mild and serum glucose is usually normal. Serum pH is usually normal.

Alcoholic Ketoacidosis

Alcoholic ketoacidosis usually occurs in advanced alcoholism when the majority of calories come from alcohol. It may be precipitated by decreased intake, pancreatitis, GI bleeding, or infection. Metabolic acidosis is usually not severe.

Metabolic Alkalosis

Textbook Presentation

The most common clinical situations that give rise to metabolic alkalosis are recurrent vomiting or diuretic treatment. The metabolic alkalosis per se is usually asymptomatic. Muscle cramping due to coexistent hypokalemia may be seen.

Disease Highlights

A. Metabolic alkalosis develops only when there is *both* an increased production of HCO_3^- *and* a renal stimulus to reabsorb $NaHCO_3$. (Since the kidney freely filters HCO_3^-, an overproduction of $NaHCO_3$ alone simply results in increased renal $NaHCO_3$ loss.) Metabolic alkalosis occurs only when concurrent mechanisms induce renal reabsorption of HCO_3^-.

B. The most common mechanism that promotes HCO_3^- reabsorption is decreased sodium delivery to

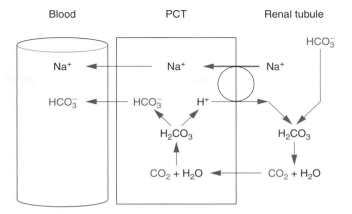

Figure 3–2. Reabsorption of HCO$_3^-$ in hypovolemia. Hypovolemia increases reabsorption of sodium in exchange for hydrogen ion at the proximal convoluted tubule (PCT). The hydrogen ion reacts with HCO$_3^-$ eventually forming CO$_2$, which crosses the cell membrane. HCO$_3^-$ is then regenerated and delivered to the bloodstream.

the nephron. This may occur in dehydration or other pathologic states associated with a decreased GFR (ie, CHF). The decreased GFR promotes avid sodium reabsorption in the proximal tubule, which in turn facilitates HCO$_3^-$ reabsorption (Figure 3–2). Hypokalemia also promotes HCO$_3^-$ reabsorption.

C. Pathologic states associated with metabolic alkalosis

   1. Vomiting or nasogastric drainage. Pathophysiology:

      a. Increased HCO$_3^-$ production by the stomach

      b. Dehydration causes increased sodium reabsorption in the nephron, which results in elevated HCO$_3^-$ reclamation.

      c. Secondary hyperaldosteronism leads to increased sodium reabsorption in exchange for potassium and hydrogen further augmenting HCO$_3^-$ production.

   2. Dehydration or other causes of reduced GFR (ie, CHF, nephrotic syndrome)

   3. Diuretics

   4. Hypokalemia

   5. Hyperaldosteronism

      a. Adrenal adenoma

      b. Licorice ingestion (licorice contains glycyrrhizic acid, an aldosterone agonist)

   6. Bartter or Gitelman syndromes

   7. Respiratory acidosis also promotes a compensatory metabolic alkalosis. Occasionally, rapid resolution of the respiratory failure will correct the hypercapnia, resulting in a transient inappropriate metabolic alkalosis (posthypercapnic metabolic alkalosis).

Treatment

A. Treatment of the underlying disorder and volume resuscitation usually results in resolution.

B. Replete potassium deficiency.

C. Carbonic anhydrase inhibitors and low bicarbonate dialysis can be used in severe cases.

Respiratory Alkalosis

Textbook Presentation

The presentation of respiratory alkalosis depends on the underlying disorder. Most causes are associated with tachypnea, which can be dramatic or subtle.

Disease Highlights

A. Hyperventilation induces hypocapnia causing respiratory alkalosis.

B. Most common causes include pulmonary disease, fever, pain, or anxiety.

C. Hypocapnia acutely reduces CNS blood flow.

D. Symptoms include paresthesias (particularly perioral), vertigo, dizziness, anxiety, hallucinations, myalgias, and symptoms reflective of underlying disorder.

E. Adverse effects include decreased cerebral blood flow, hypokalemia, hypocalcemia, lung injury, seizures, angina, and arrhythmias.

Treatment

Therapy is directed at the underlying disorder.

4

I have a patient with anemia.
How do I determine the cause?

CHIEF COMPLAINT

PATIENT 1

Mrs. A is a 48-year-old white woman who has had 2 months of fatigue due to anemia.

What is the differential diagnosis of anemia? How would you frame the differential?

CONSTRUCTING A DIFFERENTIAL DIAGNOSIS

The framework for organizing the differential diagnosis of anemia is a combination of pathophysiologic and morphologic. The first step in determining the cause of an anemia is to determine the general mechanism of the anemia, using a pathophysiologic framework. Anemia is caused by 1 of 3 processes:

1. **Acute or chronic blood loss:** Acute blood loss is clinically obvious. Chronic blood loss leads to an underproduction anemia.
2. **Underproduction** of RBCs by the bone marrow.
3. Increased **destruction** of RBCs, known as **hemolysis.**

After determining the general mechanism, the next step is to determine the cause of the underproduction or increased destruction. (This chapter will not discuss the approach to acute blood loss.) The framework for underproduction anemia is morphologic:

A. Microcytic anemias (mean corpuscular volume [MCV] < 80 mcm^3)
   1. Iron deficiency
   2. Thalassemia
   3. Anemia of chronic disease

4. Sideroblastic anemia
5. Lead exposure

B. Macrocytic anemias (MCV > 100 mcm^3)
   1. Megaloblastic anemias (abnormalities in DNA synthesis)
      a. B$_{12}$ deficiency
      b. Folate deficiency
      c. Antimetabolite drugs, such as methotrexate or zidovudine
   2. Nonmegaloblastic anemias
      a. Alcohol abuse
      b. Liver disease
      c. Hypothyroidism

C. Normocytic anemias
   1. Anemia of chronic disease
   2. Early iron deficiency
   3. Infiltration of bone marrow due to malignancy or granulomas
   4. RBC aplasia
      a. Aplastic anemia
      b. Suppression by parvovirus B19 or medications

The framework for hemolytic anemias is pathophysiologic:

A. Hereditary
   1. Enzyme defects, such as pyruvate kinase or glucose-6-phosphate dehydrogenase (G6PD) deficiency
   2. Hemoglobinopathies, such as sickle cell anemia
   3. RBC membrane abnormalities, such as spherocytosis

B. Acquired
   1. Hypersplenism
   2. Immune

    a. Autoimmune: warm IgG, cold IgM, cold IgG

    b. Drug induced: autoimmune or hapten

3. Traumatic

    a. Impact

    b. Macrovascular: shearing due to prosthetic valves

    c. Microvascular: disseminated intravascular coagulation (DIC), thrombotic thrombocytopenic purpura (TTP), and hemolytic uremic syndrome (HUS)

4. Infections, such as malaria

5. Toxins, such as snake venom and aniline dyes

6. Paroxysmal nocturnal hemoglobinuria

Mrs. A has a past medical history of obesity, reflux, depression, asthma, and arthritis. She comes to your office complaining of feeling down with progressive fatigue for the last 2 months. She has no chest pain, cough, fever, weight loss, or edema. Her only GI symptoms are poor appetite and her usual reflux symptoms; she has had no vomiting, melena, or rectal bleeding. She still has regular menses that are occasionally heavy. She brought in her medication bottles, which include ranitidine, sertraline, tramadol, cetirizine, and a fluticasone inhaler. Her physical exam shows a depressed affect, clear lungs, a normal cardiac exam, a nontender abdomen, guaiac-negative stool, no edema, and no pallor.

 How reliable is the history and physical for detecting anemia?

A. Symptoms in chronic anemia are due to decreased oxygen delivery to the tissues.

    1. Fatigue is a common but not very specific symptom.

    2. Dyspnea on exertion occurs in patients with normal or abnormal cardiac function.

    3. Exertional chest pain occurs most often in patients with underlying coronary artery disease or severe anemia or both.

    4. Palpitations or tachycardia

    5. Edema

    6. No symptoms: mild anemia is often asymptomatic

B. Symptoms of hypovolemia occur only in acute anemia due to large volume blood loss.

C. Conjunctival rim pallor

    1. Present when the anterior rim of the inferior conjunctiva is the same color as the deeper posterior aspect of the palpebral conjunctiva, rather than the normal bright red color of the anterior rim.

    2. The LR+ of conjunctival rim pallor for the presence of anemia is 16.7.

D. Palmar crease pallor has an LR+ of 7.9.

E. Pallor elsewhere (facial, nail bed) is not as useful, with LR+ < 5.

F. **No physical sign rules out anemia.**

G. The overall sensitivity and specificity of the physical exam for anemia is about 70%.

 Order a CBC if patients have suggestive symptoms, even without physical exam signs, or if you observe conjunctival rim or palmar crease pallor.

Mrs. A's initial laboratory test results show a WBC of 7100/mcL, RBC of 3.6 million/mcL, Hgb of 6.7 g/dL, Hct of 23.3%, and MCV of 76 mcm³. A CBC 6 months ago showed an Hgb of 12 g/dL, Hct of 36%, and MCV of 82 mcm³.

 At this point, what is the leading hypothesis, and what are the active alternatives? What other tests should be ordered?

ORGANIZING THE DIFFERENTIAL DIAGNOSIS

The first step is to determine the mechanism of Mrs. A's anemia. Mrs. A is not having any symptoms or signs of acute blood loss. She does have symptoms suggestive of chronic blood loss, such as reflux and occasional menorrhagia. However, it is not possible to distinguish underproduction from hemolysis based on the history. Although the **change in her CBC tells you a new process is going on**, it also does not distinguish between these 2 mechanisms.

Always look at previous CBC results to see if the anemia is new, old, or progressive.

The best test to distinguish underproduction from hemolysis is the **reticulocyte count:**

A. Low or normal reticulocyte counts are seen in underproduction anemias.

B. High reticulocyte counts occur when the bone marrow is responding normally to anemia or if there is hemolysis.

C. Reticulocyte measures include:

   1. The **reticulocyte count,** which is the percentage of circulating RBCs that are reticulocytes (normally 0.5–1.5%).

   2. The **absolute reticulocyte count,** which is the number of reticulocytes actually circulating, normally 25,000–75,000/mcL (multiply the percentage of reticulocytes by the total number of RBCs).

   3. The **reticulocyte production index (RPI),** which corrects the absolute reticulocyte count for the degree of anemia and for the increased rate of reticulocyte maturation that occurs in anemia, leading to increased numbers of circulating reticulocytes.

      a. RPI = reticulocyte% × (Hct/45) × 0.5

      b. The normal RPI is about 1.0

 The first step in evaluating anemia is checking a reticulocyte count.

 Mrs. A's reticulocyte count is 1.5%, which is an absolute reticulocyte count of 54,000/mcL, and an RPI of 0.39.

 Now that you have found that Mrs. A has an underproduction anemia, what is the leading hypothesis, and what are the active alternatives? What other tests should be ordered?

Mrs. A's MCV is 76 mcm³, so you should consider the differential diagnosis for microcytic anemia. However, it is important to keep in mind that the **MCV is not specific and should not be used to rule in or rule out a specific cause of anemia.**

A. In 1 study, normal MCVs were found in 50% of patients with abnormal serum vitamin B_{12}, folate, or iron studies.

   1. 5% of patients with iron deficiency had high MCVs

   2. 12% of patients with B_{12} or folate deficiency had low MCVs

B. What about the rest of the CBC? Do the other indices help?

   1. Other red cell indices (mean corpuscular hemoglobin [MCH] and mean corpuscular hemoglobin concentration [MCHC]) tend to trend with the MCV and are not particularly sensitive or specific.

   2. The red cell distribution width (RDW) is also not sensitive or specific in identifying the cause of an anemia.

 Use the MCV to organize your thinking, not to diagnose the cause of an anemia.

Despite this caveat about the MCV, in a patient with a microcytic anemia and symptoms suggestive of possible chronic blood loss, iron deficiency is by far the most likely cause, with a pretest probability of 80%. Therefore, the leading hypothesis for Mrs. A is iron deficiency anemia. Anemia of chronic disease, by virtue of being common, is the best active alternative; to make this diagnosis, keep in mind that the patient must have 1 of the chronic diseases known to cause anemia. Sideroblastic anemia and lead exposure are other hypotheses, and isolated thalassemia is excluded by the degree of anemia and the recently normal CBC. Because the MCV lacks specificity, the causes of normocytic and macrocytic anemia also need to be kept in mind as other hypotheses. Table 4–1 lists the differential diagnosis.

Leading Hypothesis: Iron Deficiency Anemia

Textbook Presentation

The most classic presentation would be a young, menstruating woman who has fatigue and a craving for ice. Typical presentations include fatigue, dyspnea, and sometimes edema.

Disease Highlights

A. The CBC varies with the degree of severity of the iron deficiency.

   1. In very early iron deficiency, the CBC is normal.

   2. A mild anemia then develops, with an Hgb of

Table 4–1. Diagnostic hypotheses for Mrs. A.

Diagnostic Hypotheses	Clinical Clues	Important Tests
Leading Hypothesis		
Iron deficiency anemia	Pica Blood loss (menorrhagia, melena, hematochezia, NSAID use)	Serum ferritin
Active Alternative—Most Common		
Anemia of chronic disease	History of renal or liver disease, inflammation, infection	Fe/TIBC, serum ferritin, erythropoietin level
Other Hypotheses		
Thalassemia	Ethnic background	Hgb electrophoresis
Lead poisoning	Exposure to lead	Lead level
B_{12} deficiency	Diet Autoimmune diseases Neurologic symptoms	B_{12} level
Folate deficiency	Pregnancy Sickle cell anemia Alcohol abuse	Folate level

9–12 g/dL, and normal or slightly hypochromic RBCs.

3. As the iron deficiency progresses, the Hgb continues to decrease, and hypochromia and microcytosis develop.

B. Causes of iron deficiency

1. Rapid growth (infancy, adolescence)

2. Inadequate diet (rare)

3. Malabsorption, seen in patients with gastrectomy, celiac sprue, or inflammatory bowel disease (IBD)

4. Blood loss, most commonly menstrual or GI

Evidence-Based Diagnosis

A. Bone marrow exam for absence of iron stores is the gold standard.

B. The ferritin is the best serum test.

1. The LR+ for a decreased serum ferritin is very high, with reports ranging from LR+ of 51 for a ferritin < 15 ng/mL to a LR+ of 25.5 for a ferritin < 32 ng/mL.

2. **Thus, a low ferritin rules in iron deficiency anemia.**

3. In general populations, the LR− for a serum ferritin > 100 ng/mL is very low (0.08).

4. **Thus, in general populations, a ferritin > 100 ng/mL greatly reduces the probability the patient has iron deficiency.**

5. However, because ferritin is an acute phase reactant that increases in inflammatory states, interpreting it in the presence of such illnesses is difficult.

   a. There is a wide range of reported LRs, with many studies finding ferritin is *not* helpful in diagnosing iron deficiency in the presence of chronic illness.

   b. The level at which the serum ferritin suggests iron deficiency is probably much higher in patients with chronic illness, but the level may vary depending on the underlying illness.

     (1) Ferritin < 60 ng/mL in patients with rheumatoid arthritis: LR+ = 7.2, LR− = 0.16

     (2) Ferritin < 50 ng/mL in patients with IBD: LR+ = 2.36, LR− = 0.13

     (3) Ferritin < 112 ng/mL in patients with chronic renal failure: LR+ = 15.8, LR− = 0.16

     (4) Ferritin ≤ 30 ng/mL in patients with tuberculosis: LR+ = 3.6, LR− = 0.13

6. **Thus, the ferritin cannot be used to absolutely rule in or rule out iron deficiency anemia in patients with chronic diseases.**

C. Other tests

1. The MCV, the transferrin saturation (serum iron/iron-binding capacity {Fe/TIBC}), red cell protoporphyrin, red cell ferritin, and RDW all are less sensitive and specific than ferritin.

2. The best of these is transferrin saturation ≤ 5%, with a LR+ of 10.46.

 In patients without chronic illness, the serum ferritin is the best single test to diagnose iron deficiency anemia.

MAKING A DIAGNOSIS

Since Mrs. A does not have any chronic, inflammatory diseases, the most useful test at this point is a serum ferritin. Serum iron and TIBC are often ordered simultaneously but are not necessary at this point.

You review the history, looking for symptoms of bleeding or chronic illness. She has no renal or liver disease and no symptoms of infection. Her ethnic background is Scandinavian. You order a serum ferritin, which is 5 ng/mL.

CASE RESOLUTION

With a pretest probability of 80% and an LR+ of 51 for this level of ferritin, Mrs. A is clearly iron deficient. It is not necessary to test for any other causes of anemia, but it is necessary to determine why she is iron deficient.

Always identify the source of blood loss in iron deficiency anemia. Be alert for occult malignancies.

Iron deficiency is almost always due to chronic blood loss and rarely due to poor iron intake or malabsorption of iron; menstrual and GI blood loss are the most common sources. Because GI blood loss can be occult, many patients need GI evaluations.

A. Who needs a GI work-up?

1. All men, all women without menorrhagia, and women over age 50 even with menorrhagia.

2. Women under age 50 with menorrhagia do not need further GI evaluation, unless they have GI symptoms or a family history of early colon cancer or adenomatous polyps.

3. Always ask carefully about minimal GI symptoms in young women, since celiac sprue often causes iron deficiency due to malabsorption, and the symptoms can easily be attributed to irritable bowel syndrome.

B. Which GI test should be done first?

1. In the absence of symptoms or in the presence of lower GI symptoms, do a colonoscopy first.

2. If there are upper GI symptoms, do an esophagogastroduodenoscopy (EGD) first.

3. If the first test is negative, the other one must be done.

4. Small bowel imaging rarely finds important lesions in patients with normal upper and lower endoscopies and often can be omitted. However, newer techniques to visualize the small bowel, such as video capsule endoscopy, may be useful in evaluating such patients.

5. Clinicians are sometimes unsure whether a colonoscopy is necessary when the EGD shows a definitive bleeding source. Finding colonic lesions in such cases is rare, and colonoscopy can be reserved for symptomatic patients or those who need routine colorectal cancer screening.

It is unclear from Mrs. A's history whether the menorrhagia is sufficient to cause this degree of iron deficiency anemia. In addition, she has the upper GI symptoms of anorexia and reflux. Therefore, you order an EGD, which shows severe reflux esophagitis and also gastritis. Further history reveals she has been using several hundred milligrams of ibuprofen daily for several weeks because of a back strain. The severe esophagitis and gastritis are sufficient to explain her anemia, and she has no lower GI symptoms or family history of colorectal cancer. The work-up is complete.

Treatment of Iron Deficiency Anemia

A. Iron deficiency anemia is generally treated with oral iron replacement, with IV iron therapy reserved for patients who demonstrate malabsorption.

B. Transfusion is necessary only if the patient is hypotensive; orthostatic; actively bleeding; or has angina, dizziness, syncope, or severe dyspnea.

C. The best absorbed oral iron is ferrous sulfate; the dose is 325 mg 3 times daily.

D. There are significant GI side effects including nausea, abdominal pain, and constipation; these can be reduced by taking the iron with food, and slowly titrating the dose from 1 tablet daily to 3 tablets daily over 1 to 2 weeks.

E. There should be an increase in reticulocytes 7–10 days after starting therapy, and an increase in Hgb and Hct by 30 days; if there is no response, reconsider the diagnosis.

F. It is necessary to take iron for 6 months in order to replete iron stores.

FOLLOW-UP OF MRS. A

Mrs. A stopped the ibuprofen, substituted a proton pump inhibitor for the H_2-blocker, and completed 6 months of iron therapy. She felt fine. A follow-up CBC showed an Hgb of 13 g/dL, an Hct of 39%, and a significantly elevated MCV of 122 mcm³.

 At this point, what is the leading hypothesis, and what are the active alternatives? What other tests should be ordered?

ORGANIZING THE DIFFERENTIAL DIAGNOSIS

Although Mrs. A is not anemic now, she has a marked macrocytosis. The approach to isolated macrocytosis is the same as the approach to macrocytic anemia. The degree of macrocytosis is not a reliable predictor of the cause, but in general, the higher the MCV, the more likely the patient has a B_{12} or folate deficiency. The pretest probability of vitamin deficiency with an MCV of 115–129 mcm³ is 50%, and nearly all patients with an MCV > 130 mcm³ will have a vitamin deficiency.

Since B_{12} deficiency is seen more often than folate deficiency in otherwise healthy people, that is the leading hypothesis, with folate deficiency being the active alternative. Use of antimetabolite drugs is excluded by history. Causes of nonmegaloblastic anemias need to be considered next. Hypothyroidism would be the most likely other hypothesis, with liver disease and alcohol abuse excluded by history. Table 4–2 lists the differential diagnosis.

Leading Hypothesis: B_{12} Deficiency

Textbook Presentation

The classic presentation is an elderly woman with marked anemia and neurologic symptoms such as paresthesias, sensory loss (especially vibration and position), ataxia, dementia, and psychiatric symptoms.

Disease Highlights

A. It takes years to develop this deficiency because of extensive stores of vitamin B_{12}.

B. Anemia and macrocytosis are not always present.

1. In 1 study, 28% of patients with neurologic symptoms due to B_{12} deficiency had no anemia or macrocytosis.

2. In another study, the following clinical characteristics were found in patients with B_{12} deficiency:

   a. 33% white, 41% black, 25% Latino

   b. 28% not anemic

   c. 17% normal MCV

Table 4–2. Diagnostic hypotheses for Mrs. A's follow-up.

Diagnostic Hypotheses	Clinical Clues	Important Tests
Leading Hypothesis		
B_{12} deficiency	Vegan diet Other autoimmune diseases Age (elderly) Neurologic symptoms	B_{12} level Homocysteine level Methylmalonic acid (MMA) level
Active Alternative—Most Common and Must Not Miss		
Folate deficiency	Alcohol abuse Starvation Pregnancy Sickle cell anemia	Serum folate level RBC folate level Homocysteine level
Other Hypotheses		
Hypothyroidism	Constipation Weight gain Fatigue Cold intolerance	TSH FTI

d. 17% leukopenia, 35% thrombocytopenia, 12.5% pancytopenia

e. 36% neuropsychiatric symptoms

 The CBC can be normal in B_{12} deficiency.

C. B_{12} must bind to intrinsic factor in the stomach in order to be absorbed in the terminal ileum.

D. Deficiency is rarely due to inadequate intake, and then generally in patients following a vegan diet.

E. B_{12} deficiency is most often due to inadequate absorption, either in the stomach or terminal ileum.

1. Gastric causes of malabsorption involve inadequate intrinsic factor, and include:

   a. **Pernicious anemia,** which is autoimmune gastritis due to antibodies to parietal cells and intrinsic factor

   b. Gastrectomy or gastric bypass

2. Small bowel diseases and conditions associated with inadequate absorption include

   a. Ileal resection or bypass

   b. Tropical sprue

   c. Crohn disease

   d. Blind loop syndrome

3. Sometimes agents such as colchicine, ethanol, neomycin, or fish tapeworm interfere with absorption.

4. Absorption may rarely be due to congenital disorders (transcobalamin II deficiency).

Evidence-Based Diagnosis

A. Determining whether a patient is B_{12} deficient is more complicated than it seems.

   1. B_{12} levels can be falsely low in folate deficiency, pregnancy, and oral contraceptive use.

   2. B_{12} levels can be falsely normal in myeloproliferative disorders, liver disease, and bacterial overgrowth syndromes.

   3. The sensitivity and specificity of B_{12} levels for true deficiency are not well established.

B. B_{12} is a cofactor in the conversion of homocysteine to methionine, and of methmalonyl CoA to succinyl CoA.

   1. Consequently, in B_{12} deficiency, the levels of homocysteine and MMA increase.

   2. Therefore, another way to diagnosis B_{12} deficiency is to measure **homocysteine and MMA levels.**

     a. In addition to B_{12} deficiency, MMA can be elevated in renal insufficiency and hypovolemia.

     b. Homocysteine can be elevated in folate or pyridoxine deficiency, renal insufficiency, hypovolemia, and hypothyroidism.

     c. The sensitivity of MMA for the diagnosis of B_{12} deficiency ranges from 86% to 98%. The sensitivity of homocysteine ranges from 85% to 96%. The specificities are not known.

C. **Response to therapy** is another way to establish the presence of B_{12} deficiency.

   1. MMA and homocysteine normalize 7–14 days after the start of replacement therapy.

   2. Figure 4–1 shows the response to a single IM injection of 100 mcg cobalamin on day 0 in a patient with pernicious anemia.

D. An algorithm for diagnosing B_{12} deficiency is the following:

   1. B_{12} level < 100 pg/mL, deficiency present

   2. B_{12} level 100–300 pg/mL, check MMA and homocysteine levels

     a. If both normal, deficiency unlikely

     b. If both elevated, deficiency present

     c. If either elevated, possible deficiency

   3. B_{12} > 300 pg/mL, deficiency unlikely

 Very low or very high B_{12} levels are usually diagnostic.

MAKING A DIAGNOSIS

Mrs. A's B_{12} level is 21 pg/mL, with a serum folate of 8.0 ng/mL.

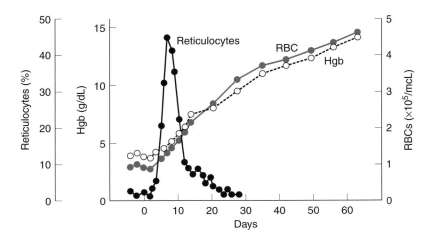

Figure 4–1. Response to B_{12} therapy.

Have you crossed a diagnostic threshold for the leading hypothesis, B_{12} deficiency? Have you ruled out the active alternatives? Do other tests need to be done to exclude the alternative diagnoses?

Alternative Diagnosis: Folate Deficiency

Textbook Presentation

The classic presentation is an alcoholic patient with malnutrition and anemia.

Disease Highlights

A. Anemia and macrocytosis are the most common manifestations; neurologic symptoms are rare.

B. Most often caused by inadequate intake (especially in alcoholic patients) or increased demand due to pregnancy, chronic hemolysis, leukemia.

C. Since absorption occurs in jejunum, malabsorption is rare in the absence of short bowel syndrome or bacterial overgrowth syndromes.

D. Some drugs can cause folate deficiency, including methotrexate, phenytoin, sulfasalazine, and alcohol.

E. Along with B_{12}, folate is a cofactor for the conversion of homocysteine to methionine, so homocysteine levels increase in folate deficiency.

Evidence-Based Diagnosis

A. The sensitivity and specificity of serum folate measurements for the diagnosis of folate deficiency are not clear.

B. Levels can decrease within a few days of dietary folate restriction, or with alcohol use, even though tissue stores can be normal; levels increase with feeding.

C. RBC folate correlates more strongly with megaloblastic changes than does serum folate; however, the sensitivity and specificity of RBC folate for the diagnosis of true deficiency are both low (about 70% each).

D. Elevated homocysteine is about 80% sensitive for the diagnosis of folate deficiency; the specificity is unknown.

E. A positive response to therapy is diagnostic.

1. Never treat folate deficiency without determining whether the patient is B_{12} deficient.

2. Folate replacement can correct hematologic abnormalities while worsening the neurologic symptoms specific to B_{12} deficiency.

F. A patient with a normal serum folate, normal RBC folate, and no response to folate replacement does not have folate deficiency.

Treatment

A. Oral folic acid 1 mg daily

B. For duration of increased demand, such as throughout pregnancy.

C. Indefinitely in patients with chronic increased demand, such as sickle cell anemia

Always check for B_{12} deficiency in a patient with folate deficiency.

CASE RESOLUTION

Mrs. A's B_{12} level is diagnostic of B_{12} deficiency. She has no conditions associated with folate deficiency, so even though the test characteristics of the serum folate are unclear, in this case the normal level is sufficient to rule out folate deficiency.

The next step is to determine the cause of the B_{12} deficiency; in most cases, this means figuring out where the malabsorption is occurring.

A. The **malabsorption is in the stomach** if:

1. The patient has had a gastrectomy or gastric bypass

2. The patient has detectable anti-intrinsic factor antibody

a. Found in about 50–80% of patients with pernicious anemia. **The presence of anti-intrinsic factor antibody rules in pernicious anemia; the absence does not rule out pernicious anemia.**

b. Antiparietal cell antibodies are found in about 85% of patients with pernicious anemia, but also in patients with other autoimmune endocrinopathies and up to 10% of normal patients. **The presence of antiparietal cell antibodies does not rule in pernicious anemia.**

3. The Schilling test stage 1 result is abnormal, with a normal stage 2 result

a. Radiolabeled oral B_{12} (1 mcg) is given, along with 1000 mcg IM; the parenteral dose saturates the binding protein, ensuring that the absorbed B_{12} is excreted in the urine.

   b. If the amount of labeled B_{12} in the urine is < 10% of the oral dose, stage 1 is abnormal, suggesting that malabsorption has occurred because there was no intrinsic factor present to bind the B_{12}.

   c. The test is then repeated (stage 2), giving oral intrinsic factor with the labeled oral B_{12}, bypassing the need for gastric production of intrinsic factor; now a normal amount should be absorbed in the ileum.

B. The **malabsorption is in the ileum** if

   1. Both Schilling test stages 1 and 2 results are abnormal.

   2. Abnormal results in both stages of the test suggest that even in the presence of adequate intrinsic factor, B_{12} is not absorbed.

However, there are many reasons for false-positive Schilling tests, including inadequate urine collection, renal insufficiency, and B_{12} deficiency–*induced* ileal dysfunction, leading to an abnormal stage 2 even in the absence of ileal disease. It is not always possible to determine the site of malabsorption, and it is acceptable to treat such patients with B_{12} replacement.

Mrs. A's intrinsic factor antibody was positive. This is a highly specific finding and is diagnostic of B_{12} deficiency due to pernicious anemia. Mrs. A began receiving B_{12} injections, and a follow-up CBC 4 months later was entirely normal.

Treatment of B_{12} Deficiency

A. IM cobalamin, 1000 mcg weekly for 8 weeks, and then monthly for life

B. Can also use oral cobalamin, 1000–2000 mcg daily

   1. Oral cobalamin is absorbed by a second, nonintrinsic factor dependent mechanism that is relatively inefficient.

   2. Compliance can be a problem.

C. Sublingual and intranasal formulations are available, but have not been extensively studied.

CHIEF COMPLAINT

PATIENT 2

Mrs. L is a 70-year-old woman with a history of squamous cell carcinoma of the larynx, successfully treated with surgery and radiation therapy 10 years ago. She has a tracheostomy and a jejunostomy tube. One week ago, she fell and fractured her right humeral head. On routine preoperative laboratory tests, her CBC was unexpectedly abnormal: WBC 11,100/mcL (63% polymorphonuclear leukocytes, 12% basophils, 2% metamyelocytes, 4% monocytes, 19% lymphocytes), Hgb 8.4 g/dL, Hct 26.3%, MCV 85 mcm³. One month ago, her Hgb was 12.0 g/dL, with a normal WBC.

What is the leading hypothesis, and what are the active alternatives? What other tests should be ordered?

ORGANIZING THE DIFFERENTIAL DIAGNOSIS

The relatively acute drop in Hct suggests either bleeding or hemolysis; these are also the "must not miss" diagnoses. The usual causes of normocytic anemia need to be considered next. Anemia of chronic disease is a common cause of normocytic anemia, with bone marrow infiltration and RBC aplasia being less common. You would also include causes of macrocytic anemia in your list of other hypotheses, especially folate deficiency since it can develop fairly rapidly. Table 4–3 lists the differential diagnosis.

She has felt feverish, with a cough productive of brown sputum. She has had no nausea or vomiting, no melena, and no hematochezia. She has been postmenopausal for a long time and has had no vaginal bleeding. The orthopedic surgeon

Table 4–3. Diagnostic hypotheses for Mrs. L.

Diagnostic Hypotheses	Clinical Clues	Important Tests
Leading Hypothesis		
Iron deficiency anemia	GI bleeding Pica Menorrhagia	Ferritin
Hemolysis	Fatigue	Reticulocyte count
Active Alternative—Must Not Miss		
Iron deficiency	GI bleeding Pica Menorrhagia	Ferritin
Hemolysis	Fatigue	Reticulocyte count
Active Alternative—Most Common		
Anemia of chronic disease	Acute infection Acute renal failure Chronic illness	Fe/TIBC, serum ferritin Erythropoetin level Bone marrow
Other Alternatives		
Marrow infiltration	Pancytopenia Bleeding Malaise	Bone marrow
RBC aplasia	Drug exposure Viral symptoms	History Bone marrow
Folate deficiency	Diet Alcohol abuse Pregnancy Sickle cell anemia	Serum or RBC folate Bone marrow

confirms it is unlikely that she has significant bleeding at the fracture site. Her rectal exam shows brown, hemoccult-negative stool. Her chest x-ray shows a new left lower lobe pneumonia.

 Is the clinical information sufficient to make a diagnosis? If not, what other information do you need?

MAKING A DIAGNOSIS

Further laboratory testing shows a reticulocyte count of 2.8% (absolute reticulocytes of 85.95/mcL, RPI of 0.38), consistent with an underproduction anemia. Her serum ferritin is 150 ng/mL.

 Have you crossed a diagnostic threshold for the leading hypotheses, iron deficiency and hemolysis? Have you ruled out the active alternatives? Do other tests need to be done to exclude the alternative diagnoses?

Alternative Diagnosis: Anemia of Chronic Disease

Textbook Presentation

Because there is such a broad spectrum of underlying causes, there is no classic presentation of anemia of chronic disease. It is most often discovered on a routine CBC.

Disease Highlights

A. Anemia of chronic disease is due to underproduction of RBCs from trapping of iron in macrophages, abnormal bone marrow response to erythropoietin, or presence of inflammatory cytokines.

B. Specific diseases associated with anemia of chronic disease

   1. Renal insufficiency: severity of anemia correlates with severity of disease

   2. Liver disease

   3. Chronic inflammation

      a. Connective tissue diseases, such as systemic lupus erythematosus, rheumatoid arthritis

      b. Chronic infections, such as subacute bacterial endocarditis, HIV

   4. Endocrinopathies, such as Addison disease, thyroid disease, panhypopituitarism

   5. "Acute" anemia of chronic disease

      a. Can occur within 24–48 hours in acute bacterial infections, with Hgb usually in the 10–12 g/dL range

      b. Occurs in as many as 90% of ICU patients,

accompanied by inappropriately mild elevations of serum erythropoietin levels and blunted bone marrow response to endogenous erythropoietin

Evidence-Based Diagnosis

A. There is no 1 test that proves or disproves a patient's anemia is from anemia of chronic disease.

B. Instead, there are several diagnostic tests that can possibly be done, sometimes simultaneously and sometimes sequentially.

 The patient must have 1 of the diseases associated with anemia of chronic disease in order for anemia of chronic disease to be diagnosed.

1. Even in the presence of a disease known to cause anemia, it is important to rule out iron, B_{12}, and folate deficiencies.

2. As discussed above, it can be difficult to interpret iron studies in the presence of chronic diseases; however, the typical pattern in anemia of chronic disease is a **low serum iron, low iron-binding capacity, normal percent saturation, and elevated serum ferritin.**

3. **Erythropoietin levels** will be low in renal insufficiency and not appropriately elevated for the degree of anemia in inflammatory conditions.

4. **Pancytopenia** suggests there is bone marrow infiltration or a disease that suppresses production of all cell lines.

 When you see pancytopenia, think about bone marrow infiltration, B_{12} deficiency, viral infection, drug toxicity, or acute alcohol intoxication.

5. **Bone marrow examination** is necessary to establish the diagnosis when pancytopenia is present, serum tests are not diagnostic, the anemia progresses, or there is not an appropriate response to empiric therapy.

CASE RESOLUTION

Mrs. L has normal liver function tests and a normal creatinine. Her B_{12} level is 400 pg/mL, and her serum folate is 10.0 ng/mL. Her iron studies show a serum iron of 25 mcg/dL, with a TIBC of 140 mcg/dL (% saturation = 18%).

Mrs. L has a very low RPI, ruling out hemolysis. She has no signs of bleeding, and iron studies consistent with an anemia of chronic disease; in the absence of a chronic inflammatory disease, a serum ferritin over 100 ng/mL generally rules out iron deficiency anemia. In addition, she has no pancytopenia to suggest bone marrow infiltration or diffuse marrow suppression, and no evidence of vitamin deficiency. She has a disease (acute bacterial pneumonia) known to be associated with "acute" anemia of chronic disease. Thus, the diagnosis is "acute" anemia of chronic disease. Her pneumonia is treated with oral antibiotics, and her CBC is normal when checked 6 weeks later.

Treatment of Anemia of Chronic Disease

A. Treat the underlying chronic disease, if possible.

B. Randomized trials have shown a benefit to administering exogenous erythropoietin in renal failure, in HIV, and in anemia associated with chemotherapy.

CHIEF COMPLAINT

PATIENT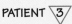

Mr. J is a 77-year-old African American man with a history of an aortic valve replacement about 2 years ago. He brought in results of tests done at another hospital: Hgb, 9.0 g/dL;

Hct, 27.4%; MCV, 90 mcm³; reticulocyte count, 6%; serum ferritin, 110 ng/mL; B_{12}, 416 pg/mL; folate 20.0 ng/mL. The RPI is 1.8.

 At this point, what is the leading hypothesis, and what are the active alternatives? What other tests should be ordered?

ORGANIZING THE DIFFERENTIAL DIAGNOSIS

The leading hypothesis is hemolysis because of the elevated reticulocyte count. Considering the normal ferritin and vitamin levels, the pretest probability of hemolysis is high. The only potential active alternative would be active bleeding, since an elevated reticulocyte count also occurs then; however, that would be clinically obvious. All other causes of anemia are other hypotheses to be considered only if the diagnosis of hemolysis is not supported by further testing. Table 4–4 lists the differential diagnosis.

Mr. J has no history of hematemesis, melena, hematochezia, or abdominal pain. His abdominal exam is normal, and rectal exam shows brown, hemoccult-negative stool.

Is the clinical information sufficient to make a diagnosis? If not, what other information do you need?

Leading Hypothesis: Hemolysis

Textbook Presentation

The presentation of hemolysis depends on the cause. Patients can be asymptomatic or critically ill.

Table 4–4. Diagnostic hypotheses for Mr. J.

Diagnostic Hypotheses	Clinical Clues	Important Tests
Leading Hypothesis		
Hemolysis	Mechanical valve Known hereditary condition Sepsis Fever	Reticulocyte count Haptoglobin Indirect bilirubin Lactate dehydrogenase
Active Alternative—Must Not Miss		
Active bleeding	Hematemesis Melena Hematochezia Vaginal bleeding Abdominal pain	

Evidence-Based Diagnosis

A. During hemolysis, RBC products are released into the circulation, and their presence (or the absence of proteins that bind them) can be measured to support the diagnosis of hemolysis.

1. Sometimes RBCs are destroyed in the **intravascular space** (impact, macrovascular trauma, some complement-induced lysis).

   a. Some incompletely hemolyzed cells reform, to be later destroyed in the spleen.

   b. Completely destroyed cells release free Hgb into the plasma, which then binds to **haptoglobin**, reducing the plasma haptoglobin level.

   c. Some Hgb is lysed intravascularly and then is filtered by the glomerulus, causing **hemoglobinuria.**

   d. Some filtered Hgb is taken up by renal tubular cells, stored as hemosiderin, and **hemosiderinuria** occurs about a week later, when the tubular cells are sloughed into the urine.

2. Deformed RBCs and those coated with complement are usually destroyed in the **extravascular space**, in the liver, or in the spleen.

   a. Most of the Hgb is degraded into biliverdin, iron, and carbon monoxide.

   b. Biliverdin is converted to **unconjugated bilirubin** and released into the plasma, increasing the unconjugated bilirubin level.

3. Some free Hgb is released, which then binds to **haptoglobin**, again reducing the plasma haptoglobin level.

B. So, what abnormalities would you expect to see during active hemolysis?

1. The reticulocyte count should be above 4–5%; in one study of autoimmune hemolytic anemia, the median was 9%.

2. The serum haptoglobin should be < 25 mg/dL (sensitivity = 83%, specificity = 96% for hemolysis, LR+ = 21, LR− = 0.18).

3. The unconjugated bilirubin may be increased (sensitivity and specificity unknown).

4. The LDH might be increased (sensitivity and specificity unknown).

5. Plasma and urine Hgb should be elevated if the hemolysis is intravascular (sensitivity and specificity unknown).

MAKING A DIAGNOSIS

Mr. J's serum haptoglobin is < 20 mg/dL, his serum bilirubin in normal, and his LDH is elevated at 359 units/L.

Have you crossed a diagnostic threshold for the leading hypothesis, hemolysis? Have you ruled out the active alternatives? Do other tests need to be done to exclude the alternative diagnoses?

The combination of the high pretest probability and the large LR+ for this level of haptoglobin confirms the diagnosis of hemolysis. Active bleeding has been ruled out by history and physical exam. At this point, any further testing should be aimed at determining the cause of the hemolysis. It is helpful to ask a series of questions to direct your search for the cause of a hemolytic anemia:

A. Does the patient have splenomegaly? The spleen is 1 of the major sites of extravascular hemolysis.

B. Is the direct antiglobulin (Coombs) test positive?

   1. Seen in autoimmune hemolytic anemias

   2. The Coombs test detects antibody or complement on the surface of the RBC

      a. The patient's RBCs are washed free of adherent proteins.

      b. They are reacted with antiserum containing anti-IgG and anti-C3.

      c. If IgG and/or C3 are present on the RBC, there will be agglutination.

      d. Over 99% of patients with warm antibody autoimmune hemolytic anemia will have a positive direct Coombs test.

   3. The indirect Coombs test detects antibodies to RBC antigens in the patient's serum.

      a. The patient's serum is incubated with normal RBCs.

      b. If the serum contains cold (IgM) antibodies, there will be agglutination.

      c. Otherwise, anti-IgG is added; if the serum contains IgG, there will be agglutination.

C. Is there concomitant thrombocytopenia and coagulopathy? This is seen in DIC.

D. Is there concomitant thrombocytopenia and renal insufficiency? This is seen in TTP and HUS.

E. Are there schistocytes on the peripheral smear? This is seen in traumatic hemolysis, both macrovascular and microvascular.

F. Has the patient been exposed to an infection, drug, or toxin known to cause hemolysis?

G. Does the patient have a mechanical valve or a disease known to be associated with hemolytic anemia?

CASE RESOLUTION

His WBC and platelet count as well as his renal function are all normal; the Coombs test is negative. He does have a few schistocytes on his peripheral smear. He has hemolysis due to his mechanical valve. Since he is asymptomatic, it is not necessary to consider removal of the valve.

Treatment of Hemolysis

Treatment depends on the underlying cause. In an autoimmune condition, immunosuppressive therapy, especially prednisone, is used. If hemolysis is associated with TTP and HUS, the treatment is plasmapheresis and immunosuppressives.

REVIEW OF OTHER IMPORTANT DISEASES

Sickle Cell Anemia

Textbook Presentation

Sickle cell anemia is often identified at birth through screening. Adult patients generally seek medical attention for pain or some of the complications (see below). Occasionally, patients have very mild disease, and sickle cell is diagnosed late in life when evidence of a specific complication, such as sickle cell retinopathy, is identified.

Disease Highlights

A. Epidemiology and prognosis

   1. Gene frequency for sickle cell or thalassemia is 0.17% of non-Hispanic white births.

   2. In African Americans, the gene frequency of Hgb S is 4%, of Hgb C is 1.5%, and of β-thalassemia is 4%.

3. Median age at death is 42 for men and 48 for women.

4. Risk factors for earlier mortality include lower Hgb F levels, episodes of acute chest syndrome, more frequent pain crises, and possibly higher WBC.

B. Clinical manifestations of sickle cell anemia

1. Hematologic

a. Hct usually 20–30%, with reticulocyte count of 3–15%

b. MCV usually high normal or high

c. Unconjugated hyperbilirubinemia, elevated LDH, and low haptoglobin are present.

d. Hgb F level usually slightly elevated.

e. WBC and platelet count usually elevated

f. Hypercoagulability: high levels of thrombin, low levels of protein C and S, abnormal activation of fibrinolysis and platelets

2. Pulmonary

a. Acute chest syndrome

(1) Defined as a new pulmonary infiltrate accompanied by fever and a combination of respiratory symptoms, including cough, tachypnea, and chest pain

(2) Most common cause of death in sickle cell patients

(3) Clinical manifestations in adults (Table 4–5)

(a) About 50% of patients in whom acute chest syndrome develops are admitted for another reason.

(b) Over 80% have concomitant pain crises

(c) Up to 25% require mechanical ventilation

(4) Etiology

(a) Fat embolism (from infarction of long bones), with or without infection in 12%

(b) Infection in 27%, with 8% due to bacteria, 5% mycoplasma, and 9% chlamydia

(c) Infarction in about 10%

(d) Unknown in about 50% of patients

(e) Hypoventilation and atelectasis due to pain and analgesia may play a role, as might fluid overload

(5) General principles of management

Table 4–5. Clinical manifestations of acute chest syndrome in adults.

Symptom or Sign	Frequency (%)
Fever	70
Cough	54
Chest pain	55
Tachypnea	39
Shortness of breath	58
Limb pain	59
Abdominal pain	29
Rib or sternal pain	30
Respiratory rate > 30 breaths per minute	38
Rales	81
Wheezing	16
Effusion	27
Mean temperature	38.8 °C

(a) Supplemental oxygen

(b) Empiric treatment with a macrolide and a cephalosporin

(c) Incentive spirometry (can be preventive)

(d) Bronchodilators for patients with reactive airways

(e) Transfusion

b. Sickle cell chronic lung disease

(1) 35–60% of patients with sickle cell disease have reactive airways.

(2) About 20% have restrictive lung disease, and another 20% have mixed obstructive/restrictive abnormalities.

(3) Up to 40% have pulmonary hypertension.

(4) The relative risk of death in sickle cell patients with pulmonary hypertension, compared with those with normal pulmonary pressures, is 10.

3. Genitourinary

a. Renal

(1) Inability to concentrate urine (hyposthenuria), with maximum urinary osmolality of 400–450 mOsm/kg

(2) Type 4 renal tubular acidosis

(3) Hematuria

    (a) Usually secondary to papillary necrosis

    (b) Renal medullary carcinoma has been reported.

(4) Proteinuria

    (a) Seen in 20–30% of patients with sickle cell disease; about 4% have nephrotic syndrome.

    (b) Progresses to chronic renal failure in about 5% of patients

    (c) ACE inhibitors reduce proteinuria.

b. Priapism

    (1) 30–40% of adults with sickle cell disease report at least 1 episode.

    (2) Bimodal peak incidences in ages 5–13 and 21–29.

    (3) 75% of episodes occur during sleep; the mean duration is 125 minutes.

    (4) Treatment approaches include hydration, analgesia, transfusion, and injection of α-adrenergic drugs.

4. Neurologic

  a. Highest incidence of first infarction is between the ages of 2 and 5, with another increase in ischemic stroke between the ages of 35 and 45.

  b. Hemorrhagic stroke can also occur.

  c. Recurrent infarction occurs in 67% of patients.

  d. Silent infarction is common (seen in 18–23% of patients by age 14); cognitive deficits also common.

  e. Patients over 2 years of age should undergo annual transcranial Doppler (TCD) screening to assess stroke risk.

    (1) Patients with elevated TCD velocities (> 200 cm/s) are at high risk.

    (2) Regular transfusions reduced the risk of stroke in such patients by 90% (10% stroke rate in control group, 1% in treatment group, number needed to treat (NNT) = 11).

5. Musculoskeletal

  a. Bones and joints often the sites of vaso-occlusive episodes.

  b. Avascular necrosis of hips, shoulders, ankles, and spine can cause chronic pain.

    (1) Often best detected by MRI

    (2) May require joint replacement

6. Other

  a. Retinopathy

    (1) More common in patients with Hgb SC disease than with sickle cell disease

    (2) Treated with photocoagulation

  b. Leg ulcers

    (1) Present in about 20% of patients

    (2) Most commonly over the medial or lateral malleoli

  c. Cholelithiasis: nearly universal due to chronic hemolysis

  d. Splenic sequestration and autosplenectomy: seen in children

  e. Liver disease: multifactorial, due to causes such as iron overload or viral hepatitis

Evidence-Based Diagnosis

A. Newborn screening

  1. Universal screening identifies many more patients than screening targeted at high-risk groups.

  2. Homozygotes have an FS pattern on electrophoresis, which is predominantly Hgb F, with some Hgb S, and no Hgb A.

  3. The FS pattern in not specific for sickle cell disease, and the diagnosis should be confirmed through family studies, DNA based testing, or repeat Hgb electrophoresis at 3–4 months of age.

B. Testing in older children and adults

  1. Cellulose acetate electrophoresis separates Hgb S from other variants; however, S, G, and D all have the same electrophoretic mobility.

  2. Only Hgb S will precipitate in a solubility test such as the Sickledex

Treatment

A. General principles

  1. All pediatric patients should receive prophylactic penicillin to prevent streptococcal sepsis.

  2. Transfusion indicated for acute chest syndrome, heart failure, multiorgan failure syndrome, stroke, splenic sequestration, and aplastic crisis.

    a. Do not transfuse above an Hgb of about 11 g/dL, to avoid hyperviscosity.

    b. Use simple transfusion if Hgb below 8 g/dL

    c. Use exchange transfusion if Hgb above 8 g/dL

3. Hydroxyurea

    a. In patients with moderate to severe sickle cell disease, hydroxyurea therapy reduced the rate of pain crises and development of acute chest syndrome by about 50%.

    b. Hydroxyurea use is associated with a lower mortality rate.

4. Stem cell transplant is an experimental therapy.

B. Management of vaso-occlusive crises

  1. The general approach should be similar to that used in patients with other causes of severe pain, such as cancer.

    a. Analgesics should be dosed regularly, rather than as needed.

    b. Patient-controlled analgesia can also be used.

    c. Remember that patients who use opiates long-term become tolerant and often require high doses for acute pain.

    d. Adding NSAIDs or tricyclic antidepressants to opiates is sometimes beneficial.

    e. Patients often need a long-acting opiate for baseline analgesia, combined with a short-acting opiate for breakthrough pain.

  2. Oral hydration is preferable to IV hydration.

  3. Oxygen is indicated only if the patient is hypoxemic.

β-Thalassemia

Textbook Presentation

β-Thalassemia major (homozygotes) presents in infancy with multiple severe abnormalities. Heterozygotes are usually asymptomatic.

Disease Highlights

A. Impaired production of β globin chains.

B. Common in patients of Mediterranean origin.

C. β-Thalassemia minor: heterozygotes with 1 normal β globin allele and 1 β thalassemic allele

D. Anemia generally milder (Hct > 30%), and microcytosis more severe (MCV < 75 mcm^3), than with iron deficiency.

E. In pregnancy, anemia can be more severe than usual.

F. Asymptomatic splenomegaly in 15–20% of patients

Evidence-Based Diagnosis

A. Iron studies should be normal; RDW usually normal; target cells abundant.

B. On Hgb electrophoresis, the Hgb A2 can be elevated, but **a normal A2 does not rule out β-thalassemia minor.**

Treatment of β-Thalassemia Minor

None.

α-Thalassemia

Textbook Presentation

Loss of 3 or 4 α globin genes causes severe disease that presents at birth or is fatal in utero. Patients with loss of 1 or 2 genes are usually asymptomatic.

Disease Highlights

A. Impaired production of α globin chains.

B. Common in patients of African or Asian origin.

C. α-Thalassemia-2 trait: loss of 1 α globin gene; CBC normal.

D. α-Thalassemia-1 trait (α-thalassemia minor): loss of 2 α alpha globin genes; mild microcytic anemia with target cells and normal Hgb electrophoresis.

Evidence-Based Diagnosis

α-Thalassemia cannot be diagnosed by clinical laboratory Hgb electrophoresis.

Treatment of α-Thalassemia Trait

None.

Diagnostic Approach: Anemia

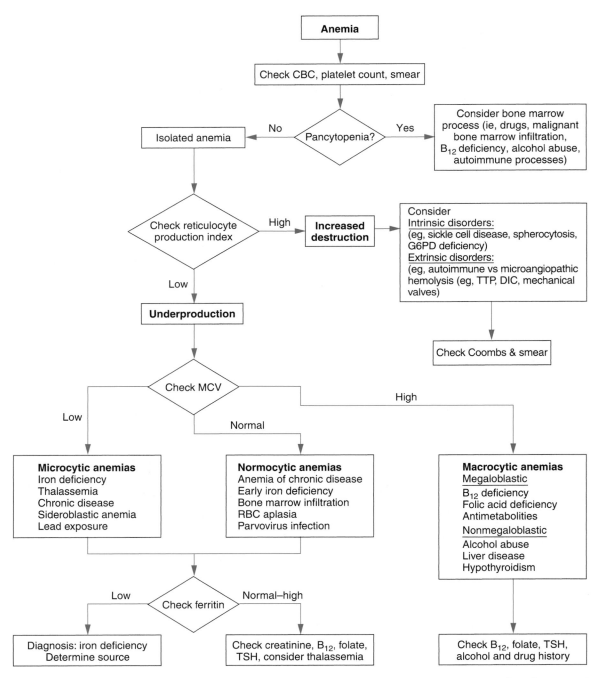

SLE, systemic lupus erythematosus; DIC, disseminated intravascular coagulation; TTP, thrombotic thrombocytic purpura; MCV, mean corpuscular volume.

I have a patient with low back pain. How do I determine the cause?

CHIEF COMPLAINT

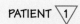

PATIENT

Mr. Y is a 30-year-old man with low back pain that has lasted for 6 days.

> What is the differential diagnosis of low back pain? How would you frame the differential?

CONSTRUCTING A DIFFERENTIAL DIAGNOSIS

Most low back pain is caused by conditions that are troublesome but not progressive or life-threatening. The primary task when evaluating a patient with low back pain is to identify those who have serious causes of back pain that require specific, and sometimes rapid, diagnosis and treatment. In practice, this means **distinguishing serious back pain (pain due to a systemic or visceral disease or pain with neurologic symptoms or signs) from nonspecific back pain** related to the musculoskeletal structures of the back (called mechanical back pain).

A. Back pain due to disorders of the **musculoskeletal** structures

  1. Nonspecific back pain

    a. In general, a specific anatomic diagnosis cannot be made.

    b. There are no neurologic signs or symptoms.

    c. It is nonprogressive.

    d. Examples include the following:

      (1) Lumbar strain and sprain

      (2) Degenerative processes of disks and facets

      (3) Spondylolisthesis (anterior displacement of a vertebra on the one beneath it)

      (4) Spondylolysis (defect in the pars interarticularis of the vertebra)

      (5) Scoliosis

  2. Specific back pain

    a. A specific anatomic diagnosis can be made.

    b. Neurologic signs and symptoms are present.

    c. It can be progressive.

    d. Examples include the following:

      (1) Herniated disk

      (2) Spinal stenosis

      (3) Cauda equina syndrome

B. Back pain due to **systemic disease** affecting the spine

  1. Serious, requiring specific and often rapid treatment

    a. Neoplasia

      (1) Multiple myeloma, metastatic carcinoma, lymphoma, leukemia

      (2) Spinal cord tumors, primary vertebral tumors

    b. Infection

      (1) Osteomyelitis

      (2) Septic diskitis

      (3) Paraspinal abscess

      (4) Epidural abscess

  2. Serious, requiring specific treatment but not necessarily immediately

    a. Osteoporotic compression fracture

    b. Inflammatory arthritis

      (1) Ankylosing spondylitis

      (2) Psoriatic arthritis

      (3) Reiter syndrome

     (4) Inflammatory bowel disease–associated arthritis

C. Back pain due to **visceral disease** is serious and often requires specific and rapid diagnosis and treatment.

   1. Retroperitoneal

     a. Aortic aneurysm

     b. Retroperitoneal adenopathy or mass

   2. Pelvic

     a. Prostatitis

     b. Endometriosis

     c. Pelvic inflammatory disease

   3. Renal

     a. Nephrolithiasis

     b. Pyelonephritis

     c. Perinephric abscess

   4. GI

     a. Pancreatitis

     b. Cholecystitis

     c. Penetrating ulcer

Mr. Y felt well until 1 week ago, when he helped his girlfriend move into her third floor apartment. Although he felt fine while helping her, the next day he woke up with diffuse pain across his lower back and buttocks. He spent that day lying on the floor, with some improvement. Ibuprofen has helped somewhat. He feels better when he is in bed and had transiently worse pain after doing his usual weight lifting at the gym.

At this point, what is the leading hypothesis, and what are the active alternatives? What other tests should be ordered?

ORGANIZING THE DIFFERENTIAL

Mr. Y's history is consistent with nonspecific mechanical back pain, which is the cause of 97% of the back pain seen in a primary care practice. History and physical exam should focus on looking for **neurologic signs and symptoms** that would suggest a specific musculoskeletal cause, such as a herniated disk, and for signs and symptoms that would suggest the presence of a **systemic disease.** The clinical clues for the alternative diagnoses listed in Table 5–1 have been associated with an increased likelihood of a serious etiology of back pain. Likelihood ratios (LRs) for these findings, when available, will be discussed later in the chapter. Table 5–1 lists the differential diagnosis.

The clinical clues listed in Table 5–1 should be assessed in all patients presenting with back pain.

Table 5–1. Diagnostic hypotheses for Mr. Y.

Diagnostic Hypotheses	Clinical Clues	Important Tests
Leading Hypothesis		
Mechanical back pain	Absence of symptoms listed below	Resolution within 3–4 weeks
Active Alternative—Most Common		
Herniated disk	Sciatica, abnormal neurologic exam, especially in L5–S1 distribution	CT or MRI
Active Alternative—Must Not Miss		
Malignancy	Duration of pain > 1 month Age older than 50 Previous cancer history Unexplained weight loss (> 10 lb over 6 months)	Spine x-ray, MRI
Infection	Fever Chills Recent skin or urinary infection Immunosuppression Injection drug use	MRI
Other Hypotheses		
Compression fracture	Age older than 70 Significant trauma History of osteoporosis Corticosteroid use	Spine x-ray, MRI

Mr. Y has no history of other illnesses. He has had no trauma, weight loss, fever, chills, or recent infections. He takes no medications and does not smoke, drink, or use injection drugs. The back pain does not radiate to his legs. On physical exam, he has mild tenderness across his lower back; lower extremity strength, sensation, and reflexes are normal. Straight leg raise test is negative.

 Is the clinical information sufficient to make a diagnosis? If not, what other information do you need?

Leading Hypothesis: Mechanical Low Back Pain

Textbook Presentation
The classic presentation is nonradiating pain and stiffness in the lower back, often precipitated by heavy lifting.

Disease Highlights
A. Can also have pain and stiffness in the buttocks and hips
B. Generally occurs hours to days after a new or unusual exertion and improves when the patient is supine
C. Can rarely make a specific anatomic diagnosis
D. Prognosis
   1. 75–90% of patients improve within 1 month
   2. 25–50% of patients have additional episodes over the next year
   3. Risk factors for persistent low back pain include a history of previous back pain, depression, substance abuse, pending or past litigation or disability compensation, low socioeconomic status, and work dissatisfaction.

Evidence-Based Diagnosis
A. Many *asymptomatic* patients will have anatomic abnormalities on imaging studies.
   1. 20% of patients aged 14–25 have degenerative disks on plain x-rays.
   2. 20–75% of patients younger than 50 years have herniated disks on MRI.

3. 40–80% of patients have bulging disks on MRI.
4. Over 90% of patients older than age 50 have degenerative disks on MRI.
5. Up to 20% of patients over age 50 have spinal stenosis.
B. Even in symptomatic patients, anatomic abnormalities are not necessarily causative, and identifying them does not influence initial treatment decisions.
C. A specific pathoanatomic diagnosis cannot be made in 85% of patients with isolated low back pain.

 Patients who have none of the clinical clues should not have any diagnostic testing done.

MAKING A DIAGNOSIS

Considering Mr. Y's history and physical exam, there is no need to consider other diagnoses at this point. Should he not respond to conservative therapy, then the alternative diagnoses would need to be reconsidered.

CASE RESOLUTION

You reassure Mr. Y that his pain will resolve within another 2–3 weeks. You recommend that he use ibuprofen as needed and be as active as possible within the limits of the pain. Rather than weight lifting, you suggest swimming or walking for exercise until his pain resolves. You also provide a handout on proper lifting techniques and back exercises, to be started after the pain resolves. He cancels a follow up appointment 1 month later, leaving a message that his pain is gone and he has resumed all of his usual activities.

Treatment of Mechanical Low Back Pain

A. Acute low back pain
   1. Nonsteroidal anti-inflammatory drugs (NSAIDs) are effective for symptomatic relief.
   2. Muscle relaxants and opioids have not been shown to be superior to NSAIDs.
   3. Specific back exercises do not help acute low back pain, but do help prevent recurrent back pain.

4. The best approach is NSAIDs during the acute phase and activity as tolerated until the pain resolves, followed by specific daily back exercises.

Bed rest does not help acute pain and may prolong the duration of pain.

B. Subacute or chronic low back pain

1. Therapeutic massage is beneficial.

2. Exercise therapy helps chronic low back pain.

3. Facet and epidural injection has not been shown to be beneficial; local injection might be helpful.

4. Acupuncture has not been shown to be beneficial.

CHIEF COMPLAINT

PATIENT 2

Mrs. H, a 47-year-old woman, was well until 2 days ago, when she developed low back pain after working in her garden and pulling weeds for several hours. The pain is a constant, dull ache that radiates to her right buttock and hip. Yesterday, after sitting in a movie, the pain began radiating to the back of the right knee. She has taken some acetaminophen and ibuprofen without much relief. Her past medical history is unremarkable, and she takes no medicines. She has no constitutional symptoms.

At this point, what is the leading hypothesis, and what are the active alternatives? What other tests should be ordered?

ORGANIZING THE DIFFERENTIAL DIAGNOSIS

Similar to the patient discussed in the first case, Mrs. H developed low back pain after an unusual exertion, and has no systemic symptoms. However, her pain is worsened by sitting and radiates down the back of her leg (which suggests sciatic pain). Both of these features increase the probability that she has a herniated disk. Table 5–2 lists the differential diagnosis.

2

On physical exam, Mrs. H is clearly uncomfortable. She has no back tenderness and has full range of motion of both hips. When her right leg is raised to about 60 degrees, pain shoots down the leg. When her left leg is raised, she has pain in her lower back. Her strength and sensation are normal, but the right ankle reflex is absent.

Is the clinical information sufficient to make a diagnosis? If not, what other information do you need?

Leading Hypothesis: Herniated Disk

Textbook Presentation

The classic presentation is moderate to severe pain radiating from the back down the buttock and leg, usually to the foot or ankle, with associated numbness or paresthesias. This type of pain is called sciatica, and it is classically precipitated by a sudden increase in pressure on the disk, such as after coughing or lifting.

Table 5–2. Diagnostic hypotheses for Mrs. H.

Diagnostic Hypotheses	Clinical Clues	Important Tests
Leading Hypothesis		
Herniated lumbar disk	Sciatica; neurologic signs or symptoms, especially in L5–S1 distribution; positive straight leg raise test	CT or MRI
Active Alternative—Most Common		
Nonspecific mechanical back pain	No neurologic or systemic symptoms	Resolution of pain

Disease Highlights

A. Disk disease is frequently asymptomatic.

B. Numbness, paresthesias, and motor weakness are found variably; any of these can occur in the absence of pain.

C. Most common site of weakness is foot plantar or dorsiflexion; proximal weakness suggests a femoral neuropathy or compression of the lumbar plexus.

D. Highest prevalence is in the 45- to 64-year-old age group.

E. Risk factors include sedentary activities, especially driving; chronic cough; lack of physical exercise; and possibly pregnancy. Jobs involving lifting and pulling have not been associated with increased risk.

F. 50% of patients recover in 2 weeks and 70% in 6 weeks.

G. L4–L5 and L5–S1 cause 98% of clinically important disk herniations, so pain and paresthesias are most often seen in these distributions.

H. There are no bowel or bladder symptoms with unilateral disk herniations.

I. Coughing, sneezing, or prolonged sitting can aggravate the pain.

J. Bilateral midline herniations can cause the **cauda equina syndrome.**

  1. Cauda equina syndrome is a rare condition caused by tumor or massive midline disk herniations.

  2. It is characterized by urinary retention with overflow incontinence (90% of patients), decreased anal sphincter tone (80%), sensory loss in a saddle distribution (75%), bilateral sciatica, and leg weakness.

 Suspected cauda equina syndrome is a medical emergency that requires immediate imaging and decompression.

Evidence-Based Diagnosis

A. History and physical exam (Table 5–3)

  1. Sciatica and positive straight leg raise have the best LRs+.

  2. Straight leg test is performed by holding the heel in 1 hand and slowly raising the leg, keeping the knee extended; a positive test reproduces the patient's sciatica when the leg is elevated between 30 and 60 degrees.

  3. Crossed straight leg test is performed by lifting the contralateral leg; a positive test reproduces the sciatica in the affected leg.

Table 5–3. History and physical exam findings in the diagnosis of herniated disk.

Finding	Sensitivity	Specificity	LR+	LR−
Sciatica	0.95	0.88	7.9	0.06
Positive crossed straight leg raise	0.25	0.90	2.5	0.83
Positive ipsilateral straight leg raise	0.80	0.40	1.3	0.50
Ankle dorsiflexion weakness	0.35	0.70	1.2	0.93
Great toe extensor weakness	0.50	0.70	1.7	0.71
Impaired ankle reflex	0.50	0.60	1.3	0.83
Ankle plantar flexion weakness	0.06	0.95	1.2	0.99

 A straight leg raise test that elicits back pain is negative.

  4. Combinations of abnormal findings (eg, positive straight leg raise and neurologic abnormalities such as absent ankle reflex, impaired plantar or dorsiflexion, impaired sensation in L5–S1 distribution) are presumably more specific than isolated findings.

B. Imaging

  1. Plain x-rays do not image the disks and are useless for diagnosing herniations.

  2. CT and MRI scans have similar test characteristics for diagnosing herniated disks.

    a. CT: sensitivity, 0.62–0.9; specificity, 0.7–0.87; LR+, 2.1–6.9; LR−, 0.11–0.54

    b. MRI: sensitivity, 0.6–1.0; specificity, 0.43–0.97; LR+, 1.1–33; LR−, 0–0.93

C. Electromyography

  1. Might be useful in assessing possible nerve root dysfunction in patients with leg symptoms lasting more than 4 weeks; not useful for isolated back pain

  2. Data regarding sensitivity and specificity are flawed but estimates are 71–100% sensitivity and 38–88% specificity.

MAKING A DIAGNOSIS

Mrs. H has sciatica, a positive straight leg raise test, and an absent ankle reflex, a combination that strongly suggests nerve root impingement at L5–S1. However, none of these findings is so specific that nonspecific mechanical back pain has been ruled out. So, one option at this point would be to order an MRI or CT scan to positively identify a herniated disk. However, there are 2 questions to consider before ordering a scan:

1. Will the scan be diagnostic? Remember that a significant percentage of asymptomatic people have herniated disks on CT or MRI.

 The abnormality on imaging studies must correlate with the findings on history and physical exam; in other words, the herniation must be in the dermatome that matches the symptoms.

2. If the scan is diagnostic, will the finding change the initial management of the patient? Conservative therapy, similar to that for nonspecific back pain, is indicated initially unless the patient has cauda equina syndrome or other rapidly progressive neurologic impairment.

CASE RESOLUTION

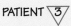

You decide not to order any imaging studies initially and prescribe ibuprofen (800 mg 3 times daily) and activity as tolerated. Mrs. H calls the next day, reporting that she was unable to sleep because of the pain. You then prescribe acetaminophen with codeine, which provides good pain relief. Two weeks later, she is using the codeine rarely, and ibuprofen 1 to 2 times a day. Two months later, she is pain free and back to her usual activities, although her ankle reflex is still absent—a common and not significant finding. She is fine until about a year later, when she develops identical pain after a bad bronchitis. Her pain resolves with a few days of acetaminophen with codeine.

Treatment of Herniated Disks

A. In the absence of cauda equina syndrome or progressive neurologic dysfunction, conservative therapy should be tried for 1 month.
  1. NSAIDs are the first choice.
  2. Opioids are often necessary.
  3. Bed rest does not accelerate recovery.
  4. Epidural corticosteroid injections may provide temporary pain relief.
B. Surgery
  1. Indications include
    a. Impairment of bowel and bladder function
    b. Gross motor weakness
    c. Evidence of increasing impairment of nerve root conduction
    d. Severe sciatic pain that persists or increases despite conservative therapy
    e. Recurrent episodes of sciatica
  2. Surgery should not be done for painless herniations or when the herniation is at a different level than the symptoms.
  3. In the absence of progressive neurologic symptoms, surgery is elective.
  4. About 60% of patients have complete resolution of symptoms after surgery.
    a. 90% if sciatic symptoms only, without back pain
    b. 6% have persistent disabling symptoms, even after surgery

CHIEF COMPLAINT

PATIENT 3

Mrs. P is a 75-year-old white woman who was well until 2 days ago when pain developed in the center of her lower back. The pain is constant and becoming more severe. There is no position or movement that changes the pain, and it is not relieved with acetaminophen or ibuprofen. It sometimes radiates in a belt like fashion across her lower back, extending around to the abdomen. She has no fever or weight loss. Her past medical history is notable for a radial fracture after falling off her bicycle 18 years ago, and breast cancer 15 years ago, treated with lumpectomy, radiation therapy, and tamoxifen. She has had annual mammograms since, all of which have been normal. She currently takes no medications.

 At this point, what is the leading hypothesis, and what are the active alternatives? What other tests should be ordered?

ORGANIZING THE DIFFERENTIAL DIAGNOSIS

Mrs. P has several clinical findings that suggest her back pain could be due to a more serious, systemic disease rather than being nonspecific, mechanical back pain. First, she is older and has a history of previous cancer; both findings are associated with malignancy as a cause of back pain. Second, her age, race, and history of a previous fracture are established risk factors for osteoporosis. Table 5–4 lists the differential diagnosis.

Table 5–4. Diagnostic hypotheses for Mrs. P.

Diagnostic Hypotheses	Clinical Clues	Important Tests
Leading Hypothesis		
Metastatic breast cancer	Duration of pain > 1 month Age older than 50 Previous cancer history Unexplained weight loss (> 10 lbs over 6 months)	Spine x-ray, MRI
Active Alternative		
Osteoporotic compression fracture	Age older than 70 Significant trauma History of osteoporosis Corticosteroid use	Spine x-ray, MRI

On physical exam, she is in obvious pain. She is 5 ft 2 in and weighs 115 lbs. There is diffuse tenderness across her lower back, with no point tenderness of the vertebrae. There is no rash, and abdominal exam is normal. Her reflexes, strength, and sensation are all normal, and straight leg raise is negative.

 Is the clinical information sufficient to make a diagnosis? If not, what other information do you need?

Leading Hypothesis: Back Pain Due to Metastatic Cancer

Textbook Presentation

The classic presentation is the development of constant, dull back pain that is not relieved by rest and is worse at night in a patient with a known malignancy.

Disease Highlights

A. Bone metastases can be limited to the vertebral body or extend into the epidural space, causing cord compression.

B. Pain can precede cord compression by weeks or even months, but compression progresses rapidly once it starts.

 Cancer + back pain + neurologic abnormalities = an emergency.

C. Malignancy causes about 1% of back pain in general but is the cause in nearly all patients with cancer who have back pain.

D. Most common sources are breast, lung, or prostate cancer.

    1. Renal and thyroid cancers also commonly metastasize to bone.

    2. Myeloma and lymphoma frequently involve the spine.

E. In most cases of cancer metastasis, the thoracic vertebrae are usually affected, while metastasis of prostate cancer most often affects the lumbar vertebrae.

F. Blastic lesions seen with prostate, small cell lung cancer, Hodgkin disease

G. Lytic lesions seen with renal cell, myeloma, non-Hodgkin lymphoma, melanoma, non–small cell lung cancer, thyroid cancer

H. Mixed blastic and lytic lesions seen with breast cancer and GI cancers

Evidence-Based Diagnosis

A. History and physical exam (Table 5–5)

 Cancer is not likely to be the cause of back pain if the patient is younger than 50 years, has no history of cancer, has not experienced unexplained weight loss, or has not failed conservative therapy.

B. Imaging
 1. Plain x-rays
  a. Must lose about 50% of trabecular bone before a lytic lesion is visible

Table 5–5. History and physical exam findings in the diagnosis of cancer as a cause of low back pain.

Finding	Sensitivity	Specificity	LR+	LR−
Previous history of cancer	0.31	0.98	14.7	0.70
Failure to improve after 1 month of therapy	0.31	0.90	3.0	0.77
Age older than 50 years	0.77	0.71	2.7	0.32
Unexplained weight loss	0.15	0.94	2.7	0.90
Duration of pain > 1 month	0.50	0.81	2.6	0.62
No relief with bed rest	0.90	0.46	1.7	0.21
Any of the following: age older than 50, history of cancer, unexplained weight loss, or failure of conservative therapy	1.00	0.60	2.5	0.0

b. Blastic lesions can be seen earlier on x-rays than lytic lesions.
  c. Sensitivity, 0.6; specificity, 0.96–0.995
  d. LR+, 12–120; LR−, 0.4–0.42
 2. CT scan: Sensitivity and specificity for diagnosing metastatic lesions are unknown.
 3. MRI
  a. Sensitivity, 0.83–0.93; specificity, 0.9–0.97
  b. LR+, 8.3–31; LR−, 0.07–0.19
 4. Bone scan
  a. Sensitivity, 0.74–0.98; specificity, 0.64–0.81
  b. LR+, 3.9; LR−, 0.32
  c. Better for blastic lesions than lytic lesions; myeloma, in particular, can be missed on bone scan.

 MRI scan is the best test for diagnosing or ruling out cancer as a cause of back pain and for determining whether there is cord compression.

C. Laboratory tests: the erythrocyte sedimentation rate (ESR) is sometimes helpful
 1. ≥ 20: sensitivity, 0.78; specificity, 0.67; LR+, 2.4
 2. ≥ 50: sensitivity, 0.56; specificity, 0.97; LR+, 19.2
 3. ≥ 100: sensitivity, 0.22; specificity, 0.994; LR+, 55.5

Treatment

A. Surgery, radiation therapy, and chemotherapy
B. Choice of therapy depends on the type of cancer and the extent of the lesion.

MAKING A DIAGNOSIS

Since Mrs. P has no neurologic abnormalities, and plain x-rays are relatively quick to perform, it is reasonable to start with lumbar spine films. However, because of the suboptimal LR− of about 0.4, it will be necessary to perform additional imaging if the plain x-rays are normal.

 The lumbar spine films show a vertebral compression fracture at L1, which is new when compared with films done several months ago.

Have you crossed a diagnostic threshold for the leading hypothesis, metastatic cancer? Have you ruled out the active alternatives? Do other tests need to be done to exclude the alternative diagnoses?

Alternative Diagnosis: Osteoporotic Compression Fracture

Textbook Presentation

The classic presentation is acute, severe pain that develops in an older woman and radiates around the flank to the abdomen, either spontaneously or brought on by trivial activity such as minor lifting, bending, or jarring.

Disease Highlights

A. Fractures are usually in mid to lower thoracic or lumbar region.

B. Fractures at T4 or higher are more often due to malignancy than osteoporosis.

 MRI scan is the best way to distinguish malignant from benign osteoporotic compression fractures.

C. Pain is often increased by slight movements, such as turning over in bed.

D. Can also be asymptomatic

E. Pain usually improves within 1 week and resolves by 4–6 weeks, but some patients have more chronic pain.

F. Osteoporosis is most commonly primary, related to menopause and aging.

G. Can occur as a complication of a variety of diseases and medications.

1. Most common diseases include thyrotoxicosis, primary hyperparathyroidism, hypogonadism, and malabsorption.

2. Medications that can lead to osteoporosis include corticosteroids (most common) and long-term heparin therapy.

H. Age is the strongest risk factor for developing osteoporosis, with a relative risk of almost 10 for women aged 70–74 (compared with women under 65), increasing to a relative risk of 22.5 for women over 80.

1. Other risk factors include personal history of rib, spine, wrist, or hip fracture; current smoking; white, Hispanic, or Asian ethnicity; weight < 132 lbs; family history of osteoporosis.

2. Risk of developing osteoporosis is decreased in women who are obese, are of African American descent, and use estrogen postmenopausally.

Evidence-Based Diagnosis

A. History and physical exam

1. Not well studied

2. Unpublished data: age > 70 has LR+ of 5.5, corticosteroid use has LR+ of 12.0 for diagnosis of osteoporotic compression fracture as a cause of back pain

B. Imaging

1. MRI is thought to be more sensitive and specific than x-rays, but data are not available.

2. MRI scan can distinguish between benign and malignant osteoporotic compression fractures, with sensitivity of 88.5–100% and specificity of 89.5–93% (LR+ = 8–14, LR– = 0–0.12).

3. Bone scan can be useful for determining acuity.

CASE RESOLUTION

 Mrs. P undergoes an MRI scan, which confirms the diagnosis of osteoporotic compression fracture. She is treated with narcotics, and her pain resolves over 3–4 weeks. Her bone density results show a spine T score of –2.1, and a hip T score of –2.6. She has no diseases or medication exposures associated with osteoporosis. She has primary osteoporosis. Treatment is started.

Regardless of Mrs. P's bone density results, the presence of a vertebral compression fracture mandates treatment for osteoporosis. Reviewing her history, she had several risk factors for osteoporosis, including her age, weight, and history of a wrist fracture.

Treatment of Osteoporosis

A. Calcium, 1200–1500 mg daily; vitamin D, 400 international units daily

B. Bisphosphonates (alendronate and risedronate) both increase bone density and reduce risk of subsequent spine and hip fractures.

C. Raloxifene reduces risk of spine fractures but not hip fractures.

D. Estrogen can prevent fractures but is no longer recommended for long-term therapy due to adverse events such as deep venous thrombosis, pulmonary embolism, myocardial infarction, and cerebrovascular accidents.

E. Calcitonin may reduce the pain from an acute vertebral compression fracture.

CHIEF COMPLAINT

PATIENT 4

Mr. F is a 65-year-old man who comes into your office complaining of several months of low back pain. It does not radiate into his buttocks, hips, or legs, but sometimes his legs feel numb after he walks. The pain is worse with walking, although he finds it goes away while he is grocery shopping if he bends a bit to push the cart. He does not have pain while in bed, and he has more pain standing than sitting. Over-the-counter ibuprofen helps somewhat, but he feels quite limited in his activity.

At this point, what is the leading hypothesis, and what are the active alternatives? What other tests should be ordered?

ORGANIZING THE DIFFERENTIAL DIAGNOSIS

The differential for back pain in a man this age is broad, but 2 historical findings suggest spinal stenosis: the sensation of numbness with exertion ("pseudoclaudication"), and the improvement in the pain when he bends forward to push a grocery cart. Other possibilities include mechanical back pain, which remains common in patients over 65, although there should be no neurologic symptoms with uncomplicated mechanical back pain. Although he does not have the unremitting pain characteristic of metastatic cancer, that is still a possibility. Disk herniation is unlikely without sciatica. Table 5–6 lists the differential diagnosis.

4

Mr. F's past medical history is notable for hypertension, diabetes, and osteoarthritis of his knees. His medications include lisinopril, glipizide, and acetaminophen or ibuprofen. He has no history of cancer, and his prostate specific antigen (PSA) was 0.9 one month ago. He has no back tenderness. Straight leg raise test is negative bilaterally; reflexes are symmetric; strength is normal; and sensation is normal, except for decreased vibratory sense in his feet.

Is the clinical information sufficient to make a diagnosis? If not, what other information do you need?

Table 5–6. Diagnostic hypotheses for Mr. F.

Diagnostic Hypotheses	Clinical Clues	Important Tests
Leading Hypothesis		
Spinal stenosis	Neurogenic claudication Age older than 65 Improvement with sitting or bending forward	MRI
Active Alternative—Most Common		
Mechanical back pain	No neurologic or systemic symptoms	Resolution of pain
Active Alternative—Must Not Miss		
Metastatic cancer	Duration of pain > 1 month Age older than 50 Previous cancer history Unexplained weight loss (> 10 lb over 6 months)	Spine x-ray, MRI

Leading Hypothesis: Spinal Stenosis

Textbook Presentation

The classic presentation is somewhat vague but persistent back and leg discomfort brought on by walking or standing that is relieved by sitting or bending forward is typically seen.

Disease Highlights

A. Leg symptoms are usually bilateral and are often described as a heaviness or numbness brought on by standing or walking ("pseudoclaudication") (Table 5–7).

B. Neurologic symptoms and signs are variable.

C. Stenosis is seen most often in lumbar spine, sometimes in cervical spine, and rarely in thoracic spine.

D. Spinal stenosis is due to hypertrophic degenerative processes and degenerative spondylolisthesis compressing the spinal cord, cauda equina, individual nerve roots, and the arterioles and capillaries supplying the cauda equina and nerve roots.

E. Pain is worsened by extension and relieved by flexion.

F. Patients with central stenosis generally have bilateral, nondermatomal pain involving the buttocks and posterior thighs.

G. Patients with lateral stenosis generally have pain in a dermatomal distribution.

H. Repeating the physical exam after rapid walking might demonstrate subtle abnormalities.

I. About 50% of patients have stable symptoms; when worsening occurs, it is gradual.

Table 5–7. Findings that differentiate vascular from neurogenic claudication.

Vascular	Neurogenic
Fixed walking distance before onset of symptoms	Variable walking distance before onset of symptoms
Improved by standing still	Improved by sitting or bending forward
Worsened by walking	Worsened by walking or standing
Painful to walk uphill	Can be painless to walk uphill because of tendency to bend forward
Absent pulses	Present pulses
Shiny skin with loss of hair	Skin appears normal

1. Lumbar spinal stenosis does not progress to paralysis and should be managed based on severity of symptoms.

2. Progression of cervical and thoracic stenoses can cause myelopathy and paralysis and requires surgery more often than lumbar spinal stenosis.

Evidence-Based Diagnosis

A. History and physical exam (Table 5–8)

B. Imaging

1. Plain x-rays can detect compromise of vertebral foramina by bone but not by soft tissue; x-ray is not as sensitive as CT or MRI.

2. CT and MRI have similar test characteristics.

   a. CT scan: sensitivity, 0.9; specificity, 0.8–0.96; LR+, 4.5–22; LR−, 0.10–0.12

   b. MRI: sensitivity, 0.9; specificity, 0.72–1.0; LR+, 3.2–∞; LR−, 0.10–0.14

   c. Up to 21% of asymptomatic patients over age 65 have spinal stenosis on MRI.

 CT and MRI scans can rule out spinal stenosis but cannot necessarily determine whether visualized stenosis is causing the patient's symptoms.

Table 5–8. History and physical exam findings in the diagnosis of spinal stenosis.

Finding	Sensitivity	Specificity	LR+	LR−
Wide based gait	0.43	0.97	14.3	0.59
No pain when seated	0.46	0.93	6.6	0.58
Abnormal Romberg test results	0.39	0.91	4.3	0.67
Symptoms improve when seated	0.52	0.83	3.1	0.58
Vibration deficit	0.53	0.81	2.8	0.58
Age older than 65	0.77	0.69	2.5	0.33
Pinprick deficit	0.47	0.81	2.5	0.65
Weakness	0.47	0.78	2.1	0.68
Absent Achilles reflex	0.46	0.78	2.1	0.94

MAKING A DIAGNOSIS

It is not clear which test, if any, needs to be done at this point. Mr. F's symptoms are suggestive of spinal stenosis, and neither history nor physical exam findings point toward another specific cause of his pain. Nevertheless, because of the overall lack of sensitivity of the history and physical exam in the diagnosis of serious causes of low back pain, it is reasonable to order plain x-rays to look for metastatic cancer. Although the LR− of 0.4 is not ideal, the pretest probability of this diagnosis is low, and normal spine films will be sufficient to rule it out. Although stenosis often cannot be diagnosed on plain films, finding significant osteoarthritis will support the diagnosis. Since initial management of lumbar spinal stenosis is always nonoperative, specifically diagnosing it on MRI will not change management at this point.

Mr. F's lumbar spine films show degenerative disk disease, spondylolisthesis, and facet joint changes, all consistent with moderate to severe osteoarthritis. There are no compression fractures or lytic or blastic lesions.

Have you crossed a diagnostic threshold for the leading hypothesis, spinal stenosis? Have you ruled out the active alternatives? Do other tests need to be done to exclude the alternative diagnoses?

The history, physical, and spine films all support the diagnosis of spinal stenosis. There is no need for further testing at this point.

CASE RESOLUTION

Mr. F begins taking 25 mg of amitriptyline at bedtime and continues using acetaminophen or ibuprofen during the day. He attends physical therapy for 8 weeks. When he returns for a follow-up appointment, he reports some improvement in his exercise tolerance, although he still has daily pain. An MRI scan, done because of his unresolved pain, confirms the presence of spinal stenosis. He continues to use ibuprofen and to do exercises at home. Several months later, he complains of worsening leg pain, especially on the right. An epidural corticosteroid injection helps quite a bit, but only for a few weeks. He asks to see a surgeon. You recommend using tramadol during the day and amitriptyline before bed, instead of acetaminophen and NSAIDs. He finds his pain is much better, and postpones the surgery consultation.

Treatment of Spinal Stenosis

A. Evidence to guide treatment decisions is minimal.

B. Nonoperative treatment is successful (defined as stable or improving symptoms) in 15–70% of patients.
   1. Medications used for pain relief include NSAIDs, tricyclic antidepressants, gabapentin, and sometimes narcotics.
   2. Physical therapy improves stamina and muscle strength in the legs and trunk.
   3. Epidural corticosteroid injection helps some patients, especially those with radicular pain.

C. Surgery
   1. Primary indication is increasing pain that is not responsive to conservative measures.
   2. More effective in reducing leg pain than back pain
   3. Reported improvement rates range between 64% and 91%.
   4. Reoperation rates range from 6% to 23%.
   5. After surgery, wait 6–12 months to determine effectiveness.

REVIEW OF OTHER IMPORTANT DISEASES

Spinal Epidural Abscess

Textbook Presentation

The classic presentation is a patient with a history of diabetes or injection drug use who has fever and back pain, followed by neurologic symptoms (eg, motor weakness, sensory changes, and bowel or bladder dysfunction).

Disease Highlights

A. Location
   1. Epidural space exists posteriorly distal to the foramen magnum; it is smallest in the cervical spine, and largest in the sacrum; the epidural space exists anteriorly only distal to L1.
   2. Spinal epidural abscess usually begins as a focal pyogenic infection involving the vertebral disk or the disk-vertebral body junction that then

spreads longitudinally, often extending 3–5 spinal cord segments.

3. 33% of cases occur in thoracic spine

B. Prevalence is 0.2–2 cases/10,000 hospital admissions

C. Microbiology

   1. *Staphylococcus aureus* is the pathogen in about 67% of cases.

   2. Gram-negative bacilli are pathogen in 16% of cases.

   3. Aerobic streptococcus is pathogen in 9% of cases.

   4. Hematogeneous spread causes disease in 33% of cases.

D. Risk factors

   1. Diabetes

   2. Injection drug use

   3. Alcohol abuse

   4. Primary infection elsewhere (especially skin, urinary tract, vertebral osteomyelitis)

 Always obtain blood cultures in patients with spinal epidural abscess, and consider endocarditis in patients with bacteremia.

   5. Invasive procedure, especially—but not exclusively—epidural anesthesia

E. Clinical manifestations

   1. Fever in 66%

   2. Back pain in 71%

   3. Local tenderness in 17%

   4. Signs of spinal irritation in 20%

   5. Muscle weakness or incontinence in 25%

   6. Paraparesis/paraplegia in 33%

Evidence-Based Diagnosis

A. ESR above 20 mm/h in 94% of patients, with average ESR of 77 mm/h

B. MRI is best imaging study.

Treatment

A. Emergent surgical decompression and drainage

B. Antibiotics

Vertebral Osteomyelitis

Textbook Presentation

The classic presentation is unremitting back pain often, but not always, with fever.

Disease Highlights

A. Pathogenesis

   1. Most commonly hematogenous spread; can also occur due to contiguous spread or direct infection from trauma or surgery.

   2. Generally causes bony destruction of 2 adjacent vertebral bodies and collapse of the intervertebral space.

B. Microbiology

   1. *S aureus* in over 50% of patients

   2. Group B and G hemolytic streptococcus, especially in diabetic patients

   3. Enteric gram-negative bacilli, especially after urinary tract instrumentation

Evidence-Based Diagnosis

A. History and physical

   1. Injection drug use, urinary tract infection, or skin infection: sensitivity, 0.40

   2. Spinal tenderness: sensitivity, 0.86; specificity, 0.60; LR+, 2.1; LR–, 0.23

   3. Fever: sensitivity, 0.52; specificity, 0.98; LR+, 26; LR– 0.49

B. Laboratory tests

   1. Leukocytosis: sensitivity, 0.43; specificity, 0.94; LR+, 7.2; LR– 0.6

   2. ESR: sensitivity and specificity unknown, but most patients in reported case series have an elevated ESR, often over 100 mm/h

   3. Blood cultures are sometimes positive (25–50% of patients); needle aspiration is necessary to establish causative organism if blood cultures are negative.

C. Imaging

   1. X-rays: sensitivity, 0.82; specificity, 0.57; LR+, 1.9; LR–, 0.32

   2. MRI: sensitivity, 0.96; specificity, 0.92; LR+, 12; LR–, 0.04

   3. Bone scan: sensitivity, 0.90; specificity, 0.78; LR+, 4.1; LR–, 0.13

Treatment

A. Primarily antibiotics for 6 weeks

B. Surgery is necessary only if neurologic symptoms suggest onset of vertebral collapse causing cord compression or development of spinal epidural abscess.

Summary table of the neurologic exam of the lower extremity nerve roots.

Root	L2	L3	L4	L5	S1
Area of pain	Across thigh diagonally	Across thigh diagonally	Down to medial malleolus; often severe at knee	Back of thigh, lateral calf, dorsum of foot and great toe	Back of thigh, back of calf, lateral foot to little toe
Sensory loss	Often none	Often none	Medial leg below knee to medial malleolus	Dorsum of foot to great toe	Behind lateral malleolus and lateral border of foot
Reflex	None	Adductor	Knee jerk	None	Ankle jerk
Motor deficit	Hip flexion, thigh adduction	Knee extension, thigh adduction	Inversion of foot	Dorsiflexion of toes and foot	Plantar flexion, eversion of foot

Summary table of motor exam of the lower extremities.

Movement	Muscle Group	Nerve Roots	Peripheral Nerves
Hip flexion	Iliopsoas	L2, 3	Femoral twigs
Hip extension	Gluteal	L4, 5	Gluteal
Hip abduction	Glutei, tensor fascia	L4, 5	None
Hip adduction	Adductor	L2, 3, 4	Obturator
Knee extension	Quadriceps	L2, 3, 4	Femoral
Knee flexion	Hamstrings	L5, S1	Tibial, peroneal
Plantar flexion	Gastrocnemius, tibialis posterior	S1, 2	Tibial
Dorsiflexion	Tibialis anterior, long extensors	L4, 5	Peroneal
Foot inversion	Tibialis anterior and posterior	L4	Tibial, peroneal
Foot eversion	Peronei longus and brevis, long extensors	S1	Peroneal

Diagnostic Approach: Low Back Pain

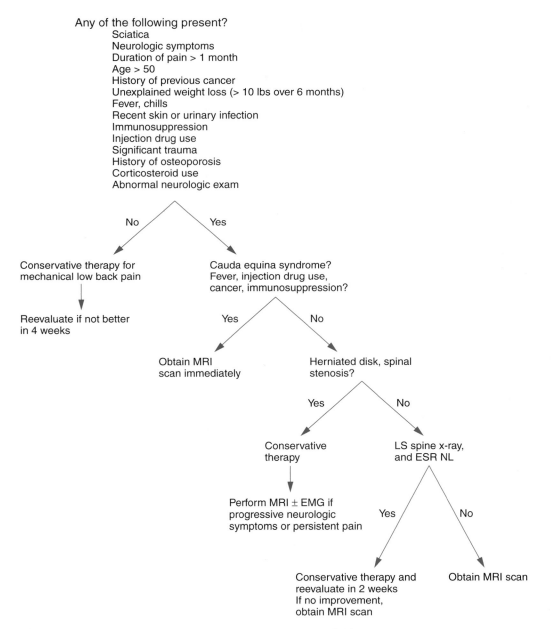

Any of the following present?
- Sciatica
- Neurologic symptoms
- Duration of pain > 1 month
- Age > 50
- History of previous cancer
- Unexplained weight loss (> 10 lbs over 6 months)
- Fever, chills
- Recent skin or urinary infection
- Immunosuppression
- Injection drug use
- Significant trauma
- History of osteoporosis
- Corticosteroid use
- Abnormal neurologic exam

No → Conservative therapy for mechanical low back pain → Reevaluate if not better in 4 weeks

Yes → Cauda equina syndrome? Fever, injection drug use, cancer, immunosuppression?

Yes → Obtain MRI scan immediately

No → Herniated disk, spinal stenosis?

Yes → Conservative therapy → Perform MRI ± EMG if progressive neurologic symptoms or persistent pain

No → LS spine x-ray, and ESR NL

Yes → Conservative therapy and reevaluate in 2 weeks. If no improvement, obtain MRI scan

No → Obtain MRI scan

LS, lumbosacral; ESR NL, normal erythrocyte sedimentation rate; EMG, electromyography.

I have a patient with chest pain. How do I determine the cause?

CHIEF COMPLAINT

Mr. W is a 56-year-old man who comes to your office with chest pain.

What is the differential diagnosis of chest pain? How would you frame the differential?

CONSTRUCTING A DIFFERENTIAL DIAGNOSIS

A patient with chest pain poses one of the most complicated diagnostic challenges. The differential diagnosis is enormous and includes diagnoses that can be imminently life-threatening if missed. The differential diagnosis of chest pain is the model for the anatomic approach to diagnosis. Consideration needs to be given to the structures from the skin to the internal organs.

A. Skin: Herpes zoster

B. Breast
  1. Fibroadenomas
  2. Gynecomastia

C. Musculoskeletal
  1. Costochondritis
  2. Precordial catch syndrome
  3. Pectoral muscle strain
  4. Rib fracture
  5. Cervical spondylosis
  6. Myositis

D. Esophageal
  1. Spasm
  2. Esophagitis
     a. Reflux
     b. Medication-related
  3. Neoplasm

E. GI
  1. Peptic ulcer disease
  2. Gallbladder disease
  3. Liver abscess
  4. Subdiaphragmatic abscess
  5. Pancreatitis

F. Pulmonary
  1. Pleura
     a. Pleural effusion
     b. Pneumonia
     c. Malignancy
     d. Viral infections
     e. Pneumothorax
  2. Lung
     a. Neoplasm
     b. Pneumonia
  3. Pulmonary vasculature
     a. Pulmonary embolism (PE)
     b. Pulmonary hypertension

G. Cardiac
  1. Pericarditis
  2. Myocarditis
  3. Myocardial ischemia

H. Vascular: Thoracic aortic aneurysm (TAA) or dissection

I. Mediastinal structures
  1. Lymphoma
  2. Thymoma

J. Psychiatric

Mr. W comes in regularly for management of hypertension and diabetes, both of which are under good control. He has been having symptoms since his last visit 4 months ago. He feels squeezing, substernal pressure while climbing stairs to the elevated train he rides to work. The pressure resolves after about 5 minutes of rest. He also occasionally feels the sensation during stressful periods at work. It is rarely associated with mild nausea and jaw pain. Medications are metformin, aspirin, and enalapril.

 At this point, what is the leading hypothesis, and what are the active alternatives? What other tests should be ordered?

Table 6–1. Diagnostic hypotheses for Mr. W.

Diagnostic Hypotheses	Clinical Clues	Important Tests
Leading Hypothesis		
Stable angina	Substernal chest pressure with exertion	Exercise tolerance test Angiogram
Active Alternative—Most Common		
GERD	Symptoms of heartburn, chronic nature	EGD Esophageal pH monitoring
Active Alternative		
Musculoskeletal disorders	History of injury or specific musculoskeletal chest pain syndrome	Physical exam Response to treatment

ORGANIZING THE DIFFERENTIAL DIAGNOSIS

Mr. W is a middle-aged man with risk factors for coronary artery disease (CAD), whose symptoms are consistent with stable angina. Given the seriousness and prevalence of CAD, it must lead the differential diagnosis. Gastroesophageal reflux disease (GERD) and musculoskeletal disorders are common causes of chest pain that can mimic angina (exacerbated by activity, sensation of pressure, radiation to back) and thus should be considered. The chronicity of the symptoms argues against many other worrisome diagnoses (eg, PE, pneumothorax, pericarditis, or TAA dissection). Pain from a mediastinal abnormality is possible. Table 6–1 lists the differential diagnosis.

Physical exam is entirely unremarkable except for mild, stable peripheral neuropathy presumably related to diabetes. The patient's ECG is remarkable only for evidence of left ventricular hypertrophy with strain.

 Is the clinical information sufficient to make a diagnosis? If not, what other information do you need?

Leading Hypothesis: Stable Angina

Textbook Presentation

Although atypical presentations are common, stable angina usually presents with classic symptoms of substernal chest discomfort precipitated by exertion. These symptoms resolve promptly with rest or nitroglycerin and do not change over the course of weeks. Affected patients usually have risk factors for CAD.

Disease Highlights

A. Stable angina is a chest pain syndrome caused by a mismatch between myocardial oxygen supply and demand.

  1. Usually a product of coronary stenosis.

  2. Can occur in the setting of normal or nearly normal coronary arteries and

  a. Anemia

  b. Aortic stenosis

  c. Hypertrophic cardiomyopathy

  d. Hyperthyroidism

 It is important to consider causes of angina other than CAD.

B. Stable angina is a common presentation for CAD.

C. Symptoms are often mild at presentation and are frequently minimized by patients.

D. Although exertional chest pain is the most common symptom of stable angina, other presentations are possible. Presentations may vary by what elicits the pain and what the symptoms are.

1. Eliciting factors other than exercise

   a. Cold weather

   b. Extreme moods (anger, stress)

   c. Large meals

2. Symptoms other than chest pain

   a. Dyspnea

   b. Nausea or indigestion

   c. Pain in areas other than the chest (eg, jaw, neck, teeth, back, abdomen)

   d. Palpitations

   e. Syncope

   f. Weakness and fatigue

E. The risk factors for CAD are important to elicit when the patient's history is suspicious. The traditional risk factors follow:

1. Male sex

2. Age > 55 years in men and > 65 years in women

3. Tobacco use

4. Diabetes

5. Hypertension

6. Family history of premature cardiovascular disease (younger than age 55 in men and younger than age 65 in women).

7. Abnormal lipid profile

   a. Elevated low-density lipoprotein (LDL)

   b. Elevated triglycerides

   c. Elevated cholesterol/high-density lipoprotein (HDL) ratio

   d. Low HDL

F. More novel risk factors are

1. Hyperhomocysteinemia

2. Elevated levels of inflammation (C-reactive protein)

3. Plasma fibrinogen

4. Microalbuminuria

Asking about the traditional cardiac risk factors should be a part of the history for any patient with possible CAD.

G. Stable angina and CAD in women

1. Although the pathophysiology of stable angina is the same in men and women, it raises some unique issues in women that deserve comment.

2. Because there is a lower prevalence of disease among women:

   a. Physicians often do not consider the diagnosis

   b. Lower pretest probability leads to worse positive predictive value of diagnostic tests (there are more false-positive results on noninvasive tests).

3. CAD presents differently in women than in men.

   a. Because CAD usually presents in women at an older age than in men, there are more comordid diseases to confuse the presentation.

   b. Women describe their chest pain differently, using terms like "burning" and "tender" more frequently.

Evidence-Based Diagnosis

A. History

1. The first step in diagnosing CAD is taking an accurate history of the patient's chest pain.

2. The vocabulary physicians use when discussing chest pain has been well validated to correlate with different risks of underlying CAD. The descriptions depend on the answers to 3 questions:

   a. Is your chest discomfort substernal?

   b. Are your symptoms precipitated by exertion?

   c. Does rest or nitroglycerin provide prompt relief of your symptoms (within 10 minutes)?

3. The number of questions to which the patient answers yes can predict the prevalence of CAD (Table 6–2).

Repeating a patient's complaint using chest pain in place of the patient's complaint (I get a feeling of heat in my ears when I climb a flight of stairs) can sometimes help identify the diagnosis of atypical angina.

Use the patient's own words when taking a history (eg, pressure, burning, aching, squeezing, piercing).

4. The remainder of the history should be aimed at collecting evidence that makes the diagnosis of CAD more likely, such as

   a. Cardiac risk factors

   b. Past history of cardiac disease

Table 6–2. Prevalence of coronary artery disease (%).[a]

Age	Asymptomatic[b]		Nonanginal Chest Pain[c]		Atypical Angina[d]		Typical Angina[e]	
	Male	**Female**	**Male**	**Female**	**Male**	**Female**	**Male**	**Female**
30–39	1.9	0.3	5.2	0.8	21.8	4.2	69.7	25.8
40–49	5.5	1.0	14.1	2.8	46.1	13.3	87.3	55.2
50–59	9.7	3.2	21.5	8.4	58.9	32.4	92.0	79.4
60–69	12.3	7.5	28.1	18.6	67.1	54.4	94.3	90.6

[a]See text for questions.
[b]Zero of 3 questions answered yes.
[c]One of 3 questions answered yes.
[d]Two of 3 questions answered yes.
[e]All 3 questions answered yes.
Source: Adapted with permisson from Diamond GA, Forrester JS. Analysis of probability as an aid in the clinical diagnosis of coronary-artery disease. *N Engl J Med.* 1979;300:1350–1358. Copyright © 1979, Massachusetts Medical Society. All rights reserved.

    c. Symptoms classic for other causes of chest pain

5. Factors that make the diagnosis of CAD less likely include

    a. Unremitting pain of prolonged duration

    b. Other explanations for the patient's symptoms

6. Initial tests should be done before testing specifically for CAD.

    a. Glucose and lipid profile can identify diseases that increase the likelihood of chest pain being ischemic in origin.

    b. Hgb and TSH can identify other diseases that may cause angina.

    c. Resting ECG looks for evidence of previous infarction.

B. Exercise testing

1. Except in very rare cases, patients with symptoms of stable angina should have an exercise test.

2. The test is used for 2 main purposes

    a. To diagnose CAD

    b. To determine whether patients should be treated with medication only, with angioplasty, or with bypass surgery.

3. All exercise tests attempt to induce and detect myocardial ischemia.

    a. Myocardial ischemia may be induced by exercise, dobutamine, adenosine, or dipyridamole.

    b. Myocardial ischemia may be detected by ECG, echocardiogram, or nuclear imaging.

4. Exercise electrocardiography is the most basic test. It requires a normal resting ECG.

    a. The sensitivity of the exercise stress test can be improved (at the cost of lower specificity) by reducing the degree of ST depression needed for a positive test.

    b. The sensitivity of an exercise test will fall if the patient does not reach an adequate degree of exercise, as measured by the rate-pressure product.

5. The sensitivity, specificity, and LRs of some of the various tests are shown in Table 6–3. (It should be noted that the test characteristics of stress thallium and dobutamine echocardiography vary among healthcare centers.)

6. The decision whether to order a routine exercise test or one with imaging is difficult. In general, reasons to obtain imaging are

    a. Abnormal resting ECG

    b. Digoxin use with > 1 mm ST depressions at baseline

    c. Previous coronary artery bypass grafting surgery (CABG) or percutaneous transluminal coronary angioplasty (PTCA)

    d. A more sensitive test is required to rule out CAD, such as in patients with a high likelihood of CAD.

7. Means of increasing coronary demand other than exercise (pharmacologic stress tests) are called for in 2 situations

Table 6–3. Test characteristics of exercise tests.

Test	Sensitivity	Specificity	LR+	LR−
Exercise ECG > 1 mm depression	45–65%	85–90%	3.0–5.0	0.56–0.65
Stress thallium	88%	91%	9.78	0.13
Dobutamine echocardiography	81%	83%	4.76	0.23

Adapted from Black ER. *Diagnostic Strategies for Common Medical Problems,* p. 52. Philadelphia: American College of Physicians, 1999.

    a. Left bundle-branch block (LBBB) or ventricular pacing

    b. Patients who are unable to exercise

8. A patient with stable angina might not undergo an exercise test if the patient has a high likelihood of disease (a test therefore does not need to be done for diagnostic purposes) and the patient would not benefit from determining the distribution or severity of the disease (usually because the patient would not or could not undergo revascularization).

9. Patients undergo angiography without first having an exercise test in a few circumstances

    a. When their symptoms are disabling despite therapy.

    b. When they have congestive heart failure (CHF).

MAKING A DIAGNOSIS

A tentative diagnosis of stable angina from CAD is made. Laboratory data is notable for normal blood counts and chemistries. There is only mild hypercholesterolemia (LDL 136 mg/dL, HDL 42 mg/dL). Mr. W is referred for an exercise tolerance test. Because of his abnormal resting ECG, a thallium treadmill test was performed. His results were normal without evidence of myocardial ischemia.

Have you crossed a diagnostic threshold for the leading hypothesis, stable angina? Have you ruled out the active alternatives? Do other tests need to be done to exclude the alternative diagnoses?

The results of the patient's exercise test are surprising. Stable angina remains high in the differential despite the normal stress test but alternative diagnoses must be considered. The intermittent nature of the pain and the lack of constitutional signs make a mediastinal lesion unlikely. The absence of a recent injury, change in activity or reproducible pain on physical exam moves musculoskeletal pain down on the differential. GERD is a common cause of chest pain and should be considered.

Alternative Diagnosis: GERD

Textbook Presentation

Heartburn is usually the presenting symptom in a patient with GERD. Other classic symptoms are regurgitation or dysphagia; chest pain is a common alternative presentation. Patients often report that their symptoms are worst at night and after large meals.

Although dysphagia is a common presentation of GERD, it should always be considered a worrisome symptom and mandates prompt evaluation, usually with upper endoscopy.

Disease Highlights

A. The symptoms of GERD are so well known that most patients diagnose themselves before visiting a physician.

B. GERD is a common cause of chest pain that may mimic that of more sinister causes.

GERD is such a common cause of acute chest pain that it should always be considered in the differential diagnosis of chest pain.

C. There are GI and non-GI complications of GERD.

    1. GI

    a. Esophagitis

    b. Stricture formation

    c. Barrett esophagus

    d. Esophageal adenocarcinoma

  2. Non-GI

    a. Chronic cough

    b. Hoarseness

    c. Worsening of asthma

D. Esophageal disorders, other than GERD, might present as chest pain.

  1. Esophagitis or esophageal ulcer

    a. Odynophagia common

    b. Multiple causes, including infection with cytomegalovirus, herpes simplex virus, and *Candida*

    c. Pill esophagitis (especially associated with certain medications)

      (1) Bisphosphonates

      (2) Tetracyclines

      (3) Anti-inflammatories

      (4) Potassium chloride

  2. Esophageal cancer

    a. Often associated with dysphagia

    b. Smoking, alcohol use, and chronic reflux are risk factors

  3. Esophageal rupture (Boerhaave syndrome). Often presents with acute pain after wretching.

  4. Esophageal spasm and motility disorders. Often presents with intermittent chest pain and dysphagia.

Evidence-Based Diagnosis

A. GERD should be high in the differential diagnosis of chest pain when heartburn, regurgitation, or dysphagia is present or when other commonly associated symptoms or complications (eg, chronic cough and asthma) are present.

B. Identifying factors that exacerbate the symptoms of GERD is helpful both in diagnosis and management.

  1. Ingesting large (especially fatty) meals

  2. Lying down after a meal

  3. Using tobacco

  4. Eating foods that relax the lower esophageal sphincter

    a. Chocolate

    b. Alcohol

    c. Coffee

    d. Peppermint

C. Historical features help differentiate esophageal from cardiac chest pain.

  1. A small study analyzed the prevalence of several historical features in 100 patients in an emergency department with either esophageal or cardiac chest pain.

  2. The differences that reached statistical significance are listed in Table 6–4. Although the study was small, the data are instructive.

  3. From these data, it is clear that history cannot differentiate esophageal chest pain from pain due to cardiac ischemia. That said, pain that is persistent, wakes the patient from sleep, is positional, and is associated with heartburn or regurgitation is more likely to be of esophageal origin.

  4. It is interesting that only 83% of patients with an esophageal cause of pain in this study had GI symptoms (ie, heartburn, regurgitation, dysphagia, or vomiting).

  5. Striking were some of the features not significantly different between the 2 groups:

    a. Radiation to the left arm

    b. Exacerbation with exercise

    c. Relief with nitroglycerin

  6. The effect of nitroglycerin in relieving chest pain has consistently been found to be useless in differentiating anginal chest pain from esophageal or other causes of chest pain.

 Response to nitroglycerin is not helpful in determining the cause of chest pain.

D. Esophageal pH testing, the gold standard for the diagnosis of GERD, is seldom necessary.

E. The combination of a suspicious history and consistent endoscopic findings has a 97% specificity for GERD.

F. Suggestive symptoms and response to therapy is generally considered diagnostic.

G. Esophagogastroduodenoscopy (EGD) should be done when

  1. Patients have symptoms of complicated disease

    a. Dysphagia

    b. Extra-esophageal symptoms

    c. Bleeding

Table 6–4. Prevalence of symptoms in patients with cardiac and esophageal chest pain.

Symptom	Prevalence (%)	
	Among Patients with Cardiac Cause	Among Patients with Esophageal Cause
Lateral radiation	69	11
More than 1 spontaneous episode per month	13	50
Pain persists as ache for several hours	25	78
Nighttime wakening caused by pain	25	61
Provoked by swallowing	6	39
Provoked by recumbency or stooping	19	61
Variable exercise tolerance	10	39
Pain starts after exercise completed	4	33
Pain relieved by antacid	10	44
Presence of heartburn	17	78
Presence of regurgitation	17	67
Presence of GI symptoms	46	83

Adapted from Davies HA, et al. Angina-like esophageal pain: differentiation from cardiac pain by history. *J Clin Gastroenterol.* 1985;7:477–481.

    d. Weight loss

    e. Chest pain of unclear etiology

  2. Patients are at risk for Barrett esophagus (long-standing symptoms of reflux).

  3. Patients require long-term therapy

  4. Patients respond poorly to appropriate therapy

H. Ambulatory pH monitoring is useful in 2 settings.

  1. In patients with symptoms of GERD and a normal endoscopy.

  2. To monitor therapy in refractory cases.

Treatment

A. Nonpharmacologic

  1. Elevate the entire head of the bed; adding extra pillows may actually worsen reflux.

  2. Avoid lying down for 3 hours after meals.

  3. Stop smoking.

  4. Stop ingesting high-risk foods and beverages.

    a. Fatty foods

    b. Chocolate

    c. Alcohol

    d. Peppermint

    e. Coffee

B. Pharmacologic

  1. Antacids

  2. H_2-blockers

  3. Proton-pump inhibitor

    a. First-line therapy in patients with reflux severe enough to prompt physician visit.

    b. Many patients require long-term therapy.

  4. Motility agents (such as metoclopramide) are useful in patients who need adjuvant therapy or who have significant symptoms of regurgitation.

  5. Surgery

    a. Antireflux surgery currently has only a very small role.

    b. May be warranted in some patients with particularly severe disease.

    c. One randomized trial has suggested that patients treated with surgery had a higher mortality rate than those treated medically at a mean follow-up of about 11 years (number needed to harm [NNH] = 8.3).

 Because GERD is a common cause of chest pain, it is appropriate to prescribe an empiric course of proton-pump inhibitors after more ominous causes of chest pain have been ruled out.

CASE RESOLUTION

Prior to the stress test, Mr. W's probability of having CAD was at least 92%. It is important to understand why the exercise test was done in this case. The diagnosis of coronary disease was essentially made by the history and physical. The exercise test was meant to guide therapy. Considering a pretest probability of 92%, and an LR– of 0.13 for the exercise test, the posttest probability is 60%. This is still well above the test threshold for a potentially fatal disease like CAD.

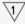

Despite the results of the stress test, stable angina was considered more likely than GERD. Mr. W was given aspirin and a β-blocker and underwent an angiogram the week after the visit. He was found to have a 90% stenosis of the mid left anterior descending artery and underwent angioplasty with stent placement.

Before ordering an exercise test, ask yourself why you are doing it: Are you trying to diagnose CAD or determine how severe the disease is.

Treatment of Stable Angina

A. The goal of treatment in patients with stable angina is to decrease symptoms and inhibit disease progression. Patients with stable angina have about a 3%/year risk of both myocardial infarction (MI) and death.

B. Nonpharmacologic
   1. Smoking cessation
   2. Exercise (intensity guided by exercise testing)
   3. Low fat, low cholesterol diet

C. Pharmacologic
   1. Symptomatic treatment
      a. Decrease oxygen demand
         (1) β-blocker
         (2) Calcium channel blocker (in those intolerant of β-blocker)
      b. Increase oxygen supply: long- and short-acting nitrates
   2. Inhibit disease progression
      a. Aspirin
      b. Risk factor modification
         (1) Lipid lowering
         (2) Glycemic control
         (3) Control of hyperhomocysteinemia

D. Interventional therapy (either via cardiac catheterization or bypass surgery) is the mainstay of treatment for the acute coronary syndromes discussed below. For stable angina, it plays a critical role for patients with more severe disease. An overview of the data is below.
   1. In **low-risk patients** (such as those with single vessel disease)
      a. There is no difference in mortality between medical management and catheter-based intervention.
      b. Patients who undergo a catheter-based intervention tend to have better control of their symptoms but undergo more procedures.
   2. In **moderate-risk patients** (such as those with multivessel disease but an otherwise normal heart)
      a. Angioplasty and CABG are about equal in terms of mortality and both are superior to medical therapy.
      b. PTCA leads to more procedures.
   3. In **high-risk patients** (such as those with disease of the left main coronary artery, 3 vessel disease, or 2 vessel disease involving the proximal left anterior descending artery)
      a. Bypass surgery is the most effective option.
      b. If a patient's anatomy is amenable to catheter-based procedures and their ejection fraction is normal, a catheter-based approach is an option.

CHIEF COMPLAINT

Mrs. G is a 68-year-old woman with a history of hypertension who arrives at the emergency department by ambulance complaining of chest pain that has lasted 6 hours. Two hours after eating, moderate (5/10) chest discomfort developed. She describes it as a burning

(continued)

sensation beginning in her mid chest and radiating to her back. She initially attributed the pain to heartburn and used antacids. Despite multiple doses over 3 hours, there was no relief. Over the last hour, the pain became very severe (10/10) with radiation to her back and arms. The pain is associated with diaphoresis and shortness of breath. The pain is not pleuritic. She called 911.

 At this point, what is the leading hypothesis, and what are the active alternatives? What other tests should be ordered?

ORGANIZING THE DIFFERENTIAL DIAGNOSIS

Mrs. G is experiencing acute, severe, nonpleuritic chest pain. This presentation is associated with multiple "must not miss" diagnoses. MI with and without ST elevations and unstable angina, as a group referred to the acute coronary syndromes, are the most common life-threatening causes of chest pain and need to be considered first. Dissection of a TAA also needs to be considered given the history of hypertension and the radiation of the patient's pain to her back. PE is another possible cause even though the chest pain is not pleuritic. Other alternative, but not life-threatening, causes of this type of pain are esophageal spasm and pancreatitis. However, it would be atypical for pancreatitis to begin so acutely. Table 6–5 lists the differential diagnosis.

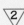

The patient takes enalapril for hypertension. She lives alone, is fairly sedentary, and smokes 1 pack of cigarettes each day. She has an 80 pack year smoking history.

On physical exam, the patient is in moderate distress related to the pain and concern that she is having a heart attack. Vital signs are temperature, 37.0 °C; BP, 156/90 mm Hg; pulse, 100 beats per minute; RR, 22 breaths per minute. Head and neck exam were normal including jugular and carotid pulsations. The lung exam was clear. Heart exam was notable for a normal S_1 and S_2 and a soft, II/VI systolic ejection murmur. Abdominal exam was unremarkable with no tenderness, hepatosplenomegaly, or bruits.

Table 6–5. Diagnostic hypotheses for Mrs. G.

Diagnostic Hypotheses	Clinical Clues	Important Tests
Leading Hypothesis		
Acute MI	Presence of cardiac risk factors, acute onset	ECG Cardiac enzymes (CK and troponin) Coronary angiography
Active Alternative—Must Not Miss		
Unstable angina	Presence of cardiac risk factors Ischemic symptoms that are new or increasing in frequency	ECG Cardiac enzymes (CK and troponin) Stress testing Coronary angiography
TAA dissection	Presence of hypertension Radiation of pain to back Signs of cardiac or neurologic ischemia	Transesophageal echocardiography CT scan
Other Alternative		
Esophageal spasm	Recurrent chest pain, often with radiation to back	Esophageal manometry and exclusion of other causes

 Is the clinical information sufficient to make a diagnosis? If not, what other information do you need?

Leading Hypothesis: Acute MI

Textbook Presentation

The classic presentation of an acute MI is crushing substernal chest pressure, diaphoresis, nausea, shortness of breath, and a feeling of impending doom in a middle-aged man with risk factors for CAD. More than most other "textbook presentations," this description is often inaccurate because it does not take into account the frequency of MIs in women, younger and older patients, and the frequency of atypical presentations.

Disease Highlights

A. MI occurs when there is a prolonged failure to perfuse an area of myocardium leading to cell death.

B. Most commonly occurs when a coronary plaque ruptures causing blockage of a coronary artery.

C. The definition of acute, evolving, or recent MI published by the American College of Cardiology is a typical rise and fall of cardiac enzymes (troponin or CK-MB) with at least 1 of the following:

1. Ischemic symptoms

2. Development of Q waves

3. ECG changes indicative of ischemia

4. Coronary artery intervention (in recognition of the frequency of myocardial injury during coronary intervention)

D. Acute MIs are classified as either with or without ST elevations.

1. ST elevations signify transmural ischemia or infarction.

2. MIs that produce abnormal cardiac enzymes but no ST elevations

   a. Are less severe, usually injuring only subendomyocardial tissue

   b. Have a higher subsequent risk for ST-segment elevation MI

3. These 2 types of MI are managed somewhat differently (discussed below).

Evidence-Based Diagnosis

A. About 15% of patients who are admitted to the emergency department with chest pain are having an MI.

B. Although historical and physical exam features are never sufficient to diagnose an MI and only rule out an MI in the lowest risk patients, a few features are fairly predictive (Table 6–6).

C. All guidelines recommend an ECG be performed within 10 minutes of a patient's arrival at a healthcare facility when an MI is suspected.

 A patient with chest pain and 1-mm ST elevations in 2 contiguous leads or a new LBBB is having an acute MI and should receive immediate therapy.

D. Prevalence rates of MI among patients with various ECG findings follow:

1. New ST elevation of 1 mm: 80%

2. New ST depression or T wave inversion: 20%

Table 6–6. Likelihood ratios of historical features and physical exam findings and effect on posttest probability.

Feature or Finding	LR+	Posttest Probability[a]
Radiation to left arm	2.3	29%
Radiation to right shoulder	2.9	34%
Radiation to both arms	7.1	56%
Nausea and vomiting	1.9	25%
Diaphoresis	2.0	26%
3rd heart sound	3.2	36%
Hypotension	3.1	35%
Rales	2.1	27%

[a]Assuming 15% pretest probability.

Adapted from Panju AA, et al. The rational clinical examination. Is this patient having a myocardial infarction? *JAMA.* 1998;280:1256–1263. Copyright © 1998. American Medical Association. All rights reserved.

3. No new changes in a patient with known CAD: 4%

4. No new changes in a patient without known CAD: 2%

E. Table 6–7 shows the test characteristics for ECG findings in patients with acute chest pain. Because there are a range of numbers from various studies, these numbers should be treated as estimates.

F. When an MI is suspected, cardiac enzymes are ordered.

1. These tests are highly reliable in diagnosing MI. (Note that the American College of Cardiology definition of MI is based on enzyme results.)

2. Our ability to diagnose MI and risk stratify patients on the basis of enzyme results continues to improve.

3. Table 6–8 lists the test characteristics for serial CK-MB and troponin I according to time after symptom onset.

4. CK-MB and troponin should be ordered and processed immediately.

5. Although troponin levels are higher in patients with renal insufficiency, higher levels are still predictive of poor outcomes.

G. MI in women

Table 6–7. Test characteristics for ECG findings in patients with chest pain for the diagnosis of acute MI.[a]

ECG Finding	LR+	LR–
New ST elevation > 1 mm	5.7–53	
New Q wave	5.3–24.8	
Any ST elevation	11.2	
New Q or ST elevation	11	0.24
New conduction defect	6.3	
Any Q wave	3.9	
T wave peaking	3.1	
Any conduction defect	2.7	
Any ECG abnormality	1.3	0.04

[a]Data are unavailable when not given.
Adapted from Panju AA, et al. The rational clinical examination. Is this patient having a myocardial infarction? *JAMA.* 1998;280:1256–1263. Copyright © 1998. American Medical Association. All rights reserved.

1. Acute MIs present differently in women than in men.
   a. Women often report prodromal symptoms such as fatigue, dyspnea, and insomnia.
   b. Chest pain is only present in 57% of women at the time of MI.
   c. Dyspnea, weakness, and fatigue are the other common presenting symptoms.
2. Women who suffer an MI are more likely to die. The cause of this disparity is multifactorial.
   a. Compared with men, women are older when they have their first MI and have more comorbid conditions.

   b. Historically, women have been less likely to undergo revascularization procedures.
3. Women who do undergo bypass surgery and catheter-based intervention have higher complication rates than men who undergo these same procedures.

H. Unrecognized MI
   1. Although the combination of symptoms, ECG findings, and enzymes make most MIs easy to diagnose, about 2% of patients with acute MI are discharged from the emergency department.
   2. Failure to recognize an MI results in worse outcomes for patients and serious medicolegal issues.
   3. MIs most commonly go unrecognized when they present in unusual ways or in people not expected to have an MI.
   4. A patient with an MI or unstable angina who is mistakenly discharged is most likely to:
      a. Be a woman younger than age 55
      b. Be non-white
      c. Have a chief complaint of shortness of breath
      d. Have a nondiagnostic ECG
   5. MI may present without chest pain; patients tend to be older women or have diabetes mellitus or a history of CHF.
   6. The most common alternative presentations of MI are listed below. MI should at least be considered in patients being discharged from the emergency department with one of these diagnoses.
      a. CHF
      b. Stable angina
      c. Arrhythmia
      d. Atypical location of pain

Table 6–8. Test characteristics for the diagnosis of acute MI by time after symptom onset.

Test	Time Frame	Sensitivity (%)	Specificity (%)	LR+	LR–
Serial CK-MB	< 24 h	99	98	50	0.01
	> 24 h	55	97	18	0.46
Troponin I	9 h	95	98	47	0.03
	> 24 h	95	98	47	0.03

Adapted from Black ER. *Diagnostic Strategies for Common Medical Problems,* p. 64. Philadelphia: American College of Physicians, 1999.

e. CNS manifestations (symptoms of cerebrovascular accident)

f. Nervousness

g. Mania or psychosis

h. Syncope

i. Weakness

j. Indigestion

 MI can present in many different ways. A high index of suspicion should always be present. Certain groups of patients (elderly, women, minorities, diabetics) are most likely to be misdiagnosed.

MAKING A DIAGNOSIS

 Mrs. G's ECG shows ST depression in leads II, III, AVL, and V3–V6. The chest x-ray is normal.

Have you crossed a diagnostic threshold for the leading hypothesis, acute MI? Have you ruled out the active alternatives? Do other tests need to be done to exclude the alternative diagnoses?

The ECG is consistent with cardiac ischemia but does not make the diagnosis of an acute MI; the diagnosis will be confirmed when the laboratory results for the enzymes are available. The abnormal ECG certainly makes the alternative diagnosis, unstable angina, quite likely if an MI is excluded. Dissections of TAAs often cause cardiac ischemia, so this too must remain in the differential.

Alternative Diagnosis: Unstable Angina

Textbook Presentation

Patients with unstable angina classically present with new or worsening symptoms of CAD. Unstable angina and an acute MI that presents without ST elevation may be identical in their presentation, only differentiated by the presence or absence of myocardial enzyme elevation.

Disease Highlights

A. Unstable angina is defined as angina that is new or worsening in severity or frequency.

B. Pathophysiology

1. Primarily caused by acute plaque rupture followed by platelet aggregation.

   a. 67% of episodes occur in arteries with < 50% stenosis.

   b. 97% occur in arteries with < 75% stenosis.

2. Caused less commonly by changes in oxygen demand or supply (eg, hyperthyroidism, anemia, high altitude).

C. The diagnosis of unstable angina can be difficult, often depending on a careful history to differentiate stable from unstable angina.

D. The job of the clinician who sees a patient with unstable angina or a non–ST-elevation MI is to

1. Immediately recognize that the patient has an acute coronary syndrome

2. Institute care

3. Determine the patient's risk of progressing to an MI or death

4. Treat accordingly

E. Vasospastic angina

1. Vasospastic angina (also called Prinzmetal or variant angina) is a phenomenon that is related to unstable angina in presentation.

2. Patients with vasospastic angina periodically have episodes of cardiac ischemia with ST elevation.

3. The attacks

   a. Are often associated with chest pain or other ischemic symptoms

   b. Resolve spontaneously or with nitroglycerin

   c. May occur in normal or diseased coronary arteries

   d. Can result in MI or death (often secondary to arrhythmia)

   e. Often occur at the same time each day

4. Vasospastic angina is usually diagnosed clinically but can also be diagnosed by inducing it with ergonovine infusion in the catheterization lab.

5. Vasospastic angina is treated effectively with calcium channel blockers and nitrates.

 Vasospastic angina should be considered in patients whose symptoms are consistent with cardiac ischemia and occur at about the same time each day. The diagnosis should also be considered when transient ST elevations develop.

Evidence-Based Diagnosis

The diagnostic considerations for a patient in whom unstable angina is suspected are 2-fold:

A. Diagnose unstable angina.

1. This is done clinically; does the patient have new or progressive angina?

2. Stress testing may clarify the diagnosis in patients at the lowest risk, in whom the diagnosis is unclear.

B. Risk-stratify the patient.

1. Risk stratification of patients with unstable angina is one of the fastest changing fields in cardiology as new markers for risk are developed.

2. There is a trend toward progressively greater numbers of patients found to benefit from early invasive strategies.

3. Clinically, increasing risk can be determined by the patient's presentation.

4. The classes of angina shown in Table 6–9 represent increasing risk of MI.

Treatment

A. Initial stabilization

1. Patients presenting with unstable angina require immediate stabilization.

2. The following treatments should be started as soon as the diagnosis is made:

a. Heparin (unfractionated or low-molecular-weight)

b. Aspirin

c. β-Blockers

d. Nitrates

B. Definitive treatment

1. Patients at very low risk for complications of unstable angina (MI or death) can be managed medically and undergo stress testing to determine their risk strata.

2. A number of other factors speak for higher risk and indicate an early invasive strategy. Some are listed below:

a. Angina at rest despite antianginal regimen

b. Elevated cardiac enzymes (which make the diagnosis of MI)

c. New ST depression

d. CHF or low ejection fraction

e. Hemodynamic or electrophysiologic instability

f. Previous CABG or recent PTCA

3. Patients who do not fulfill any of these criteria but have worrisome findings on noninvasive testing (exercise test) should also undergo invasive testing.

Alternative Diagnosis: Dissection of the Thoracic Aorta

Textbook Presentation

The textbook presentation of a thoracic aorta (TA) dissection is an older man with a history of hypertension and possibly atherosclerotic disease who complains of "tearing" chest or back pain. The pain might be associated with vascular complications such as syncope, stroke, cardiac ischemia, or CHF secondary to acute aortic regurgitation. On physical exam, there is asymmetry in the upper extremity BPs, and the chest x-ray shows a widened mediastinum.

Disease Highlights

A. Risk factors for development of TAA are numerous.

1. Hypertension is the most common, present in at least 80% of patients.

2. Inflammatory diseases of the vessel wall (eg, giant cell arteritis and syphilitic aortitis) are present in about 10% of patients.

3. Disorders of vascular structure

a. Cystic medial necrosis (in about 6% of patients)

Table 6–9. Classes of unstable angina.

Class	Description	Risk of MI
IA	Accelerated angina without ECG changes	2.7%
IB	Accelerated angina with ECG changes	5.6%
II	New-onset exertional angina	5.7%
III	New-onset rest angina	8.8%
IV	Protracted rest angina with ECG changes	17.7%

Adapted from Simons M. Classification of unstable angina and non-ST elevation (non-Q wave) myocardial infarction. In: *UpToDate*, Rose, BD (Ed), UpToDate, Wellesley, MA, 2003. Copyright © 2003 UpToDate, Inc. For more information visit UpToDate.com.

b. Marfan syndrome and Ehlers-Danlos syndrome (rare)

B. Patients with TAA without dissection commonly present with an abnormal chest film.

C. Other modes of presentation are via aortic regurgitation, pain related to mass effect, or through mass effects on other structures.

  1. Hoarseness due to compression of the recurrent laryngeal nerve

  2. Airway compression

  3. Esophageal compression

D. Dissection of TA

  1. A rapidly fatal disease as well as a very difficult diagnosis.

  2. A high clinical suspicion is necessary to differentiate this diagnosis from the more common causes of life-threatening chest pain, such as cardiac ischemia and PE.

  3. Dissection begins with a tear in the aortic intima allowing blood to dissect the aorta between the intima and media.

  4. The risk factors for dissection of the TA are the same as for development of aneurysms and about 15% of patients with dissections have TAA.

  5. An additional risk factor for TA dissection is cocaine use. This is associated with dissections in younger patients (mean age 41).

 TA dissection should be considered in the differential of a young hypertensive patient who has chest pain after using cocaine.

  6. The symptoms of dissection include pain as well as symptoms of vascular complications of the dissection. The type of complication depends on what type of dissection occurs.

  a. Type A dissections involve the ascending aorta with or without the descending aorta

  b. Type B dissections involve only the descending aorta

  7. Type A dissections tend to be more complicated leading to:

  a. Acute aortic insufficiency

  b. Myocardial ischemia due to coronary occlusion.

  c. Neurologic deficits

  d. Cardiac tamponade due to hemopericardium

Evidence-Based Diagnosis

A. The diagnosis of a dissection of the TA is reliably difficult. There are no signs or symptoms that are consistently associated with very high or very low LRs.

B. A study of 464 patients with aortic dissection helps describe the common presenting signs and symptoms of people with this diagnosis. This study included patients with aortic dissection diagnosed at any time during their hospitalization as well as patients in whom the diagnosis was made postmortem.

  1. 62% of the patients had a type A dissection.

  2. The demographic findings were not surprising:

  a. Mean age ≈ 63 years

  b. 73% of patients had hypertension

  3. The presenting signs and symptoms were notable for the infrequency of some classic findings.

  a. Pulse deficit was noted in only 15% of patients, syncope in 9%, cerebrovascular accident in 5%, and CHF in 7%.

  b. Some of the more common symptoms are shown in Table 6–10.

  4. Chest film and ECG were found to be very insensitive diagnostic tools.

 The aorta is normal on the chest film in about 40% of patients with a dissection of the TA.

C. Another study looked at independent predictors of aortic dissection: aortic type pain (pain of acute onset or tearing or ripping character), aortic or mediastinal widening on chest film, and pulse or BP differentials.

  1. Patients were stratified by these risk factors.

  a. Low-risk patients had none of the characteristics.

  b. Intermediate-risk patients had only consistent pain or consistent chest film.

  c. High-risk patients had pulse or BP differentials or any combination of 2 or 3 of the variables.

  2. Low-risk patients had a 7% risk of dissection.

  3. Intermediate-risk patients had a 30–40% risk of dissection.

  4. High-risk patients had a > 84% risk of dissection.

Table 6–10. Prevalence of various findings and symptoms in patients with thoracic aortic dissection (type A).

Finding or Symptom	Prevalence Among Patients with Type A Dissection
Abrupt onset pain	85%
Chest pain	79%
Back pain	47%
Severe or worst ever pain	90%
Sharp pain	62%
Tearing pain	51%
Normal chest film	11%
Widened mediastinum	63%
Normal mediastinum and aortic contour	17%
Nonspecific ST-segment or T-wave changes	43%

D. Summarizing the clinical diagnosis of dissection: Patients with dissections are likely to have a history of hypertension and experience severe, acute pain. Patients with chest pain are unlikely to have a dissection if they do not have any of the following: acute or tearing or ripping pain; aortic or mediastinal widening; and asymmetric pulse or BPs.

E. The gold standard for diagnosis is angiography but most patients undergo only noninvasive tests.

F. All the commonly used noninvasive tests have sensitivities and specificities above 95%.

G. The most commonly used tests are CT scans and transesophageal echocardiography.

H. Angiography is recommended to help guide therapy if there is evidence of organ ischemia.

Treatment

A. Because dissection is associated with extremely high mortality, the ideal is to identify and repair the aneurysm prior to rupture.

B. TAA

1. When aneurysms are detected prior to rupture,

the goal of therapy is to slow their growth and operate prophylactically when the aneurysm reaches a certain size.

2. Patients with aneurysms should have tight BP control.

3. Patients should be closely monitored for increasing aneurysm size.

4. Indications for surgery are based on the size of the aneurysm:
   a. 5.5 cm for ascending TAAs
   b. 6.5 cm for descending TAAs
   c. Rapid growth

5. There is growing enthusiasm for using intravascular stents to repair some aneurysms.

C. TA dissection

1. Dissection of the TA is a medical emergency.

2. Type A dissections are generally operated on immediately.

3. Type B dissections usually are managed medically.

4. The mortality of dissection is high. In a recent study, the inhospital mortality was about 35% for type A dissections and 15% for type B dissections.

CASE RESOLUTION

Mrs. G's initial troponin was elevated at 3.5 ng/mL with a CK of 750 units/L and positive MB fraction. The final diagnosis is acute MI. Following stabilization in the emergency department, she was taken directly to the cardiac catheterization laboratory. There she was found to have a left dominant system and an acute thrombosis of the branch of the left circumflex artery. This was opened with intracoronary thrombolysis and a stent was placed.

The patient's troponin and CK make the diagnosis of an acute MI. It should be realized that the presence of an MI does not rule out dissection of the TA. Between 3% and 5% of patients with dissections have associated MIs. Even before the catheterization the subacute onset of the pain, the normal chest film, the lack of "tearing pain," and symmetric pulses all make dissection less likely.

Treatment of MI

A. A patient with an acute MI needs to receive immediate treatment with antianginals and pain medications. The initial treatment is outlined below:

1. Oxygen
2. IV nitroglycerin
3. Aspirin
4. β-blocker
5. Anticoagulation is generally recommended although data are not as strong as for those above.
6. Other therapy based on presentation
    a. Narcotics for patients in pain
    b. Atropine for patients with pathologic bradycardia
    c. Antiarrhythmic agents

B. The next and most important step is opening the culprit vessel. The 2 options are systemic thrombolysis or primary angioplasty.

1. Although less widely available, primary angioplasty is the preferred option.
2. Primary angioplasty is associated with
    a. Lower mortality (even in patients who must be transferred—albeit quickly—to a hospital with the capability)
    b. Significantly lower risk of serious bleeding complication. Hemorrhagic stroke is not a potential complication as it is with systemic thrombolysis.
3. The ability to do primary angioplasty depends on the presence of a skilled team of interventional cardiologists who can rapidly bring the patient to the catheterization laboratory.
4. Primary angioplasty with stent placement is probably the most efficacious treatment.

5. Both primary angioplasty and thrombolysis are most effective when completed within 12 hours of symptom onset.

C. Once the culprit vessel has been opened, various medications have been shown to improve survival after acute MI.

1. Unfractionated heparin
    a. For all patients having primary angioplasty
    b. Will likely be replaced by low-molecular-weight heparin
2. β-Blockers
3. ACE inhibitors
4. Aspirin
5. HMG-coa reductase inhibitors, dosed to achieve an LDL at least < 100 mg/dL
6. Glycoprotein IIB/IIIA inhibitors are recommended for high-risk patients with non–ST-elevation MIs.

D. An exercise test is also recommended within 3 weeks of an MI for information on prognosis, functional capacity, and risk stratification.

Four days after her MI, Mrs. G underwent a submaximal exercise test. This was essentially normal except for a mildly depressed ejection fraction of 45%. She was discharged with prescriptions for the following medications:

1. Atorvastatin 20 mg
2. Enalapril 20 mg
3. Atenolol 100 mg
4. Aspirin 81 mg
5. Hydrochlorothiazide 25 mg

CHIEF COMPLAINT

PATIENT 3

Mr. H is a 31-year-old man, previously in excellent health who arrives at the emergency department complaining of chest pain. He reports that the pain began 10 days earlier. It was initially mild and is accompanied by mild cough and shortness of breath that the patient attributes to his asthma. Five days earlier, he had come to the emergency department and musculoskeletal chest pain was diagnosed; he was given nonsteroidal anti-inflammatory drugs (NSAIDs) and discharged.

Now he reports more severe pain that is worst when he takes a deep breath. He says it

(continued)

is located over the right lateral lower chest wall. His dyspnea is still only mild. He also has noted low-grade fevers with temperatures running about 38 °C.

 At this point, what is the leading hypothesis, and what are the active alternatives? What other tests should be ordered?

ORGANIZING THE DIFFERENTIAL DIAGNOSIS

This is a healthy young man presenting with an acute illness. He reports pleuritic chest pain, cough, dyspnea, and fevers. The first diagnoses to consider are infectious disease that could cause pleuritic chest pain. Pneumonia or pleural effusion could cause these symptoms, either individually or as part of the same process. (Pleural effusions will be discussed below while pneumonia will be diagnosed in Chapter 7). Pericarditis can also cause pleuritic chest pain and can be associated with fevers. PE is a classic cause of pleuritic chest pain and shortness of breath and may be associated with fever (see Chapter 11, Dyspnea). Intra-abdominal processes, such as subdiaghragmatic abscess should be kept in mind as causes of pleuritic chest pain. The combination of fever, dyspnea, and chest pain places pneumonia or pleural effusion at the top of the list. Table 6–11 lists the differential diagnosis.

During further history taking, Mr. H reports no radiation of the pain. He denies abdominal pain, nausea, vomiting, or change in appetite. Deep breathing and sudden movements tend to worsen the pain. There are no other palliative or provocative features.

On physical exam, Mr. H is a healthy appearing man who appears in mild distress. He moves somewhat gingerly because of the pain and is dyspneic. He coughs occasionally during the history. This causes great pain. Vital signs are temperature, 38.9 °C; BP, 130/84 mm Hg; pulse, 110 bpm; RR, 26 breaths per minute. Head and neck exam is normal; there is no jugular venous distention. Lung exam is notable for dullness to percussion and decreased breath sounds at the right base. There is an area of egophony just superior to the decreased

Table 6–11. Diagnostic hypotheses for Mr. H.

Diagnostic Hypotheses	Clinical Clues	Important Tests
Leading Hypothesis		
Pleural effusion or pneumonia	Cough and shortness of breath with associated physical exam findings	Chest film Thoracentesis for pleural effusion
Active Alternative		
Pericarditis	Pain relieved by leaning forward Friction rub ECG changes	ECG Echocardiogram
Active Alternative—Must Not Miss		
Pulmonary embolism	Risk factors Tachycardia	Ventilation-perfusion scan Helical CT Pulmonary angiogram
Other Alternative		
Subdiaghragmatic abscess	Intra-abdominal process Fevers	Abdominal ultrasound or CT

breath sounds and normal breath sounds superior to this. All these findings are consistent with a pleural effusion. The left chest is clear. Heart exam is normal as are the abdomen and extremities.

 Is the clinical information sufficient to make a diagnosis? If not, what other information do you need?

Leading Hypothesis: Pleural Effusion

Textbook Presentation

Small effusions are usually asymptomatic while large effusions reliably cause dyspnea with or without pleuritic chest pain. Presentation depends on the cause of the effusion. Parapneumonic effusions will be accompanied by the signs and symptoms of pneumonia while neoplastic effusions will usually present with dyspnea alone and symptoms of the underlying cancer. Pleural effusions related to rheumatologic disease are usually accompanied by signs of the specific illness. Physical exam reveals dullness to percussion and decreased breath sounds over the area of effusion.

Disease Highlights

A. Pathophysiology of pleural effusions vary by etiology but may be due to 1 or any combination of the following:

1. Increased capillary permeability
2. Increased hydrostatic pressure
3. Decreased oncotic pressure
4. Increased negative intrapleural pressure
5. Disruption of pulmonary lymphatics

B. The differential diagnosis of a pleural effusion is enormous. The most common causes with their approximate yearly incidence are listed in Table 6–12.

C. The differential diagnosis is mainly broken down into exudative and transudative effusion.

1. Exudative effusions are caused by increased capillary permeability or disruption of pulmonary lymphatics.
2. Transudative effusions are caused by increased hydrostatic pressure, decreased oncotic pressure, or increased negative intrapleural pressure.

D. Exudative effusions commonly complicate the following diagnoses:

1. Pneumonia

   a. Any effusion associated with pneumonia, lung abscess, or bronchiectasis is considered a parapneumonic effusion.
   b. Empyemas are parapneumonic effusions that have become infected.
   c. Empyemas, and certain parapneumonic effusions called complicated parapneumonic effusions, are more likely to form fibrotic, pleural peels. The diagnostic criteria for these types of effusions are given below.
   d. Parapneumonic effusions accompany 40% of all pneumonias while empyemas occur 2% of the time, at most.
   e. Effusions are more likely to form and more likely to become infected if the treatment of the underlying pneumonia is delayed.
   f. The bacteriology of parapneumonic effusions is shown in Table 6–13.

2. Malignancy

   a. Most common cancers leading to effusions are
      (1) Lung
      (2) Breast
      (3) Lymphoma
      (4) Leukemia
      (5) Adenocarcinoma of unknown primary
   b. The effusion may occur as the presenting symptom of the cancer or occur in patients with a previously diagnosed malignancy.

Table 6–12. The incidences of several causes of pleural effusion.

Etiology	Incidence
CHF	500,000
Pneumonia	300,000
Malignancy	200,000
Pulmonary embolism	150,000
Viral disease	100,000
Coronary artery bypass surgery	60,000
Cirrhosis with ascites	50,000

Less common but prevalent causes, including uremia, tuberculosis, chylothorax, and rheumatologic disease (RA and SLE)

RA, rheumatoid arthritis; SLE, systemic lupus erythematosus.
Adapted with permission from Light RW. Clinical practice. Pleural effusion. *N Engl J Med.* 2002;346:1971–1977. Copyright © 2002, Massachusetts Medical Society. All rights reserved.

Table 6–13. Bacteriology of parapneumonic effusions.

Bacteria	Percentage of Pneumonias with Effusion	Percentage of Effusions that Are Empyemas
Streptococcus pneumoniae	40–60	< 5
Anaerobes	35	90
Staphylococcus aureus	40	20
Haemophilus influenzae	50	20
Escherichia coli	~50	~99

c. The presence of a malignant effusion is generally a very poor prognostic sign.

3. PE

  a. Effusions are present in 26–56% of patients with PE.

  b. Effusions accompany PE most commonly in patients with pleuritic pain or hemoptysis.

4. Viral infections

  a. Considered to be a common cause of effusions

  b. Difficult to diagnose; definitive diagnosis is rarely made

  c. Usually diagnosed in patients with febrile or nonfebrile illness with transient effusion and negative work-up.

  d. Other clues such as atypical lymphocytes, monocytosis, and leukopenia are helpful in diagnosing viral infection.

 Viral pleural effusions should only be diagnosed in an appropriate clinical setting when more serious causes of effusion have been ruled out.

5. CABG surgery

  a. Pleural effusions develop in up to 90% of patients immediately following CABG.

  b. Can be left sided or bilateral

  c. Usually resolve spontaneously

6. Other diseases that are not uncommon causes of pleural effusions include:

  1. Uremia

  2. Tuberculosis (TB)

  3. Chylothorax

  4. Rheumatologic disease (eg, rheumatoid arthritis and systemic lupus erythematosus)

E. The most common causes of transudative effusions are:

1. CHF

  a. Most common cause of transudative effusions in the United States

  b. Effusions are accompanied by other findings of left heart failure.

  c. Effusions are usually small and resolve with diuresis alone.

  d. Effusions are usually bilateral; unilateral effusions can occur, but they are less common.

2. Cirrhosis with ascites

  a. About 6% of patients with ascites have pleural effusions.

  b. Effusion is thought to be secondary to ascites moving into the thorax via defects in the diaphragm.

  c. Extremely rare to have pleural effusions on the basis of cirrhosis without ascites.

Evidence-Based Diagnosis

A. The diagnosis of a pleural effusion itself is based on the recognition of fluid in the pleural space on physical exam.

  1. The sensitivity and specificity of dullness to chest percussion for detecting pleural effusions is very good.

   a. Sensitivity, 96%; specificity, 95%

   b. LR+, 18.6; LR−, 0.04

  2. There is often an area of egophony just superior to the effusion.

  3. Once detected, a pleural effusion is confirmed on chest x-ray, ultrasound, or other form of chest imaging.

B. After diagnosing a pleural effusion, the next step is to determine the cause. If the effusion is clinically significant (usually considered > 1 cm on a chest film), it should be sampled.

  1. A cause should be determined for any new pleural effusion.

  2. The only exception to this is in the case of CHF. If the clinical suspicion for CHF as the sole cause of the effusion is very high, the effusion can be observed while the patient is treated. If the effusion persists or the diagnosis becomes unclear, the effusion should then be sampled.

 Pleural effusions are abnormal; any new pleural effusion should be evaluated.

C. The first step in determining the cause of an effusion is to differentiate transudative from exudative effusions.

D. The sensitivity and specificity of the various tests for distinguishing exudates from transudates are given in Table 6–14. Light's criteria (1 or more positive results of the preceding 3 criteria in the table) is by far the most commonly used.

E. The most common transudative and exudative effusions are shown in Table 6–15.

F. Once the diagnosis of a transudate or exudate is made, various other tests will help determine the exact diagnosis. Besides lactate dehydrogenase (LDH) and protein, certain tests are routinely sent when pleural fluid is sampled.

Table 6–14. Test characteristics for methods that distinguish transudative from exudative effusions.

Method	Sensitivity (%)	Specificity (%)	LR+	LR−
Pleural fluid protein/serum protein > 0.5	86	84	5.37	0.17
Pleural fluid LDH/serum LDH > 0.6 units/L	90	82	5.00	0.12
Pleural fluid LDH > ²/₃ upper limits of normal serum LDH	82	89	7.45	0.20
Light's criteria	98	83	5.76	0.02
Pleural fluid cholesterol > 60 mg/dL	54	92	6.75	0.50
Serum albumin-pleural fluid albumin < 1.2 g/dL	87	92	10.88	0.14

Adapted with permission from Light RW. Clinical practice. Pleural effusion. *N Engl J Med.* 2002;346:1971–1977. Copyright © 2002, Massachusetts Medical Society. All rights reserved.

1. Gram stain and culture help make the diagnosis of an empyema.
2. Fluid pH. A low pH is commonly seen with:
   a. Empyemas
   b. Malignant effusions
   c. Esophageal rupture
3. Cell count
   a. Neutrophil count over 50% argues for an acute process
      (1) Parapneumonic effusion (sensitivity = 91%)
      (2) PE

Table 6–15. Common transudative and exudative effusions.

Transudative Effusions	Exudative Effusions
Congestive heart failure	Parapneumonic effusions
Cirrhosis with ascites	Malignancy
Pulmonary embolism (¼)	Pulmonary embolism (¾)
Nephrotic syndrome	Viral infections
Severe hypoalbuminemia	Post CABG Subdiaphragmatic infections and inflammatory states Chylothorax, uremia, connective tissue diseases

CABG, coronary artery bypass grafting.

   b. High neutrophil count is rarely seen in other diseases, such as TB and malignancy.
   c. Lymphocyte predominant exudative effusions are almost always caused by TB or malignancy (positive predictive value = 97%).
   d. Pleural fluid eosinophilia is a nonspecific finding. It is seen frequently with inflammatory diseases, pneumococcal pneumonia, viral pleuritis, TB, and even repeated thoracentesis.
   e. A low mesothelial cell count (< 5%) count is highly suggestive of TB.
4. Cytology
   a. Highly specific for the diagnosis of cancer
   b. Sensitivity is 70% at best, with significantly lower values for some cancers.
G. Other tests are done if the clinical suspicion for certain diseases is high.
   1. TB
      a. Usually suspected based on clinical presentation and pleural fluid lymphocytosis
      b. Polymerase chain reaction (100% specificity) and adenosine deaminase levels most commonly used tests. See Chapter 7, Acute Respiratory Complaints.
   2. Glucose levels < 60 mg/dL are helpful and are seen in:
      a. Empyema
      b. TB
      c. Rheumatoid arthritis and systemic lupus erythematosus
   3. Triglycerides are greater than 110 mg/dL in patients with chylothorax. The fluid is also a milky white.

4. Thoracoscopy with pleural biopsy often used when suspicion for malignancy is high and cytology is negative.

MAKING A DIAGNOSIS

A posteroanterior, lateral, and decubitus chest film were done that revealed an effusion. The effusion was tapped and yielded pale, turbid fluid. The initial results are glucose, < 20 mg/dL; LDH = 38,400 units/L; protein = 4.4 g/dL; fluid pH, 6.2; RBC, 3200/mcL; WBC, 144,000/mcL; Gram stain positive for gram-positive cocci in pairs and chains. Serum values at the time included total protein of 7.8 g/dL and LDH 141 units/L.

Have you crossed a diagnostic threshold for the leading hypothesis, pleural effusion? Have you ruled out the active alternatives? Do other tests need to be done to exclude the alternative diagnoses?

Mr. H has a pleural effusion. Given the size of the effusion on the chest film, a thoracentesis was clearly indicated. The results of the tap are diagnostic. The fluid is an exudate and the low glucose, low pH, high WBC, and positive Gram stain make the diagnosis of an empyema.

It is worth noting that Mr. H's previous diagnosis of musculoskeletal chest pain was incorrect. A chest x-ray done on his previous visit to the emergency department may have made the correct diagnosis and treatment could, potentially, have prevented the development of an empyema. There are many indications for chest films, one is to diagnose a cause for chest pain.

A chest film should be performed in any patient with chest pain and no clear diagnosis.

Alternative Diagnoses: Acute Pericarditis

Textbook Presentation

Acute pericarditis typically presents in young adults, with 1 week of viral symptoms and chest pain that improves when the person leans forward. Physical exam reveals a 3-part friction rub. ECG reveals ST elevations and PR depressions in all leads.

Disease Highlights

A. Pericarditis is the most common cause of pericardial effusions.

B. Although the causes of pericarditis are extremely varied, most (around 80%) are caused by viruses or are considered idiopathic.

1. Idiopathic

2. Viral

   a. Coxsackievirus

   b. Echovirus

   c. Adenovirus

3. Other infections

   a. TB (historically the most common)

   b. HIV and related diseases

4. Post myocardial injury (may be early or late in onset)

   a. Post MI

   b. Postcardiac surgery

5. Rheumatologic (systemic lupus erythematosus and rheumatoid arthritis most common)

6. Drug-induced (procainamide and hydralazine most common)

7. Neoplasm

   a. Malignancy metastatic to the pericardium

   b. Pericarditis can also be caused by exposure of the chest to radiation.

8. Uremia

Evidence-Based Diagnosis

A. The diagnosis of pericarditis is made based on a characteristic history as well as physical exam and ECG findings. Most studies require 2 of the 3 to make a diagnosis.

1. History

   a. Chest pain is almost always present.

   b. The pain is usually pleuritic.

   c. It classically radiates to the trapezius ridge.

   d. Pain improves with sitting and worsens with reclining.

2. Physical exam

   a. The pericardial friction rub is insensitive but nearly 100% specific.

   b. The rub is usually triphasic.

      (1) Triphasic in 58% of cases

(2) Biphasic in 24% of cases

(3) Monophasic in 18% of cases

c. Although the physical exam is insensitive for effusions, it is good for detecting tamponade.

(1) Sensitivity of jugular venous distention to detect tamponade is 100%.

(2) Sensitivity of tachycardia to detect tamponade is 100%.

(3) Pulsus paradoxus > 12

(a) Sensitivity, 98%; specificity, 83%

(b) LR+, 5.9; LR−, 0.03

3. ECG

a. The ECG most commonly shows widespread ST elevations and PR depressions. This finding is highly specific but the sensitivity is only about 60%.

b. The differentiation of pericarditis from acute MI on ECG can be difficult. Some of the key differentiating factors are:

(1) ST elevation in pericarditis is usually diffuse while in MI it is usually localized.

(2) ST elevations in MI are often associated with reciprocal changes.

(3) PR depression is very uncommon in acute MI.

(4) Q waves are not present with pericarditis.

 Pericarditis can mimic MI. The presence of a rub and careful analysis of the ECG should enable their distinction.

4. Other diagnostic tests

a. Echocardiogram

(1) An echocardiogram is always done when pericarditis has been diagnosed to evaluate the presence of a significant pericardial effusion and exclude the presence of tamponade.

(2) About 50% of patients with pericarditis have pericardial effusions.

b. Cardiac enzymes are frequently positive and are therefore not helpful for distinguishing the chest pain for pericarditis from that of cardiac ischemia.

B. Once the diagnosis of pericarditis is made, the cause needs to be determined.

1. Because most patient's pericarditis is either idiopathic or viral, requiring only supportive care, extensive work-up is generally not indicated.

2. After a thorough history, most experts recommend only a few diagnostic tests.

a. Chest x-ray

b. BUN and creatinine

c. PPD

d. Antinuclear antibodies

e. Blood cultures

3. More extensive evaluation is appropriate for patients with refractory or recurrent disease.

a. Even the most invasive diagnostic studies, pericardiocentesis and pericardial biopsy, are generally not helpful. Their diagnostic yield is only about 20%.

b. It should be noted that both tests are more effective in making a diagnosis if done for therapeutic reasons (to relieve tamponade) rather than for diagnostic reasons only.

Treatment

A. Because most patients have viral or idiopathic disease, the treatment of acute pericarditis is supportive.

1. NSAIDs are the treatment of choice, usually providing good pain relief.

2. The addition of colchicine may improve response to therapy.

B. Prednisone is effective in patients with refractory disease but only after excluding the presence of diseases (such as TB) that are potentially exacerbated by corticosteroids.

C. Pericardiocentesis is required in patients with tamponade.

CASE RESOLUTION

Mr. H underwent chest tube drainage of the effusion. Three tubes were placed with thoracoscopic guidance because the effusion was loculated. He was given a third-generation cephalosporin while sensitivities of his presumed pneumococcus were pending. He became afebrile after 2 days of antibiotics and chest tube drainage. The tube output declined over 5 days and the tubes were removed on day 6. Total output was about 3 L.

He was discharged and given oral antibiotics for 6 weeks for treatment of an empyema.

Empyemas are a medical emergency. They are closed space infections that need to be drained in order to cure them and preserve future lung function. As soon as one is detected, steps should be taken to drain it.

Treatment of Pleural Effusion

A. Pleural effusions are treated by treating the underlying disease (eg, pneumonia, uremia, and CHF). Specific treatment of the effusion is called for in certain circumstances.

B. Complicated parapneumonic effusions

1. Evacuation by chest tube drainage prevents pleural scarring and the development of restrictive pleural disease.

2. Indications for chest tube placement are:

a. Purulent fluid or positive Gram stain

b. pH < 7.2

c. LDH > 1000 units/L

d. Glucose < 40 mg/dL

e. Small effusions that are close to the above 3 cutoffs can sometimes be carefully monitored.

C. Malignant pleural effusions

1. Usually managed by treating the underlying disease and periodic therapeutic thoracentesis.

2. If thoracentesis is required frequently and the patient's life expectancy is long, pleurodesis is indicated.

3. Pleurodesis obliterates the pleural space, therefore preventing reaccumulation of fluid.

4. Pleurodesis is usually done with talc.

D. Chylothorax

1. Caused by nontraumatic (primarily lymphoma) or traumatic (usually surgical) disruption of the thoracic duct.

2. In nontraumatic cases, the underlying disease is treated.

3. In both nontraumatic and traumatic disease, the pleural space is evacuated with chest tube drainage.

4. A diet of medium chain fatty acids or a trial of total parenteral nutrition is used to decrease flow through the thoracic duct.

5. Pleurodesis and surgical management reserved for refractory cases.

I have a patient with acute respiratory complaints of cough and congestion. How do I determine the cause?

CHIEF COMPLAINT

PATIENT 1

Ms. L is a 22-year-old woman who comes to your office in August complaining of cough and fever. She reports that she was in her usual state of health until 3 days ago when a cough developed. Two days ago, a low-grade fever (37.2 °C) developed, which increased to 38.8 °C yesterday. She reports that her sputum is yellow and that she has no chest pain or shortness of breath.

CONSTRUCTING A DIFFERENTIAL DIAGNOSIS

The framework for the differential diagnosis of acute respiratory complaints is anatomic and microbiologic. Although there are a myriad of viral and bacterial (and occasional mycobacterial) infections that infect the respiratory tree, a practical approach addresses 3 issues:

1. Where is the infection (sinuses, tracheobronchial tree, alveoli)?
2. Will the patient benefit from antibiotics?
3. Among patients with pneumonia, clinicians must separate the common community-acquired pneumonias (CAPs) from the less common but important pneumonias due to aspiration, tuberculosis (TB), and opportunistic infections.

Differential Diagnosis of Acute Cough and Congestion

A. Common cold
B. Sinusitis
C. Bronchitis
D. Influenza
E. Pneumonia
  1. CAP
  2. Aspiration pneumonia
  3. Severe adult respiratory syndrome (SARS)
  4. TB
  5. Opportunistic (eg, *Pneumocystis* pneumonia [PCP])

On physical exam, Ms. L is in no acute distress. Vital signs are RR, 18 breaths per minute; BP, 110/72 mm Hg; pulse, 92 bpm; temperature, 38.6 °C. Pharynx is unremarkable; lung exam reveals normal breath sounds without crackles, dullness, bronchophony, or egophony.

At this point, what is the leading hypothesis, and what are the active alternatives? What other tests should be ordered?

ORGANIZING THE DIFFERENTIAL DIAGNOSIS

The differential diagnosis for Ms. L includes acute bronchitis, influenza, aspiration pneumonia, SARS, and CAP. Acute bronchitis is usually *not* associated with significant fever (unless caused by influenza). Influenza can cause high fevers and chest symptoms but almost always occurs between December and May. Aspiration pneumonia usually occurs in patients with impaired mentation due to neurologic disease or substance abuse. SARS, an epidemic in 2003, would be a consideration if the endemic or epidemic recurs. Risk factors for SARS include travel to an endemic area or contact with a sick traveler or known case. Finally, although Ms. L's lung exam is normal, the high fever raises the possibility of CAP. The high fever makes this the leading diagnosis. Table 7–1 lists the differential diagnosis.

A high fever should raise the suspicion of pneumonia.

Influenza occurs from December to May; it is highly unlikely at other times.

Ms. L reports drinking only an occasional glass of wine and denies recent intoxication, loss of consciousness, or substance abuse. She reports no travel history and no sick contacts.

Table 7–1. Diagnostic hypotheses for Ms. L.

Diagnostic Hypothesis	Clinical Clues	Important Tests
Leading Hypothesis		
CAP	Cough Shortness of breath High fever Crackles or dullness on lung exam	Chest x-ray Blood culture Sputum Gram stain and culture (occasionally)
Active Alternatives—Most Common		
Acute bronchitis	Cough Absence of high fever Normal lung exam	Chest x-ray (if abnormal lung exam, shortness of breath, or high fever)
Influenza	Sudden onset, high fever Severe myalgias December to May	Diagnosis is usually clinical; direct immuno-fluorescence or ELISA can be used
Aspiration pneumonia	Impaired menta-tion (dementia, prior stroke, sub-stance abuse)	Chest x-ray

Is the clinical information sufficient to make a diagnosis of CAP? If not, what other information do you need?

Leading Hypothesis: CAP

Textbook Presentation

Productive cough and fever are often the presenting symptoms in patients with pneumonia. Symptoms may worsen over days or develop abruptly. Pleuritic chest pain, shortness of breath, chills, and rigors may also de-velop.

Disease Highlights

A. Most common cause of infectious death in the United States

B. Most common identified pathogens

   1. *Streptococcus pneumoniae*

   2. *Mycoplasma pneumoniae*

     a. More common in younger patients

     b. Cannot be distinguished from other pyo-genic infections based on clinical presenta-tion or chest x-ray

   3. *Chlamydia*

   4. Influenza

   5. Polymicrobial infection

   6. *Haemophilus influenzae*

   7. *Legionella*

   8. *Staphylococcus aureus* infection may develop post influenza.

C. 3.4% of pneumonias are associated with underlying malignancy

D. Complications

   1. Respiratory failure

   2. Death

   3. Empyema (See Chapter 6, Chest Pain)

E. Prognosis is good overall.

   1. 8% hospitalization rate

   2. 95% radiographic cure in 1 month

   3. Mortality 1.2%

     a. Any of the following increase the risk of death: older age, dyspnea, confusion, neuro-logic disease, cancer, renal disease, congestive heart failure (CHF), hypotension (systolic

BP < 100 mm Hg), tachypnea, hypothermia, WBC > 10,000 cells/mcL, BUN > 20 mg/dL, multilobar infiltrates on chest film

b. Models have been created and validated that predict risk and need for hospitalization (PORT score; see Figure 7–1)

Evidence-Based Diagnosis

A. Diagnosis is usually clinical, based on constellation of cough, fever, and infiltrate on chest film

B. Prevalence of symptoms in patients with pneumonia

1. Cough, 96%
2. Fever, 81%
3. Chills, 59%
4. Headache, 58%
5. Dyspnea, 46–66%
6. Pleuritic chest pain, 37–50%

 Nineteen percent of patients with pneumonia do not have a history of fever.

C. Physical exam

1. Fever absent ≥ 27%
2. Table 7–2 lists the LRs for physical exam findings for pneumonia.
   a. No single finding is very sensitive. Therefore, the absence of any single finding does not rule out pneumonia.

 A normal lung exam *does not* rule out pneumonia.

   b. Normal vital signs make pneumonia less likely (LR 0.18)
   c. Combination of normal vital signs and normal chest exam make pneumonia highly unlikely.
   d. Egophony and dullness are fairly specific and significantly increase the likelihood of pneumonia when they are present.

 Pneumonia should be considered in the differential diagnosis of elderly patients who have changes in their mental status.

D. Sputum cultures are insensitive and are often unreliable due to contamination by oral flora. Occasionally, the cultures help determine the resistance pattern.

E. Sputum Gram stain

1. Often unreliable (due to poor quality, preparation, and interpretation)
2. Sensitivity, 63–82%; specificity, 63–77%
3. LR+, 1.4–3.5; LR−, 0.9–0.23

F. Pneumococcal urinary antigen

1. Sensitivity for pneumococcal pneumonia, 50–80%
2. Sensitivity in patients with pneumococcal bacteremia, 70–90%
3. Specificity, 90% (false-positives may occur secondary to colonization)

G. WBC > 10,400 cells/mcL: LR+, 3.7; LR−, 0.6

H. Chest film

1. Sensitivity is lower in dehydrated patients.
2. Compared with high-resolution chest CT scan, chest film sensitivity is 69%.

 Because chest x-ray is not completely sensitive for the diagnosis of pneumonia, consider antibiotic therapy in patients with high pretest probability of pneumonia despite normal chest film (ie, crackles and temperature > 38.0 °C).

3. 94% of infiltrates are in the lower and middle regions.

 CAP rarely affects the upper lobes; consider TB or aspiration pneumonia when upper lobe involvement is seen.

I. Blood cultures are positive in 4% of patients.

MAKING A DIAGNOSIS

Ms. L does not have risk factors for aspiration pneumonia or SARS. Influenza is highly unlikely in August. The differential diagnosis is narrowed to CAP and acute bronchitis.

 Have you crossed a diagnostic threshold for the leading hypothesis, CAP? Have you ruled out the active alternatives? Do other tests need to be done to exclude the alternative diagnosis?

Step 1. Is the patient low risk (class I) based on history and physical examination and not a resident of a nursing home?
• Age 50 years or younger, and
• None of the coexisting conditions or physical examination findings listed in step 2

NO   ☐▶   Go to step 2

YES   ☐▶   Outpatient treatment is recommended

Step 2. Calculate risk score for classes II–V

Patient Characteristics	Points Assigned	Patient's Points
Demographic factors		
Age (in years)		
Males	Age	
Females	Age – 10	
Nursing home resident	+10	
Coexisting conditions		
Neoplastic disease	+ 30	
Liver disease	+ 20	
Congestive heart failure	+ 10	
Cerebrovascular disease	+ 10	
Renal disease	+ 10	
Initial physical examination findings		
Altered mental status	+ 20	
Respiratory rate ≥ 30/min	+ 20	
Systolic BP < 90 mm Hg	+ 20	
Temperature < 35° or ≥ 40°C	+ 15	
Pulse ≥ 125 bpm	+ 10	
Initial laboratory findings (score zero if not tested)		
pH < 7.35	+ 30	
BUN > 30 mg/dL	+ 20	
Sodium < 130 mEq/L	+ 20	
Glucose ≥ 250 mg/dL	+ 10	
Hct < 30%	+ 10	
PO_2 < 60 mm Hg or O_2 sat < 90%	+ 10	
Pleural effusion	+ 10	
Total score (sum of patient's points):		

30-Day Mortality Data by Risk Class

Total Score	Risk Class	Recommended Site of Treatment	Mortality Range Observed in Validation Cohorts, %
None (see step 1)	I	Outpatient	0.1
≤ 70	II	Outpatient	0.6
71–90	III	Outpatient	0.9–2.8
91–130	IV	Inpatient	8.2–9.3
> 130	V	Inpatient	27.0–29.2

Figure 7–1. Application of Pneumonia Patient Outcomes Research Team (PORT) severity index to determine initial site of treatment. (Reproduced with permission from *Annals of Internal Medicine.* Metlay JP. Testing strategies in the initial management of patient's with community acquired pneumonia; 2003;138:109–118.)

Table 7–2. Likelihood ratios for selected physical findings in pneumonia.

Finding	LR+	LR−
Fever > 37.8 °C	1.4–4.4	0.8–1.0
Crackles	1.6–2.7	0.6–0.7
Egophony	2.0–8.6	0.8–1.0
Dullness to percussion	2.2–4.3	0.8–0.9

Modified with permission from *Annals of Internal Medicine*. Metlay, JP. Testing strategies in the initial management of patient's with community acquired pneumonia; 2003;138:109–118.

Alternative Diagnosis: Acute Bronchitis

Textbook Presentation

Acute bronchitis presents in the healthy adult primarily as a cough of 1–3 weeks duration. Myalgias and low-grade fevers may be seen. This is distinct from an acute exacerbation of chronic obstructive pulmonary disease (COPD) (See Chapter 23, Wheezing & Stridor).

Disease Highlights

A. Etiology
1. Viruses
   a. Influenza
   b. Parainfluenza
   c. Respiratory syncytial virus
   d. Adenovirus
   e. Rhinovirus
   f. Coronavirus
2. Bacterial
   a. < 10% of cases are caused by bacteria
   b. Organisms include *Bordetella pertussis, Mycoplasma,* and *Chlamydia*
3. Noninfectious
   a. Asthma
   b. Pollution
   c. Tobacco
   d. Cannabis

B. Symptoms
1. Initial phase: Cough and systemic symptoms secondary to infection are seen.
2. Fever may be low grade. Consider pneumonia in patients whose fever is high-grade or persistent.
3. Protracted phase
   a. In 26% of patients, cough persists secondary to bronchial hyperresponsiveness and lasts 2 weeks.
   b. 40–65% of patients without prior pulmonary disease show evidence of reactive airway disease during acute bronchitis.

Evidence-Based Diagnosis

A. Sputum may be clear or discolored. Discoloration arises from WBCs and is *not* indicative of bacterial infection.

> *Purulent* sputum is not an indication for antibiotic therapy in patients with acute bronchitis.

B. Chest film is not routine. Consider in elderly patients and in those with high fever, focal findings on chest exam, COPD, CHF, cancer, or immunocompromised state.

Treatment

A. Antibiotics
1. Antibiotics do not provide major clinical benefit and are *not* recommended in the treatment of acute bronchitis.
2. No trials have studied the efficacy of antibiotics in smokers with acute bronchitis. Subgroup analysis of other trials does not suggest that smokers with acute bronchitis benefit from antibiotic treatment. (This is distinct from acute exacerbations of COPD.)

B. Bronchodilators significantly reduce cough compared with placebo, particularly in patients with bronchial hyperreactivity.

C. Antitussives and mucolytics are useful symptomatic measures.

CASE RESOLUTION

At this point, obtaining a chest x-ray is critical. WBCs and sputum studies are too imprecise, and blood cultures are too insensitive to rule out pneumonia.

A chest film reveals a left lower-lobe infiltrate, confirming the diagnosis of pneumonia.

25–50% of patients with pneumonia do not have crackles on auscultation. Chest film is required when pneumonia is suspected.

WBC is 10,200 cells/mcL with 67% neutrophils and 5% bands. Her SaO_2 is 96% on room air. You elect to send sputum for Gram stain and culture. Antibiotics must be chosen and a decision must be made to admit or discharge Ms. L.

Treatment of CAP

A. Prevention: Indications for polyvalent pneumococcal vaccine follow:

1. Patients older than 65 years
2. Diabetes mellitus
3. Cardiovascular disease
4. Lung disease
5. Liver disease
6. Renal failure or nephrotic syndrome
7. Alcohol abuse
8. Cerebrospinal fluid leak
9. Sickle cell disease
10. Immunosuppression (including HIV)

B. Determine need for hospitalization

1. Prospective validated clinical tools can help determine the need for admission (see Figure 7–1).
2. Absolute indications for admission include hypoxia, confusion, unable to tolerate oral intake, unreliable social situation.

C. Evaluation

1. Chest film is recommended in the evaluation of all patients with CAP.
2. Evaluate oxygenation in all patients with CAP (ABG or SaO_2)
3. An ABG is required in patients with respiratory distress, particularly those with preexistent COPD.

A normal SaO_2 does not exclude respiratory insufficiency, hypercarbia, or respiratory failure. A blood gas to check $PaCO_2$ is required for patients with respiratory distress.

4. Two sets of blood cultures, sputum culture, and Gram stain are recommended for all patients hospitalized for CAP.
5. HIV testing is recommended for all adults aged 15–54 years who have CAP.
6. Consider testing urine for legionella antigen.

D. Antibiotics

1. Treatment must cover atypical (*Mycoplasma* and *Chlamydia*) and pyogenic organisms.
2. Penicillin-resistant *S pneumoniae* (PRSP)

   a. Increasing resistance in United States
   b. Marked geographic variability in frequency of resistance but up to 65% in some areas
   c. PRSP often resistant to cephalosporins and macrolides but not quinolones with extended activity against *S pneumoniae.*

3. Empiric therapy

   a. Outpatients are usually treated with an advanced macrolide (clarithromycin, azithromycin) or a respiratory quinolone (moxifloxacin, gatifloxacin, levofloxacin, or gemifloxacin).
   b. Inpatients should be treated with respiratory quinolone or advanced macrolide with β-lactam (cefotaxime, ceftriaxone, or ampicillin-sulbactam).

Ms. L's blood cultures showed no growth and HIV test is negative. Review of the PORT score (Figure 7–1) reveals that she is in class 1 with a very low risk of mortality with outpatient treatment. She is treated with azithromycin. She is instructed to call immediately if her fever increases or increasing shortness of breath or chest pain develop.

One week later, she reports feeling much better. A follow-up chest film 6 weeks later shows resolution of the pneumonia.

A follow-up chest x-ray is indicated in patients with pneumonia to exclude an underlying obstructing mass.

CHIEF COMPLAINT

PATIENT 2

Mr. P is a 32-year-old African American man with cough and progressive shortness of breath over the last 4 weeks. He complains of a persistent cough productive of purulent sputum and low-grade fever. His past medical history is unremarkable. Social history: Mr. P reports that he is homeless. He admits to drinking 1 pint of gin per day. He reports no history of recreational or injection drug use. He reports that he has rarely used paid sex workers. He has no history of sex with men. He denies using condoms.

On physical exam he appears disheveled and smells of alcohol and urine. Vital signs are pulse, 95 bpm; temperature, 37.0 °C; RR, 20 breaths per minute; BP, 140/90 mm Hg. There is temporal wasting. Lung exam reveals diffuse fine crackles in the lower lung fields bilaterally. Cardiac exam is normal. His chest x-ray demonstrates bilateral lower lobe infiltrates. No cardiomegaly is seen. A CBC is normal. SaO_2 is 88%.

 At this point, what is the leading hypothesis, and what are the active alternatives? What other tests should be ordered?

ORGANIZING THE DIFFERENTIAL DIAGNOSIS

The clinical findings of cough, shortness of breath, crackles on pulmonary exam, and infiltrates on chest film all suggest pneumonia. CAP is possible, although the duration of symptoms is unusually long. Aspiration pneumonia is another possibility. Aspiration pneumonia is more common in patients with a history of substance abuse or neurologic disorders. His alcoholism makes aspiration pneumonia the leading diagnosis. The duration of his complaints and temporal wasting also raise the possibility of more chronic pneumonias caused by TB, fungi, or PCP. TB is more common in alcoholic patients and malnourished patients. Given the public health risks, TB is a must not miss possibility. PCP primarily affects HIV-infected patients. It is important to consider PCP even in patients without a history of *known* HIV infection because PCP can be the first sign of HIV infection. A history of injection drug use or high-risk sex-

ual exposures increases the probability of HIV infection and PCP. The sexual history makes PCP (or another HIV-related pneumonia) an active alternative diagnosis. Finally, uncomplicated influenza does not persist for 4 weeks, although a postinfluenza pneumonia could be considered in the proper season. Table 7–3 lists the differential diagnosis.

Is the clinical information sufficient to make a diagnosis? If not what other information do you need?

Table 7–3. Diagnostic hypotheses for Mr. P.

Diagnostic Hypothesis	Clinical Clues	Important Tests
Leading Hypothesis		
Aspiration pneumonia	Impaired mentation (dementia, prior stroke, substance abuse)	Chest x-ray
Active Alternatives—Most Common		
CAP	Cough Shortness of breath High fever Crackles or dullness on lung exam	Chest x-ray Blood culture Sputum culture and Gram stain (occasionally)
HIV-related pneumonia	Injection drug use, men who have sex with men, engaging in sex with paid sex workers	HIV CD4 count Chest x-ray demonstrating diffuse bilateral infiltrates
Active Alternatives—Must Not Miss		
TB	Long duration of symptoms Risk factors for TB (alcoholism, HIV infection, use of corticosteroids, diabetes mellitus, cancer, foreign-born persons, end-stage renal disease, homeless persons, incarceration)	Chest x-ray shows upper lobe, cavitary, or reticulonodular disease Sputum for acid-fast stain and culture

Leading Hypothesis: Aspiration Pneumonia

Textbook Presentation

Aspiration pneumonia typically develops in patients with impaired mentation (ie, the demented elderly patient or alcoholic). Classic symptoms include fever, cough, chest pain, and putrid sputum. The syndrome most commonly evolves over days to weeks rather than acutely.

Disease Highlights

A. Aspiration of gastric acid may result in chemical damage (aspiration *pneumonitis*) or subsequent infection (aspiration *pneumonia*).

B. Risk factors for aspiration

1. Neurologic disease (dementia, cerebrovascular accident, seizures)

2. Sedation (drug overdose, general anesthesia)

3. Impaired oral pharyngeal clearance (status post [S/P] head and neck surgery)

4. Gastroesophageal reflux disease, vomiting

5. Endoscopy, tracheostomy, bronchostomy, nasogastric feeding

C. Aspiration *pneumonitis*

1. Lower pHs and larger volumes leads to more damage

2. Clinical syndrome

a. Usually follows large volume aspiration (ie, during anesthesia)

b. Cyanosis and shortness of breath develop within 2 hours

c. Fever is usually low grade

d. Outcome varies from rapid recovery within 24–36 hours (62%) to acute respiratory distress syndrome (12%)

3. Complications

a. Bacterial superinfection may complicate aspiration pneumonitis (26%).

b. Acute respiratory distress syndrome

c. Pulmonary fibrosis

d. Death

D. Aspiration *pneumonia* refers to infection due to aspirated organisms.

1. Accounts for 5–15% of pneumonias

2. Poor dentition increases the risk of aspiration pneumonia.

3. Aspiration is usually not witnessed.

4. Clinical features include cough, fever, sputum production, and shortness of breath, which may progress over days to weeks.

5. Organisms

a. Community-acquired aspiration pneumonia may be caused by anaerobes, *S pneumoniae, S aureus,* and *H influenzae.*

b. Nosocomial aspiration pneumonias may be caused by anaerobes, gram-negative organisms (including *Pseudomonas*), and *S aureus.*

Evidence-Based Diagnosis

A. Often presumptive based on aspiration risk factors and typical chest film.

B. Swallowing evaluations can identify patients at risk.

C. Rigors and acute onset suggest more virulent organisms (ie, *S pneumoniae* and *S aureus*)

D. Chest film

1. The classic location of infection is in the basal segment of lower lobes, but it can involve upper lobes if aspiration occurred while the patient was recumbent.

2. Cavitation is more common in aspiration pneumonia than in CAP.

MAKING A DIAGNOSIS

At this point, it is appropriate to order blood cultures, sputum cultures, and Gram stain. The patient's chest x-ray does not have any features that suggest TB (see below), which makes TB less likely. Nonetheless, PPD placement and obtaining sputum for acid-fast bacillus (AFB) stain and culture would be reasonable. Finally, given his sexual history, testing for HIV is mandatory. Although the patient's PORT score is only 42 (32 points for age, 10 for SaO$_2$ < 90%) his hypoxia and lack of a reliable social structure make admission mandatory. Antibiotics that cover both CAP and aspiration pneumonia should be started.

Mr. P is admitted to an isolation bed on the general medical floor. He is empirically treated with clindamycin (for presumed aspiration pneumonia), azithromycin, and ceftriaxone. The PPD test is done and is negative. Blood cultures are negative and sputum cultures reveal normal flora.

 Have you crossed a diagnostic threshold for the leading hypothesis, aspiration pneumonia? Have you ruled out the active alternatives tuberculosis and PCP? Do other tests need to be done to exclude the alternative diagnosis?

Alternative Diagnosis: PCP

Textbook Presentation

Patients with PCP typically have diagnosed or *undiagnosed* advanced HIV disease with CD4 counts < 200 cells/mcL. Patients commonly complain of progressive shortness of breath and dry cough of 1 to 3 week duration.

 PCP is often the presenting manifestation of AIDS. Suspect PCP in patients with diffuse bilateral pneumonia, particularly of subacute onset.

Disease Highlights

A. The exact classification of the organism is unclear.

B. PCP presents as diffuse bilateral pneumonia.

C. PCP is most common cause of acute diffuse lung disease in immunocompromised patients.

D. PCP occurs most commonly in patients with advanced HIV disease and CD4 counts below 200 cells/mcL.

E. PCP may also develop in patients undergoing organ transplantation or chemotherapy and in patients with idiopathic CD4 lymphocytopenia.

Evidence-Based Diagnosis

A. History

   1. Patients may *or may not* already carry diagnosis of HIV or AIDS.

   2. Fever is present in 79–100% of cases.

   3. Cough is present in 95% of cases. It is usually (but not always) nonproductive.

   4. Progressive dyspnea is present in 95% of cases.

B. Physical exam: Chest auscultation is normal in 50% of cases.

C. Chest film

   1. May show diffuse symmetric bilateral alveolar or interstitial infiltrates (81–93% of cases)

   2. Isolated upper lobe disease may be seen in patients taking inhaled pentamidine.

   3. Occasionally shows pneumothorax

   4. Normal in 10–25% of cases

 PCP should be considered in dyspneic patients with HIV and CD4 counts < 200 cells/mcL even when the chest exam and chest x-ray are normal.

D. Lactate dehydrogenase (LDH)

   1. Elevated in 90% of cases; specificity is low.

   2. Helpful, but some patients with PCP have normal LDH levels.

E. High-resolution chest CT scan

   1. Patchy or nodular ground-glass appearance; ground glass most marked in perihilar regions. Cystic lesions may be seen.

   2. 100% sensitive, 83–89% specific

   3. LR+, 5.9; LR−, 0

F. Pulmonary function tests

   1. Carbon monoxide diffusing capacity of the lungs (DLCO) is highly sensitive for PCP.

   2. Likelihood of PCP is < 2% if DLCO is > 75% predicted

G. Some centers have successfully used induced sputums for diagnosis.

   1. 55–92% sensitive, 100% specific.

   2. Sensitivity is lower at centers without expertise in induced sputums.

H. Bronchoalveolar lavage (BAL) is the test of choice.

   1. Diagnosis is based on staining the fluid obtained during BAL.

   2. Silver staining and monoclonal antibodies have been used.

   3. Sensitivity is 86–97%.

   4. Sensitivity of BAL is lower (62%) after inhaled pentamidine prophylaxis.

I. Clinical diagnosis (without BAL) is incorrect in 43% of patients.

Treatment of PCP

A. Antimicrobial therapy

   1. Trimethoprim-sulfamethoxazole (TMP-SMX) is initial treatment of choice.

   2. Therapy may markedly *worsen* preexistent hypoxia. Some patients require concomitant glucocorticoids (see below).

   3. IV pentamidine and TMP-SMX have similar efficacy.

4. Occasional resistance to TMP-SMX has been reported.

5. Both TMP and pentamidine may cause hyperkalemia.

6. Patients with allergic reactions to TMP-SMX may be desensitized.

7. Other options limited to patients with mild to moderate PCP infections include clindamycin plus primaquine, dapsone plus TMP, atovaquone, or trimetrexate plus leukovorin.

B. Glucocorticoids

1. Reduce the mortality and respiratory failure rate in patients with severe PCP treated with TMP-SMX.

2. Initiate at time of PCP therapy if room air PaO_2 < 70 mm Hg

3. Prednisone 40 mg twice daily for 5 days, then 40 mg daily for 5 days, then 20 mg daily for 11 days

Concomitant glucocorticoid therapy is lifesaving for patients with PCP whose PaO_2 is < 70 mm Hg.

C. Prophylaxis

1. Indications

a. Prior PCP

b. CD4 counts < 200 cells/mcL

c. HIV-infected patients with unexplained persistent fevers or oral candidiasis for more than 2 weeks

2. TMP-SMX is superior to pentamidine (and also covers toxoplasmosis).

3. Dapsone and atovaquone have similar efficacy to inhaled pentamidine.

4. Prophylaxis may be safely discontinued when CD4 count rises above 200 cells/mcL (for approximately 3 months).

Alternative Diagnosis: TB

Textbook Presentation

Clinical TB usually develops due to reactivation of latent mycobacteria. Symptoms, including cough, fever, weight loss, and night sweats, are chronic. By the time patients seek medical attention, they may have had these symptoms for weeks or months. The weight loss and duration of symptoms often suggest cancer. Pulmonary TB is the most common manifestation, typically affecting the upper lobes.

Disease Highlights

A. Obligate aerobe has predilection for lung apices.

B. The organism is slow growing; the generation time is 12–18 hours, resulting in slow progression.

C. Common and serious

1. Infects 33% of the world's population

2. 8 million new cases per year and 2 million deaths (worldwide)

D. Epidemiology

1. 7% of US population is PPD positive.

2. 67% of cases occur in the nonwhite population.

3. In the nonwhite population, the median age is 39. In whites, the median age is 62.

4. Reactivation TB accounts for 90% of TB in older patients and 67% of TB in younger patients.

5. High risk groups

a. HIV

(1) HIV-infected patients are at highest risk for TB (200× increased incidence).

(2) TB may be the first manifestation of HIV.

Patients with TB should be tested for HIV.

(3) Extrapulmonary TB without pulmonary disease is more common in patients with AIDS (30%) than in those without AIDS (15%).

(4) In early HIV infection, TB is fairly typical. However, in advanced HIV infection, pulmonary TB is much more often atypical.

b. Alcoholics

c. Other high-risk groups include foreign-born persons; patients taking corticosteroids or immunosuppressives; patients with cancer, diabetes mellitus, end-stage renal disease, transplants, or malnutrition; PPD-positive patients; patients with evidence of prior TB on chest film; economically disadvantaged, inner city residents; nursing home residents; Hispanics; African Americans; drug-dependent persons; homeless persons; prison inmates.

E. Pathophysiology

1. Inhaled organism lands in the middle and lower lobes (due to increased ventilation).

2. Multiplies over next 3 weeks, spreads to hilar nodes and often bloodstream.

3. Organism grows preferentially in areas of high PaO_2 (lung apices, renal cortex, vertebrae).

4. In 90% of patients, the immune system then contains the organism resulting in typical scarring (Ghon complex). However, the chest film can be normal.

5. Above sequence usually asymptomatic.

6. In some patients a few viable organisms remain. This is referred to as **latent TB infection** (LTBI). Latent TB can reactivate later (**reactivation TB**).

7. The PPD is positive 6–8 weeks after the initial infection. These patients are resistant to subsequent *exogenous* infection.

8. Primary TB

   a. In approximately 10% of patients (higher in immunocompromised patients and children), the initial infection is not controlled and causes primary TB.

   b. Primary TB accounts for 23–34% of adult cases.

   c. Chest x-ray shows patchy lower lobe pneumonia.

      (1) Disease is usually unilateral.

      (2) Lymphadenopathy is seen in 10–65% of adults.

      (3) Often occurs in those unable to mount a sensitized macrophage response

      (4) PPD may be negative in these patients.

      (5) Most cases of primary TB resolve spontaneously without treatment.

      (6) Pneumonia progresses without treatment in 15% of patients

   d. Alternatively, primary infection may produce tuberculous empyema.

      (1) Rare

      (2) Pleural fluid characterized by numerous TB organisms

9. Reactivation TB

   a. 3–5% of patients LTBI experience reactivation due to declining immune function

   b. Reactivation TB results in 90% of adult non–AIDS-related TB.

   c. 71% of cases occur in foreign-born patients

   d. Symptoms are usually insidious and include weight loss, night sweats, anorexia, cough, and low- or high-grade fevers.

   e. Reactivation TB progresses unless patient is treated.

10. Tuberculous effusions

   a. Reactivation TB may present as tuberculous effusions

   b. Tuberculous effusions should be distinguished from tuberculous empyema. Tuberculous effusions result from a delayed hypersensitivity reaction to mycobacterial antigens in the pleural space.

   c. Typical features include acute high fever, cough (94%), and pleuritic chest pain (78%)

   d. Chest x-ray shows unilateral effusion in 95% of cases. Parenchymal infiltrate is seen in 50% of cases.

   e. PPD is usually positive (69–93%).

11. Extrapulmonary TB may involve the spine, kidney, pericardium, and CNS.

Evidence-Based Diagnosis

A. History

   1. 50% of patients with TB have fever and night sweats or night sweats alone.

   2. Only 31–62% of patients with TB have fever.

 The lung exam is frequently normal.

   3. Cough may be mild, nonproductive, purulent, or bloody.

   4. Hemoptysis develops in 25% of TB patients. (TB accounts for 5–15% of cases of hemoptysis in the United States.)

   5. 33% of TB cases are diagnosed after admission for an unrelated complaint.

   6. Symptoms and risk factors for disease tend to vary between older patients who often have reactivation TB and younger patients in whom primary TB is more common. Compared with older patients, younger patients have a higher incidence of alcoholism (66% vs 37%). In addition, younger patients more frequently have fever (62% vs 31%), night sweats (48% vs 6%), and hemoptysis (40% vs 17%).

B. PPD

   1. Immune response to 0.1 mL intradermal PPD

   2. Turns positive 4–7 weeks after primary infection

   3. Test results are determined by measuring the maximal diameter of *induration* (not redness).

4. Maximal induration occurs 48–72 hours after injection.

5. *Significant* reaction suggests prior infection, not necessarily active disease. Patients with positive tests who do not have active TB are classified as having LTBI.

6. Sensitivity (for active TB) 70–80%

   a. Primary TB: PPD is often negative

   b. Reactivation TB: PPD is positive in 80% of cases

   c. Tuberculous pleurisy: PPD usually positive

   d. AIDS patients with TB: PPD is positive in 50% of cases

 A negative PPD does *not* rule out active TB.

7. Specificity 98–99%

8. Table 7–4 lists the criteria for a positive reaction.

9. Annual PPD

   a. Useful to determine if patient has recently converted

   b. Recent converters at higher risk for developing active TB

   c. Conversion defined as *increase* in induration of ≥ 10 mm

   d. Therapy is indicated for patients who have recently converted due to high risk of developing active TB.

   e. Indications for annual PPD

      (1) HIV infection

      (2) Health care workers

      (3) Prison workers

      (4) Residents in long-term care facilities

      (5) Medical conditions that carry an increased risk of active TB (diabetes mellitus, corticosteroid therapy, end-stage renal disease, hematologic malignancy, injection drug use, silicosis, malnutrition)

      (6) Homeless persons

Table 7–4. Criteria for a positive PPD test.

Diameter of Induration	Population
≥ 5 mm	Patients with marked impaired immune response or high pretest probability 　HIV infection 　Immunosuppressed patients[a] 　Close contact with person with infectious TB 　Chest x-ray consistent with prior TB[b]
≥ 10 mm	Patients with modest impaired immunity of moderate pretest probability 　Medical condition that carries an increased risk of active TB in patients with latent TB infection[c] 　Foreign-born persons who arrive from high prevalence area within 5 years 　Injection drug abuse 　Homeless persons 　Residents and staff of long-term care facilities (including prisons and nursing homes) 　Health care workers 　Children younger than 4 years 　Recent PPD converters (within 2 year period)
≥ 15 mm	Patients with normal immunity and low pretest probability 　All others[d]

[a]Equivalent to ≥ 15 mg prednisone per day ≥ 1 month.
[b]Chest x-ray findings suggestive of TB include fibrotic opacities occupying more than 2 cm of upper lobe; pleural thickening or isolated granuloma suggestive of TB.
[c]End-stage renal disease, malnutrition (or > 10% loss of ideal body weight), diabetes mellitus, immunosuppressive therapy, lymphoma, leukemia, carcinoma of head and neck, silicosis, gastrectomy, or jejunoileal bypass.
[d]These patients should not be screened.

10. Indications for single PPD test
   a. Clinical suspicion of active TB
   b. Immigrants from high-incidence areas (eg, Africa, Asia, Latin America)
   c. S/P exposure to TB
   d. Fibrotic lung lesion
11. Bacillus Calmette-Guérin (BCG)
   a. Vaccine used in some countries to prevent TB
   b. BCG does *not* usually result in significant PPD reactions in adults (only 8% of BCG recipients have a positive PPD test 15 years later).

 Positive PPD reactions in adult recipients of BCG should be treated without consideration to their BCG status (ie, as though they had *not* received BCG).

12. Booster phenomenon
   a. In patients with latent TB, the PPD may revert to negative many years after exposure.
   b. In such patients, the *initial* PPD may be negative but stimulate immune memory cells such that *subsequent* PPD tests may be positive.
   c. Subsequent positive tests may be *misinterpreted* as recent conversion.
   d. Misinterpretation can be avoided by performing the 2-step skin tests in patients scheduled for annual PPD.
      (1) Patients with initial negative PPD are retested 1 week later.
         (a) Patients in whom the second PPD test is negative are truly negative. Subsequent positive reactions in these patients should be considered recent conversions.
         (b) Patient in whom the second PPD test is positive should be treated as though the first test was positive.
C. Diagnosis of active TB
   1. Chest x-ray and clinical features on admission
      a. Chest films typically demonstrate unilateral or bilateral *apical* disease (OR for TB, 5.0)
      b. Cavitation is seen in 19–50% of cases (OR for TB 3.9). The walls are usually thick and irregular. Air-fluid levels are rare and may indicate anaerobic abscess or superinfection.

   c. Endobronchial spread may result in nodular disease that cluster in the dependent portion of the lung.
   d. Calcification can be seen in active lesions. Demonstrating stability requires comparison of prior films.
   e. 5% of patients with reactivation pulmonary TB have normal chest x-rays.
   f. The chest x-ray in TB usually presents in 1 of 3 patterns: apical disease, cavitary disease, or reticular nodular pattern. Such patterns are *consistent* with TB.
      (1) Sensitivity, 86%; specificity, 83%
      (2) LR+, 5.0; LR−, 0.16
      (3) Negative predictive value 0.2%

 TB should be considered in patients with apical, cavitary, or reticulonodular patterns on chest x-ray. TB is unlikely if none of these features are present.

2. AFB stain and culture
   a. Culture is the gold standard and is specific.
   b. Sensitivity depends on the number of specimens (Table 7–5).
   c. Negative smears decrease the likelihood of contagion even in patients with positive TB cultures; 35% of family members of persons with positive smears are PPD positive compared with 9% of family members when patients are smear negative
   d. Other mycobacteria may lead to false-positive smears.

Table 7–5. Sensitivity of test according to the number of sputum specimens sent to the laboratory.

Number of Specimen	Sensitivity		
	Culture Alone	Sputum Stain Alone	Either
1	79%	58%	81%
2	96%	82%	97%
3	99%	93%	99%

Reprinted with permission from Scott B. Early identification and isolation of inpatients at high risk for tuberculosis. *Arch Intern Med* 1994;154:326–330.

e. Specific nucleic amplification tests of sputum are specific for TB and can help distinguish TB from other mycobacteria.

3. BAL

a. Smears: 38% sensitive, 100% specific

b. Culture or smear: 74% sensitive, 75% specific

c. Comparable to data for a single induced sputum

d. Not routine or superior to induced sputums

e. Use when induced sputums are unavailable.

D. Tuberculous pleurisy with effusion

1. Pleural fluid

a. Exudative effusion

b. Pleural fluid glucose variable

c. Pleural fluid pH always < 7.4

d. WBC 1000–6000 cells/mcL with neutrophilic predominance early and lymphocytic predominance later. Pleural fluid eosinophils > 10% suggests alternative diagnosis (unless prior thoracentesis).

2. Sensitivity of tests for diagnosis of tuberculous pleurisy

a. Pleural fluid culture, 42%

b. Pleural biopsy culture, 64%

c. Pleural biopsy histology (caseating granulomas), 70–80%

d. Histology and pleural tissue culture > 90%

e. Sputum culture, 20–50%

3. Adenosine deaminase: Utility unclear due to different cut points and different isoenzymes.

Treatment of TB

A. Isolation

1. Only 1% of all patients tested for TB are proven to have TB. Consider isolation of hospitalized patients with upper lobe, cavitary, or reticulonodular disease.

2. Highest risk of contagion among household contacts, schoolmates, or other close contacts.

3. Patients with cavitary disease, HIV, or watery sputum have the highest infectivity.

B. Principles of therapy

1. Resistance is a significant problem.

2. Precise drug recommendations evolve due to resistance.

3. Susceptibility testing is critical to ensure an appropriate regimen is used.

4. Premature discontinuation and nonadherence promotes drug resistance and must be avoided. Direct observed therapy (DOT) is an option when adherence is an issue.

5. Effective regimens require at least 2 drugs to which the organism is susceptible.

6. Effective therapy takes many months.

7. Infectious disease consultation is advised.

C. There are many therapeutic options.

1. Initiate therapy (in patients at low risk for multidrug resistant TB) with isoniazid, rifampin, pyrazinamide, and ethambutol.

2. Ethambutol may be discontinued if the organism is fully susceptible.

3. After 2 months, the regimen is simplified (again provided the organism is susceptible) to just isoniazid and rifampin for an additional 4 months.

D. Multidrug resistant TB (MDR-TB)

1. Defined as organisms that are resistant to isoniazid and rifampin

2. Suspect MDR-TB in patients previously treated for TB, in patients who are HIV positive, in close contacts of patients with MDR-TB, and in patients who have not responded to therapy.

3. Therapy should last 18–24 months and requires at least 3 drugs to which the organism is susceptible.

4. DOT should be used for patients with MDR-TB.

5. Surgery is occasionally used for patients with localized disease and persistently positive sputums. Antituberculous therapy is continued.

6. Expert consultation is mandatory.

E. The median duration of fever after the institution of antituberculous drugs was 10 days but ranged from 1 to 109 days. For patients with tuberculous effusion, resorption can take 4 months.

F. Pleural fluid drainage does not improve outcome in patients with tuberculous effusions (nonempyema).

G. Latent TB

1. Definition of positive PPD test depends on the population (see Table 7–4).

2. Prior to treatment for LTBI, active infection must be ruled out with a careful history, physical exam, and chest x-ray.

3. Expert consultation is recommended if exposure to drug-resistant TB is likely.

4. Isoniazid

    a. Drug most commonly used for latent TB

    b. Dose is 300 mg/d for 6–9 months or 900 mg twice a week with DOT in noncompliant patients.

    c. Side effects

        (1) Hepatitis

            (a) Defined as transaminase elevation ≥ 5× normal

            (b) Reported incidence is 0.1–2.3%

            (c) Incidence may be higher in older patients.

            (d) Alcohol may increase the risk. Patients who are taking isoniazid should avoid drinking alcohol.

            (e) Monthly monitoring for *clinical* symptoms of hepatitis is recommended.

            (f) Obtain baseline liver function tests in patients with risk factors for hepatitis.

            (g) Repeat liver function tests in symptomatic patients (right upper quadrant pain, anorexia, or nausea)

        (2) Peripheral neuropathy develops in 2% of patients taking isoniazid and can be prevented with pyridoxine (10–25 mg/d).

5. Rifampin

    a. Alternative to isoniazid for LTBI

    b. Efficacy similar to isoniazid

    c. Preferred medication in patients from Vietnam, Haiti, and Philippines due to isoniazid resistance

    d. Dose 10 mg/kg (max 600 mg) for 4 months

    e. Side effects include hepatitis, rash, thrombocytopenia, fever, orange bodily fluids (urine, tears, sweat, and stool).

    f. Monthly monitoring for *clinical* symptoms of hepatitis is recommended.

    g. Obtain baseline liver function tests in patients with risk factors for hepatitis. Repeat in symptomatic patients.

6. Rifampin and pyrazinamide

    a. Alternate regimen

    b. Duration 2 months

    c. Not routinely recommended due to increased incidence of severe hepatotoxicity

CASE RESOLUTION

Fortunately, Mr. P's HIV result was negative. His PPD and AFB smears were negative. On day 3 of his hospitalization, he became agitated, tachycardic, and complained of visual hallucinations. He was treated for delirium tremens with high doses of IV benzodiazepines. By day 5, he was improving. He was afebrile and his appetite improved. He was given a prescription for oral antibiotics and discharged to an outpatient alcohol treatment center.

 Patients with a history of alcohol abuse must be monitored for withdrawal during any hospitalization.

Treatment of Aspiration Pneumonia

A. Prevention

    1. Soft diets and feeding strategies can reduce subsequent aspiration.

    2. Tube feedings may decrease aspiration from eating. However, gastroesophageal reflux disease, vomiting, and aspiration of saliva may still result in aspiration.

B. Supportive treatment

    1. Suction any material in airway.

    2. Intubation if necessary for ventilation, oxygenation, or to protect airway in patients with altered level of consciousness.

C. Aspiration *pneumonitis*

    1. Antibiotics are recommended if the infiltrates do not resolve within 48 hours or if the patient likely has gastric colonization (H_2 blockers, proton pump inhibitors, bowel obstruction).

    2. Corticosteroids are controversial.

D. Aspiration *pneumonia*

    1. Antibiotics indicated

        a. Community-acquired aspiration

            (1) Clindamycin is drug of choice.

            (2) Other options include amoxicillin/clavulanate, ceftriaxone, cefotaxime, moxifloxacin, gatifloxacin

        b. Nosocomial aspiration: Coverage requires addition of an antibiotic that is effective against gram-negative organisms.

REVIEW OF OTHER IMPORTANT DISEASES

Influenza

Textbook Presentation

Although there is a wide range of severity of influenza symptoms, patients typically complain of a severe, febrile, respiratory illness that began abruptly. Complaints include the abrupt onset ("like being hit by a train"), severe myalgias (even their eyes hurt when they look around), diffuse pain (they may complain that their hair or skin hurts), respiratory symptoms (cough, rhinitis, pharyngitis), and fever that is often pronounced and peaks within 12 hours (occasionally as high as 40–41 °C). Influenza typically occurs between December and May. Patients may have rigors (frankly shaking chills) and headache (Figure 7–2).

 Influenza is an unlikely diagnosis in the late spring, summer, or early fall.

Disease Highlights

A. Pathogenesis

  1. Influenza virus A or B infects respiratory epithelium.

  2. Antigenic change in the virus surface glycoprotein (hemagglutinin or neuraminidase) renders populations susceptible to the virus. Antigenic shifts are most common with influenza virus A and are associated with epidemics. The pandemic of 1918 is believed responsible for 40 million deaths.

B. Manifestations

  1. History

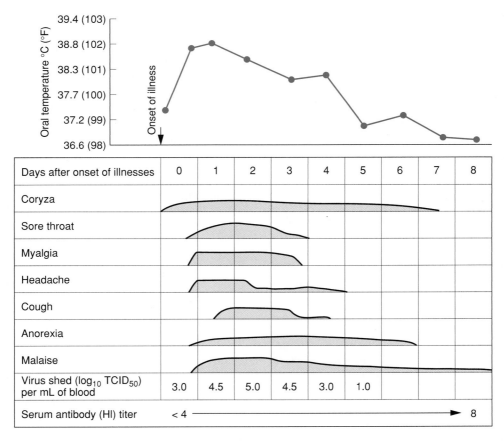

Figure 7–2. The typical clinical course of influenza. (Reproduced with permission from Montalto NJ: An office based approach to influenza: Clinical diagnoses and laboratory testing. *Am Fam Physician* 2003;67:111–118. Copyright © 2003. American Academy of Family Physicians.)

a. Onset is sudden in 75% of cases.

b. Fever present in 51% of cases.

    (1) Peaks within 12–24 hours of onset of illness

    (2) Typically spikes between 38.0 °C and 40.0 °C. May reach 41.0 °C.

    (3) Typical duration is 3 days but may last 1–5 days.

High fever within 12–24 hours of symptom onset is typical of influenza but not other viral respiratory pathogens.

Fever that *increases* over several days is *not* characteristic of influenza.

c. Prevalence of other symptoms in influenza

    (1) Headache, 58%

    (2) Cough, 48%

    (3) Sore throat, 46%

    (4) GI symptoms are not characteristic of influenza.

Patients with significant diarrhea or vomiting should be evaluated for an alternative diagnosis.

d. Symptoms help distinguish influenza from acute bronchitis or pneumonia (Table 7–6).

2. Crackles seen in < 25% of patients.

C. Complications

  1. Pneumonia

a. High-risk groups for pneumonia and death include

    (1) Elderly. Mortality rates are 100× greater in patients over age 65 than in patients aged 15–44 years

    (2) Patients with CHF, COPD

    (3) Immunocompromised patients

    (4) Patients with renal disease, diabetes mellitus, or hemoglobinopathies

    (5) Pregnant women

b. Two types of pneumonia are seen in influenza patients.

    (1) Influenza pneumonia *per se.*

    (2) *Post*-influenza bacterial pneumonia

c. Influenza pneumonia

    (1) Often develops within 1 day of influenza and represents direct progression of disease.

    (2) Most frequent in patients with underlying cardiopulmonary disease, diabetes, immunodeficiency states, and pregnancy.

    (3) Patients with influenza pneumonia complain of shortness of breath more often than patients with uncomplicated influenza (82% vs 17%)

Obtain a chest film in patients with influenza and shortness of breath to rule out pneumonia.

    (4) Associated with tachycardia, tachypnea, cyanosis, and crackles on pulmonary exam

    (5) Hypoxemia and leukocytosis may be seen

Table 7–6. A comparison of features in influenza, community-acquired pneumonia, and acute bronchitis.

Infection	High Fever[a]	Localized Lung Findings[b]	Shortness of Breath[c]	Season
Community-acquired pneumonia	Common	Common	Variable	Anytime
Influenza	Common	Uncommon	Uncommon	December–May
Acute bronchitis	Uncommon	Uncommon	Uncommon	Anytime

[a]Indication for chest film (unless flu season *and* patient has normal lung exam).
[b]Findings include crackles, dullness, bronchophony, or egophony. All such findings are indications for chest film.
[c]Indication for chest film.

(6) Chest film shows bilateral or lobar pulmonary infiltrates.

(7) 29% mortality

(8) Treatment: Antiviral therapy, empiric antibacterial agents pending culture, oxygen, intubation, and positive end-expiratory pressure as necessary. Antibiotics should cover methicillin-resistant *S aureus* in endemic regions

d. Postinfluenza (secondary) bacterial pneumonia

(1) Suspect when initial improvement is following by worsening cough, purulent sputum, and increasing fever.

(2) Among patients hospitalized for influenza pneumonia, 30% have concomitant bacterial pneumonia caused by *S aureus* or *S pneumoniae*

(3) Chest film may show either bilateral or lobar infiltrates.

(4) *S pneumoniae* is most common (29–48%)

(5) *S aureus* is next most common (7–40%), highly destructive and associated with significant incidence of empyema and death.

(6) *Haemophilus* and *Moraxella* may also cause secondary pneumonia.

2. Exacerbation of asthma or COPD

3. Less common complications include CHF, myositis, meningo-encephalitis, Guillain-Barré syndrome

Evidence-Based Diagnosis

A. History

1. Current prevalence of influenza helps determine risk

a. www.cdc.gov/flu/weekly/fluactivity.htm

b. 888/232-3228

2. Cough and fever (during influenza season)

a. Sensitivity, 63–78%; specificity, 55–71%

b. LR+, 1.9; LR–, 0.5

c. Posttest probability, 79% (80–85% if temperature ≥ 39.0 °C)

B. Laboratory results

1. Confirmation is usually not required.

2. During influenza outbreaks, empiric therapy is appropriate.

3. Rapid testing is most appropriate in *non*influenza periods.

4. Confirming influenza may help exclude SARS from consideration.

5. Various methods available. For rapid diagnosis, enzyme linked immunosorbent assay (ELISA) is test of choice.

6. Institutionalized patients are at higher risk for respiratory syncytial virus, which can mimic influenza. Testing may be useful in such patients.

Treatment

A. Prevention

1. Options include vaccination or chemoprophylaxis with neuraminidase inhibitors.

2. Trivalent inactivated influenza vaccine (TIIV)

a. Prophylactic strategy of choice

b. IM vaccine uses inactivated viruses that are currently prevalent.

c. 50% fewer cases of influenza, associated pneumonia, and hospitalizations.

d. 68% decrease in all cause mortality

e. Contraindications

(1) Egg allergy

(2) First trimester of pregnancy

(3) Significant febrile illness (Patients may be vaccinated during mild nonfebrile upper respiratory tract infections)

(4) History of Guillain-Barré syndrome following prior vaccination

f. Adverse effects

(1) Soreness at injection site occurs in 25% of patients

(2) Low grade fever and myalgias occur in < 5% of patients

(3) Guillain-Barré may increase by 1 case per million recipients.

(4) Upper respiratory tract infection symptoms are *not* more common than placebo.

(5) TIIV cannot *cause* influenza.

g. Indications (adults)

(1) Patients older than 50 years

(2) Residents of long-term care facilities

(3) Cardiopulmonary disease (including asthma)

(4) Diabetes

      (5) Renal disease

      (6) Hemoglobinopathy

      (7) HIV

      (8) Women who will be in the second or third trimester of pregnancy during flu season

      (9) Health care personnel

      (10) Employees or household members having contact with high-risk groups

      (11) Any individual wishing to reduce their chance of influenza

3. Live-attenuated intranasal vaccine

    a. Uses live-attenuated strains that replicate poorly in the warmer lower respiratory tract

    b. Effective in children but may increase the risk of asthma in children 18–35 months of age

    c. Approved for children 5- to 17-years-old and adults 18- to 49-years-old

    d. Still under study in older adults

4. Chemoprophylaxis

    a. Significantly more costly than vaccination

    b. Amantadine and rimantadine prevent influenza virus A but not influenza virus B.

    c. Oseltamivir also is approved as chemoprophylaxis; it is active against influenza viruses A and B.

    d. Indications for chemoprophylaxis: Persons at high risk, vaccinated after influenza exposure (treat for 2 weeks after vaccination)

B. Treatment of influenza

    1. Amantadine and rimantadine are active against influenza virus A but not influenza virus B.

      a. Amantadine

        (1) Renal excretion; decrease dose in patients with renal insufficiency.

        (2) Avoid giving to women who are nursing

        (3) Adverse effects include confusion, anxiety, jitteriness, and insomnia.

      b. Rimantadine

        (1) 10× more active than amantadine

        (2) Less CNS side effects than amantadine

        (3) Avoid giving to women who are nursing

    2. Neuraminidase inhibitors zanamivir and oseltamivir are effective against influenza viruses A and B.

      a. When given within 48 hours of symptom onset, neuraminidase inhibitors reduce the symptom severity over the course of the illness and the duration of symptoms approximately 1–2 days.

      b. Safety during pregnancy is unknown.

      c. Neuraminidase inhibitors should not be started > 48 hours after symptom onset.

    3. Oseltamivir

      a. Route of administration is oral. Taking the drug with food decreases nausea and vomiting, which occurs in 10% of patients.

      b. Reduce the dose if creatinine clearance < 30 mL.

      c. Studies suggest empiric therapy with oseltamivir is cost effective for several groups.

      d. Rapid influenza testing is recommended if the prevalence of influenza is low.

    4. Zanamivir

      a. Route of administration is inhalation; can cause bronchospasm.

      b. Not recommended in patients with asthma or COPD.

      c. Studies suggest that empiric therapy with zanamivir is cost effective for several groups.

      d. Rapid influenza testing is recommended if prevalence of influenza is low.

    5. Indications for treatment

      a. All people at high risk for complications in whom influenza develops, regardless of their vaccination status

      b. Persons with severe influenza

      c. Consider for persons with influenza who wish to shorten the duration of illness.

Diagnostic Approach: Acute Respiratory Infections[a]

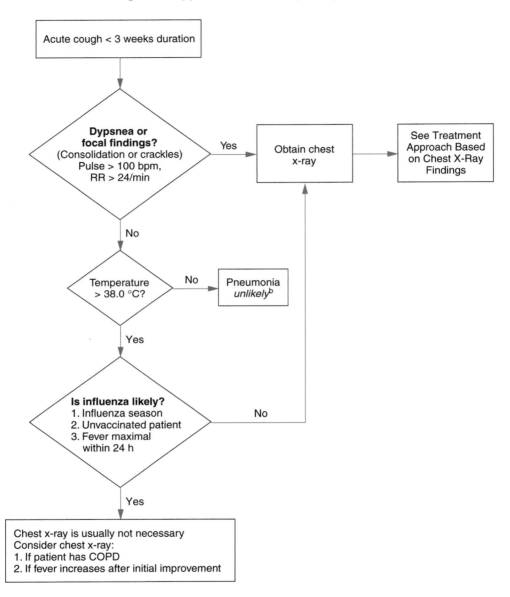

[a]In HIV-negative patients
[b]Certain clinical characteristics make pneumonia more difficult to clinically detect. Consider chest x-ray in the elderly or in patients with CHF, COPD, or immunosuppression.
COPD, chronic obstructive pulmonary disease; CHF, congestive heart failure.

Treatment Approach Based on Chest X-Ray Findings

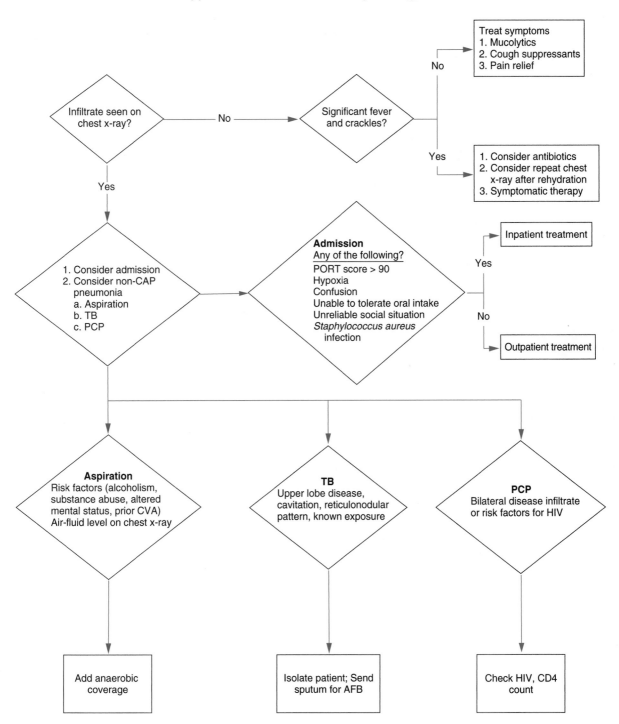

CAP, community-acquired pneumonia; TB, tuberculosis; PCP, *Pneumocystis* pneumonia; CVA, cerebrovascular accident; AFB, acid-fast bacilli.

I have a patient with delirium or dementia. How do I determine the cause?

CHIEF COMPLAINT

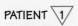

PATIENT 1

Mr. B is a previously healthy 70-year-old man who underwent elective right upper lobectomy for localized squamous cell lung cancer 5 days ago. On morning rounds, he comments that he is in a military barracks and that he is ready to go home.

What is the differential diagnosis of delirium and dementia? How would you frame the differential?

CONSTRUCTING A DIFFERENTIAL DIAGNOSIS

Delirium and dementia are both syndromes of neurologic dysfunction. Both present as a "change in mental status." Their similarities end here. Whereas delirium is acute and sometimes reversible, dementia is chronic and seldom reversible. The definitions of these syndromes, as included in the DSM-IV follow:

A. Delirium
  1. Reduced level of consciousness and difficulty focusing, shifting, or sustaining attention.
  2. Cognitive change (deficit of language, memory, orientation, perception) that a dementia cannot better explain.
  3. Symptoms develop rapidly (hours to days) and tend to vary during the day.
  4. History, physical exam, or laboratory data suggest that a general medical condition has directly caused the condition.

B. Dementia
  1. Impaired memory: Inability to learn new information or recall previously learned information plus 1 of the following:
     a. Aphasia (inability to produce or comprehend language)
     b. Apraxia (inability to execute purposeful movements)
     c. Agnosia (inability to recognize objects by feel)
     d. Impaired executive functioning (eg, abstracting and organizing)
  2. Symptoms must also impair work, social, or personal functioning.

Because any illness can cause delirium in a susceptible patient (primarily those of advanced age or with underlying neurologic disease), the differential diagnosis of delirium is nearly infinite. The differential diagnosis of dementia, although long, is finite and disorders have been listed in order of their approximate prevalence as etiologic factors.

A. Delirium
  1. Metabolic
     a. Dehydration
     b. Electrolyte abnormalities
     c. Hyperglycemia or hypoglycemia
     d. Acidosis or alkalosis
     e. Liver disease
     f. Hypoxia or hypercarbia
     g. Thyroid disease
     h. Azotemia
  2. Infectious disease
     a. CNS infection
     b. Systemic infection of any kind

3. Cerebrovascular event
   a. Ischemic stroke
   b. Hemorrhagic stroke
   c. Vasculitis
4. CNS mass
   a. Tumor
   b. Subdural hematoma
5. Cardiovascular
   a. Myocardial infarction
   b. Congestive heart failure
   c. Arrhythmia
6. Drugs
   a. Alcohol withdrawal
      (1) Delirium tremens
      (2) Wernicke encephalopathy
   b. Diuretics
   c. Anticholinergics
      (1) Antihistamines (H_1 or H_2)
      (2) Antipsychotics
   d. Nonsteroidal anti-inflammatory drugs
   e. Corticosteroids
   f. Digoxin
   g. Narcotics
   h. Antidepressants
   i. Anxiolytics
7. Miscellaneous
   a. Fecal impaction
   b. Urinary retention
   c. Sensory deprivation
   d. Severe illness

B. Dementia
   1. Alzheimer dementia
   2. Dementia with Lewy bodies
   3. Multi-infarct dementia
   4. Frontotemporal dementia
   5. Alcohol-related
   6. Uncommon dementias
      a. Subdural hematoma
      b. Hypothyroid
      c. Vitamin B_{12} deficient
      d. Infectious
         (1) Syphilis
         (2) Prion disease
      e. Normal-pressure hydrocephalus

 Almost any illness can cause delirium in a susceptible patient.

 Mr. B was previously healthy with only mild chronic obstructive pulmonary disease. His surgery went well but was complicated by transient hypotension and excessive blood loss. He was extubated on postoperative day 3. On postoperative day 4, his wife noted some confusion. The medical team did not detect any abnormalities when they evaluated him.

Today, postoperative day 5, he is more confused. Besides his disorientation to place, evaluation revealed he is disoriented to time as well. He is unable to answer any minimally complicated questions.

 At this point, what is the leading hypothesis, and what are the active alternatives? What other tests should be ordered?

ORGANIZING THE DIFFERENTIAL DIAGNOSIS

Based on his history, Mr. B's subacute mental status change appears to fulfill the definition of delirium. His symptoms seem to vary with time of day; he is disoriented and possibly inattentive. He certainly has many potential causes of delirium. Although Mr. B does not have a history of alcohol abuse, alcohol withdrawal is always a possible diagnosis for acute mental status changes in the hospital and should not be missed. Stroke and seizure, although commonly considered in the differential diagnosis of mental status change, are rare causes of delirium. Table 8–1 lists the differential diagnosis.

 On physical exam, Mr. B is lying in bed. He is irritable and somewhat hypervigilant, becoming frustrated during questioning. His vital signs are temperature, 37.0 °C; BP, 146/90 mm Hg; pulse, 80 bpm; RR, 18 breaths per minute. General physical exam reveals a healing surgical

(continued)

Table 8–1. Diagnostic hypotheses for Mr. B.

Diagnostic Hypotheses	Clinical Clues	Important Tests
Leading Hypothesis		
Delirium caused by postsurgical state, fluid and electrolyte abnormalities, hypoxia or hypercarbia	Subacute onset and fluctuating course	Confusion Assessment Method Basic metabolic panel ABG Urinalysis Review of medications
Active Alternative—Must Not Miss		
Alcohol withdrawal	History of alcohol use Predictable syndrome with systemic and neurologic symptoms	Improvement with benzodiazepines
Other Alternative		
Delirium caused by stroke, seizure, or meningitis	Focal neurologic exam Seizure activity Fever or meningismus	CNS imaging EEG Lumbar puncture

scar, normal lung, heart, and abdominal exam. On neurologic exam, he scores a 14 on a Mini-Mental Status Exam (MMSE) based on poor orientation, inability to do serial sevens, and inability to recall items. The rest of the neurologic exam is nonfocal.

Initial laboratory data including basic metabolic panel, liver function tests (LFTs), and urinalysis are normal.

 Is the clinical information sufficient to make a diagnosis? If not, what other information do you need?

Leading Hypothesis: Delirium

Textbook Presentation

Delirium commonly manifests as confusion (often referred to as mental status change). It is usually seen in older patients with severe illness. Clouding of consciousness has classically been used to describe a patient's symptoms.

Disease Highlights

A. Almost any illness can present as delirium in a susceptible patient.

B. Delirium often complicates medical or surgical hospitalizations.

C. The most important clue to delirium is the acuity of onset and fluctuation in course.

D. It is most common in the elderly and in patients with underlying neurologic disease.

 There is always a cause of delirium. Clinicians must recognize delirium and then identify the cause.

E. Several diseases are more likely to cause delirium than others.

1. Fluid and electrolyte disturbances (hyponatremia and azotemia)

2. Infections

3. Drug toxicity

4. Severe illness

5. Hypothermia or hyperthermia

F. Delirium is very common in sick patients over the age of 65.

1. 10% of emergency department patients

2. 12–25% of medical patients

3. 20–50% of surgical patients (highest in patients after hip replacement)

 Assume that a sick, elderly patient with a deterioration in mental status is delirious until proved otherwise.

G. The prognosis of delirium is poor.

1. Although there are generally no mortality differences when patients with delirium are compared with matched controls, patients in whom delirium develops will have worse functional status and less independence at discharge.

2. Patients with dementia and delirium have the worst prognosis.

3. Delirium is also very persistent. Many studies show that less than 10% of patients will recover by the end of the hospitalization and up to 50% will have persistent symptoms 1 year later.

 Only in the minority of patients will delirium resolve completely with cure of the underlying disease or returning home.

Evidence-Based Diagnosis

A. Pretest probability

1. Predictors of delirium have been identified in various studies. These help provide pretest probabilities.

2. Predictors identified in a study that outlined a model to stratify patients by their risk of developing delirium while in the hospital include:

   a. Vision impairment

   b. Severe illness

   c. Cognitive impairment

   d. High BUN/creatinine ratio

3. In a patient population with a mean age of 78, a patient with

   a. No risk factors had a 3% chance of becoming delirious.

   b. 1 or 2 risk factors had a 14% chance of becoming delirious.

   c. 3 or 4 risk factors had a 26% chance of becoming delirious.

4. Several predictors from another study, with odds ratios for association with delirium, are listed in Table 8–2.

 Consider a patient's risk for delirium upon hospital admission; a priori identification both lessens the likelihood of delirium occurring and promotes a more appropriate response if it does.

B. Diagnosis

1. Doctors are generally not very good at recognizing delirium.

Table 8–2. Predictors for delirium.

Predictor	Odds Ratio
Abnormal sodium level	6.2
Severe illness	5.9
Chronic cognitive impairment	5.3
Hypothermia or hyperthermia	5.0
Moderate illness	4.0
Psychoactive drug use	3.9
Azotemia	2.9

Modified from Francis J, Martin D, Kapoor WN. A prospective study of delirium in hospitalized elderly. *JAMA*. 1990;263: 1097–1101. Copyright © 1990, American Medical Association. All rights reserved.

2. A routine exam is very specific but not very sensitive for the diagnosis of delirium.

3. The confusion assessment method (CAM) is one of the best-validated and most widely used tools for diagnosing delirium. A patient with a positive CAM fulfills points a and b and either c or d:

   a. Acute onset and fluctuating course

      (1) Is there evidence of an acute change in mental status from the patient's baseline?

      (2) Does the behavior fluctuate during the day?

   b. Inattention: Does the patient have difficulty focusing his or her attention (eg, is the patient easily distracted or have trouble following the conversation)?

   c. Disorganized thinking: Is the patient's thinking disorganized or incoherent (such as rambling or irrelevant conversation, unclear or illogical flow of ideas, or unpredictable switching from subject to subject)?

   d. Altered level of consciousness: Anything other than alert (vigilant, lethargic, stupor)

 When using the CAM, make use of information from family members and medical staff; do not rely on a single mental status exam.

4. Table 8–3 compares the test characteristics of the CAM with those from a routine evaluation in the emergency department.

Table 8–3. Test characteristics for the CAM and emergency department evaluation in the diagnosis of delirium.

Criteria	Sensitivity	Specificity	LR+	LR−
Evaluation in emergency department	17–35	98–100	8.5–∞	0.65–0.85
CAM	94–100	90–95	9.4–20	0.00–0.07

CAM, Confusion Assessment Method.

C. Etiology

1. Common causes

   a. The search for a cause of delirium involves a review of the processes that most commonly cause delirium in hospitalized patients.

   b. Repeat a full physical exam, focusing on sources of infection (pneumonia, decubitus ulcers).

   c. Review medications in detail.

   d. Always order basic laboratory tests, such as a CBC, basic metabolic panel, LFTs, and urinalysis.

   e. Always check ECG, chest x-ray, ABG, and blood and urine cultures.

 Medication toxicity, even at therapeutic doses, is a common cause of delirium and is particularly common in elderly patients. Review all medications, especially psychoactive ones.

2. Uncommon causes

   a. Common questions when evaluating a patient with delirium are: How extensive should the evaluation be? If the initial work-up outlined above is negative, when is it reasonable to assume the delirium is related to the acute illness and when is further assessment for diseases that directly affect the CNS—stroke, seizure, and meningitis or encephalitis—necessary?

   (1) Stroke

      (a) Very rare cause of delirium

      (b) Best study has only about 7% of cases of delirium caused by stroke.

      (c) 97% of these patients had focal abnormalities on a good neurologic exam.

   (2) Seizure

      (a) Nonconvulsive seizures such as temporal lobe epilepsy are usually recognized by their intermittent nature.

      (b) Nonconvulsive status epilepticus is very rare but could cause mental status consistent with severe delirium. Patients with nonconvulsive status epilepticus almost always have risk factors for seizures or abnormal eye movements, defined as eye jerking, hippus (unprovoked changes in pupil size), repeated blinking, and persistent eye deviation.

   (3) Meningitis: Fever and mental status change may be the only presenting symptoms.

   b. In the work-up of delirium, consider neuroimaging, electroencephalogram (EEG), and lumbar puncture only in certain conditions.

   (1) **Neuroimaging** is only necessary if delirium is associated with a focal neurologic exam or if there is a very high suspicion of a cerebrovascular event.

   (2) **EEG** is only necessary if there is no other explanation for delirium and the patient has either risk factors for seizure or abnormal eye movements.

   (3) **Lumbar puncture** is only necessary if there is fever with no other source or a suspicion for a CNS infection.

MAKING A DIAGNOSIS

Review of Mr. B's medication list revealed that 0.5 mg doses of lorazepam ordered to be given as needed, were being given every 8 hours. Laboratory data was normal with the exception of an ABG: 7.36/46/70.

Have you crossed a diagnostic threshold for the leading hypothesis, delirium? Have you ruled out the active alternatives? Do other tests need to be done to exclude the alternative diagnoses?

Considering the CAM, Mr. B is clearly delirious. The onset of his symptoms were acute and his mental status is fluctuating. He displays inattention on his MMSE. His level of consciousness is described as hypervigilant. He has recently undergone a major surgery, he is taking medications known to cause delirium, and he is found to be hypoxic. Despite his intraoperative blood loss and hypotension there are no signs of cerebrovascular accident and no anemia.

Alternative Diagnosis: Alcohol Withdrawal

Textbook Presentation

A typical presentation of alcohol withdrawal in the medical setting is in a hospitalized patient who no longer has access to alcohol. Agitation with hypertension and tachycardia often develop during the first 2 days after admission. Seizures may soon follow with delusions and delirium occurring during the first 3–5 days.

Disease Highlights

A. Symptoms of alcohol withdrawal are stereotypical, occurring on a predictable time line as outlined in Figure 8–1.

B. The predominant symptoms of minor withdrawal are irritability, hypertension, and tachycardia.

C. Alcoholic hallucinosis is a syndrome of hallucinations, usually visual, with a clear sensorium that makes this easily distinguishable from delirium.

D. Major withdrawal is synonymous with delirium tremens.

1. Occurs in older patients with history of severe alcohol abuse.

2. Confusion, disorientation, and autonomic hyperactivity are the hallmarks of this disorder.

3. Delirium tremens can be fatal if the patient does not receive appropriate supportive care.

E. Wernicke encephalopathy

1. Caused by administration of glucose to a person with thiamine deficiency.

2. Alcohol abuse is the most common cause of thiamine deficiency.

3. Symptoms include the triad of confusion, disorders of ocular movement, and ataxia. The confusion manifests predominantly as disorientation and indifference.

4. Korsakoff syndrome is the chronic form of Wernicke encephalopathy. Korsakoff syndrome presents with memory problems and resulting confabulation and develops when Wernicke encephalopathy is not recognized.

Evidence-Based Diagnosis

A. Delirium tremens and Wernicke encephalopathy are the alcohol withdrawal syndromes most likely to be confused with nonalcohol-related delirium. Various features clearly differentiate these syndromes.

B. Wernicke encephalopathy

1. Generally requires long-term alcohol use. (Rare cases of Wernicke encephalopathy with hyperemesis gravidarum or after bariatric surgery do occur.)

2. Eye findings or ataxia are usually present.

3. Fluctuation that characterizes nonalcohol-related delirium is absent.

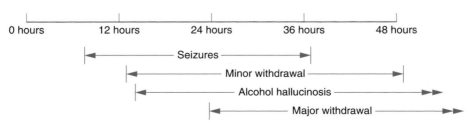

Figure 8–1. Symptoms of alcohol withdrawal. (Reproduced with permission from the Virtual Naval Hospital web site. http://www.vnh.org/EmergPsychHB/WDSyndrome.gif)

C. Delirium tremens
1. Always follows minor withdrawal.
2. Minor withdrawal is sometimes overlooked in the hospital if a patient is critically ill, sedated, or anesthetized.
3. History of heavy alcohol use required.
4. Adrenergic overactivity always present unless masked by medications.
    a. Hypertension
    b. Tachycardia
    c. Fever

D. The diagnoses of delirium tremens and Wernicke encephalopathy are clinical. They are based on suggestive clinical signs in the setting of a history of alcohol use. An appropriate response to treatment is helpful. There are specific MRI findings that are seen in Wernicke encephalopathy.

 Because of the frequency and potential dangers of alcohol withdrawal in hospitalized patients, every patient should have an alcohol history taken on admission.

 If a clinical syndrome suggestive of alcohol withdrawal occurs in a patient who denied alcohol use, information about alcohol use should be sought from other sources.

Treatment

A. Both Wernicke encephalopathy and delirium tremens are preventable.
B. Wernicke encephalopathy
1. Any patient in whom thiamine deficiency is suspected should receive 100 mg of IV thiamine prior to receiving glucose-containing fluids.
2. Patients suspected of having Wernicke encephalopathy should receive thiamine until symptoms resolve.
C. Alcohol withdrawal and delirium tremens
1. Supportive care
2. Benzodiazepines
    a. Benzodiazepines decrease the symptoms of withdrawal and can prevent delirium tremens, seizures, and death.
    b. Outpatient benzodiazepines can be used in some patients.

c. Indications for inpatient therapy
    (1) Moderate to severe withdrawal
    (2) Prior history of seizures or delirium tremens
    (3) Patient unable to cooperate with outpatient therapy
    (4) Comorbid psychiatric or medical conditions
    (5) Unsuccessful outpatient detoxification
d. Inpatient management
    (1) The optimal dose of benzodiazepines cannot be determined in advance and must be titrated to the particular needs of the patient.
    (2) Dosing options include fixed-scheduled and symptom-triggered therapy. Both strategies require careful patient monitoring and medication adjustment.
    (3) The Addiction Research Foundation Clinical Institute Withdrawal Assessment for Alcohol (CIWA-Ar) has developed a tool that predicts the level of withdrawal better than just BP or pulse.
        (a) The tool scores the severity of symptoms in various categories such as tremor, anxiety, and sensory disturbances.
        (b) A higher score (> 8–12) generally calls for active pharmacologic management, whether using a fixed-dose or symptom-triggered protocol.
        (c) An easily printable version of the tool is available at http://addiction-medicine.org/files/15doc.html
    (4) Fixed-schedule therapy
        (a) Delivers regular fixed doses of benzodiazepines to the patients.
        (b) Careful monitoring still required to avoid undertreatment or oversedation.
        (c) Fixed-schedule therapy may provide a slight margin of safety if careful monitoring cannot be performed adequately.
    (5) Symptom-triggered therapy
        (a) Avoids unnecessary medications in the group of patients who will not need them.
        (b) Careful monitoring is required to avoid withdrawal and delirium tremens.

Careful monitoring and prompt patient-specific adjustment of the benzodiazepine dose is the key to successful management of the alcoholic patient.

3. β-Blockers

   a. β-Blockers can decrease sympathetic overactivity in patients during withdrawal.

   b. β-Blockers can serve as useful adjuncts but can mask sympathetic signs that alert the clinician to increasingly severe withdrawal and thereby lead to inadequate use of benzodiazepines.

CASE RESOLUTION

On the afternoon of the fifth postoperative day, Mr. B pulled out his IV and attempted to climb out of bed while his chest tube was still attached. Around the clock observation was ordered.

Further history revealed no history of alcohol use. Mr. B was placed on oxygen with near normalization of his blood gas. The benzodiazepines were discontinued.

By postoperative day 8 (3 days after the onset of his delirium) Mr. B's mental status had returned nearly to baseline. He was still occasionally disoriented to time.

He was discharged on postoperative day 14. His wife noted him to still be occasionally "spacey" at the time of discharge. The patient was completely back to normal at a postoperative visit 14 days later.

The patient's delirium was severe for 3–4 days and persisted for at least 1 week. The delirium was assumed to be a symptom of hypoxia, the postsurgical state, and medication complication. No specific therapy was given. The patient's safety was ensured with a "sitter"

and the reversible factors (hypoxia, medication dosing mistakes) were addressed.

Treatment of Delirium

A. Prevention

  1. Because of the poor prognosis of delirium, prevention is the goal.

  2. Multidisciplinary intervention helped prevent delirium in a recent study; the rate of delirium decreased from 15% to 9.9% (number needed to treat ≅ 20).

  3. The intervention addressed the risk factors in the following ways:

    a. Cognitive impairment: Repeated orientation of the patient and performance of cognitively stimulating activity (eg, discussion of current events).

    b. Sleep deprivation: Noise reduction and minimizing of nighttime activities.

    c. Immobility: Early mobilization.

    d. Visual and hearing impairment: Visual and hearing aids as well as adaptive devices.

    e. Dehydration: Aggressive volume repletion.

B. Treatment

  1. Once delirium occurs, the causes must be addressed and then supportive measures must be instituted.

    a. Administer fluids to prevent dehydration.

    b. Avoid sleep deprivation.

    c. Provide quiet environment.

    d. Keep nighttime awakenings to a minimum.

    e. Protect from falls or self-inflicted injury.

      (1) "Sitters" fare better than restraints

      (2) Sitters can also provide constant reorientation and reassurance.

      (3) Occasionally, medications such as low doses of neuroleptics (haloperidol, risperidone) and low doses of benzodiazepines are necessary for safety.

CHIEF COMPLAINT

PATIENT 2

Mr. R is a 75-year-old man who comes to see you in clinic accompanied by his wife because

she is concerned that his memory is getting worse. She states that, for the last few months, he has been getting lost driving 20 miles from his home to his local VA hospital

(continued)

where he volunteers. He has done this job twice weekly for 25 years.

At this point, what is the leading hypothesis and what are the active alternatives? What other tests should be ordered?

ORGANIZING THE DIFFERENTIAL DIAGNOSIS

Mr. R has had a decline in functional status. He is unable to do a higher-level task that he used to do. Given that this patient is exhibiting functional decline, dementia—most commonly Alzheimer disease (AD)—has to be included in the differential diagnosis. The subacute onset of this patient's symptoms with loss of visuospatial function (getting lost) makes AD likely. Another common cause of dementia in the elderly is vascular dementia (VaD). It will be important to determine whether this patient has risk factors for cerebrovascular disease. In an older person, clinicians have to consider the normal cognitive decline that comes with aging, but normal aging never causes functional compromise. An alternative diagnosis is mild cognitive impairment (MCI), a syndrome of memory loss more severe than the memory loss that occurs with normal aging. MCI, however, also does not cause functional decline. Delirium and depression should always be considered in an elderly patient with cognitive decline be-

cause they are highly treatable. Table 8–4 lists the differential diagnosis.

A patient who is unable to successfully live independently because of cognitive issues always has an abnormality.

Mr. R's past medical history is notable for chronic leg pain resulting from a war injury. He also has a history of ischemic bowel, which has been asymptomatic since a hemicolectomy 3 years ago, and gout.
His medications are

1. Paroxetine, 20 mg daily
2. Methadone, 20 mg 3 times a day
3. Meloxicam, 7.5 mg daily, orally
4. Acetaminophen with codeine (300/60), 2 tablets 3 times a day
5. Allopurinol 300 mg daily, orally

His physical exam reveals an alert, pleasant man. His vital signs are normal. He answers about half the history questions himself but turns to his wife for assistance with details about doctors he has seen, medications he takes, and the timing of his surgery. He and his wife deny any symptoms

Table 8–4. Diagnostic hypotheses for Mr. R.

Diagnostic Hypotheses	Clinical Clues	Important Tests
Leading Hypothesis		
Dementia, most commonly Alzheimer type	Memory loss with impairments in instrumental activities of daily living	MMSE Neuropsychiatric testing
Active Alternative		
Vascular dementia	Risk factors for vascular disease, acute onset	Evidence of vascular disease, positive ischemia score
Active Alternative—Must Not Miss		
Delirium	Altered level of consciousness with variation during the day	Confusion Assessment Method
Depression	May present as patient-reported memory loss	Fulfillment of DSM-IV criteria

of depression. His physical exam is normal except for evidence of bilateral knee osteoarthritis. His initial neurologic exam, including motor, sensory, and reflex exam, is normal.

Is the clinical information sufficient to make a diagnosis? If not, what other information do you need?

Leading Hypothesis: AD

Textbook Presentation

Typically, a family member brings in an elderly patient because of confusion, memory loss, or personality change. The patient may deny that a problem exists and detection of dementia during casual conversation may be difficult. Alternatively, a patient may present with somatic complaints with no clear origin.

Dementia, especially early in its course, is sometimes difficult to detect on casual questioning; more formal assessment is frequently necessary.

Disease Highlights

A. AD commonly occurs after the age of 65.

B. Earlier presentations are possible.

C. AD may present with memory loss, behavioral or personality change, functional impairments, or social withdrawal.

D. Language disturbances are usually present early in the course of disease and often become severe with time.

E. Eventually, global cognitive impairment develops and patients become unable to independently accomplish the most basic activities of daily living.

Memory loss may not be the presenting symptom in patients with AD; rather, behavioral or personality changes, functional impairments, social withdrawal, and language disturbances may be the initial symptoms.

F. AD accounts for about 67% of cases of dementia.

G. Early symptoms of AD include memory loss, social withdrawal, and language disturbances.

1. Language disturbances are often the most obvious finding.

2. As the disease progresses, fluent aphasia, paraphasias, and word substitutions may develop.

H. Strictly speaking, the diagnosis of AD can only be made pathologically. That said, the diagnosis of AD is always made clinically.

I. All definitions of AD include the deterioration in a person's ability to function independently. A patient's level of functioning can be evaluated by assessing his ability to do the instrumental activities of daily living (IADLs):

1. The IADLs include
   a. Cooking
   b. House cleaning
   c. Laundry
   d. Management of medications
   e. Management of the telephone
   f. Management of personal accounts
   g. Shopping
   h. Use of transportation

2. Late in the disease, a patient's ability to perform the activities of daily living (ADLs) often becomes compromised. These ADLs are:
   a. Bathing
   b. Eating
   c. Walking
   d. Continence
   e. Dressing
   f. Grooming

J. The prognosis of AD is poor.

1. Estimates of median survival have traditionally ranged from 5 to 9 years with more recent data suggesting median survival close to 3 years with a range of 2.7 to 4 years.

2. Patients with AD also have much worse prognosis after an acute illness. Mortality after an episode of pneumonia or a hip fracture is about 4 times that of matched controlled (~50% vs ~15%).

Evidence-Based Diagnosis

A. Diagnosing AD can be challenging because patients often have subtle symptoms early in the disease course.

1. AD presents with self-reported memory loss in only a minority of patients.
   a. Memory loss reported by a spouse, relative, or close friend is more predictive of dementia.
   b. Memory loss reported by a patient is more predictive of depression.

2. Behavioral changes are commonly recognized by family members and may include delusions, hallucinations, and mood changes.

3. Physicians may recognize behavioral changes as increased anxiety, increased somatic complaints, or delusional thinking regarding illness.

B. The most efficient way to diagnose AD is to follow these 3 steps:

   1. Consider the probability that a patient has dementia.

   2. Then diagnose dementia.

   3. Then diagnose AD by ruling out other causes and ensuring that the presentation fits.

C. Diagnosing dementia

   1. The prevalence of dementia in the older population is very high. The prevalence at different ages is given in Table 8–5.

   2. The MMSE is the most commonly used test to diagnose dementia. The test characteristics for this test and some of its components are listed in Table 8–6.

      a. An important point about the MMSE is that its performance is influenced by the patient's level of education.

      b. The exam tends to underestimate the level of dementia in highly educated people and overestimate it in the poorly educated.

   3. Another test, the Memory Impairment Screen (MIS) seems to be less affected by the level of education and may perform better than the 3-item recall.

      a. In this test, patients are given 4 words.

      b. They are then asked to match them to a category (for example apple and fruit) and then asked to recall the words 2–3 minutes later.

      c. Patients receive 2 points for words remembered without prompting and 1 point for those remembered after prompting with the category.

      d. A positive test is a score of less than 5 points. The test characteristics are given below:

         (1) Sensitivity, 86%; specificity, 97%

         (2) LR+, 28.67; LR−, 0.14

   4. Neuropsychiatric testing

      a. When the diagnosis of dementia is especially difficult, neuropsychiatric testing can be very helpful.

   b. Some of the situations in which neuropsychiatric testing is commonly used are:

      (1) When there is disagreement between the clinical suspicion and in-office tests.

      (2) To specifically gauge deficits in order to recommend ways of compensating.

      (3) When present or suspected psychiatric disease complicates the diagnosis.

      (4) When a more definitive diagnosis would be helpful for the patient or family members.

D. The diagnosis of AD is a clinical one based on the diagnosis of dementia and the presence of features consistent with AD.

   1. Various office-based tests are useful in making this diagnosis. The National Institute of Neurological and Communicative Disorders and Stroke and the Alzheimer's Disease and Related Disorders Association (NINCDS-ADRDA) criteria for probable AD are currently the most commonly used.

   2. Criteria for the clinical diagnosis of probable AD

      a. Dementia

      b. Deficits in 2 or more areas of cognition

         (1) Orientation

         (2) Registration

         (3) Visuospatial and executive functioning

         (4) Language

         (5) Attention and working memory

         (6) Memory

      c. Progressive worsening of memory and other cognitive functions

      d. No disturbance of consciousness

      e. Onset between ages 40 and 90, most often after age 65

      f. Absence of other disorders that could account for the symptoms

   3. The NINCDS-ADRDA also gives factors that support the diagnosis. These are very helpful clinically. Some of these are included below:

      a. Progressive deterioration of specific cognitive functions

         (1) Aphasia

         (2) Apraxia

         (3) Agnosia

      b. Impaired ADLs and altered patterns of behavior.

      c. Family history of dementia

      d. Normal lumbar puncture, normal or non-specific EEG findings, and cerebral atrophy on neuroimaging

Table 8–5. Prevalence of dementia by age.

Age	Prevalence Outpatient	Prevalence Inpatient
65–75	2.1%	6.4%
> 75	11.7%	13%
> 85	–	31.2%

Table 8–6. Test characteristics for the MMSE and some of its components.

Test	Sensitivity	Specificity	LR+	LR–
MMSE score < 24	87%	82%	4.83	0.16
Unable to name month			16	0.4
Unable to name year			37	0.5
Unable to do serial 7s to 79			1.9	0.06
3-item recall < 2	65%	85%	4.33	0.41
Clock drawing				
Normal				0.2
Almost normal				0.8
Abnormal			24	

MMSE, Mini-Mental Status Exam.

4. The test characteristics for these criteria are:
   a. Sensitivity, 83%; specificity, 84%
   b. LR+, 5.19; LR–, 0.2
5. Because these criteria are not perfect in the diagnosis of AD, patients in whom dementia or AD is suspected but who do not meet the criteria should be monitored closely or referred for more detailed neuropsychiatric testing.

E. Reversible dementias
   1. An important issue that comes up when diagnosing AD is how much more of a work-up should be done? The concern is that when making a clinical diagnosis, potentially reversible dementias might be missed. These reversible dementias include:
      a. CNS infections
      b. Hypothyroidism
      c. B_{12} deficiency
      d. CNS masses
         (1) Neoplasms
         (2) Subdural hematomas
      e. Normal-pressure hydrocephalus
      f. Medications
   2. Current practice is to order the following tests:
      a. CBC
      b. TSH
      c. Basic metabolic panel and LFTs
      d. Vitamin B_{12} level
      e. Rapid plasma reagin
      f. Consider neuroimaging (MRI or CT)
         (1) Imaging is not required in most patients with dementia.
         (2) In practice, most patients will undergo imaging both to assess for diagnoses other than AD and to detect brain atrophy that may support the diagnosis of AD.

MAKING A DIAGNOSIS

Mr. R's exam thus far reveals some difficulty with recalling recent events. Given his age, his baseline risk of dementia is at least 10%. The first step in his work-up would be to diagnose dementia with the MMSE. If this is positive, an effort should be made to see if he fulfills the NINCDS-ADRDA criteria for probable AD.

2

Further history revealed that the patient's wife had taken over bookkeeping because a few bills had gone unpaid during the last 3 months. The patient was given the MMSE and

(continued)

scored a 20 out of 30. He was not able to give the day of the month, could only register 2 of 3 items and recalled 0 of 3. He only got 1 of the serial 7s and could not draw pentagons.

Consideration of the NINCDS-ADRDA criteria showed him to have dementia with deficits in 2 or more areas of cognition (orientation, visuospatial and executive functioning, attention and working memory, and memory). At the time of the visit, it was not clear whether his cognitive functioning was worsening and there were no disturbances in consciousness.

The plan was made for initial laboratory work to be done and for a 3-month follow-up visit. Given that he was taking multiple psychoactive medications, his regimen was scaled back to the minimum doses necessary to control his pain.

 Have you crossed a diagnostic threshold for the leading hypothesis, AD? Have you ruled out the active alternatives? Do other tests need to be done to exclude the alternative diagnoses?

Alternative Diagnosis: Multi-infarct Dementia (Vascular Dementia, VaD)

Textbook Presentation

A patient with VaD usually has an abrupt onset dementia or worsening of a previously mild and stable dementia. The patient usually has risk factors for vascular disease or has previously diagnosed vascular disease. The patient often has difficulty walking or a focal neurologic exam.

Disease Highlights

A. Generally considered to be the most common cause of dementia after AD.

B. Disease seen most commonly in patients with risk factors for vascular disease or embolic stroke.

C. Patients have dementia and evidence that cerebrovascular disease has caused the dementia.

1. Classic clue is a "step-like deterioration" related to intermittent cerebrovascular accidents.

2. Other clues may be a focal neurologic exam or evidence of strokes on neuroimaging.

D. Clues to the diagnosis of VaD are gait disturbance, urinary symptoms, and personality changes.

Evidence-Based Diagnosis

A. The criteria for the clinical diagnosis of VaD include:

1. Dementia without another cause and cerebrovascular disease (defined clinically or by neuroimaging) and

2. A causal relationship between the 2 disorders because

   a. The onset of dementia was within 3 months of a stroke

   b. There was an abrupt deterioration in cognitive function

   c. There is fluctuating, stepwise progression of cognitive deficits

B. Features consistent with the diagnosis of VaD are

1. Early presence of a gait disturbance.

2. History of unsteadiness and frequent, unprovoked falls.

3. Early urinary frequency, urgency, and other urinary symptoms not explained by urologic disease.

4. Pseudobulbar palsy (pathologic laughing, crying, grimacing; and weakness of the muscles associated with cranial nerves V, VII, IX, X, XI, and XII).

5. Personality and mood changes, abulia (loss of ability to perform voluntary actions), depression, emotional lability, or other subcortical deficits including psychomotor retardation and abnormal executive function.

C. The ischemia score is helpful in the clinical diagnosis of VaD.

1. 2 points are given for each of the following features

   a. Abrupt onset

   b. Fluctuating course

   c. History of stroke

   d. Focal exam

2. 1 point is given for each of the following features

   a. Stepwise deterioration

   b. Nocturnal confusion

   c. Preservation of personality

   d. Depression

   e. Somatic complaints

   f. Emotional lability

   g. Hypertension

   h. Atherosclerosis

3. A score of greater than 5 carries a LR+ of 5.

Treatment

A. All means of modifying risk factors for cerebrovascular disease and preventing recurrent vascular events should be used.

1. Smoking cessation

2. Control of hypertension

3. Control of diabetes mellitus

4. Cholesterol lowering (to an LDL < 100 mg/dL)

5. Aspirin therapy

6. Anticoagulation is indicated for
    a. Atrial fibrillation
    b. Severe ventricular dysfunction

7. Carotid endarterectomy when indicated

B. Disease-specific therapy

1. VaD is treated similar to AD.

2. Trials of more specific therapy for VaD have generally been inconclusive although there is some evidence that the cholinesterase inhibitors may have some effect.

CASE RESOLUTION

2

Initial laboratory evaluation, including CBC, TSH, basic metabolic panel and LFTs, vitamin B_{12} level, and rapid plasma reagin was normal. He was able to wean his medications and felt like he had a little more energy. On a follow-up visit 3 months later, the patient's wife reported that he was no longer driving to his job as it had become too difficult. On physical exam, his language skills had worsened, and he frequently answered questions with short affirmative phrases and nods that were often contradicted by his wife. (He would subsequently agree with her.) A CT scan with contrast was ordered and showed only cerebral atrophy.

AD can be confidently diagnosed in this patient. His only risk factor for VaD is a history of ischemic bowel. His ischemia score is only 2. Dementia was diagnosed at his previous visit; since his symptoms have progressed, he now fulfills the criteria for AD. Reversible causes of dementia are unlikely given the normal evaluation. The patient's functional limitations exclude MCI as a cause. The patient has no symptoms of delirium or depression.

Treatment of AD

A. Counseling

1. When the diagnosis of AD is made, patients and families should be educated on course, complications, and prognosis of the disease.

2. Decisions need to be made regarding health care proxies, financial and estate planning, and end-of-life care.

3. It is crucial to make these decisions while the patient is still a competent decision maker.

B. Safety

1. At some point in the disease, patient safety often becomes an issue.

2. Driving, wandering, and cooking are often early concerns.
    a. Driving is usually the most difficult to address because patients lack insight into the dangers they pose and resist the loss of independence that not driving brings.
    b. Physicians should raise this issue since it is often difficult for caregivers to bring up.
    c. Patients with even mild dementia should be told not to drive, or they should undergo frequent performance evaluations.

C. Behavioral

1. Caregivers should be told to expect behavioral and personality changes.

2. Maintenance of routines is important.

3. Situations likely to be stressful to patients, such as those in which a patient's deficits interfere with his functioning, should be avoided.

The fact that medications are only moderately effective in treating AD does not mean that the physician's role is limited.

D. Pharmacotherapy

1. Cholinesterase inhibitors
    a. 4 cholinesterase inhibitors are approved for treatment
        (1) Donepezil
        (2) Tacrine
        (3) Rivastigmine
        (4) Galantamine
    b. These medications have been shown to have modest effects on objective measures of dementia and functional status.

2. Vitamin E

    a. One study demonstrated effectiveness of vitamin E in treating patients with moderate AD.

    b. The combined endpoint in the study was a delay in the time to the occurrence of any of the following:

        (1) Death

        (2) Institutionalization

        (3) Loss of the ability to perform at least 2 of the following: eating, grooming, or toileting

        (4) Severe dementia

3. Associated neuropsychiatric symptoms

    a. May include agitation (60–70%) or either delusions or hallucinations (30–60%)

    b. Often treated well with atypical neuroleptics, such as olanzapine and risperidone; neither of these drugs are approved for this indication.

4. Depression

    a. Very common in patients with AD

    b. Present in up to 50% of patients

    c. Usually treated well with selective serotonin reuptake inhibitors

5. Caregiver care

    a. Taking care of a friend or relative with AD can be extremely challenging.

    b. Caregivers should be counseled on the importance of taking time off.

    c. They should be counseled that behavioral difficulties are a result of the disease and not the patient's anger or heartlessness.

    d. Caregiver support groups can be extremely helpful.

REVIEW OF OTHER IMPORTANT DISEASES

Mild Cognitive Impairment (MCI)

Textbook Presentation

Usually presents in an older patient complaining of memory loss. Common complaints are difficulty remembering names and appointments or solving complex problems. Detailed testing shows abnormal memory, but patients have no functional impairment.

Disease Highlights

A. Memory complaints are very common in the elderly.

B. Concern for AD is also very common.

C. The definition of MCI includes the lack of any functional impairment and

    1. Memory complaint

    2. Normal ADLs

    3. Normal general cognitive function

    4. Abnormal memory for age

    5. No dementia

D. Patients with this disorder are not neurologically normal.

    1. Their memory is worse than age-matched controls.

    2. They have a higher rate of progression to dementia than those without memory impairments (12% per year vs 1–2% per year).

Evidence-Based Diagnosis

The diagnosis of this disease is made by the above criteria. The memory deficits are sometimes difficult to detect and distinguish from normal, age-related changes. If it is desirable to obtain a definite diagnosis, neuropsychiatric testing is helpful.

Treatment

Presently, there is no proven treatment for MCI. Patients should be monitored closely for development of more severe cognitive or functional decline.

Dementia with Lewy Bodies (DLB)

Textbook Presentation

DLB is typically seen in a patient with Parkinson disease who has dementia. The predominant symptoms of the dementia are a fluctuating course and the presence of hallucinations. In patients without a previous diagnosis of Parkinson disease, motor symptoms similar to those seen in Parkinson disease are often present.

Disease Highlights

A. Lewy bodies are seen in the cortex of about 20% of patients with dementia.

    1. Includes some patients with a clinical diagnosis of AD

    2. Probably among the most common types of dementia after AD. It may coexist with AD.

B. The most important features of DLB are included in the Evidence-Based Diagnosis section below.

C. The fluctuating course can mean that early in the disease patients may seem nearly normal at times and demented at other times. Because of the fluctuation in symptoms, delirium needs to be included in the differential diagnosis.

D. Visual hallucinations are common in DLB, unlike in most other types of dementia.

E. Mild extrapyramidal motor symptoms (rigidity and bradykinesis) are often seen. These may occur late in the course of other dementias but occur early with DLB.

Diagnosis

The diagnostic criteria for DLB are presented below.

A. There is dementia that might be mild at the onset of disease.

B. Two of the following are essential for a diagnosis of probable DLB:

1. Fluctuating cognition with pronounced variations in attention and alertness

2. Recurrent visual hallucinations that are typically well formed and detailed

3. Spontaneous motor features of parkinsonism

C. The following features are supportive of the diagnosis of DLB

1. Repeated falls

2. Syncope

3. Transient loss of consciousness

4. Neuroleptic sensitivity

5. Systematized delusions and hallucinations

Treatment

A. Supportive treatment of patients with DLB is the same as for patients with AD.

B. Anticholinergic medications have also been shown to be effective.

C. Neuroleptics can be dangerous, potentially worsening symptoms.

Patients with dementia with parkinsonian features, a fluctuating course and visual hallucinations should be evaluated for DLB before they are treated with neuroleptics.

I have a patient with acute diarrhea. How do I determine the cause?

CHIEF COMPLAINT

PATIENT 1

Mr. C is a 35-year-old man who comes to your outpatient office complaining of 1 day of diarrhea.

What is the differential diagnosis of diarrhea? How would you frame the differential?

CONSTRUCTING A DIFFERENTIAL DIAGNOSIS

Although the presence of diarrhea is actually defined by stool weight, it is more useful to define acute diarrhea clinically. Diarrhea can be thought of as bowel movements of a looser consistency than usual that occur more than 3 times a day. Acute diarrhea develops over a period of 1–2 days and lasts for less than 4 weeks. The differential diagnosis below organizes diagnoses by the presenting symptoms. This structure is easy to remember, focuses history taking, allows prognosticating, and is also a good framework on which to consider therapy. (This chapter will not address chronic or intermittent diarrhea.)

Noninfectious diarrhea is recognized by the lack of constitutional symptoms. Infectious diarrhea that presents with large volume (often watery) stool, constitutional symptoms, nausea and vomiting, and often abdominal cramps can be categorized as gastroenteritis. The inflammatory diarrheas are infections that present with infectious symptoms and often with dysentery (fever, tenesmus, and stools with blood and mucus). Many organisms can cause both gastroenteritis and inflammatory diarrhea.

A. Noninfectious diarrhea
1. Medications and other ingestible substances (some with osmotic effect)
    a. Sorbitol (gum, mints, pill fillers)
    b. Mannitol
    c. Fructose (fruits, soft drinks)
    d. Fiber (bran, fruits, vegetables)
    e. Lactulose
2. Magnesium-containing medications
    a. Nutritional supplements
    b. Antacids
    c. Laxatives
3. Malabsorption
    a. Lactose intolerance
    b. Pancreatitis
4. Medications causing diarrhea through nonosmotic means
    a. Metformin
    b. Antibiotics
    c. Colchicine
    d. Digoxin
    e. Selective serotonin reuptake inhibitor antidepressants
B. Infectious diarrhea: gastroenteritis
1. Viral (most common)
    a. Norwalk virus
    b. Rotovirus
2. Bacterial (commonly food-borne)
    a. *Cholera*
    b. *Escherichia coli*
    c. *Shigella* species
    d. *Salmonella* species
    e. *Campylobacter* species
    f. *Yersinia enterocolitica*

3. Toxin-mediated
   a. *Staphylococcus aureus*
   b. *Clostridium perfringens*
   c. *Bacillus cereus*
C. Infectious diarrhea: inflammatory colitis
   1. Bacterial
      a. *Shigella* species
      b. *E coli*
      c. *Campylobacter* species
      d. *Salmonella* species
      e. *Y enterocolitica*
   2. Antibiotic-associated
      a. *Clostridium difficile*
      b. Non-*C difficile*–related

The patient was in good health until the morning before he comes to your office. After a morning jog he picked up breakfast at a local coffee shop. He was unable to finish a cup of coffee and a scone because of a poor appetite. During his 20-minute drive to work he developed nausea and diaphoresis. Upon arriving at work

he developed low-grade fever, abdominal cramping, and vomiting. Over the next 12 hours, diarrhea developed. He describes the stool being watery and brown without any blood.

At this point, what is the leading hypothesis and what are the active alternatives? What other tests should be ordered?

ORGANIZING THE DIFFERENTIAL DIAGNOSIS

Mr. C seeks medical attention within about 24 hours of the onset of diarrhea. Notable findings in the history are:

1. Onset of symptoms over about 60 minutes
2. Exposure to foods prepared outside the home
3. Early predominance of nausea
4. Low-grade fever
5. Watery brown stool

This presentation certainly speaks for an infectious cause. The low-grade fever and absence of dysentery make it likely that the diagnosis is in the category of gastroenteritis. Table 9–1 lists the differential diagnosis.

Table 9–1. Diagnostic hypotheses for Mr. C.

Diagnostic Hypotheses	Clinical Clues	Important Tests
Leading Hypothesis		
Norwalk virus	Hyperacute onset Vomiting usually present	Resolution in 24–48 hours
Active Alternative		
Toxin-mediated gastroenteritis, such as *Staphylococcus aureus*	Common food poisoning Onset 1–8 hours after exposure Vomiting is predominant	Rapid resolution, within 12 hours
Bacterial gastroenteritis, such as *Salmonella* infection	Usually food-borne; fairly specific clinical syndromes; high fevers possible	Stool cultures can be diagnostic
Other Alternative		
Rotavirus	Contact with children Vomiting common and constitutional signs present	Resolution in 24–72 hours

Mr. C is otherwise in good health. He reports no recent illnesses or antibiotic exposures. There have been no recent changes in his diet and, other than the noted breakfast, he has eaten food prepared at home for the last week. He lives alone with wife and reports no known sick contacts. He works as a bus driver.

The physical exam is notable for temperature, 38.2 °C; BP is 110/80 mm Hg and pulse is 100 bpm while lying down; BP is 90/72 mm Hg and pulse is 126 bpm while standing; RR, 12 breaths per minute. Sclera and conjunctiva are normal. The abdomen is soft and diffusely tender with hyperactive bowel sounds. The rectal exam shows brown, heme-negative stool.

Is the clinical information sufficient to make a diagnosis? If not, what other information do you need?

Leading Hypothesis: Norwalk Virus

Textbook Presentation

Acute vomiting is usually the presenting symptom. Mild diarrhea begins after the vomiting. Mild abdominal cramping is common. Low-grade fever and dehydration are usually present. All symptoms resolve completely by 3 days.

Disease Highlights

A. Norwalk virus and closely related viruses account for about 90% of adult nonbacterial gastroenteritis.

B. Most commonly occurs in winter.

C. High attack rate (~50%) means that exposure history is often identifiable.

    1. Most commonly transmitted by person-to-person contact

    2. Food-borne transmission also occurs.

D. Incubation is 1–2 days, so exposure typically is recent.

E. Constitutional symptoms and vomiting are common.

Evidence-Based Diagnosis

A. There are no diagnostic tests available for routine clinical use.

B. Diagnosis is made by clinical presentation.

MAKING A DIAGNOSIS

At the time of the patient's visit he was feeling better than he had previously. He still noted an "upset stomach" and was having soft watery diarrhea every 2–3 hours. He had not had any vomiting in about 6 hours and was therefore able to keep down fluids.

Have you crossed a diagnostic threshold for the leading hypothesis, Norwalk virus? Have you ruled out the active alternatives? Do other tests need to be done to exclude the alternative diagnoses?

Unlike many of the diseases diagnosed in the outpatient setting, an exact diagnosis in a patient with diarrhea often need not be made. The clinical syndrome in Mr. C is consistent with viral gastroenteritis. By recognizing this syndrome, you are able to reassure him that he would be better in the next 24–48 hours. Even if a diagnostic test for Norwalk virus were available for routine use in clinical practice, the usefulness would be low because treatment is only supportive.

Most evaluations for diarrhea are negative. In a selected population in which cultures have been done, only 2–12% of stool cultures are positive and 0.4–0.7% of ova and parasite tests are positive.

In most patients with an acute diarrheal illness, diagnostic testing is not helpful to the patient but may be important from a public health standpoint.

Alternative Diagnosis: Toxin-Mediated Gastroenteritis

Textbook Presentation

The presentation of these illnesses is usually acute, with vomiting and crampy abdominal pain. Vomiting is the predominant symptom with diarrhea being mild and watery and fever being low grade. Because of the very short lag between ingestion and illness (2–8 hours), the culpable meal is usually the last one eaten. Recovery is very rapid (12–48 hours). This syndrome is most commonly caused by *S aureus* or *C perfringens*.

Disease Highlights

A. Toxin-mediated gastroenteritis caused by *S aureus, C perfringens,* or *B cereus* is essentially always food-borne; these organisms are not the most common causes of food-borne infection.

B. *Campylobacter, Giardia, Salmonella,* and *Shigella* are the most common bacterial and parasitic causes of food-borne infections according to the most recent CDC data (Table 9–2).

C. Viral causes are almost certainly even more common.

D. *S aureus, C perfringens,* and *B cereus* can often be recognized through the clinical and exposure history.

　1. This recognition can enable the physician to provide prognosis, avoid unnecessary testing, and prevent further infection from a common source.

　2. Table 9–3 describes the clinical syndromes of these infections.

 Illnesses presenting with the acute onset of vomiting and constitutional symptoms, often with abdominal cramping, are usually caused by viruses or bacteria that elaborate toxins.

Evidence-Based Diagnosis

A. There are no diagnostic tests available for routine clinical use.

B. Diagnosis is by clinical presentation.

Treatment

Treatment is supportive. See below for details of supportive care for diarrhea.

Alternative Diagnosis: Infection with *Salmonella* Species

Textbook Presentation

The onset of disease is usually subacute with nausea, fever, and diarrhea. Fever and nausea often resolve over 1–2 days while diarrhea persists for 5–7 days. Patients usually have watery diarrhea with 6–8 bowel movements each day. Dysentery is possible. Bacteria commonly remains in the stool for 4–5 weeks. This syndrome may cause higher fevers than viral or preformed toxin disease.

Disease Highlights

A. *Salmonella* species cause 3 major types of disease.

　1. Diarrheal illnesses

　　a. Gastroenteritis

　　b. Dysentery (discussed later in the chapter)

　2. Bacteremia with the potential for focal infectious complication.

　　a. Usually a secondary complication of gastroenteritis

　　b. Bacteremia develops in ~5% of patients and focal infections develop in a small percentage of these patients.

Table 9–2. Common causes of food-borne illness.

Organism	Approximate % Total Food-Borne Infections	% Infections with a Given Organism That Are Food-Borne
Norwalk-like viruses	60.0	40
Campylobacter species	6.0	80
Giardia lamblia	5.2	10
Salmonella species	3.7	95
Shigella species	1.2	20
Clostridium perfringens	0.6	100
Staphylococcus aureus	0.5	100

Table 9–3. Clinical syndromes of toxin-mediated gastroenteritis.

Organism	Pathogenesis	Incubation	Source	Clinical Syndrome
Staphylococcus aureus	Preformed toxin	1–6 hours	Protein rich food	Acute onset, vomiting predominant, resolves within 2 hours
Clostridium perfringens	Elaborated toxin	8–16 hours	Meats	Diarrhea with abdominal cramping, lasts 1–2 days
Bacillus cereus	Preformed toxin	1–6 hours	Grains	Very similar to *S aureus*

3. Typhoid fever

  a. Not a diarrheal illness and not discussed in detail here.

  b. Seen almost exclusively in nonvaccinated travelers.

  c. Should be considered in the differential diagnosis of a traveler with a febrile illness.

B. Although typhoid fever is a common public health problem worldwide, gastroenteritis is the most common salmonella-related disease in the United States.

C. Salmonella is transmitted by:

  1. Food

    a. Eggs and poultry are most common sources.

    b. There are reports of infection from almost any type of food.

  2. Fecal-oral contact with infected patients

    a. Patients shed bacteria for weeks after infection

    b. Animals also carry salmonella (reptiles most classically).

Evidence-Based Diagnosis

The gold standard for diagnosis of salmonella gastroenteritis remains stool culture results. There are tests with greater sensitivity, but none are used in routine clinical practice.

Treatment

A. Prevention

  1. Easily preventable

  2. Because salmonella is heat sensitive, cooking food well and good hand washing practices prevent most infections.

B. Treatment

  1. Most salmonella infections require no treatment.

2. The patients who should receive therapy beyond supportive care are those who have

  a. Severe disease

  b. Immunocompromised status, probably including the very elderly

  c. Elevated risk of focal infection

    (1) Prosthetic joints or hardware

    (2) Sickle cell anemia

  d. Typhoid fever

3. Although most patients shed bacteria for weeks after infection, antibiotics should not be used in attempts to prevent transmission. Antibiotics do not shorten the duration of carriage.

4. In a patient who is being treated for bacteremia, the treatment is

  a. First-line: ceftriaxone, 2 g IV daily for 7–14 days

  b. Second-line: ciprofloxacin 400 mg IV twice daily for 7–14 days

5. Treatment for dysentery is discussed below.

CASE RESOLUTION

Mr. C was sent home with directions for oral rehydration. He reported sleeping for most of the afternoon and was well enough to return to work the next day. By the following day (day 4 of the presentation), the patient was completely better. He reported that none of his close contacts became ill.

The patient's symptoms lasted 48–72 hours. He required no specific therapy. There were no suspicious food exposures and nobody else became ill. The case is consistent with a viral gastroenteritis such as Norwalk virus. A toxin-induced food-borne illness is possible. The preformed toxins are less likely because of the rapid onset of symptoms. (Mr. C's symptoms developed within 15 minutes of eating, rather than the 1–8 hours expected with preformed toxins.) *C perfringens* food poisoning is possible, although the lack of suspicious food ingestion the previous evening make this less likely.

Treatment of Norwalk Virus

A. Supportive care

  1. The majority of cases of patients with acute diarrhea require only supportive care. Supportive care is meant to provide rehydration and symptom relief.

  2. Rehydration

    a. Oral rehydration is the most important means of rehydration. All commercially available oral rehydration solutions contain NaCl, KCl, HCO_3 or citrate, and glucose.

      (1) A liter of the World Health Organization product contains

        (a) 3.5 g of NaCl

        (b) 2.5 g of $NaHCO_3$

        (c) 1.5 g of KCl

        (d) 20 g of glucose

      (2) If this solution is not available, patients can be instructed to mix the following in 1 L of water

        (a) one-half teaspoon of salt

        (b) one-quarter teaspoon of baking soda

        (c) 8 teaspoons of sugar

      (3) Most "clear liquid replacements" are inadequate for replenishing lost electrolytes but are still adequate for mild diarrhea.

    b. IV fluids (lactated Ringer solution or normal saline) are reasonable until the patient can take fluid orally

  3. Antidiarrheals (usually an opioid with or without an anticholinergic) are safe and effective for patients without dysentery.

    a. Loperamide

    b. Atropine/diphenoxylate

  4. Antiemetics

  5. Diet

    a. BRAT diet (banana, rice, applesauce, toast) is often recommended.

    b. Avoid dairy products (see below).

Antidiarrheals are very effective for control of symptoms. They should never be used for patients with dysentery or signs of invasive infection (tenesmus, blood or mucus in stool, high fever, and severe abdominal pain).

B. Specific treatments

  1. Treatment other than supportive care is not necessary for Norwalk virus-like illnesses.

  2. Specific treatment is recommended for diarrheal infections only in limited circumstances.

  3. The indications depend on severity of the clinical illness, individual patient risk factors, and specific indications based on organism.

  4. These indications are discussed with each disease and summarized in the algorithm at the end of the chapter.

  5. Below are some situations in which to consider empiric therapy:

    a. Presentation specific

      (1) Severe disease

        (a) Fever

        (b) Abdominal pain

      (2) Dysentery

      (3) High band count

    b. Patient specific

      (1) Immunosuppressed

      (2) Prosthetic device

    c. Contact specific

      (1) Healthcare worker

      (2) Daycare worker

      (3) Food handler

Empiric therapy for diarrhea is reasonable for patients with severe symptoms, those patients at high risk for complication, and those patients most likely to infect others.

FOLLOW-UP OF MR. C

Two weeks later Mr. C comes to see you again. He attributes his recovery to antibiotics that

(continued)

he took on the day he saw you. They were left over from an old dental infection. About 5 days after his recovery, he began to feel poorly again. For the last 10 days he has had diarrhea, abdominal bloating, and belching. He denies fever, chills, nausea, vomiting, or tenesmus. There has been no blood in his stool.

 At this point, what is the leading hypothesis and what are the active alternatives? What other tests should be ordered?

ORGANIZING THE DIFFERENTIAL DIAGNOSIS

There are 3 important aspects of this presentation:

1. The patient has recently experienced what was almost certainly an infectious GI illness.
2. The patient has recently taken antibiotics.
3. The patient's symptoms have been present for 10 days. This is prolonged when considering acute infectious diarrhea.

The recent gastroenteritis should raise the possibility of recurrent disease or lactose intolerance. Many of the bacterial causes of diarrhea can recur as they persist in the stool after clinical symptoms have resolved. This prolonged bacterial shedding also accounts for spread of the illness. This is especially common with *Salmonella* and *Campylobacter*. Lactose intolerance is also common after gastroenteritis due to injury to the small bowel mucosa. Antibiotic-associated diarrhea is a common entity. The prolonged nature of the illness should prompt consideration of the less typical pathogens, such as parasites. Table 9–4 lists the differential diagnosis.

The patient describes 3–4 soft bowel movements a day. He also notes a fair amount of abdominal discomfort. There is no real pain, but there is bloating and belching. He says he goes to the bathroom 3 or 4 additional times each day just to pass gas.

The patient took 3 doses of amoxicillin on the day he first came to see you. He ran out after these 3 doses. He has not been out of the city since his infection and does not note any

Table 9–4. Diagnostic hypotheses for Mr. C's repeat visit.

Diagnostic Hypotheses	Clinical Clues	Important Tests
Leading Hypothesis		
Lactose intolerance	Ethnic predisposition Recent illness Relation to diet	Resolution with dietary changes
Active Alternative		
Antibiotic-associated diarrhea	Only caused by *Clostridium difficile* about 15–20% of time	Usually resolves with discontinuation of antibiotic Specific tests for *C difficile* toxin
Recurrent infection	Similar symptoms as initial illness Most common with bacterial pathogen	Stool cultures
Other Alternative		
Parasitic infection	Exposure history common (often with travel) Consider especially in immunosuppressed patients	Stool ova and parasites may be diagnostic

unusual exposures. He reports that his diet has been a little more simple than usual with a lot of cereal, rice, potatoes, and milk to "soothe his stomach."

 Is the clinical information sufficient to make a diagnosis? If not, what other information do you need?

Leading Hypothesis: Lactose Intolerance

Textbook Presentation

Lactose intolerance most commonly presents as chronic symptoms in a person of susceptible ethnic background. The symptoms may be subacute or acute in the setting of infection or dietary changes. The predominant symptom may be belching, bloating, flatulence, diarrhea, or abdominal pain. A suspicious dietary history should be present.

Disease Highlights

A. Lactose intolerance is very common.

B. Predictable by ethnic background, worsens with age.

C. Episodes of small bowel infection can cause transient lactose intolerance in anyone but is more apt to cause symptoms in people with low levels of lactase activity at baseline.

D. Ethnic groups and native populations most likely to have low levels of lactase activity come from the following regions:

1. Middle East and Mediterranean

2. Asia

3. Africa

4. Native American

E. Milk, ice cream, and yogurt have the highest levels of lactose.

F. Foods with high lactose and low fat (skim milk) tend to cause the most symptoms as these foods deliver lactose to the small intestine the fastest.

Evidence-Based Diagnosis

The diagnosis of lactose intolerance is generally a clinical one based on a suspicious history in a patient with a susceptible background whose symptoms resolve on a lactose-free diet. More definitive tests, the lactose tolerance test or lactose breath hydrogen test, can be performed in patients in whom the diagnosis is likely but not clear historically.

 Because of the high prevalence of mild lactose intolerance and the frequent exacerbation following gastroenteritis, patients with acute gastroenteritis should be advised to avoid dairy products for 2 weeks after recovery.

MAKING A DIAGNOSIS

 On exam he appears well. Vital signs are all normal. His abdominal exam reveals hyperactive bowel sounds with minimal distention. It is soft and nontender. Rectal exam reveals soft, brown, heme-negative stool.

 Have you crossed a diagnostic threshold for the leading hypothesis, lactose intolerance? Have you ruled out the active alternatives? Do other tests need to be done to exclude the alternative diagnoses?

The patient does not appear to have an infectious cause of his diarrhea—at least not a bacterial or viral cause. This fact makes recurrence of his previous infection very unlikely. Antibiotic-associated diarrhea or diarrhea caused by a parasitic infection are still possible.

Alternative Diagnosis: Antibiotic-Associated Diarrhea

Textbook Presentation

Patients with antibiotic-associated diarrhea usually have symptoms of gastroenteritis or dysentery during antibiotic therapy. Upper abdominal symptoms of nausea and vomiting are rare.

Disease Highlights

A. Complicates between 2% and 25% of antibiotic courses, the level of risk varies with antibiotic.

B. There are really 2 distinct types of antibiotic-associated diarrhea: *C difficile*–associated and non-*C difficile*–associated. The antibiotics most commonly responsible for both types of diarrhea are:

1. Clindamycin

2. Cephalosporins

3. Ampicillin, amoxicillin, amoxicillin-clavulanate

C. Only about 20% of the episodes are related to *C difficile*.

D. Hospitalized or institutionalized patients are at higher risk if *C difficile* is endemic in the setting.

E. *C difficile* causes diarrhea via toxin-mediated effects on the large bowel. This can present as severe diarrhea, often presenting with symptoms of colonic inflammation and a high WBC count.

F. Patients with antibiotic-associated diarrhea not related to *C difficile* usually have mild disease that occurs either during or immediately after a course of antibiotics. It is usually mild. Possible causes of this type of diarrhea are numerous:

1. Change in intestinal flora

2. Nonantimicrobial effect of antibiotics such as the promotility effects of erythromycin

3. Enteric infections other than *C difficile*

Evidence-Based Diagnosis

A. The diagnosis of antibiotic-associated diarrhea not associated with *C difficile* is usually easy—diarrhea temporally associated with antibiotic use that resolves following the removal of the causative agent.

B. *C difficile* colitis

1. Diagnosed by identification of either the toxin or by demonstration of the classic pseudomembranous colitis on sigmoidoscopy or colonoscopy.

2. Culture, although highly sensitive and specific is used less because there are nontoxin-producing strains of *C difficile* that are not clinically important.

3. The test characteristics of the toxin assay are listed below. Because of the lower sensitivity, 3 samples are recommended.

    a. Sensitivity, 70–95%; specificity, 95–99%

    b. LR+, 14–95; LR–, 0.05–0.32

C. If a clinical syndrome consistent with *C difficile* colitis persists despite negative toxin assay, sigmoidoscopic exam of the colon is recommended. If symptoms do not resolve and evaluation for *C difficile* is negative, stool cultures to rule out another antibiotic-associated enteric infection are reasonable.

Treatment

A. Antibiotic-associated diarrhea not related to *C difficile* infection usually resolves with discontinuation of antibiotics. Other useful treatments include:

1. Probiotic agents such as yogurt

2. Antidiarrheals

B. The treatment of *C difficile* is as follows

1. First-line treatment: 500 mg of oral metronidazole 3 times daily for 10 days

2. Second-line treatment: 125 mg of oral vancomycin 4 times daily for 10 days

3. Avoid antidiarrheals

Alternative Diagnosis: *Giardia lamblia*

Textbook Presentation

Giardiasis can present as either acute or chronic diarrhea. It usually occurs in patients with exposure to infected water supplies, although person-to-person transmission can occur. Symptoms usually include diarrhea, nausea, abdominal cramps, bloating, flatulence, and foul-smelling stools.

Disease Highlights

A. *Giardia* is the most common cause of parasitic diarrhea acquired in the United States.

B. Most infections in the United States result from drinking infected water.

C. Classic exposures occur while a person is camping or while traveling to countries where the infection is endemic.

D. Common symptoms

1. Diarrhea occurs in 96% of cases.

2. Weight loss is present in 62% of cases.

3. Abdominal cramps occur in 61% of cases.

4. Greasy stools are present in 57% of cases.

5. Belching, flatulence, and foul-smelling stools are commonly reported.

E. Fever is uncommon.

F. Chronic infection occurs in about 10% of untreated patients.

G. If evaluation for *Giardia* is negative and there is no response to empiric therapy, other organisms should also be considered.

1. This is especially true in patients who are immunocompromised.

2. Other organisms commonly seen are:

    a. *Cryptosporidium*

    b. *Cyclospora cayetanensis*

    c. *Isospora belli*

Evidence-Based Diagnosis

A. *Giardia lamblia*

1. Sensitivity of stool ova and parasites for *Giardia* is 50–70% for 1 stool sample.

2. Sensitivity is over 90% for 3 samples.

3. Antigen assays sensitive to over 90%.

4. Classic "string test" is seldom used.

B. Other organisms

    1. *Cryptosporidium* can be identified on antigen assay.

    2. *C cayetanensis* and *I belli* can be identified on acid-fast stain.

Treatment

The treatment of choice for *G lamblia* infection is 250 mg of oral metronidazole 3 times daily for 5 days. Empiric therapy is often recommended.

CASE RESOLUTION

A lactose-free diet was recommended for the patient. Three stool samples were tested for *C difficile* toxin; results were negative. The suspicion for a recurrent bacterial infection or a parasitic infection was very low.

The patient began a lactose-free diet and was better within 3 days. After 2 weeks, he slowly reintroduced his usual diet without symptoms.

Treatment of Lactose Intolerance

A. In general, lactose intolerance is treated by decreasing lactose intake.

B. Because people have variable levels of lactase activity, levels of tolerance differ from person to person.

C. Enzyme supplements, available over the counter, are often helpful.

D. In acquired illness (eg, post gastroenteritis), lactase levels will eventually recover when the intestinal brush border regenerates.

E. It is usually reasonable to suggest waiting 2 weeks before reintroducing lactose-containing products.

CHIEF COMPLAINT

PATIENT 2

Ms. V is a 45-year-old woman who comes to see you in the office; she complains of 4 days of diarrhea. She reports feeling tired and weak. She is moving her bowels about 6–8 times a day. She says that she has significant abdominal pain. She came in today because she has begun to pass bloody stools.

On physical exam, her vital signs are temperature, 38.3 °C; BP, 130/84 mm Hg; pulse, 90 bpm; RR, 12 breaths per minute. She is orthostatic.

Her abdomen has hyperactive bowel sounds. It is diffusely tender, without peritoneal signs. Her stool is a mixture of soft brown stool and blood.

At this point, what is the leading hypothesis and what are the active alternatives? What other tests should be ordered?

ORGANIZING THE DIFFERENTIAL DIAGNOSIS

Ms. V has bloody stools, abdominal pain, and fever. This symptom complex makes diarrhea caused by a bacterial infection likely. The organisms that commonly cause bloody diarrhea are *Shigella* species, *Campylobacter* species, and *E coli. Salmonella* species, *Y enterocolitica,* and *C difficile* also occasionally cause bloody diarrhea. Noninfectious causes, such as bowel infarction or ulcerative colitis, should also be considered.

It is impossible to clinically differentiate between the bacterial diarrheas. That said, it is important to know organisms' recognizable symptom complexes because these can give clues to the causative organism. Because treatment decisions are often made before the specific organism is identified by culture, these clues can help guide appropriate therapy. Table 9–5 lists the differential diagnosis.

The patient first felt sick on Monday with fever and lethargy. She felt terrible for the entire day and thought she was getting the flu. On

(continued)

Table 9–5. Diagnostic hypotheses for Ms. V.

Diagnostic Hypotheses	Clinical Clues	Important Tests
Leading Hypothesis		
Bacterial diarrhea caused by *Campylobacter* infection	Constitutional prodrome Diarrhea with significant abdominal pain Occasional dysentery	Stool culture
Active Alternative		
Bacterial diarrhea, caused by infection with *Shigella* species	Varies by species but classically colonic predominant symptoms—-dysentery	Stool culture High bandemia common
Active Alternatives—Must Not Miss		
Bacterial diarrhea, caused by infection with *Escherichia coli* 0157:H7	Diarrhea, usually bloody Fever uncommon Right-sided abdominal pain	Stool culture for organism must be specifically requested. Toxin can be identified.
Other Alternative		
Ulcerative colitis	Usually subacute to chronic	Endoscopic diagnosis

Tuesday, she began to have diarrhea and feel diffuse abdominal pain. Today is Thursday and she comes to your office because she began to have blood in her stool.

She reports that her husband is also sick with similar symptoms. His diarrhea developed the day before hers did but he has not noticed blood in his stool. He refused to come in because he figured it was "just a virus."

 Is the clinical information sufficient to make a diagnosis? If not, what other information do you need?

Leading Hypothesis: *Campylobacter* Infection

Textbook Presentation

Presenting symptoms of *Campylobacter* infection are usually diarrhea and abdominal pain. The diarrhea is often profuse and watery and the pain can be severe, often mimicking appendicitis or other abdominal disease that may require surgery. The fever usually resolves over the first 2 days of the illness, while the diarrhea and abdominal pain may last 4–6 days.

Disease Highlights

A. *Campylobacter* species are among the most commonly isolated pathogens in patients with diarrhea and are a common cause of bloody stool.

B. Incidence in 2001 was 13.8 cases/100,000 persons.

C. In 1 recent study of patients presenting to emergency departments with bloody diarrhea, the breakdown of diagnoses were:

   1. *Shigella* in 15.3% of patients
   2. *Campylobacter* in 6.2% of patients
   3. *Salmonella* in 5.2% of patients
   4. Shiga toxin–producing *E coli* in 2.6% of patients
   5. Other cause in 1.6% of patients

D. Common aspects of the presentation are

   1. Constitutional symptoms before GI disease
   2. Bloody diarrhea beginning after 2–3 days watery diarrhea

E. There can be rare late complications.

   1. Reactive arthritis
   2. Guillain-Barré

F. Bacteria commonly remain in the stool for 4–5 weeks and reinfection might occur.

Evidence-Based Diagnosis

A. Although stool cultures are most likely to be negative (even in patients with bloody diarrhea), they need to be done because the results are useful in guiding specific therapy.

   1. Overtreatment carries risk of inducing resistance organisms.

   2. *Campylobacter* and *Shigella* infections clearly benefit from treatment.

   3. Treatment can worsen the outcome of some diseases causing prolonged salmonella carriage and increasing the risk of hemolytic uremic syndrome with *E coli*.

   4. Culture results are very useful from a public health standpoint.

B. Stool cultures are really the only way to distinguish organisms.

   1. A representative study that looked at the clinical characteristics of patients with diagnostic stool cultures showed the overlap of the clinical syndromes.

   2. Table 9–6 lists the percentage of patients with various characteristics by organism.

C. In order to increase the yield of the cultures (both in terms of positive results and clinical usefulness), it is useful to consider the following questions:

   1. Is there a clinical suspicion for a specific disease that requires treatment?

      a. Severely ill patient (fever, dysentery, abdominal pain); about 30% of patients with dysentery have positive cultures (compared with 2–12% of all patients).

      b. Suspicious exposure (travel, high risk sexual behavior, antibiotics)

         (1) Travelers diarrhea (usually *E coli*) can usually be treated empirically.

         (2) Other infections associated with travel (*Entamoeba histolytica*, *G lamblia*) benefit from treatment.

   2. Does the patient have an underlying disease that makes treatment more necessary?

      a. Immunosuppression

      b. Inflammatory bowel disease

   3. Are there public health reasons that a diagnosis needs to be made?

      a. Possible outbreak of food-borne illness

      b. Patient might potentially spread disease (health-care worker, daycare worker, food handler)

D. Is there a reason not to culture?

   1. In-hospital stool cultures and ova and parasite exams are particularly unrevealing.

   2. Consider limiting in-hospital cultures to the following circumstances:

      a. Onset of diarrhea within 3 days of admission

      b. Onset > 3 days but

         (1) Patient is older than 65 years and has co-morbidities.

         (2) Patient has HIV infection.

Table 9–6. Percentages of patients with various clinical characteristics by organism.

Characteristic	Organism			
	Shigella	*Campylobacter*	*Salmonella*	*E coli*
Bloody diarrhea	54.3%	37.0%	33.8%	91.3%
Abdominal pain	77.9%	79.5%	69.7%	90.5%
Abdominal tenderness	33.5%	45.4%	28.8%	72.0%
Subjective fever	78.6%	58.7%	72.0%	35.0%
Objective fever	69.4%	50.9%	69.4%	41.4%
Visible blood in stool sample	14.7%	7.8%	4.8%	63.0%
Occult blood	59.1%	52.0%	43.4%	82.8%
Fecal leukocytes	37.8%	42.9%	29.4%	70.5%
Leukocytes > 10,000/mcL	58.0%	42.0%	45.3%	70.9%

Modified from Slutsker L et al. Escherichia coli O157:H7 diarrhea in the United States: clinical and epidemiologic features. *Ann Intern Med.* 1997;126:505–513.

(3) Neutropenia is present.

(4) Extraintestinal manifestations are present.

(5) There is an outbreak of diarrhea in the hospital.

Patients with more severe clinical presentations, including high fever, abdominal pain, and dysentery, should always have stool cultures taken.

E. Diagnostic tests other than stool cultures are useful only in limited situations.

1. *C difficile* toxin for patients with antibiotic exposure

2. Shiga toxin to identify *E coli* 0157:H7 or related strains

3. Fecal occult blood and fecal leukocytes not predictive of invasive infections. Sensitivities and specificities range from 20% to 80%.

4. WBC

   a. WBC is neither sensitive nor specific for the presence of invasive bacterial infections.

   b. A marked left shift, especially if band count is > neutrophil count, suggests bacterial etiology.

MAKING A DIAGNOSIS

The patient is given IV fluids in the office. After receiving acetaminophen and 2 L of fluid she is feeling somewhat better. Stool cultures are sent. A CBC and Chem-7 are normal.

Have you crossed a diagnostic threshold for the leading hypothesis, **Campylobacter** infection? Have you ruled out the active alternatives? Do other tests need to be done to exclude the alternative diagnoses?

Alternative Diagnosis: *Shigella* Infection

Textbook Presentation

Shigella infection often begins with fever and constitutional symptoms. Diarrhea is initially watery and may become bloody. The diarrhea can be very frequent. There are often predominant colonic symptoms (tenesmus).

Disease Highlights

A. *Shigella* can cause classic bacterial dysentery.

B. Although there is a spectrum of disease (some of the species can cause milder disease), a patient who is systemically ill with classic dysentery (frequent bloody stools with tenesmus) is most likely to have *Shigella* infection.

C. Presenting symptoms are noted below:

   1. Fever occurs in 30–40%.

   2. Abdominal pain is present in 70–93%.

   3. Mucoid diarrhea is seen in 70–85%.

   4. Bloody diarrhea occurs in 35–55%.

   5. Watery diarrhea is present in 30–40%.

   6. Vomiting is seen in 35%.

D. *Shigella* is a highly infectious organism with as few as 10 organisms causing disease. It can be transmitted by anyone of the 4 Fs: (1) fingers, (2) food, (3) flies, and (4) feces.

Evidence-Based Diagnosis

A. Because of the highly invasive nature of *Shigella*, some of the tests that reveal colonic inflammation are more useful in detecting *Shigella* than other organisms.

   1. Sensitivity of band count > 1% = 85%.

   2. Sensitivity of fecal leukocytes is at least 70%.

B. Stool culture is gold standard.

Treatment

A. *Shigella* dysentery clearly benefits from treatment.

B. Patients who should receive treatment are those who are sick enough to warrant treatment and those with special reasons to be treated for more mild disease (immunosuppressed, healthcare workers).

C. Patients may be treated prior to culture results if suspicion is high.

D. The drug of choice is 500 mg of oral ciprofloxacin twice daily for 3 days.

Alternative Diagnosis: *E coli* Infection

Textbook Presentation

The presentation of *E coli* depends on the type. Enterohemorrhagic *E coli* (EHEC), which is discussed below, usually presents with diarrhea and abdominal pain. The pain is often worse in the right lower quadrant. Bloody diarrhea is very common, while nausea, vomiting, and fever are not.

Disease Highlights

A. There are 3 types of *E coli* that commonly cause diarrheal illnesses in adults.

  1. Enterotoxigenic *E coli* (ETEC)

     a. Symptoms caused by toxin

     b. Watery diarrhea

     c. Common cause of traveler's diarrhea

  2. EHEC

     a. Secretes *Shiga* toxin that is primarily responsible for disease.

     b. Causes a bloody diarrhea in most infected patients

     c. Frequently associated with severe abdominal pain

     d. Fever often absent

     e. Association with hemolytic uremic syndrome. This occurs mainly in children.

  3. Enteroinvasive *E coli* (EIEC) causes bloody diarrhea with tenesmus similar to *Shigella.*

B. EHEC is discussed below. EIEC is the least common and does not differ significantly from other pathogens. ETEC will be discussed at the end of the chapter.

Evidence-Based Diagnosis

A. Patients infected with EHEC are significantly more likely than patients infected with other pathogens to

  1. Report bloody diarrhea

  2. Provide visibly bloody specimens

  3. Not report fever

  4. Have abdominal tenderness

  5. Have a WBC > 10,000/mcL

B. If an organism is isolated from a patient with bloody diarrhea, it is most likely to be *Shigella* or *Campylobacter.*

C. On the other hand, a patient infected with EHEC is more likely to have bloody diarrhea than a patient with *Shigella* or *Campylobacter* infection.

D. Positive culture and detected Shiga toxin are considered diagnostic.

E. Culture for *E coli* O157:H7 must be specifically requested.

F. If culture is negative but toxin is positive, samples need to be submitted to infection control centers to isolate the strain producing this toxin.

Treatment

A. Treatment of EHEC is controversial.

B. Studies have reported no effect of antibiotics, an increase in risk of hemolytic uremic syndrome with some antibiotics (trimethoprim-sulfamethoxazole), and beneficial effects of other antibiotics (fluoroquinolones).

C. The general thinking is that antibiotics are probably not beneficial but that fluoroquinolones are not dangerous.

CASE RESOLUTION

The patient was treated with supportive therapy. Antidiarrheals were withheld because of her bloody diarrhea. Ciprofloxacin was prescribed empirically. Her stool was sent for culture.

Her stool cultures were negative, and her symptoms resolved within 3 days.

The resolution of this case is not surprising. The decision to treat the patient was based on 2 things: she appeared quite ill and the presentation was thought to be consistent with *Campylobacter* infection. Even though stool cultures have the highest yield in patients with bloody stool, about 67% of the cultures will still be negative. Also not surprising is her rapid improvement since this is generally the course of infectious diarrhea.

Treatment of Bacterial Diarrhea and *Campylobacter* Infection

A. Severe diarrhea with bloody stool is sometimes treated empirically while cultures are pending.

B. Ciprofloxacin 500 mg twice daily for 3–5 days is the usual treatment. A few points should be kept in mind when deciding on therapy.

  1. There is evidence that antibiotics improve the outcome of *Shigella* and *Campylobacter* infections.

  2. There is quinolone resistance in some strains of *Campylobacter.* Oral erythromycin (500 mg twice daily for 5 days) is the preferred treatment.

  3. It is controversial whether antibiotics are beneficial for EHEC.

  4. Antibiotics are not beneficial for salmonella.

REVIEW OF OTHER IMPORTANT DISEASES

Travelers' Diarrhea

Textbook Presentation

Patients with traveler's diarrhea usually become ill in the first 5 days of their trips from a temperate climate to a tropical one. They usually have mild symptoms of a gastroenteritis-like illness. Patients are often better by the time they return home.

Disease Highlights

A. Up to 10 million cases yearly

B. May occur with travel to any environment more contaminated than one's home.

C. Disease usually occurs in the first 5 days and resolves in 1–5 days.

D. Predominant cause is *E coli* (ETEC).

E. Symptoms are usually of mild to moderate diarrhea but more severe symptoms can occur.

F. Although ETEC is classic, it is important to consider infections particularly common in certain locations.

   1. St. Petersburg: *G lamblia*

   2. Wilderness streams in Western US: *G lamblia*

   3. Nepal: *Cyclospora, G lamblia*

   4. India: *E histolytica*

G. Because these infections usually occur far from the patient's physician, the doctor's role is usually advisory.

   1. Prevention

      a. Ensure clean water

         (1) Boiled, filtered, or chemically purified local water.

         (2) Carbonated beverages and bottled water

      b. Bismuth before meals

         (1) Decreases risk of diarrhea

         (2) Need to balance against the risk of included salicylates

      c. Prophylactic antibiotics are not recommended unless traveler is at special risk.

      d. Gastric acidity is natural prevention, temporarily discontinue proton pump inhibitors or H_2-blockers, if safe.

      e. CDC website has very useful information for patients.

   2. Advise patients of common mistakes.

      a. Ice and mixed drinks are often made with contaminated water.

      b. Ensure bottled water is sealed and not just bottled tap water.

      c. As the renowned parasitologist Dr. B. H. Kean once said, "The only way to clean lettuce is with a blowtorch."

      d. Any food heated for a prolonged time is potentially dangerous.

      e. Fruit is only safe if the traveler peels it.

Treatment

A. Supportive care

B. Avoid antidiarrheals if dysentery is present.

C. Antibiotics are warranted.

   1. ETEC

      a. Quinolones are the preferred treatment.

      b. Decrease symptoms (from 3 days to 1 day)

   2. Ciprofloxacin, 250 mg twice daily for 3 days

   3. Consider causes of travelers' diarrhea other than ETEC (such as giardiasis, amebiasis), which require different therapies.

Diagnostic Approach: Diarrhea

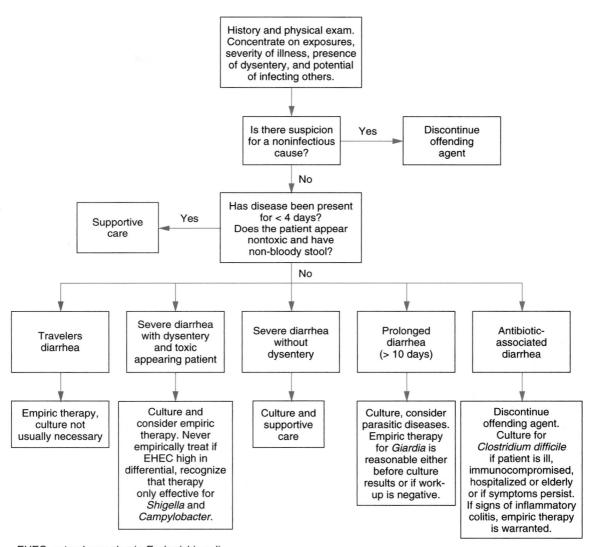

EHEC, enterohemorrhagic *Escherichia coli*.

I have a patient with dizziness. How do I determine the cause?

CHIEF COMPLAINT

PATIENT 1

Mr. J is a 32-year-old man who comes to your office complaining of dizziness.

What is the differential diagnosis of dizziness? How would you frame the differential?

CONSTRUCTING A DIFFERENTIAL DIAGNOSIS

The framework for dizziness recognizes that most patients who complain of dizziness are actually complaining of 1 of 4 distinct sensations (Figure 10–1):

1. Vertigo
2. Near syncope or
3. Disequilibrium
4. Lightheadedness

The first step in evaluating the dizzy patient is to clarify the patient's symptom, since each of the above sensations has its own distinct differential diagnosis and evaluation. Therefore, the first and most important question is "What does it feel like when you are dizzy?" At this point, patients must be given enough time, *without interruptions or suggestions,* to describe their dizziness as clearly as possible. Commonly used descriptions, their precipitants, and differential diagnosis are listed in Table 10–1. The patient's description of the symptom and precipitant helps select the proper sensation, which is crucial to the remainder of the evaluation.

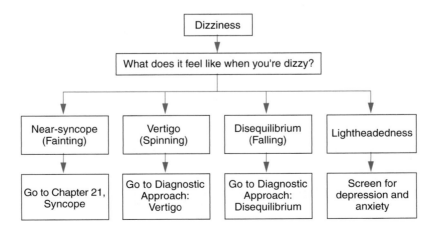

Dizziness Framework

Figure 10–1.

Table 10–1. Classification and characteristics of dizziness.

	Vertigo	Near Syncope	Disequilibrium	Lightheaded
Chief complaint	Spinning or "merry-go-round"	Nearly fainting	Falling Loss of balance	Woozy Floating Vague
Typical precipitants	Turning over in bed Looking up to shelf	Standing	Walking	Stress
Important historical features	Attack duration *CNS signs or symptoms* (eg, dysarthria, ataxia, diplopia, headache, neck pain) Peripheral symptoms (eg, hearing loss, tinnitus)	CAD CHF History of syncope Palpitations Medications Melena or rectal bleeding	Diabetes Neuropathy Visual problems Imbalance Medications	Multiple somatic complaints Feeling down or hopeless Anhedonia
Key physical exam findings	Cranial nerve exam Gait Finger-to-nose exam Dix-Hallpike maneuver	Orthostatic blood pressure and pulse Cardiac exam	Gait Sensation Position sense Cranial nerve exam	
Differential diagnosis	**Peripheral:** BPPV, Vestibular neuritis, Meniere disease **Central:** CVA, MS, cerebellar hemorrhage	Dehydration Hemorrhage Orthostatic hypotension Vasovagal Arrhythmias Hypoglycemia Aortic stenosis PE	Multiple sensory deficits Parkinson disease Cerebellar degeneration or stroke B_{12} deficiency Tabes dorsalis Myelopathy	Depression Generalized anxiety disorder Panic attacks Somatization disorder

CAD, coronary artery disease; CHF, congestive heart failure; BPPV, benign paroxysmal positional vertigo; CVA, cerebrovascular accident; MS, multiple sclerosis; PE, pulmonary embolism.

Differential Diagnosis of Dizziness

A. Vertigo is the most common cause of dizziness. Vertigo may arise from diseases of the inner ear (peripheral) or diseases of the brainstem (central). About 90% of patients with vertigo have a peripheral etiology.

   1. Peripheral

      a. Benign paroxysmal positional vertigo (BPPV)

      b. Labyrinthitis or vestibular neuritis

      c. Meniere disease

      d. Uncommon etiologies: head trauma, herpes zoster, acoustic neuroma, aminoglycosides

   2. Central

      a. Cerebrovascular disease

         (1) Vertebrobasilar insufficiency

         (2) Cerebellar or brainstem stroke

         (3) Cerebellar hemorrhage

         (4) Vertebral artery dissection

      b. Cerebellar degeneration

      c. Migraine

      d. Multiple sclerosis (MS)

      e. Alcohol intoxication

      f. Tumors of the brainstem or cerebellum

B. Near syncope is the cause of dizziness in 6% of cases, and up to 28% in elderly patients with severe dizziness. (See Chapter 21, Syncope.)

C. Disequilibrium is diagnosed in 5% of patients with dizziness.

   1. Multiple sensory deficits

   2. Parkinson disease

   3. Normal-pressure hydrocephalus

   4. Cerebellar disease (degeneration, tumor, infarction)

5. Peripheral neuropathy (ie, diabetes)

6. Dorsal column lesions

    a. B$_{12}$ deficiency

    b. Syphilis

    c. Compressive lesions

7. Drugs (alcohol, benzodiazepines, anticonvulsants, aminoglycosides, antihypertensives, muscle relaxants, cisplatin)

D. Lightheadedness is seen in 16% of dizzy patients.

1. Psychological

    a. Major depression

    b. Anxiety, panic disorder

    c. Somatization disorder

2. Recently corrected vision (new glasses, cataract removal)

Mr. J reports that when he is dizzy, it feels as though the room is spinning. His first episode occurred 3 days ago when he rolled over in bed. The spinning sensation was very intense, causing nausea and vomiting. It lasted less than 1 minute.

At this point, what is the leading hypothesis, and what are the active alternatives? What other tests should be ordered?

ORGANIZING THE DIFFERENTIAL DIAGNOSIS

Clearly, Mr. J is describing vertigo, the most common complaint in patients with dizziness. Patients with vertigo complain that either they or their surroundings are spinning. Vertigo develops secondary to disorders in either the peripheral nervous system or the CNS. Peripheral vertigo usually stems from disease in the semicircular canals or cochlear and is far more common than central vertigo. Central vertigo occurs in patients with disorders involving the brainstem. While less common, central vertigo is serious and may be caused by stroke, hemorrhage, tumors, and MS. Therefore, the first step in the evaluation of a patient with vertigo is to distinguish peripheral from central vertigo. Features that suggest central vertigo include *CNS signs or symptoms, headache, significant imbalance,* and *cerebrovascular risk factors* (Figure 10–2). Central vertigo is suggested by ab-

normalities in the neurologic exam (particularly gait or cranial nerve findings) and nystagmus that is vertical, persistent (> 1 minute), or fails to stop with repetition. Table 10–2 summarizes the differences between peripheral and central vertigo.

On further questioning, Mr. J reports that he had a similar episode 5 years ago. Other than nausea, he has no other symptoms. Specifically, he has not noticed any diplopia (double vision), imbalance, dysarthria (slurred speech), ataxia, incoordination, or headaches. He has no risk factors for cerebrovascular disease (diabetes mellitus, hypertension, coronary artery disease, peripheral vascular disease). He has no prior history of neurologic complaints (eg, unilateral vision loss of optic neuritis or motor weakness). On physical exam, he appears anxious. His vital signs are BP, 110/70 mm Hg; RR, 16 breaths per minute; pulse, 84 bpm; temperature, 37.0 °C. HEENT exam reveals extraocular muscles intact with 15 beats of horizontal nystagmus on left lateral gaze. This stops after repeating the maneuver several times. Optic disks are sharp and visual fields are intact to confrontation. Cardiac, pulmonary, and abdominal exams are normal. On neurologic exam, cranial nerves are intact (except for nystagmus). Hearing is grossly normal. Gait and finger-to-nose testing are normal.

Is the clinical information sufficient to make a diagnosis? If not, what other information do you need?

Fortunately, Mr. J's symptoms and exam point to a peripheral rather than central etiology. You strongly suspect peripheral vertigo. The leading hypothesis is benign paroxysmal positional vertigo. Vestibular neuronitis and Meniere disease are active alternatives (Table 10–3).

Leading Hypothesis: BPPV

Textbook Presentation

BPPV typically presents with acute onset of severe dizziness. Patients describe it as feeling like the room is spinning, which began when they rolled over in bed, looked up (to get something out of a closet), or bent down to tie their shoe. Each episode is *brief* (lasting

Diagnostic Approach: Vertigo

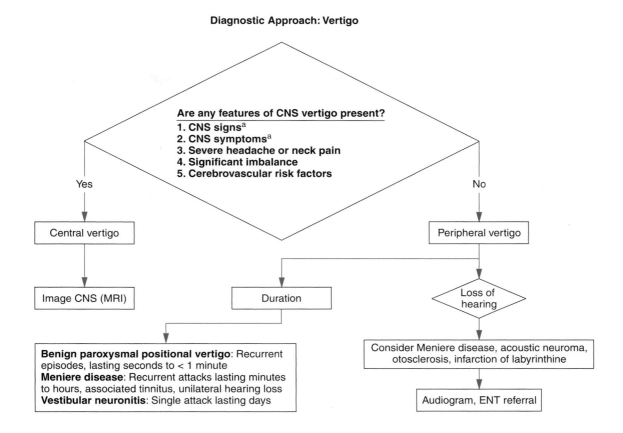

^a**CNS symptoms**: dysarthria, diplopia, abnormal gait, weakness, incoordination
CNS signs: cranial nerve abnormalities, ataxia, positive Romberg, abnormal nystagmus
(eg, nystagmus seen on leftward and rightward gaze, does not fatigue with repetition
of maneuver, lasts > 1 minute, is not suppressed by visual fixation or is purely vertical)

Figure 10–2.

10–20 seconds) rather than *persistent* (as in vestibular neuronitis). However, since the episodes occur in clusters, patients often complain of vertigo that occurs for days or weeks. A careful history can help make this distinction. Symptoms may recur years later (again for a few weeks).

 Determining the duration of a single episode of vertigo is critical to establish the correct diagnosis.

Disease Highlights

A. Most common cause of vertigo

B. Vertigo precipitated by positional changes

C. Vertigo is brief, usually lasting < 15 seconds but may last as long as 90 seconds.

D. Secondary to free-floating canalith within posterior semicircular canal

E. Usually idiopathic; may follow labyrinthitis or head trauma

Table 10–2. Features distinguishing central from peripheral vertigo.

Finding	Peripheral Vertigo	Central Vertigo
CNS symptoms and signs (eg, dysarthria, diplopia [double vision], ataxia, cranial nerve palsies)	Rare	Common
Imbalance	Mild to moderate[a]	Severe
Nystagmus characteristics	Inhibited by fixation Unidirectional Horizontal with torsional component Lasts < 1 minute Fatigues with repetition	Not inhibited by fixation May change direction May be purely vertical or torsional Lasts > 1 minute Does not fatigue
Duration of single episode	Seconds to days	Minutes to indefinite
Risk factors for vascular disease	May be present or absent	Commonly present
Nausea and vomiting	Severe	Variable, may be minimal
Severity of vertigo	Severe	Less severe to none
Hearing loss	May be present in otosclerosis, Meniere disease, and acoustic neuromas	May occur in infarctions involving labyrinth

[a]Patients with peripheral lesions can usually walk, whereas those with central lesions may have great difficulty.

Evidence-Based Diagnosis

A. Positional nystagmus is mixed rotary and vertical component and can be precipitated by the Dix-Hallpike maneuver.

   1. Nystagmus fatigues with repetition of maneuver.
   2. Sensitivity, 42–78%; specificity 94%

B. CNS imaging should be performed in patients with *atypical* findings.

MAKING A DIAGNOSIS

Mr. J's history is characteristic of BPPV. At this point, the Dix-Hallpike maneuver should be performed to evaluate positional nystagmus.

Mr. J reports intense vertigo with the maneuver. Horizontal nystagmus with a rotary component is noted, which lasts for 20 seconds. After repeating the maneuver, the nystagmus disappears.

Have you crossed a diagnostic threshold for the leading hypothesis, BPPV? Have you ruled out the active alternatives? Do other tests need to be done to exclude the alternative diagnoses?

The clinical history and exam point strongly to peripheral rather than central causes. The brief episodes strongly suggest BPPV. Other peripheral causes of vertigo should be considered.

Alternative Diagnoses: Acute Vestibular Neuronitis

Textbook Presentation

Acute vestibular neuronitis typically presents acutely with severe *constant* vertigo and nausea made worse by head turning that lasts for days. Subsequently, patients may complain of *intermittent* vertigo that occurs for weeks to months and is precipitated by head movement.

Table 10–3. Diagnostic hypotheses for Mr. J.

Diagnostic Hypotheses	Clinical Clues	Important Tests
Leading Hypothesis		
Benign paroxysmal positional vertigo	Vertigo lasts seconds, precipitated by rolling over in bed or looking up to shelf Peripheral type nystagmus	Thorough neurologic history and physical exam (to exclude CNS lesions)
Active Alternatives—Most Common		
Vestibular neuronitis	Vertigo lasts for days Peripheral type nystagmus	Thorough neurologic history and physical exam (to exclude CNS lesions)
Meniere disease	Vertigo lasts for minutes to hours Tinnitus, intermittent hearing loss Peripheral type nystagmus	Thorough neurologic history and physical exam Audiogram

Disease Highlights

A. Acute vestibular neuronitis may follow viral infection involving the vestibular nerve.

B. Nausea and vomiting are common.

C. Vertigo typically lasts 2–3 days and may last up to 1 week.

D. Hearing is preserved.

E. Ramsay Hunt syndrome is a variant of vestibular neuronitis: Varicella zoster reactivation involving cranial nerves VII and VIII produces vestibular neuronitis *with* hearing loss and facial weakness. Vesicles are seen in the external auditory canal.

Evidence-Based Diagnosis

A. Diagnosis is usually made clinically.

B. Perform MRI if features suggest CNS lesion.

Treatment

A. Meclizine (antihistamine) and scopolamine (anticholinergic) are drugs of choice in most patients.

B. Promethazine (especially for severe nausea, vomiting)

C. Benzodiazepines have also been used.

D. Medications are sedating. Driving should be avoided.

E. In chronic peripheral vertigo, drugs should be discontinued when vomiting ceases to allow CNS adaptation.

F. Vestibular rehabilitation using exercises that stimulate the labyrinth can promotes CNS adaptation.

Alternative Diagnosis: Meniere Disease

Textbook Presentation

Patients complain of intermittent spells of vertigo. They may note associated ear fullness, unilateral hearing loss, and tinnitus. Spells typically last for minutes to hours (rarely longer than 4–5 hours) and occasionally up to a day.

Disease Highlights

Secondary to excess fluid in the endolymphatic spaces of the inner ear.

Evidence-Based Diagnosis

A. Diagnostic criteria of the American Academy of Otolaryngology and Head and Neck Surgery requires the following for a definite diagnosis

  1. Two spontaneous episodes of vertigo lasting > 20 minutes

  2. Confirmed sensorineural hearing loss

  3. Tinnitus or perception of aural fullness, or both

B. Audiometry should be performed.

  1. Early Meniere disease is characterized by low frequency sensorineural hearing loss.

  2. Hearing can be normal between attacks.

C. Test should be done to rule out syphilis (fluorescent treponemal antibody absorption [FTA-Ab]).

D. Some authors recommend an MRI to rule out CNS lesions (tumors, Arnold-Chiari malformations, MS)

Treatment

A. Specialty consultation is advised.

B. Low salt diet

C. Anecdotal evidence suggest restriction of caffeine and tobacco

D. Diuretics reduce vertigo

E. Surgical therapies are available for patients with refractory incapacitating symptoms.

CASE RESOLUTION

Mr. J's history, physical exam, and response to Dix-Hallpike maneuver are entirely consistent with peripheral vertigo. There are no alarm features to suggest central vertigo. The duration of each vertiginous episode suggests BPPV rather than vestibular neuronitis or Meniere disease. There is no tinnitus or hearing loss to suggest Meniere disease. Further testing is not indicated.

An Epley maneuver is performed resulting in resolution of Mr. J's symptoms (see below). One month later he returns and is feeling well.

Treatment of BPPV

A. Most patients recover regardless of therapy.

B. Epley maneuver allows a canalith to be repositioned and stop vertigo; it is 85–95% effective with 1 treatment. Recurrences can be treated with the same maneuver.

C. Vestibular suppressants (meclizine and benzodiazepines) may delay CNS adaptation and should be used only when necessary.

D. Surgical options are available for patients with refractory symptoms but are rarely necessary.

CHIEF COMPLAINT

PATIENT 2

Mr. D. is a 29-year-old white man who complains of dizziness. Detailed questioning reveals that he has had a constant spinning sensation for the last several weeks. He has no history of similar episodes or hearing loss. Although head movement exacerbates the symptom, it is persistent even when he is still. He has not experienced diplopia (double vision), dysarthria (garbled speech), arm or leg weakness, or visual loss. He has no history of hypertension, diabetes, or cocaine use. He has a prior history of headaches for several years described as unilateral pounding headaches that may last for several hours. These occur approximately 1–2 times per month. Occasionally, the headaches are preceded by scintillating scotomata. Vertigo has never preceded or accompanied the headache. On physical exam his vital signs are BP, 126/82 mm Hg; pulse, 74 bpm; RR, 16 breaths per minute; temperature, 37.0 °C. HEENT exam reveals horizontal nystagmus on leftward and rightward gaze that lasts 1–2 minutes. The nystagmus does not fatigue with repetition of the maneuver. Pupils are equal, round, react to light and accommodation (PERRLA). Cardiac, pulmonary, and abdominal exams are normal. Neurologic exam reveals normal gait, motor strength, sensation, negative Romberg, and intact cranial nerves with the exception of the nystagmus noted above.

At this point, what is the leading hypothesis, and what are the active alternatives? What other tests should be ordered?

ORGANIZING THE DIFFERENTIAL DIAGNOSIS

Again, the first task in the dizzy patient is to properly identify whether the patient has vertigo, near syncope, disequilibrium, or ill-defined lightheadedness. Mr. D is clearly suffering from vertigo. Our next step is to determine whether the disease process is central or peripheral. Mr. D's persistent vertigo, lasting weeks, argues strongly for a central cause. BPPV, Meniere disease, and vestibular neuronitis are not associated with vertigo of such long duration. Furthermore, Mr. D's prolonged nystagmus, which does not fatigue and is bidirectional, strongly suggests a central process.

Possible diagnoses include migraine, cerebrovascular disease, MS, and CNS tumors (Table 10–4). The prior history of headaches and the patient's young age make migraine the leading hypothesis.

 Is the clinical information sufficient to make a diagnosis? If not, what other information do you need?

Leading Hypothesis: Migraine & Vertigo

Textbook Presentation

Classically, migraine sufferers complain of intermittent attacks of severe unilateral throbbing headache associated with photophobia, phonophobia, nausea and vomiting (see Chapter 15, Headache). Headaches may be preceded by a visual aura (scotoma or scintillating lights). Occasionally, an associated symptom is vertigo.

Table 10–4. Diagnostic hypotheses for Mr. D.

Diagnostic Hypotheses	Clinical Clues	Important Tests
Leading Hypothesis		
Migraine	History of recurring throbbing headaches with or without aura Temporal association of headache and vertigo	Thorough neurologic history and physical exam (to exclude CNS lesions) MRI
Active Alternatives—Most Common		
Vertebrobasilar insufficiency	*Risks:* Hypertension, diabetes mellitus, peripheral vascular disease, coronary artery disease, tobacco use, older age, atrial fibrillation, valvular heart disease *CNS signs or symptoms:* diplopia, dysarthria, weakness, ataxia	MRI/MRA Transcranial doppler Angiogram
Cerebellar hemorrhage	*Risks:* HTN, cocaine use, warfarin therapy *Other symptoms:* Severe headache at onset, vomiting, ataxia	Head CT scan or MRI/MRA (see below)
Vertebral artery dissection	*Risks:* Trauma or spinal manipulation *Other symptoms:* Severe headache or neck pain at onset, progressive neurologic deficit with cranial neuropathies, ataxia, weakness	MRA or angiogram
Subclavian steal	Asymmetric arm BP, symptoms with arm exercise, diplopia, dysarthria, weakness, ataxia	Duplex exam, MRA, angiography
Active Alternatives—Must Not Miss		
Multiple sclerosis	CNS lesions developing at different times and places: prior episodes of visual loss (optic neuritis), weakness, diplopia	Brain MRI Oligoclonal bands in cerebrospinal fluid Antibodies to MBP or MOG
Cerebellar tumor	Ataxia, headache	MRI

MBP, myelin basic protein; MOG, myelin oligodendrocyte glycoprotein.

Disease Highlights

A. Migraine affects 11 million people in the United States.

B. Peak age is 30–46 years.

C. Brainstem signs are rare.

D. Vertigo may last minutes to days.

Evidence-Based Diagnosis

A. In patients with vertigo due to migraine, vertigo may precede, be concurrent with, or temporally unrelated to headache.

1. Vertigo was regularly associated with headache in 45% of patients.

2. Vertigo occurred with *and* without headache in 48% of patients.

3. Vertigo and migraine did not occur together in 6% of patients.

B. Consider migraine as an etiology of vertigo in patients with migraine disorder, particularly if temporal association exists between headache and vertigo.

C. Migraine should be considered as a *possible* etiology in patients with a history of migraine and vertigo without a clear temporal association. Other possibilities should be explored.

Treatment

See Chapter 15, Headache.

MAKING A DIAGNOSIS

Have you crossed a diagnostic threshold for the leading hypothesis, migraine? Have you ruled out the active alternatives? Do other tests need to be done to exclude the alternative diagnoses?

Although Mr. D's history suggests a migraine disorder, there is no temporal association of Mr. D's vertigo and migraine. Furthermore, the continuous vertigo is atypical for migraine, and the abnormal neurologic exam (nonfatiguing, bidirectional nystagmus) raises the possibility of a serious CNS disorder, such as cerebrovascular disease, MS, and CNS tumors. You wonder if Mr. D has suffered from a cerebrovascular event.

Alternative Diagnosis: Cerebrovascular Disease

Textbook Presentation

Cerebrovascular disease encompasses a multitude of diseases in which disordered blood supply results in CNS damage. The neurologic symptoms may be transient if blood supply is reestablished within 24 hours (transient ischemic attack [TIA]) or permanent if blood flow is not reestablished within this period (stroke). (Patients with symptoms lasting > 1 hour but < 24 hours often have subclinical infarction.) The location within the brain and the mechanism of the event determine the type of symptoms, their rapidity of onset, and severity.

Disease Highlights

A. Thrombosis

1. Large intracranial or extracranial vessels (ie, middle cerebral artery, carotid artery)

a. Risk factors include older age, hypertension, tobacco use, and diabetes.

b. Occasionally, secondary to hypercoagulable states, vasculitis (ie, Takayasu arteritis, giant cell arteritis), or sickle cell anemia.

2. Small penetrating vessels: Small arteries that penetrate at right angles and are obstructed by arteriolar sclerosis resulting in small cavitary infarcts (lacunar infarcts). Usually secondary to hypertension and involve basal ganglia, internal capsule, thalamus, and pons.

3. May progress in sputtering manner

4. Unusual in patients younger than age 40

5. Headache unusual at onset of symptoms (< 20%)

B. Embolization

1. Sources include left atrium, left ventricle (myocardial infarction), heart valves, aortic arch, and carotid or vertebral arteries.

2. Symptoms maximal at onset and may involve multiple vascular territories.

3. Risk factors include atrial fibrillation, myocardial infarction, congestive heart failure, valvular heart disease, endocarditis, and carotid stenosis.

C. Hypotension may result in symmetric damage to watershed areas including occipital cortex (resulting in blindness), motor strips (resulting in shoulder and hip weakness).

D. Hemorrhage (15%)

1. Intraparenchymal

a. Usually secondary to hypertension

b. Other causes include trauma, amyloid angiopathy, bleeding diathesis (warfarin) or cocaine use. Cocaine may be associated with spasm and thrombosis or intracranial hemorrhage.

   c. Neurologic symptoms and headache progress over minutes to hours.

   d. Headache is present at the onset of symptoms in 50–60% of cases.

   e. Focal deficits common

  2. Subarachnoid (See Chapter 15, Headache)

The remainder of the discussion will focus on the subset of cerebrovascular disorders that frequently involve the brainstem and cerebellum and may result in vertigo or imbalance. This includes vertebrobasilar insufficiency (thrombosis of the large basilar or vertebral arteries), cerebellar hemorrhage or infarction, subclavian steal, and vertebral artery dissection.

1. Vertebrobasilar Insufficiency (VBI)

Textbook Presentation

The classical presentation of VBI is intermittent spells of vertigo associated with other neurologic symptoms, such as diplopia, dysarthria, or ataxia, in the elderly patient who has hypertension or diabetes or both.

Disease Highlights

A. Risk factors include male sex, increased age, hypertension, and diabetes mellitus.

B. Thrombosis accounts for > 80% of episodes. Embolism is the next most common cause.

C. Vertigo is the sole complaint in 25% of patients with VBI. Headache is the most common associated symptom.

D. Dizziness in patients with VBI may be described as tilting rather than spinning.

E. Most patients complain of concurrent diplopia, drop attacks, ataxia, dysarthria, Horner syndrome, other motor problems, or crossed face and body numbness.

F. Symptoms usually last for minutes with VBI (but may persist in patients with stroke or cerebellar hemorrhage).

G. In patients with infarction of the territory supplied by the basilar artery, cranial neuropathies, hemiparesis, and coma may be found.

Evidence-Based Diagnosis

A. 50% of patients have CNS *symptoms* and a normal neurologic exam between the episodes

B. Most common symptom is visual dysfunction (eg, diplopia, field defects, hallucinations, and blindness).

C. Transcranial Doppler, magnetic resonance angiography (MRA), and angiography have been used.

  1. Transcranial Doppler is operator dependent.

  2. Angiography is invasive, but it is the gold standard.

  3. MRI with MRA is procedure of choice:

    a. Noninvasive

    b. 95–97% sensitive and 99% specific for posterior circulation disorders

Treatment

A. Aspirin, clopidogrel, aspirin plus dipyridamole, and warfarin have been used.

B. Warfarin is preferred for patients with stroke and atrial fibrillation.

C. Some clinicians use warfarin for significant vertebral or basilar artery stenosis.

D. Ticlopidine is a second-line drug due to the risk of hematologic toxicity.

E. Modify risk factors

2. Subclavian Steal

(See Chapter 21, Syncope.)

3. Lacunar Infarction of the Pons or Cerebellum

Textbook Presentation

Typically, the presenting symptoms are rapid onset of ataxia or hemiparesis (or both) and sensory symptoms.

Disease Highlights

A. Small, white matter infarcts secondary to obstruction of the small penetrating arteries are present; occasionally, they are cardioembolic in origin.

B. Typically involves basal ganglia, internal capsule, thalamus, and pons.

C. Hypertension and diabetes are risk factors.

D. Incidence in the black population is approximately twice that in the white population.

E. Cortical signs (aphasia, agnosia, hemianopsia) are absent.

F. Symptoms depend on stroke location (Table 10–5).

Evidence-Based Diagnosis

A. CT scan is 30–44% sensitive

B. MRI scan is 86% sensitive.

Table 10–5. Lacunar strokes: Location and associated symptoms.

Location	Typical Symptoms
Internal capsule	Pure unilateral motor stroke involving face, arm, and leg Dysarthria without associated aphasia
Thalamus	Pure sensory stroke (unilateral)
Pons	Ataxia-hemiparesis: (ipsilateral weakness and limb ataxia) Dysarthria, clumsy hand syndrome

C. MRA is unable to visualize small vessel occlusion but can be useful to exclude occlusion of large feeding vessel.

D. Other tests may be useful

  1. Echocardiogram (to look for embolic etiology)

  2. Erythrocyte sedimentation rate (elevated in certain vasculitides).

Treatment

A. Antihypertensive therapy reduces stroke 35–40%.

B. Recombinant tissue-type plasminogen activator (rt-PA) improves outcomes in *carefully selected* stroke patients *only if given within 3 hours of symptom onset. Guidelines for the use of rt-PA have been published and must be followed carefully to avoid intracranial hemorrhage.*

C. Secondary prevention with aspirin or other antiplatelet medication is recommended.

D. Risk factor management (control of diabetes mellitus, hypertension, smoking, and dyslipidemia)

4. Cerebellar Hemorrhage

Textbook Presentation

The textbook presentation of cerebellar hemorrhage is the abrupt onset of headache associated with vomiting, ataxia, and vertigo. The hemorrhage may occur with exertion or at rest. Patients may have incoordination and ataxia. Brainstem compression may produce weakness, cranial nerve abnormalities, coma, and death. Patients with cerebellar infarctions have similar symptoms.

Disease Highlights

A. Cerebellar hemorrhage accounts for 5–16% cases of intracerebral hemorrhages.

B. Etiologies heterogeneous:

  1. Most common: Hypertensive hemorrhage, subarachnoid hemorrhage, amyloid angiopathy, and arteriovenous malformations

  2. Less common: Blood dyscrasias, hemorrhagic infarction, septic emboli, anticoagulant and thrombolytic therapy, neoplasms, cocaine use

C. Demographics

  1. 60% occur in men

  2. Mean age is 61 years

  3. 36% of patients have diabetes mellitus

  4. 32% of patients have hypertension

  5. 14% of patients have coagulation disorders

  6. 16% of patients have liver disease

D. Presentation

  1. Headache is the initial symptom in 80% of patients.

  2. 60% of patients are comatose at admission.

E. Complications

  1. Hydrocephalus (48%)

  2. Chronic disability

  3. Herniation and death

  4. Other: Pneumonia, myocardial infarction, ventricular arrhythmias

F. Poor prognostic factors include

  1. Marked hydrocephalus

  2. Deteriorating consciousness

  3. Stupor and coma (100% mortality without surgery)

Evidence-Based Diagnosis

A. Brainstem findings are common (100% in 1 small study).

B. Laboratory evaluation should include platelet count, INR, partial thromboplastin time

C. Cross sectional imaging is critical.

  1. Noncontrast CT scan is test of choice.

  2. MRI scans have been used.

  3. MRA can demonstrate saccular aneurysms and arteriovenous malformations.

    a. Consider aneurysms and arteriovenous malformations in patients with cerebellar hemorrhage who are younger than age 60 who do not have a convincing history of hypertension. Also consider in patients with a history of cocaine use.

    b. Abnormal results on MRA can be evaluated with cerebral angiography.

  4. Prompt imaging is vital.

Treatment

A. Craniotomy and evacuation can be lifesaving in appropriate patients.

B. Emergent neurosurgical consultation is advised.

C. ICU monitoring is critical.

D. BP should be maintained to optimize cerebral perfusion pressure.

E. Anticoagulation should be reversed, if present.

F. Acute intracranial hypertension can be treated with mannitol, barbiturates, and hyperventilation as temporizing measures to prevent herniation.

5. Vertebral Artery Dissection

Textbook Presentation

Unlike patients with atherosclerotic disease, patients with vertebral artery dissection are usually younger (mean age 48) and complain of severe neck pain, occipital headache, and evolving neurologic symptoms due to progressive involvement of the brainstem. Numbness, hemiparesis, quadriparesis, coma, a locked-in syndrome, or death can result from this uncommon but devastating illness.

Disease Highlights

A. The vertebral artery passes through the transverse process of C1–C6. As C1 rotates on C2, the vertebral artery can be stretched and can be injured initiating dissection and thrombosis. Thrombosis may extend to involve the basilar artery compromising the entire brainstem.

B. Pain (from the dissection) is a common feature.

C. Risk factors differ from patients with typical ischemic stroke. May occur spontaneously or following trauma, chiropractic manipulation, or sporting activity. When secondary to chiropractic manipulation, symptoms develop within 1 hour of procedure in 85% of patients.

Evidence-Based Diagnosis

A. Warning symptoms are present in 54% of cases; the most common are occipital headache and neck pain. These symptoms are usually sudden, severe, and persistent until other neurologic signs develop. Headache preceded other neurologic signs and symptoms by 1–14 days.

B. Signs and symptoms

   1. Pain (neck, head, or both) occurs in 85% of cases.

   2. Vertigo is seen in 57% of cases.

   3. Nausea and vomiting occurs in 53% of cases.

   4. Unilateral facial numbness occurs in 46% of cases.

   5. Unsteadiness is seen in 42% of cases.

   6. Diplopia is present in 23% of cases.

   7. Limb weakness occurs in 11% of cases.

   8. Cerebellar findings are present in 35% of cases.

   9. Isolated vertigo and headache are present in 12% of cases.

C. Neuroimaging: Infarction is seen in 65% of scans.

Treatment

A. A variety of treatments have been used including thrombolysis for associated thrombosis, anticoagulation, and antiplatelet medications.

B. Anticoagulation has been associated with lower mortality than placebo in uncontrolled trials.

C. In various series, 20–50% of patients had no or minor residual defect, 10–56% had major sequelae, and 10–24% died.

 In patients who complain of vertigo *and headache*, migraine, subarachnoid hemorrhage, cerebellar hemorrhage, and vertebral artery dissection should be considered.

 Mr. D reiterates that he has no history of hypertension, cocaine use, known heart disease, neck pain, trauma, or neck manipulation. His only headaches have been those typical of his prior migraines (and do not suggest intracranial hemorrhage). These headaches have not been associated with vertigo.

 Have you ruled out the active alternatives of cerebrovascular disease or MS? Do other tests need to be done to exclude alternative diagnoses? If so, which ones?

Although cerebrovascular disease is common, Mr. D's young age and absence of hypertension, diabetes, and tobacco use make thrombotic cerebrovascular disease unlikely. Subarachnoid or intraparenchymal hemorrhage is unlikely without a history of severe headache, hypertension, or cocaine use. There is no history of neck pain or spinal manipulation to suggest vertebral artery dissection.

However, Mr. D's nystagmus still suggests central vertigo. You wonder if Mr. D may in fact have MS. Although less common in men than women, no other diagnosis is suggested by the clinical features and exam. You order an MRI.

Alternative Diagnosis: MS

Textbook Presentation

The hallmark of MS is CNS lesions that develop in *different CNS locations* and at *different times.* Typically, symptoms worsen in warm environments (ie, in the shower and during exercise). Relapsing-remitting MS, characterized by attacks followed by remission with re-myelination, is usually the presenting form of the disease. Eventually, this form of the disease transforms into the progressive form, characterized by progressive deterioration and axonal loss.

Disease Highlights

A. Women are affected 3 times more than men.

B. Affects 2–4% of first-degree relatives

C. Patients are usually between 18- and 45-years-old at onset.

D. Etiology: Idiopathic inflammatory CNS demyelination

E. Vertigo is the presenting symptom in 5% of patients with MS and is reported in 30–50% of patients with MS; it is commonly associated with other cranial nerve dysfunction.

F. Some studies suggest that Epstein-Barr virus infection may predispose patients to MS.

G. Prognosis at 10 years
   1. 50% of patients require a cane
   2. 15% of patients are wheelchair-dependent

H. Common initial syndromes include
   1. Partial spinal cord syndromes
      a. Band like sensation
      b. Varying degrees of pain, light touch, and proprioceptive loss
      c. Bilateral sensory loss from a certain level downwards
      d. Weakness associated with spasticity and hyperreflexia
      e. Electrical sensation from spine into the limbs that occurs with neck flexion (Lhermitte sign)
   2. Optic neuritis
      a. Patients complain of unilateral visual loss (scotoma)
      b. Pain with extraocular movement is common (92%)
      c. Fundascopic exam is usually normal.
      d. With long-term follow-up, MS develops in up to 60% of patients with optic neuritis (MS develops in 50–80% of patients if the MRI scan is abnormal compared with 6–16% of patients if the MRI scan lacks disseminated features of MS).
   3. Intranuclear ophthalmoplegia (INO)
      a. A lesion interrupts the medial longitudinal fasciculus pathway in the brainstem, which coordinates conjugate eye movement.
      b. On lateral gaze, adduction is impaired and nystagmus develops in the abducting eye.
      c. INO is seen in 33–50% of patients with MS.
      d. INO is not specific for MS; it may develop secondary to vascular disease.

Evidence-Based Diagnosis

A. Diagnosis is primarily clinical, resting on the demonstration of ≥ 2 attacks separated in space and time. Complex criteria have been established.

B. 30% of patients with isolated syndrome progress to MS

C. Brain MRI test of choice
   1. Demonstrates periventricular white matter lesions (lesions may also be seen in other white matter locations)
   2. Sensitivity > 84–90%
   3. Specificity
      a. 71–74%
      b. Ischemia, systemic lupus erythematosus, sarcoidosis and other vasculitides may look similar

D. Spinal MRI is 75% sensitive and is more specific than brain MRI.

E. Cerebrospinal fluid (CSF)
   1. Cell counts are usually normal.
   2. Immunoglobulin (oligoclonal bands) may be elevated
      a. 85–95% sensitive; 92% specific
      b. LR+, 11.3; LR−, 0.11
      c. 25% of patients with oligoclonal bands and 1 event progressed to MS, compared with 9% without bands (at 3 years)

F. Evoked potentials
   1. Visual evoked potentials are 85% sensitive but not specific for MS.
   2. Somatosensory evoked potentials
      a. 77% sensitive

b. Abnormal in 50% of MS patients without sensory signs or symptoms

G. Antibodies against basic myelin protein (BMP) or myelin oligodendrocyte glycoprotein (MOG)

1. These antibodies predict progression to clinically definite MS among patients with an isolated syndrome consistent with MS, an abnormal MRI, and oligoclonal bands.

2. MS develops in 83–95% of patients who have 1 or both anti-MOG and anti-BMP antibodies, while it develops in only 23% of patients in whom both of the antibodies are absent.

H. Differential diagnosis includes other inflammatory CNS diseases ie, acute disseminated encephalomyelitis, transverse myelitis, CNS vasculitis, systemic lupus erythematosus, syphilis, HIV, HTLV 1, neurosarcoidosis, cerebrovascular disease, antiphospholipid syndromes, Lyme disease, migraine

I. Clues to alternative etiology include:

1. Single CNS lesion

2. Unusual age of presentation

3. Spinal lesion in absence of intracranial disease

CASE RESOLUTION

▽2

Mr. D's MRI reveals multiple periventricular and brainstem white matter lesions strongly suggestive of MS. A lumbar puncture is performed and is positive for oligoclonal bands. Antibodies to MOG and MBP proteins are positive. Although the patient has suffered from only 1 clinical event, you are reasonably confident that he has MS. Mr. D refuses initial therapy. He returns 6 months later with unilateral visual loss and eye pain. A diagnosis of optic neuritis is made. This confirms the diagnosis of MS. Mr. D agrees to see a neurologist who initiates interferon therapy. One year later, he is doing well, without any new or persistent symptoms.

Treatment of MS

A. Corticosteroids for acute attacks associated with disability have been demonstrated to be superior to placebo.

B. Disease modifying agents can slow the rate of progression and relapse in relapse-remitting MS. Approved drugs include interferons, glatiramer, and mitoxantrone.

C. Some studies suggest IV immune globulin and anti-integrin antibodies may also be useful in the therapy of MS.

D. Neuropathic pain can be treated with gabapentin, carbamazepine, and valproic acid.

E. Bone mineral density should be monitored in patients with diminished activity or requiring corticosteroids.

F. Specialty consultation is advised.

CHIEF COMPLAINT

PATIENT ▽3

Mrs. P is an 85-year-old woman with diabetes who complains of dizziness. She reports that she has noticed dizziness for several years but that her symptoms seem to be progressing.

When asked to describe her symptoms in more detail, she reports that she feels (and worries) that she might fall. She reports no rotational or spinning sensation. She also reports no history of near or actual fainting.

 At this point, what is the leading hypothesis, and what are the active alternatives? What other tests should be ordered?

ORGANIZING THE DIFFERENTIAL DIAGNOSIS

Mrs. P is complaining of disequilibrium. Disequilibrium can arise from abnormalities of the brain, cerebellum, spinal cord, or peripheral nerves. Possible causes include Parkinson disease, normal-pressure hydrocephalus, cerebellar degeneration (ie, from alcohol), cerebellar stroke, B_{12} deficiency, tabes dorsalis, and multiple sensory deficits. Finally, a multitude of drugs can cause disequilibrium including benzodiazepines, tricyclic antidepressants, alcohol, and aminoglycosides. The neurologic exam is critical in such patients. The cranial nerve exam, gait, and sensory exams may provide critical clues to the diagnosis. Gait disturbances may suggest Parkinson disease (shuffling gait) or cerebellar disease (wide-based gait). Stocking glove sensory deficits are typical of diabetic neuropathy, whereas loss of proprioception suggests posterior column disease (ie, B_{12} deficiency, tabes dorsalis, and some compressive spinal lesions) (Figure 10–3).

> 3
>
> Mrs. P reports that her symptoms occur almost exclusively when she gets up from her bed during the night to go to the bathroom. She has stumbled twice but has never fallen. She reports a long history of cataracts (but has declined surgery). In addition, she has experienced tingling and numbness in her hands and feet for several years. She reports a history of hypertension but no known stroke. She fervently denies any history

> of sexually transmitted disease and was monogamous with her husband. She drinks alcohol rarely. Her medications include hydrochlorothiazide, metformin, triazolam (for sleep), and aspirin. On physical exam, her BP while sitting is 142/70 mm Hg and pulse is 76 bpm; while standing, her BP is 125/55 mm Hg and pulse is 82 bpm. She has bilaterally dense cataracts. Neurologic exam reveals decreased sensation to the monofilament in a stocking glove distribution. She has no resting or intention tremor. Her face is quite expressive. Gait is hesitant but not wide based. She is unsteady during Romberg testing. Finger-to-nose testing is normal.

The key features of Mrs. P's history and physical are her stocking glove neuropathy, diabetes mellitus, cataracts, and nocturnal pattern of symptoms (when the room is dark). In combination, these features suggest multiple sensory deficits, which should be the leading diagnosis. Active alternatives include medications, in particular the triazolam. The history of diabetes mellitus and hypertension increase the possibility of cerebellar stroke, although her neurologic exam does not suggest this or Parkinson disease. Since treatment is available for B_{12} deficiency and tabes dorsalis, they are "must not miss" possibilities. The differential diagnosis is summarized in Table 10–6.

 Is the clinical information sufficient to make a diagnosis? If not, what other information do you need?

Diagnostic Approach: Disequilibrium

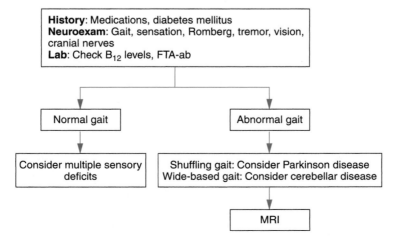

Figure 10–3.

Table 10–6. Diagnostic hypotheses for Mrs. P.

Diagnostic Hypotheses	Clinical Clues	Important Tests
Leading Hypothesis		
Multiple sensory deficits	Symptoms occur in dark environment Visual impairment (cataracts) Peripheral neuropathy Diabetes Orthopedic disorder	Careful neurologic exam
Active Alternatives—Most Common		
Medications	Benzodiazepines Tricyclic antidepressants Aminoglycosides	Discontinue medication
Cerebellar stroke	*Risks:* Hypertension, diabetes mellitus, peripheral vascular disease, coronary artery disease, tobacco use, older age, atrial fibrillation, valvular heart disease *Other symptoms:* Ataxia	MRI/MRA Transcranial doppler Angiogram
Active Alternatives—Must Not Miss		
B_{12} deficiency	Megaloblastic anemia Pancytopenia Vibratory and positional sense deficits	See Chapter 4, Anemia Vitamin B_{12} level MMA level
Tabes dorsalis	Vibratory and position sense deficits History of primary syphilis (painless single ulcerated lesion), secondary syphilis (rash involving palms and soles)	FTA antibody

Leading Hypothesis: Multiple Sensory Deficits

Textbook Presentation

The typical patient is an elderly diabetic who complains of symptoms when arising from their bed during the night. Patients may fall or simply feel as though they are going to fall. Multiple sensory losses and physical deconditioning create imbalance and an unsteady gait. Orthostatic hypotension (aggravated by many medications) and benzodiazepines for sleep may contribute to the symptoms.

Disease Highlights

A. Multiple systems are involved.

B. Typically, at least 2 or more of the following are present:

   1. Visual loss (secondary to myopia, presbyopia, cataracts, macular degeneration)

   2. Priorioceptive loss (neuropathy from diabetes, myelopathy from cervical spondylosis)

   3. Chronic bilateral vestibular damage (from ototoxic drugs)

   4. Orthopedic disorder impairing ambulation

Evidence-Based Diagnosis

A. Ataxia is uncommon (0/14 in one series).

B. Patients with significant ataxia or cerebellar findings should undergo MRI to exclude alternative diagnoses.

MAKING A DIAGNOSIS

Obtaining CNS imaging is often a matter of judgment in patients with disequilibrium. Definite indications for MRI include cerebellar signs on physical exam (ataxia), cranial neuropathies, or history of cerebrovascular accident. Possible indications for CNS imaging include multiple risk factors for cerebrovascular disease.

An MRI reveals mild atrophy, appropriate to age without discrete evidence of prior infarction. Vitamin B_{12} level is normal and FTA-antibody testing for syphilis is negative.

Have you crossed a diagnostic threshold for the leading hypothesis, multiple sensory deficits? Have you ruled out the active alternatives? Do other tests need to be done to exclude the alternative diagnoses?

Alternative Diagnosis: Vitamin B_{12} Deficiency

See Chapter 4, Anemia.

CASE RESOLUTION

Mrs. P's normal MRI effectively rules out cerebellar stroke as a cause of her disequilibrium. She has no findings that suggest Parkinson disease (shuffling gait, resting pill rolling tremor, bradykinesia, or masked facies) and her normal B_{12} level and FTA-antibody exclude the diagnoses of B_{12} deficiency and tabes dorsalis. You conclude that the disequilibrium is caused by multiple sensory deficits.

Treatment of Disequilibrium

A multifaceted approach is often necessary; elements include:

A. Visual correction

B. Night lighting

C. Instructing patients to sit at the edge of the bed prior to standing

D. Modifying medications to minimize orthostatic hypotension (ie, α-blockers, diuretics)

E. When possible, eliminating benzodiazepines, neuroleptics, and any unnecessary medications.

F. Home visits can identify fall risks (electric and telephone cords, loose rugs, etc).

G. Lower limb strength training and balance training have been demonstrated to reduce falls.

H. Hip protectors have been demonstrated to reduce fractures in some studies.

I. Bisphosphonates reduce the risk of fractures in patients with osteoporosis.

Mrs. P's hydrochlorothiazide is reduced by half. In addition, the triazolam is discontinued, and she reluctantly agrees to cataract surgery. A home visit reveals multiple risk factors for falls (including loose rugs), which are removed. Nightlights are installed. One year later Mrs. P reports that she remains unsteady on standing but has not fallen or sustained a hip fracture.

REVIEW OF OTHER IMPORTANT DISEASES

Other Dizziness

Textbook Presentation

Patients with a variety of psychiatric disorders including panic disorder, generalized anxiety disorder, depression, and somatization disorder may complain of ill-defined dizziness. The dizziness is often of long duration (years) and poorly defined. Patients may complain of lightheadedness, fogginess, feeling woozy, mental fuzziness, loss of energy, or a wobbly or a floating sensation. Patients may complain of other associated symptoms particularly if they have panic attacks including chest pain, shortness of breath, perioral paresthesias, tingling in the hands and feet, and lightheadedness.

Disease Highlights

A. 20–38% of patients attending a specialty dizzy clinic demonstrated panic disorder.

B. Psychiatric symptoms may develop without any identifiable organic cause or develop after episodes of true vertigo or syncope.

C. Symptoms are, in part, secondary to hyperventilation, which leads to hypocapnia resulting in decreased cerebral blood flow.

D. Patients may complain of lightheadedness or near syncope.

E. Depression is reviewed in Chapter 22, Unintentional Weight Loss

F. Milder variants of somatization disorder are more common than the full-blown entity. Such variants may be precipitated by stress or minor physiologic disturbances. Paradoxically, such patients are often disturbed by negative test results rather than reassured.

Evidence-Based Diagnosis

A. *Continuous sensation of vertigo > 1–2 weeks* without daily variation is likely psychogenic. This is to be distinguished from intermittent vertigo, recurring for weeks, precipitated by motion.

B. One study reported 62% of patients with hyperventilation had other significant psychiatric disorders.

C. Symptom reproduction by induced hyperventilation is nonspecific.

D. Care must be taken before ascribing dizziness to a psychiatric etiology.

1. Multiple studies have demonstrated a high prevalence of anxiety (22–67%) among patients with well-defined *organic* etiologies to their dizziness.

2. Anxiety scores were as high in patients with acute labyrinthine failure and vestibular dysfunction as among patients with no vestibular diagnosis.

3. This suggests that dizziness from an organic etiology leads to significant psychiatric distress in many patients and that the psychiatric symptoms may be sequelae of the dizziness rather than the cause of the dizziness.

4. A fear response, symptom focus or abnormal mood that progresses to panic disorders, somatization disorders, or major depression may develop.

E. In some patients an initial episode of vertigo or near syncope precipitates intense fear, which magnifies normal physiologic sensations. The history should review the first episode whenever possible.

F. Certain physical findings suggest a psychogenic disturbance.

1. Moment-to-moment fluctuations in impairment

2. Excessive slowness or hesitation

3. Exaggerated sway on Romberg, improved by distraction

4. Sudden buckling of knee, typically without falling

5. A cautious "walking on ice" pattern

Treatment

A. Appropriate evaluation considers organic etiologies and evaluates appropriate possibilities.

B. Discuss patient's concerns and fears about the diagnosis.

C. Educate patient not to overly restrict physical activities since this impairs CNS compensation and may worsen the physical symptoms.

D. For patients with hyperventilation, breathing in and out of paper bag, increases inspired $PaCO_2$, and thereby arterial $PaCO_2$. This increases cerebral blood flow and improves symptoms.

E. Selective serotonin reuptake inhibitors (SSRIs) and benzodiazepines are used in patients with panic attacks and anxiety disorders. SSRIs are preferred due to potential problems with benzodiazepines (eg, dependence, tolerance, exacerbation of symptoms on discontinuation, sedation, interference with cognition in the elderly, and exacerbation of depression).

F. Cognitive and behavioral therapy have also been effective.

I have a patient with dyspnea. How do I determine the cause?

CHIEF COMPLAINT

PATIENT 1

Mr. C is a 64-year-old man who comes to see you complaining of shortness of breath.

What is the differential diagnosis of dyspnea? How would you frame the differential?

CONSTRUCTING A DIFFERENTIAL DIAGNOSIS

The differential diagnosis of dyspnea is long and can be difficult to remember. However, since most causes of dyspnea can impair oxygen delivery, the differential diagnosis can be organized by considering the components of oxygen delivery. The determinants of oxygen delivery are the cardiac output, (determined by stroke volume and heart rate), Hgb, and oxygen saturation. Abnormal oxygen saturation (hypoxia) is usually secondary to some pulmonary pathology, either in the alveoli, airways, blood vessels, pleura, or interstitium. Looking at each item in turn allows us to deduce a fairly comprehensive differential diagnosis of dyspnea.

Differential Diagnosis of Dyspnea

A. Stroke volume
   1. Congestive heart failure (CHF)
   2. Coronary ischemia
   3. Valvular heart disease (ie, aortic stenosis, mitral regurgitation [MR], aortic regurgitation, mitral stenosis)

B. Heart rate
   1. Tachycardia
      a. Atrial fibrillation (AF) and other supraventricular arrhythmias
      b. Ventricular tachycardia
   2. Bradycardia

C. Hgb (anemia)

D. Oxygen saturation
   1. Alveolar diseases
      a. Pulmonary edema
      b. Pneumonia
   2. Airway diseases
      a. Suprathoracic narrowing
         (1) Laryngeal edema
         (2) Epiglottitis
         (3) Croup
      b. Intrathoracic narrowing
         (1) Asthma
         (2) Chronic obstructive pulmonary disease (COPD) (see Chapter 23, Wheezing & Stridor)
   3. Vascular disease
      a. Pulmonary emboli
      b. Pulmonary hypertension
   4. Pleural disease
      a. Pneumothorax
      b. Pleural effusions
         (1) Transudative
            (a) CHF
            (b) Cirrhosis
            (c) Nephrotic syndrome
            (d) Pulmonary embolism

(2) Exudative

    (a) TB

    (b) Cancer

    (c) Parapneumonic effusions

    (d) Connective tissue diseases

    (e) Pulmonary embolism

5. Interstitial diseases

    a. Edema

    b. Inflammatory

      (1) Organic exposures (eg, hay, cotton, grain)

      (2) Mineral exposures (eg, asbestos, silicon, coal)

      (3) Idiopathic diseases (eg, sarcoidosis, scleroderma, systemic lupus erythematosus, Wegeners)

    c. Infectious (ie, *Pneumocystis* pneumonia)

Over the last 2 years, Mr. C has noticed worsening dyspnea on exertion. He complains of shortness of breath with minimal exertion. He is unable to walk around his house without resting. Several years ago, Mr. C could walk several blocks without any difficulty. He notes that he is unable to sleep lying flat due to shortness of breath (orthopnea), and he sleeps on a recliner for the last 6 months. Occasionally, he awakes from sleep acutely short of breath (paroxysmal nocturnal dyspnea). He complains that his feet are swollen.

Always quantify the increase in dyspnea *from baseline*. Significant changes suggest serious disease and warrant thorough evaluations.

Past medical history is notable for a myocardial infarction 2 years ago. Vital signs are temperature, 37.0 °C; RR, 24 breaths per minute; pulse, 110 bpm; BP, 120/78 mm Hg. His pulse is regular with an occasional irregularity. Cardiac exam reveals JVD to the angle of the jaw in the upright position, a grade II/VI systolic murmur at

the apex, and a positive S_3 gallop. Lung exam reveals crackles half of the way up from the bases bilaterally. He has 2+ pretibial edema to the knees.

At this point, what is the leading hypothesis, and what are the active alternatives? What other tests should be ordered?

ORGANIZING THE DIFFERENTIAL DIAGNOSIS

Although the differential diagnosis of dyspnea is broad, the patient has numerous signs and symptoms that point to a cardiac etiology. The jugular venous distention (JVD), S_3 gallop, and peripheral edema are all consistent with cardiac disease. The leading hypothesis with these signs and symptoms is CHF secondary to his previous myocardial infarction. Alternative diagnoses include valvular heart diseases (ie, MR, aortic stenosis, or aortic regurgitation). This particular murmur is most consistent with MR. Mr. C's irregular pulse also raises the possibility of AF. Finally, cardiac ischemia presenting as dyspnea rather than pain is a must not miss possibility. Table 11–1 lists the differential diagnosis.

Pursue highly specific positive physical findings (in this case the S_3 gallop and JVD); they should help drive the diagnostic search.

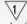

A chest x-ray and ECG are performed.

A chest x-ray often provides key information and is *always* indicated in the evaluation of patients with dyspnea.

Is the clinical information sufficient to make a diagnosis of CHF? If not, what other information do you need?

Table 11–1. Diagnostic hypotheses for Mr. C.

Diagnostic Hypothesis	Clinical Clues	Important Tests
Leading Hypothesis		
Congestive heart failure	History of myocardial infarction, poorly controlled hypertension S_3 gallop, JVD Crackles on lung exam Peripheral edema	Echocardiogram ECG
Active Alternatives—Most Common		
Valvular disease Mitral regurgitation	Blowing systolic murmur at apex radiating to axilla	Echocardiogram
Aortic stenosis	Systolic murmur at right upper sternal border radiating to neck Loss of A2	Echocardiogram
Aortic regurgitation	Early diastolic murmur left sternal border	Echocardiogram
Atrial fibrillation	Irregularly irregular pulse	ECG Echocardiogram
Active Alternatives—Must Not Miss		
Angina	Exertional symptoms History of CAD or risk factors (diabetes mellitus, male sex, tobacco use, hypertension, hypercholesterolemia)	ECG Stress test Coronary angiogram

Leading Hypothesis: CHF

Textbook Presentation

CHF refers to a syndrome in which any of several structural or functional cardiac disorders impair cardiac output. Patients typically have fatigue, dyspnea on exertion, orthopnea, paroxysmal nocturnal dyspnea, and edema. Often, there is an antecedent history of either myocardial infarction or poorly controlled hypertension.

Disease Highlights

A. Pathophysiologic classification: CHF may be secondary to either systolic dysfunction or diastolic dysfunction. CHF may also be classified based on whether the primary process affects the left ventricle (LV) or the right ventricle (RV).

   1. Systolic failure

      a. Most common pathophysiology underlying CHF.

      b. Coronary artery disease (CAD) accounts for 2/3 of all cases of CHF.

   c. Other causes include longstanding hypertension, alcohol abuse, or viral cardiomyopathy.

   d. Less common causes include postpartum cardiomyopathy, drug toxicity (ie, doxorubicin), and idiopathic cardiomyopathy.

   2. Diastolic heart failure

      a. Diastolic heart failure accounts for 20–50% of all CHF cases.

      b. Diastolic *dysfunction* occurs when LV wall thickness increases and LV compliance decreases. The increased LV pressure is transmitted to the pulmonary capillaries.

      c. Decreased LV compliance impairs LV filling and lowers cardiac output.

      d. The increasing pulmonary capillary pressures and decreased cardiac output can cause dyspnea and fatigue.

      e. Symptomatic patients are classified as having diastolic heart failure. This can occur despite normal LV systolic function.

f. The most common cause of diastolic dysfunction is hypertension.

g. A less common cause is aortic stenosis.

h. Uncommon causes include infiltrative cardiomyopathies (eg, hemochromatosis, amyloidosis)

3. Right- versus left-sided CHF

    a. CHF may involve the LV, the RV, or both.

    b. Common causes of LV failure include CAD, hypertension, and alcoholic cardiomyopathy.

    c. Common causes of RV failure include severe pulmonary disease (especially COPD) and advanced LV failure.

    d. Peripheral edema, JVD, and fatigue may be seen in LV or RV failure, but pulmonary edema is seen only in LV failure.

B. Functional classification (NYHA): Descriptively useful. May be limited prognostically by the ability of patients to move from 1 class to another with therapy.

    1. Class I: Asymptomatic

    2. Class II: Symptoms on ordinary exertion (ie, climbing stairs)

    3. Class III: Symptoms with less than ordinary exertion (ie, walking on flat surface)

    4. Class IV: Symptoms at rest

C. Complications

    1. Electrical: Heart block, ventricular tachycardia, AF, sudden death

    2. Stroke and thromboembolism

        a. 2–4% annual incidence.

        b. Risk increases if AF coexists

    3. Structural: MR

    4. Death

        a. Symptomatic mild to moderate CHF: 20–30%/y

        b. Symptomatic severe CHF: up to 50%/y

        c. Mechanism of death

            (1) Sudden in 50% (secondary to ventricular tachycardia or asystole)

            (2) Progressive heart failure in 50%

Evidence-Based Diagnosis

A. History and physical

    1. Overview

        a. Clinical signs and symptoms are affected by

            (1) Patient's current volume status

            (2) Chronicity. In *chronic* heart failure, many signs and symptoms are often absent despite marked impairment of LV function *and* marked volume overload.

        b. Clinical findings are not sensitive for CHF

        c. CHF cannot be ruled out by the absence of clinical findings.

        d. Certain findings (S_3 and JVD) are highly specific and significantly increase the likelihood of CHF when present.

    2. Orthopnea

        a. Orthopnea is nonspecific. It is found in patients with CHF and pulmonary disease.

        b. Sensitivity for CHF varies depending on patient's clinical condition. Sensitivity is 91% in patients with severe CHF.

    3. S_3 gallop

        a. An S_3 gallop occurs when a large volume of blood rushes from the left atrium (LA) into the LV at the start of diastole. (Just after S_2.)

        b. Virtually pathognomonic of volume overload and occurs most commonly in patients with decompensated CHF.

        c. Highly specific for CHF (approximately 95%)

        d. Low sensitivity

            (1) 69% sensitive when pulmonary capillary wedge pressure (PCWP) > 22 mm Hg

            (2) 89% sensitive when PCWP > 34 mm Hg

        e. Associated with increased risk of hospitalization and death

    4. S_4 gallop

        a. Occurs when the LA contracts and sends blood into the LV (just before S_1).

        b. An S_4 gallop may be heard in some normal patients and in many patients with hypertension and LV hypertrophy.

        c. S_4 is *not* specific for CHF (approximately 50%)

    5. JVD

        a. Defined as $\geq$ 3 cm of elevation above the sternal angle (Figure 11–1)

        b. Highly specific for CHF (> 95%); may occur in RV or LV failure

        c. Not sensitive for CHF

            (1) < 50% for all patients with CHF

            (2) 21% among patients with CHF and normal PCWP

            (3) 68% among patients with markedly increased PCWP (mean 34 mm Hg)

        d. Associated with increased risk of hospitalization and death

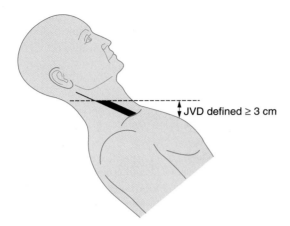

JVD defined ≥ 3 cm

Figure 11–1. Measurement of jugular venous distention. (Modified from McGee S. *Evidence Based Physician's Diagnosis*, p. 402. Copyright © 2001. With permission from Elsevier.)

6. Crackles
   a. Crackles are not specific for CHF. They may be heard in cases of alveolar edema secondary to CHF, acute respiratory distress syndrome, pneumonia, and other diseases.
   b. Sensitivity is low (16%) in severe, chronic, stable CHF.
   c. Sensitivity is only 67% in patients with marked elevation in PCWP (mean 34 mm Hg).
7. Combined findings: 42% of patients with severe chronic CHF (mean ejection fraction [EF] 18%) and PCWP > 22 mm Hg had none of following: crackles, increased JVP, or edema.

 The absence of clinical findings (S_3, JVD) does not exclude CHF. Patients may have severe CHF despite the absence of crackles, increased JVP, or edema.

B. The chest x-ray is *not* highly sensitive for CHF.
   1. Cardiomegaly
      a. 53–58% sensitive for moderate CHF; 87% sensitive for severe CHF
      b. 90% specific
   2. Pulmonary edema is seen in only 25–63% of patients with CHF.
C. ECG can provide evidence of prior myocardial infarction or LV hypertrophy. It can neither rule in nor rule out CHF.

D. Brain natriuretic peptide (BNP)
   1. Secreted by LV or RV in response to increased volume or pressure or both
   2. Often elevated in patients with increased LV end-diastolic pressure as cause of their dyspnea
   3. Levels increase proportionately to the degree of CHF
   4. BNP does not distinguish CHF secondary to systolic dysfunction from CHF secondary to diastolic dysfunction.
   5. BNP is elevated in patients with right-sided CHF (ie, due to cor pulmonale or pulmonary embolism [PE]), limiting its ability to distinguish dyspnea from left heart failure versus pulmonary disease.
   6. Low BNP helps rule out CHF as a cause of dyspnea.
      a. BNP 100 pg/mL
         (1) Sensitivity 90% specificity 76%
         (2) LR+, 3.8; LR−, 0.13
      b. BNP < 50 pg/mL is 97% sensitive for CHF.
   7. Some authorities use the following criteria to interpret BNP levels:
      a. < 100 pcg/mL: CHF unlikely
      b. 100–500 pcg/mL: Indeterminate
      c. > 500 pcg/mL: CHF most likely diagnosis
E. 2-D echocardiogram is the test of choice to diagnose CHF
   1. Systolic and diastolic function can be evaluated.
   2. Regional systolic dysfunction suggests an ischemic etiology.
   3. Valvular function can be assessed.
F. Radionuclide tests can quantify EF but cannot access LV wall thickness or valvular abnormalities.

MAKING A DIAGNOSIS

Mr. C has several features that are highly specific for CHF. His history of prior myocardial infarction, orthopnea, and most importantly the clinical findings of JVD and an S_3 gallop are highly specific for CHF.

 Have you crossed a diagnostic threshold for the leading hypothesis, CHF? Have you ruled out the active alternatives? Do other tests need to be done to exclude the alternative diagnoses?

Alternative Diagnosis: MR

Textbook Presentation

Patients with MR may be identified due to an asymptomatic holosystolic murmur at the apex or during an evaluation of such symptoms as shortness of breath, dyspnea on exertion, orthopnea, and fatigue. Alternatively, it may be discovered during the evaluation of patients with AF.

Disease Highlights

A. Trivial symptomatic MR is commonly discovered on echocardiogram (80% of patients). The remainder of the discussion will focus on patients with more significant regurgitation.

B. Etiologies: MR develops secondary to damaged mitral leaflets (primary) or a dilated mitral annulus (secondary).

   1. Primary MR

      a. Causes include mitral valve prolapse, rheumatic heart disease, and endocarditis.

      b. Although most patients with mitral valve prolapse never require valve replacement, it is the most common cause of MR and the need for valve replacement.

   2. Secondary MR

      a. CHF: LV dilatation leads to mitral annular dilatation and MR.

      b. Ischemic MR: Leaflet tethering shortens the mitral apparatus, resulting in MR.

C. Pathophysiology

   1. Chronic regurgitation may lead to LV dilatation and irreversible LV impairment.

   2. LA dilatation may lead to AF.

D. Disease progression is slow. Average delay from diagnosis to symptoms is 16 years. However, in patients with severe MR, the annual mortality is 5%.

E. Complications include dyspnea, pulmonary edema, AF, and sudden death.

Evidence-Based Diagnosis

A. Physical exam: The typical murmur is a blowing, holosystolic murmur heard at the apex that radiates to the axilla. S_2 may be inaudible.

   1. Grade 3 or louder systolic murmur

      a. 85% sensitive, 81% specific for moderate to severe MR

      b. LR+, 4.5; LR−, 0.19

   2. S_3 gallops may be heard due to increased flow across the mitral valve.

B. ECG and chest x-ray may demonstrate LA enlargement or LV hypertrophy. Neither is sensitive or specific for the diagnosis.

C. Echocardiography is the test of choice to diagnosis and quantify MR. Transesophageal echocardiography provides more precise details on valve anatomy and may help determine whether valve repair (vs replacement) is an option.

Treatment

A. Serial echocardiography

   1. Serial echocardiography is important to detect signs of *LV dysfunction, which may occur despite the absence of symptoms.*

   2. Echocardiography can be performed every 5 years for patients with mild MR and annually for patients with moderate MR.

   3. For patients with severe MR and decreased LV function, echocardiography has been recommended every 6 months.

B. Afterload reduction has not been shown to delay the need for valve replacement. It may be useful in the subset of patients with MR secondary to CHF (see below). In these patients, the reduction in LV volume may decrease MR.

C. Treat underlying ischemia.

D. Endocarditis prophylaxis

E. Valve repair or replacement

   1. Indicated for patients with symptoms or evidence of LV dysfunction. Criteria for LV dysfunction include LV end-systolic diameter ≥ 45 mm or EF of ≤ 60%. Valve repair or replacement is also considered in patients with AF or pulmonary hypertension.

   2. Surgical outcome is poor in patients with an EF < 30% or LV end-systolic diameter > 55 mm.

      a. Mitral valve repair or replacement decreases regurgitation from the LV, leading to increased LV afterload.

      b. Surgery may precipitate heart failure.

      c. Predicting which patients will benefit from valve replacement is difficult.

   3. Valve repair versus replacement: Valve repair is superior to valve replacement (when technically feasible). Valve repair is associated with substantially decreased operative mortality (1–2% vs 5–10%), does not require subsequent anticoagulation, and is associated with a significantly better EF.

Alternative Diagnosis: Chronic Aortic Regurgitation

Textbook Presentation

Patients with chronic aortic regurgitation typically complain of progressive dyspnea on exertion or the sensation of a pounding heart. Alternatively, the diagnosis may be suspected when an early diastolic murmur is detected by a careful examiner.

Disease Highlights

A. Secondary to damaged aortic leaflets or dilated aortic root

B. Etiologies

1. Valvular abnormalities: Rheumatic carditis, bacterial endocarditis, congenital bicuspid valves, collagen vascular disease, fenfluramine and phentermine

2. Aortic root dilatation: Ascending aortic aneurysm, Marfan syndrome, aortic dissection, syphilitic aortitis

C. Pathophysiology

1. Regurgitation results in LV remodeling and LV hypertrophy to maintain wall stress. Eventually, the LV dilates to maintain effective stroke volume.

2. The increasing preload and afterload may eventually result in LV dysfunction and a falling EF. LV end-diastolic pressure increases and pulmonary congestion and dyspnea result.

3. Significant LV dysfunction can be irreversible. Valve replacement should be performed before irreversible LV dysfunction and CHF develop (see below).

4. Progression to LV dysfunction or symptoms in patients with normal LV function develops in 4% of patients per year.

5. Regurgitation results in a rapid drop of BP during diastole, as blood flows back into the LV. This results in a wide pulse pressure (pulse pressure = systolic BP − diastolic BP).

6. The wide pulse pressure results in many of the classic physical findings, such as bounding pulses and head bobbing.

7. A systolic murmur suggesting aortic *stenosis* may be heard.

   a. Regurgitation results in increasing end-diastolic volumes.

   b. Stroke volumes increase to maintain forward flow.

c. The increased cardiac output may exceed the capacity of even a normal aortic valve to accommodate flow, resulting in "functional" aortic stenosis.

Evidence-Based Diagnosis

A. Wide pulse pressures are not specific for aortic regurgitation. Other causes include anemia, fever, pregnancy, cirrhosis, thyrotoxicosis, and patent ductus arteriosa.

B. Auscultation

1. May demonstrate an early decrescendo *diastolic* murmur following S_2. Best heard at the left sternal border.

   a. Auscultation is more sensitive for moderate to severe aortic regurgitation.

   b. Sensitivity is 0–64% among students and residents.

   c. Sensitivity is 80–95% among experienced cardiologists.

2. Austin Flint murmur

   a. Aortic regurgitant streams may impact the mitral valve leaflets during diastole resulting in functional mitral stenosis and a late diastolic murmur over the apex.

   b. Sensitivity varies from 0% to 100%.

   C. Doppler echocardiography is the test of choice.

D. Exercise testing can help access LV function during stress.

E. Echocardiography is the test of choice.

Treatment

A. Echocardiography is recommended every 6 months in asymptomatic patients with moderate to severe aortic regurgitation to assess LV function and aid in the determination of the need for and timing of valve replacement.

B. Asymptomatic patients with moderate to severe aortic regurgitation

1. Afterload reduction reduces regurgitation, the rate of progression of cardiac enlargement, and the need for valve replacement.

2. Indications for afterload reduction include moderate to severe aortic regurgitation with either LV enlargement or hypertension.

3. Options include nifedipine or ACE inhibitors.

4. β-Blockers are relatively contraindicated. Prolonged diastole increases regurgitation and accelerates progression.

C. Endocarditis prophylaxis

D. Valve replacement corrects aortic regurgitation but results in problems associated with a mechanical or bioprosthetic valve. Careful consideration as to the appropriate timing of replacement is critical. Valve replacement should be undertaken before irreversible LV dysfunction develops. (However, even patients with EF < 35% benefit from surgery.) Indications are based on symptoms and LV dysfunction:

1. Class III or IV CHF regardless of EF

2. Class II CHF in patients with normal LV function but progressive LV dilatation or falling EF

3. Moderate to severe aortic regurgitation undergoing coronary artery bypass grafting

4. LV EF < 50%

5. LV end-systolic diameter > 50–55 mm or end-diastolic diameter > 70–75 mm

6. Some authorities recommend valve replacement for patients with class II CHF and no evidence of LV dysfunction or dilatation.

7. Aortic root dilatation: Patients with root sizes > 50–55 mm in men or > 40 mm in women should have valve replacement.

8. Replacement valves may be either mechanical or bioprosthetic (eg, porcine valves). Mechanical valves are more durable and are often chosen for young patients to minimize the need for subsequent aortic valve replacement. However, patients with mechanical valves require lifelong anticoagulation. Older patients (> 70 years) with shorter life expectancies and higher bleeding risks while receiving anticoagulation therapy often receive bioprosthetic valves.

Alternative Diagnosis: Aortic Stenosis

See Chapter 21, Syncope.

Alternative Diagnosis: AF

Textbook Presentation

Classically, patients with AF seek medical care for palpitations. Patients may complain of shortness of breath and dyspnea on exertion. The abrupt onset of palpitations and tachycardia may prompt patients to be seen emergently. In other patients, AF may be detected during a routine office visit when an irregularly irregular pulse is noted and evaluated.

Disease Highlights

A. AF is the most common clinical arrhythmia.

1. Seen in 1% of patients who are 60 years old

2. Seen in 5% of patients who are 70–75 years old

3. Seen in 10% of patients older than 80 years

B. May be episodic or persistent

C. Secondary to multiple wavelets of excitation that meander around the atria

D. Etiologies

1. Most common etiologies are hypertension, CAD, and CHF.

2. Other etiologies include alcoholic heart disease, valvular heart disease, cor pulmonale, thyrotoxicosis, and PE.

E. Complications

1. Worsening CHF due to loss of atrial kick; especially important in patients with stiff LV (ie, diastolic dysfunction)

2. Stasis promotes thrombus formation. Subsequent embolization results in stroke and other systemic emboli.

   a. AF accounts for 1/6 strokes at an annual cost of $6.6 billion.

   b. Stroke is more common in patients with AF who have other clinical risk factors:

      (1) Valvular heart disease

      (2) Prior transient ischemic attack or stroke

      (3) Increasing age

      (4) Hypertension

      (5) Diabetes

      (6) CHF

      (7) Gender (women affected 1.5–3.0 times more than men)

 Elderly patients with AF are at higher risk for stroke but are also at higher risk for falls and complications from warfarin therapy.

Evidence-Based Diagnosis

A. Easily recognized on ECG (Figure 11–2)

B. Episodic AF can be detected with Holter monitoring or event recorders.

Treatment

A. Evaluation

1. Baseline echocardiogram to assess LV function and stroke risk

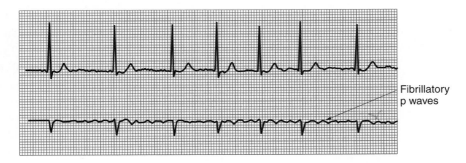

Figure 11–2. ECG of atrial fibrillation demonstrating irregularly spaced QRS complexes and fibrillatory p waves.

2. Obtain baseline thyroid function tests to rule out hyperthyroidism.

3. Electrolyte testing is recommended.

4. Consider evaluation for other etiologies (eg, PE)

B. Rhythm control versus rate control

1. Cardioversion should be performed immediately in unstable patients.

2. In stable patients, 2 options exist: rhythm control or rate control

   a. Rhythm control attempts to restore normal sinus rhythm using cardioversion and antiarrhythmic agents.

   b. Rate control allows persistent AF. The *ventricular* response is controlled with atrioventricular nodal blocking agents (eg, β-blockers, diltiazem, verapamil, or digoxin).

   c. Rhythm control and rate control results in similar outcomes and stroke rates.

   d. Rate control is the recommended strategy in most patients. Patients with symptoms or exercise intolerance may choose rhythm control.

   (1) Uses β-blockers, diltiazem, verapamil, or digoxin

   (2) Digoxin

      (a) Less effective at controlling ventricular response during activity

      (b) Useful in patients with decreased LV function

      (c) Second-line drug

   e. Rhythm control therapy

   (1) AF < 48 hours duration: Administer heparin at presentation followed by cardioversion. Maintain anticoagulation therapy for 4 weeks after cardioversion.

(2) AF > 48 hours duration:

   (a) Anticoagulation therapy for 3 weeks and then perform cardioversion or perform transesophageal echocardiography. If there is no evidence of LA thrombus or spontaneous contrast on transesophageal echocardiography, administer heparin and perform cardioversion.

   (b) For either strategy, maintain anticoagulation therapy for 4 weeks after cardioversion.

(3) The probability of conversion to normal sinus rhythm decreases the longer the AF lasts.

(4) Multiple antiarrhythmic drugs have been used to convert patients to normal sinus rhythm. Flecainide should be avoided in patients with a history of CAD or LV dysfunction. Cardiac consultation is advised.

(5) Surgery (MAZE procedure) can dissect the atrium into pieces too small to allow AF to persist and is used in a few centers.

C. Stroke prevention in chronic AF

1. Aspirin reduces risk by 22% compared with placebo

2. Warfarin reduces risk by 68% compared with placebo

3. Indications for warfarin in patients with AF include factors that increase risk of cerebrovascular accident

   a. Valvular heart disease

   b. Prior transient ischemic attack or cerebrovascular accident

   c. CHF (Even asymptomatic patients, with moderate to severe LV function and AF, have a markedly increased stroke rate [9.3%/y].)

d. Hypertension

e. Diabetes mellitus

f. Age > 75 years

g. Transesophageal echocardiogram demonstrating LA thrombus or spontaneous contrast.

4. Low risk patients

a. Young patients without valvular heart disease, transient ischemic attack or cerebrovascular accident, CHF, hypertension, or diabetes mellitus are at lowest risk for cerebrovascular accident on aspirin therapy (1%/year).

b. Risk of hemorrhage in patients taking warfarin is approximately 1.3%/y.

c. Such patients should have careful discussions to decide between aspirin and warfarin therapy.

5. Contraindications to warfarin therapy include recent GI or CNS hemorrhage, uncontrolled hypertension, noncompliance, syncope, or alcoholism.

Alternative Diagnosis: CAD

See Chapter 6, Chest Pain.

CASE RESOLUTION

Mr. C undergoes a transthoracic echocardiogram, which reveals marked systolic dysfunction and an EF of 18%. There are regional wall motion abnormalities. The anterior wall is very hypokinetic. There is no significant aortic stenosis or aortic regurgitation. MR is mild. An EKG reveals normal sinus rhythm with evidence of prior myocardial infarction.

Mr. C's echocardiogram confirms CHF. The regional wall motion abnormalities suggest an ischemic etiology, likely secondary to his prior infarction. A stress test to rule out reversible ischemia would be appropriate. The echocardiogram rules out significant valvular heart disease as the primary etiology of his dyspnea.

A stress thallium study is performed. This reveals a large prior myocardial infarction but no reversible ischemia. The EF is 20%.

The stress test confirms prior myocardial infarction as the cause of Mr. C's CHF without evidence of active ischemia.

Mr. C is admitted for treatment of his CHF. He starts a salt-restricted diet and is given diuretics, ACE inhibitors, and β-blockers (when his CHF is controlled). The diuresis results in a 20-lb weight loss, and his dyspnea on exertion improves markedly. His orthopnea resolves. He remains stable at follow-up 5 years later.

Treatment of CHF

A. Prevention: Hypertension therapy decreases the incidence of CHF by 30–50%.

B. Initial laboratory tests: BUN, creatinine, electrolytes, CBC, and TSH

C. Multiple therapies have been demonstrated to reduce morbidity and mortality in patients with systolic dysfunction and CHF.

1. ACE inhibitors

a. Indicated in symptomatic and asymptomatic patients

b. Angiotensin receptor blockers (ARBs) may be used when a troublesome cough develops in patients taking ACE inhibitors.

c. ARBs may cause angioedema in patients who had angioedema while taking ACE inhibitors

d. Hydralazine and nitrates may be used in patients who had angioedema while taking ACE inhibitors

2. β-Blockers

a. β-Blockers reduce morbidity and mortality for all stages of CHF, including severe CHF (EF < 25%).

b. Carvedilol has been shown to be superior to metoprolol.

c. Initiate therapy when patients are euvolemic.

3. Spironolactone

a. Reduces mortality in patients with class IV CHF.

b. Contraindications include creatinine > 2.0 mg/dL, serum potassium > 5.0 mEq/L

D. Digoxin

1. Reduces hospitalizations but not mortality.

2. Low serum concentrations are as effective as higher concentrations.

3. ACC/AHA guidelines restrict digoxin to symptomatic patients.

E. Diuretics (loop or thiazides)

1. Mainstay of therapy to treat edema and pulmonary congestion.

2. The clinical assessment of volume status is critical. Increasing weight, edema, JVD, pulmonary edema, or an S_3 gallop suggests patients are volume overloaded.

3. However, multiple studies demonstrate that patients with severe chronic CHF and marked volume overload (by PCWP) may have no signs of CHF.

4. Therefore, patients with dyspnea should undergo aggressive diuresis while monitoring renal function.

F. Daily weights

G. Sodium restriction

H. Control of hypertension

I. Asymptomatic patients status post MI or with decreased EF should be treated with an ACE inhibitor and a β-blocker.

J. Nonsteroidal anti-inflammatory drugs increase fluid retention and have been associated with worsening CHF and precipitating CHF.

K. Automatic implantable cardiac defibrillator (AICD)

1. A substantial proportion of deaths in patients with CHF are sudden, presumably secondary to ventricular tachycardia and ventricular fibrillation.

2. AICDs are indicated in select patients with CHF, especially in patients who have survived cardiac arrest and in patients with syncope and sustained ventricular tachycardia.

L. Influenza and pneumococcal vaccination

M. ACC/AHA guidelines recommend the detection and correction of underlying cardiac ischemia in patients with angina or risk factors for CAD. Options include catheterization or stress tests to detect reversible ischemia. In CHF patients who do not have known CAD, angina, or risk factors for CAD, consensus is less clear about the usefulness of noninvasive imaging.

N. Heart transplantation is an option for a few patients with severe CHF refractory to intensive medical therapy.

O. Treatment of diastolic dysfunction

1. Most clinical trials focus on patients with systolic dysfunction

2. ACC/AHA treatment guidelines for diastolic dysfunction

    a. Control hypertension

    b. Control ventricular rate for patients with AF

    c. Diuretics to control peripheral and pulmonary edema

    d. Coronary revascularization for patients with reversible ischemia

    e. The effectiveness of ACE inhibitors, β-blockers, or ARBs is less well established. Recent studies suggest ARBs decrease hospitalizations in patients with diastolic heart failure.

CHIEF COMPLAINT

PATIENT 2

Mrs. L is a 58-year-old woman who arrives at the emergency department with a chief complaint of shortness of breath. She reports that this has developed gradually over the last 3–6 months. Six months ago, she was able to walk as far as she wanted without any shortness of breath. Now she is experiencing dyspnea even walking around her house. She denies any episodes of acute shortness of breath, chest pain, or hemoptysis. She denies wheezing. She has no history of myocardial infarction, hypertension, or known heart disease. She smoked 1 pack of cigarettes per day for 10 years and quit when she was 28 years old. She drinks 1 glass of wine per week. She works as an accountant and spends her free time with her grandchildren. She has no unusual hobbies.

 At this point, what is the leading hypothesis, and what are the active alternatives? What other tests should be ordered?

ORGANIZING THE DIFFERENTIAL DIAGNOSIS

Mrs. L's shortness of breath is not only severe but markedly worse than baseline. Both of these features should prompt a thorough investigation. Unfortunately, the clinical information does not suggest a specific diagnosis. There is no history of CAD, hypertension, or alcohol abuse to suggest CHF nor is there a significant tobacco history to suggest COPD. A careful exam is vital to look for helpful clues.

On physical exam, the patient appears comfortable at rest, but becomes markedly dyspneic with ambulation. Vital signs are BP, 140/70 mm Hg; pulse, 72 bpm; temperature, 37.1 °C; RR, 20 breaths per minute. Conjunctiva are pink. Lung exam is clear to percussion and auscultation. There are no crackles or wheezes. Cardiac exam reveals a regular rate and rhythm. S_1 and S_2 are normal. There is no JVD, S_3, S_4, or murmur. There is only trace peripheral edema. Abdominal exam is normal. A chest x-ray is normal. A CBC is normal.

Despite a thorough exam, the leading diagnosis is unclear. In such cases, it is particularly important to systematically review the differential diagnosis in order to arrive at the correct diagnosis. Each item on the list should be reviewed in light of the history and physical to determine whether it remains in the differential and should be explored further, or whether the existing information makes it highly unlikely.

Refer to the differential diagnosis listed at the beginning of the chapter. CHF is not particularly suggested by the history and physical exam, but it cannot be excluded given the low sensitivity of the S_3 gallop and JVD. The patient denies any history of chest pain, but dyspnea is occasionally an anginal equivalent, thus CAD remains a possibility. The absence of a murmur makes MR and aortic stenosis unlikely, since the clinical exam is 85–90% sensitive for these conditions. The clinical exam is less sensitive for aortic regurgitation (see above). Therefore, aortic regurgitation remains on the differential diagnosis. An arrhythmia is essentially ruled out by the patient's normal heart rate during symptoms. Anemia is ruled out by the normal CBC. Pneumonia seems highly unlikely given the absence of cough, fever, or infiltrate on chest film. Alveolar diseases are unlikely given the normal chest x-ray. Asthma remains a possibility although this is not particularly suggested by the history or physical. COPD is effectively ruled out by the trivial smoking history. PE cannot be excluded by the current information and remains on the list, although the presentation is not particularly classic for PE. Since PE is associated with a high mortality, it should be considered a must not miss possibility. A significant pleural effusion or pneumothorax are ruled out by the normal chest x-ray, which also makes interstitial disease unlikely (al-

though not impossible). We can now focus on the clinical clues and diagnostic tests for these remaining possible diagnoses (CHF, CAD, aortic regurgitation, asthma, and PE). Table 11–2 lists the differential diagnosis.

A methodical approach to the differential diagnosis is vital whenever the leading diagnosis is unclear or when the leading hypothesis cannot be confirmed.

In terms of CAD, she denies any history of exertional chest pain or pressure and has minimal coronary risk factors. (Her last cholesterol level was normal [180 mg/dL] with an HDL of 70 mg/dL. She has no history of diabetes mellitus, no family history of CAD, and no recent tobacco use.) With respect to asthma, she denies any history of wheezing or worsening cough associated with cold, exercise, pets, or dust. With respect to PE, she denies any history of chest pain with inspiration, hemoptysis, immobilization, surgery, or family history of venous thromboembolism. She does take hormone replacement therapy (HRT).

An echocardiogram reveals normal LV function and a normal aortic valve. Pulmonary function tests reveal normal peak flows and a methacholine challenge test is also normal.

Considering each diagnosis in turn, the patient's physical exam and echocardiogram exclude CHF. The patient's pretest probability of CAD is quite low given her age, sex, and risk factors (3.2%; see Chapter 6, Chest Pain). In addition, the Framingham data suggest the likelihood of a coronary event in a female patient with these CAD risk factors to be < 1% over the ensuing 8 years. The normal echocardiogram also excludes significant aortic regurgitation and the history as well as the normal PFTs with methacholine challenge make asthma very unlikely. Although her history sounds atypical for PE, she is taking HRT, a known risk factor for venous thromboembolism. Given the exclusion of the other diagnoses, PE becomes more probable. You revise your differential diagnosis and make PE both your leading and must not miss diagnosis.

Is the clinical information sufficient to make a diagnosis of PE? If not, what other information do you need?

Table 11–2. Diagnostic hypotheses for Mrs. L.

Diagnostic Hypothesis	Clinical Clues	Important Tests
Active Alternatives—Most Common		
Congestive heart failure	Poorly controlled hypertension or history of myocardial infarction S_3 gallop, JVD Crackles on lung exam Peripheral edema	Echocardiogram
Coronary artery disease	History of symptoms with exertion (eg, chest pain, pressure) Risk factors for	Exercise stress tests coronary artery disease
Aortic regurgitation	Early diastolic murmur left sternal border	Echocardiogram
Asthma	History of wheezing, chest tightness, worsening cough with cold, exercise, pets, mold	Peak flow Pulmonary function tests Methacholine challenge Response to treatment
Active Alternatives—Must Not Miss		
Pulmonary embolism	Pleuritic chest pain Risk factors (immobilization, postoperative or postpartum states, estrogen therapy, cancer, thrombophilia)	Helical CT scan Ventilation-perfusion scan Pulmonary angiography Duplex leg exam

Leading Hypothesis: PE

Textbook Presentation
Classically, sudden onset of shortness of breath and severe chest pain that increases with inspiration are the presenting symptoms. Patients may complain of hemoptysis and associated leg swelling.

Disease Highlights
A. Pathophysiology: Most commonly occurs when a lower extremity venous thrombosis embolizes to the lung. Upper extremity thrombi may cause PE.
   1. 80% of patients with PE have deep venous thrombosis (DVT)
   2. 48% of patients with DVT have PE (often asymptomatic)
B. Symptoms vary markedly from asymptomatic to death. Massive obstruction may result in RV failure and death.
C. 3-month mortality is 17.5%
D. Diagnosis is difficult. PE is eventually ruled out in 80% of patients who are evaluated.
E. Risk factors for venous thromboembolism

1. Age (2 × increased risk per decade)
2. Estrogenic factors
   a. Obesity
   b. Oral birth control pill (OBCP) (3 × increased risk)
   c. HRT (2 × increased risk)
3. Immobilization
4. Postoperative or postpartum states
5. Cancer
6. Thrombophilia
   a. Antiphospholipid antibodies: Present in 2–8.5% of patients with venous thromboembolism
   b. Factor V Leiden
      (1) Most common thrombophilia
      (2) Mutation in factor V causes resistance to cleavage by activated protein C
      (3) 11% of patients with DVT
      (4) 2.7 × increased risk of venous thromboembolism in patients with factor V Leiden mutation

(5) Combined with OBCP, mutation increases risk 35 times

c. Prothrombin gene mutation

d. Protein C or S deficiency (rare)

    (1) Protein C and S are naturally occurring anticoagulants

    (2) Deficiency is associated with hypercoagulability.

    (3) Synthesis of protein C and S requires vitamin K.

    (4) Warfarin decreases synthesis of both factors

    (5) Assays for protein C and S must be performed while patients are not taking warfarin.

e. Antithrombin III deficiency (also rare): Assay must be done while patient is not taking heparin.

f. Hyperhomocysteinemia: 3 × increased risk of venous thromboembolism

Evidence-Based Diagnosis

A. No clinical finding is sensitive for PE

  1. Prevalence of various findings in patients with PE

    a. Risk factor for PE, 80%

    b. Sudden onset of dyspnea, 73%

    c. Pleuritic pain, 44–74%

    d. Hemoptysis, 13–28%

    e. Pleural rub, 3%

    f. Tachycardia, 30–70%

    g. Shortness of breath, chest pain, and hemoptysis, 33%

    h. Isolated dyspnea, 25%

    i. Syncope, 5%

    j. Leg swelling, 17%

    k. $PaO_2 < 80$ mm Hg on room air, 74%

 Patients with PE are often *not* hypoxic. Therefore, normal oxygen does not rule out PE. (On the other hand, unexplained hypoxia, particularly in the company of a normal chest x-ray, may raise the suspicion of PE.)

B. A few findings are highly specific and increase the likelihood of PE in patients evaluated for PE.

  1. Pleural rubs, 98% specific

  2. Hemoptysis, 92% specific

 The classic presentation of PE is actually the exception. Patients may have very few symptoms. A low index of suspicion must be maintained for the diagnosis of PE.

C. Chest film

  1. Normal in 50% of patients with PE

  2. May reveal focal oligemia, wedge-shaped infiltrate, or pleural effusions

D. ECG

  1. Useful to diagnose other conditions (ie, myocardial infarction)

  2. Certain findings suggest PE but are unusual (50% sensitive, 88% specific)

    a. S1Q3T3

    b. T wave inversion in V1–V4

    c. Transient right bundle-branch block

E. D-dimers

  1. Fibrin breakdown products

  2. Elevated in many conditions: surgery, trauma, cancer, end-stage renal disease, and venous thromboembolism

  3. Nonspecific. Elevated levels do not diagnose venous thromboembolism

  4. Sensitivity to rule out venous thromboembolism depends on assay used.

    a. Enzyme-linked immunosorbent assay (ELISA) and quantitative rapid ELISA are more sensitive than other assays (95–98%; LR–, 0.05–0 .11).

    b. Other D-dimer assays are not sensitive enough to rule out venous thromboembolism.

    c. A negative quantitative rapid ELISA markedly decreases the likelihood of PE and effectively rules out PE in patients with a low to moderate pretest probability of PE.

F. Angiography

  1. Gold standard

  2. Invasive; serious complications occur in 0–3% of patients

  3. Usually reserved for patients in whom there is a high index of suspicion in whom other tests are nondiagnostic

G. Ventilation-perfusion scan ($\dot{V}/\dot{Q}$)

  1. Radio-isotope infused and inhaled

  2. Ventilation images and perfusion images are compared.

  3. *High probability scan*

    a. Multiple areas of absent perfusion with normal ventilation

b. 60% sensitive, 96% specific

c. LR+, 15; LR−, 0.4

d. The probability of PE is 88% in patients with a high probability scan

4. *Normal or near normal perfusion scan*

  a. Seen in 0–2% of patients with PE

  b. A normal scan effectively rules out PE

5. *Nondiagnostic scan (low or intermediate)*

  a. Matched areas of ventilation and perfusion abnormality

  b. 67% of patients who undergo V̇/Q̇ testing have this pattern

  c. Neither rules in or out PE

H. Helical CT scan

  1. Noninvasive

  2. May demonstrate filling defects in proximal pulmonary arteries

  3. Positive findings highly specific for PE

  4. Makes alternative diagnosis in 25% of patients (lymphadenopathy, tumor, aortic dissection)

  5. Insensitive for peripheral pulmonary emboli

  6. Overall sensitivity is 70%.

I. Helical CT scan combined with duplex exam of the legs

  1. 1 study suggests that the combined study is 99% sensitive

  2. Limited follow-up weakens conclusions

J. Diagnostic algorithm (Figure 11–3)

  1. Patients pretest probability can help determine extent of work-up.

  2. Initial study is usually helical CT scan or V̇/Q̇ scan. V̇/Q̇ scan has higher negative predictive value but is less useful in patients with underlying lung disease and an abnormal chest film. Local expertise may also determine initial test of choice.

Diagnosis of DVT

A. Given the overlap of PE and DVT (and the same therapy), the diagnosis of DVT is often taken as evidence of concomitant PE.

B. Leg swelling is found in only 50% of patients with DVT.

The clinical exam is insensitive for the diagnosis of DVT. Clinicians must have a low threshold for ordering duplex studies.

1. Clinical prediction rule can help predict risk (Table 11–3).

  a. Unlikely risk group: Incidence of DVT 5.5%

  b. Likely risk group: Incidence of DVT 27.9%

2. Duplex ultrasonography

  a. Test of choice

  b. 95–99% sensitive for symptomatic proximal DVT; 96% specific

  c. LR+, 24; LR−, 0.05

  d. 75% sensitive for DVT below the knee

  e. Incidence of symptomatic DVT < 1% in patients with initial negative color duplex exam.

  f. Patients with increasing symptoms should be reevaluated.

3. Other options include venography (invasive) and magnetic resonance direct thrombus imaging (accurate but costly).

MAKING A DIAGNOSIS

A helical infused chest CT scan or V̇/Q̇ scan would be an appropriate choice at this time. A V̇/Q̇ scan is ordered.

The ventilation reveals normal homogeneous ventilation. The perfusion demonstrates multiple perfusion deficits. The combination of multiple perfusion defects with normal ventilation qualifies as a high probability for PE scan.

Have you crossed a diagnostic threshold for the leading hypothesis, PE? Have you ruled out the active alternatives? Do other tests need to be done to exclude the alternative diagnoses?

The high probability scan is very predictive of PE. At this point, PE is ruled in and further confirmation is unnecessary. There is no need for further testing to exclude alternative diagnoses.

Alternative Diagnosis: Asthma

See Chapter 23, Wheezing & Stridor.

Diagnostic Approach: Pulmonary Embolism

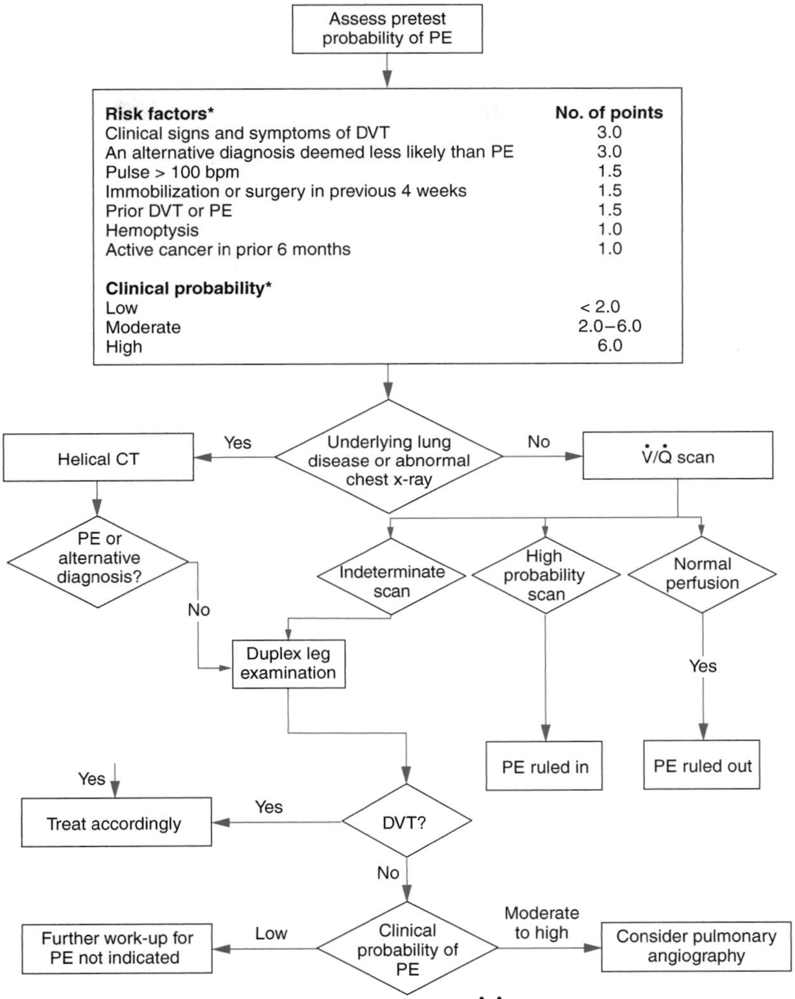

PE, pulmonary embolism; DVT, deep venous thrombosis; V̇/Q̇, ventilation-perfusion.

Figure 11–3. (*This box is reproduced with permission by Wells PS, Anderson DR, Rojer M, et al. Derivation of a simple clinical model to categorize patients probability of pulmonary embolism: Increasing the models validity with the simplified D-dimer. *Thromb Haemosc* 2000;83:416–420.)

Alternative Diagnosis: CAD

See Chapter 6, Chest Pain.

CASE RESOLUTION

2

A hypercoagulable work-up is sent to assess future risk of recurrence (prior to heparin and warfarin therapy). Her HRT is stopped. Mrs. L is started on low-molecular-weight (LMW) heparin and warfarin. At follow-up 6 months later, she reports feeling better. Her anticoagulation therapy has been uncomplicated.

Treatment of PE

A. Initiate treatment with LMW heparin, unfractionated IV heparin, or adjusted-dose subcutaneous heparin.

Table 11–3. Clinical prediction rule for DVT.[a]

Clinical Characteristic	Score
Active cancer (patient receiving treatment for cancer within the previous 6 months or currently receiving palliative treatment)	1
Paralysis, paresis, or recent plaster immobilization of the lower extremities	1
Recently bedridden for 3 days or more, or major surgery within the previous 12 weeks requiring general or regional anesthesia	1
Localized tenderness along the distribution of the deep venous system	1
Entire leg swollen	1
Calf swelling at least 3 cm larger than that on the asymptomatic side (measured 10 cm below tibial tuberosity)	1
Pitting edema confined to the symptomatic leg	1
Collateral superficial veins (nonvaricose)	1
Previously documented DVT	1
Alternative diagnosis at least as likely as DVT	−2

[a]A score of 2 or higher indicates that the probability of DVT is likely; a score of less than 2 indicates that the probability of DVT is unlikely. In patients with symptoms in both legs, the more symptomatic leg is used. DVT, deep venous thrombosis.

Reproduced with permission from Wells PS. Evaluation of D-dimer in the diagnosis of suspected deep-vein thrombosis. *N Engl J Med* 2003;349:1227–1235. Copyright © 2003. Massachusetts Medical Society. All rights reserved.

B. LMW heparin is more convenient and may result in slightly less recurrent venous thromboembolism than standard unfractionated heparin. LMW heparin may offer a survival benefit in patients with cancer. The bioavailability of LMW heparin is difficult to predict in morbidly obese patients and patients with renal insufficiency. Consultation is recommended for such patients.

C. Warfarin is started at the same time as heparin or LMW heparin. Heparin is discontinued when the INR has been therapeutic for 2 consecutive days.

D. An initial warfarin dose of 10 mg/d for 2 days is superior to 5 mg/d in well-nourished outpatients not taking antibiotics.

E. The target INR is 2.0–3.0.

F. Patients with venous thromboembolism secondary to the antiphospholipid syndrome may require more intensive anticoagulation. The optimal target INR is uncertain.

G. Patients with venous thromboembolism secondary to active cancer have a high rate of recurrence during warfarin therapy. LMW heparin is superior.

H. For massive PE or severe iliofemoral thrombosis, heparin therapy should be continued for approximately 10 days.

I. Long-term anticoagulation: Duration of therapy

1. Warfarin is effective *during* therapy. For many patients, the risk of recurrence returns when warfarin is discontinued.

2. The risk of recurrence varies depending on the precipitating risk factor for the initial venous thromboembolism. From lowest to highest risk (Table 11–4):

   a. Postoperative or postpartum patients

   b. Other short-term risk factors (immobilization)

   c. Idiopathic venous thromboembolism (no clinical risk factors or thrombophilia)

   d. Thrombophilic states

   e. Antiphospholipid syndrome

   f. Active cancer

3. The risk of recurrence is also affected by the persistence of DVT at the completion of therapy.

4. Patients with venous thromboembolism secondary to postoperative or postpartum states should be treated for 6 months.

5. Consider long-term therapy for patients with venous thromboembolism and any of the following:

   a. Recurrent venous thromboembolism

   b. Cancer

   c. Thrombophilia

Table 11–4. Recurrence rate of VTE.

Risk Category	Annual Recurrence Rate (%)	
Postpartum or postoperative state	0	
Short-term risk factor	Duplex[a] (−)	Duplex (+)
	0	7.1
Idiopathic VTE	4.4	7.5
Thrombophilic state	10	23
Cancer (on active therapy)	18–34[b]	
Men	6.1%	
Women	1.7%	
D-dimer measured after completion of therapy		
< 250	2.4%	
≥ 250	5–6%	

[a]Duplex result at the completion of 3 months of anticoagulation.
[b]Recurrence rates for patients with active cancer are despite active therapy. The recurrence rate was 18% on low-molecular-weight heparin and 34% on warfarin.
VTE, venous thromboembolism.

6. The optimal duration for patients with idiopathic venous thromboembolism is unclear.

   a. Whether subsequent duplex exams or D-dimer levels should guide therapy is unproven.

   b. One study reported a higher rate of recurrence in men than in women after a first idiopathic venous thromboembolism (6.1%/y vs 1.7%/y)

   c. One study reported a higher recurrence rate in patients with elevated D-dimer levels at the completion of therapy (Table 11–4)

7. Ximelagatran is a new oral thrombin inhibitor anticoagulant under study.

   a. Requires no monitoring of anticoagulation

   b. Markedly reduces risk of recurrent venous thromboembolism compared with placebo in patients who have been treated for 6 months with warfarin (1.9%/y vs 8.4%/y)

   c. Not associated with increased risk of hemorrhage

   d. Increased transaminases in 6% of patients; 1 liver fatality

8. Patients with symptomatic isolated calf vein thrombosis should be treated with anticoagulation for at least 6–12 weeks. If for any reason anticoagulation is not administered, serial noninvasive studies of the lower extremity should be performed over the next 10–14 days to assess for proximal extension of thrombus.

J. Inferior vena caval procedures: Indications for placement

   1. Contraindication or complications of anticoagulant therapy

   2. Recurrent venous thromboembolism that occurs despite adequate anticoagulation

   3. Chronic recurrent embolism with pulmonary hypertension

   4. Inferior vena cava filters are associated with an increased risk of subsequent DVT (but not PE).

K. Prevention of venous thromboembolism

   1. Many hospitalized patients benefit from prophylactic anticoagulation to decrease the risk of venous thromboembolism.

   2. The intensity of the prophylaxis depends on the risk. At particularly high risk are patients undergoing hip replacement. Guidelines are updated frequently by the American College of Chest Physicians and printed in the journal *Chest.*

L. Work-up for thrombophilia: Duration of therapy may be affected by presence of underlying thrombophilia. Clear guidelines for routine testing not determined. Consider tests for thrombophilic states listed above particularly in patients without clear precipitant of venous thromboembolism.

Diagnostic Approach: Dyspnea

History: HPI: **Quantify magnitude, change and time course.** *Asthma*: Wheezing, coughing, cold-induced symptoms; *CHF*: Orthopnea, PND, history of HTN or MI; *CAD*: DM, hypercholesterolemia, HTN, tobacco use, family history of premature CAD or exertional chest pain; *Pneumonia*: Cough, fever, sputum production; *PE*: Hemhoptysis, pleuritic chest pain, leg swelling, immobilization, recent surgery, active cancer, family history of VTE; history of connective tissue disease
Social history: Tobacco use, high-risk sexual behavior, lifetime occupational and vocational work exposures
Medications: HRT, OBCP, bleomycin, amiodarone
Physical exam: Vital signs, lung exam (wheezing, crackles), cardiac exam (rhythm, edema, JVD, S_3, S_4, murmur), FOBT
Baseline lab tests: Hct, chest x-ray, ECG

Clues		Consider This Diagnosis	Tests
History	Physical		
MI, CAD, HTN, alcohol abuse, orthopnea, PND, history of CHF	S_3, **JVD, bilateral lung crackles**	CHF	Echocardiogram
Exertional chest pain, MI, CAD, DM, other CAD risk factors		Coronary ischemia	Stress test, angiography
Rheumatic heart disease	Significant **murmur**	Valvular heart disease	Echocardiogram
Tobacco use, wheezing, cold or exercise-induced cough	Wheezing, decreased breath sounds	COPD or asthma	PFTs, bronchodilator response, methacholine challenge test
Pleuritic chest pain, immobilization, cancer, estrogen therapy, postoperative or postpartum, leg swelling	JVD, hypotension, loud S_2, **pleural rub,** unilateral leg edema	PE	$\dot{V}/\dot{Q}$ scan, helical CT scan, leg dopplers, angiography
Connective tissue disease, Raynaud, vocational or occupational exposures	Arthritis, erythema nodosum, malar rash, **diffuse lung crackles**	Interstitial lung disease	PFTs, high-resolution chest CT scan
High-risk sexual exposures, injection drug use	Kaposi sarcoma, **thrush,** skin pop marks, bilateral crackles	HIV-associated infection: (PCP, TB, bacterial pneumonia)	HIV test, CD4, bronchoscopy
Palpitations	**Irregular pulse**	Arrhythmia	ECG, holter, event monitor
Fever, productive cough, alcohol or drug abuse	Fever, crackles	Pneumonia (bacterial, TB, aspiration)	Chest x-ray
Melena, rectal bleeding, menorrhagia	Conjunctival pallor	Anemia	Hct
Nephrotic syndrome, cancer, cirrhosis, CHF	Dullness to percussion, ↓ breath sounds	Pleural effusion	Chest x-ray

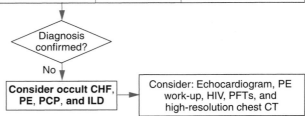

Diagnosis confirmed?

No

Consider occult CHF, PE, PCP, and ILD → Consider: Echocardiogram, PE work-up, HIV, PFTs, and high-resolution chest CT

HPI, history of present illness; CHF, congestive heart failure; PND, paroxysmal nocturnal dyspnea; HTN, hypertension; MI, myocardial infarction; DM, diabetes mellitus; CAD, coronary artery disease; PE, pulmonary embolism; VTE, venous thromboembolism; HRT, hormone replacement therapy; OBCP, oral birth control pills; JVD, jugular venous distention; FOBT, fecal occult blood test; PCP, *Pneumocystis* pneumonia; TB, tuberculosis; PFTs, pulmonary function tests; $\dot{V}/\dot{Q}$, ventilation-perfusion.

12

I have a patient with edema.
How do I determine the cause?

CHIEF COMPLAINT

PATIENT 1

Mrs. V is 62-year-old woman with leg edema for the past 2 weeks.

What is the differential diagnosis of edema? How would you frame the differential?

CONSTRUCTING A DIFFERENTIAL DIAGNOSIS

Edema is defined as an increase in the interstitial fluid volume and is generally not clinically apparent until the interstitial volume has increased by at least 2.5–3 L. It is useful to review some background pathophysiology before discussing the differential diagnosis:

A. Distribution of total body water

   1. 67% intracellular; 33% extracellular

   2. Extracellular water: 25% intravascular; 75% interstitial

B. Regulation of fluid distribution between the intravascular and interstitial spaces

   1. Constant exchange of water and solutes at the arteriolar end of the capillaries

   2. Fluid is returned from the interstitial space to the intravascular space at the venous end of the capillaries and via the lymphatics.

   3. Movement of fluid from the intravascular space to the interstitium

      a. Capillary hydrostatic (hydraulic) pressure pushes fluid out of the vessels

      b. Interstitial oncotic pressure pulls fluid into the interstitium

      c. Increased capillary permeability allows fluid to escape into the interstitium

   4. Movement of fluid from the interstitium to the intravascular space

      a. Intravascular (plasma) oncotic pressure from plasma proteins pulls fluid into the vascular space

      b. Interstitial hydrostatic pressure pushes fluid out of the interstitium

   5. In skeletal muscle, the capillary hydrostatic pressure and the intravascular oncotic pressure are the most important.

   6. There is normally a small gradient favoring filtration out of the vascular space into the interstitium; the excess fluid is removed via the lymphatic system.

C. Edema formation occurs when there is

   1. An increase in capillary hydrostatic pressure (for example, increased plasma volume due to renal sodium retention)

   2. An increase in capillary permeability (for example, burns, angioedema)

   3. An increase in interstitial oncotic pressure (for example, myxedema)

   4. A decrease in plasma oncotic pressure (for example, hypoalbuminemia)

   5. Lymphatic obstruction

Although it is possible to construct a pathophysiologic framework (Figure 12–1) for the differential diagnosis of edema, it is more useful clinically to combine anatomic, pathophysiologic, and organ/system frameworks:

A. Generalized edema due to a systemic cause and manifested by bilateral leg edema, with or without presacral edema, ascites, pleural effusion, pulmonary edema, periorbital edema

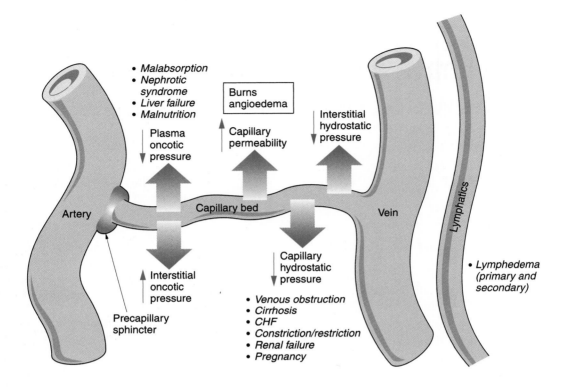

Figure 12–1. Pathophysiology of edema. (Adapted with permission from Cho S et al: Peripheral edema. *American Journal of Medicine* V113: 581. Copyright © 2002 *Excerpta Medica,* Inc.)

1. Cardiac
   a. Systolic or diastolic dysfunction, or both
   b. Constrictive pericarditis
   c. Pulmonary hypertension
2. Hepatic (cirrhosis)
3. Renal
   a. Advanced renal failure of any cause
   b. Nephrotic syndrome

 The most common systemic causes of edema are cardiac, renal, and hepatic diseases.

4. Nutritional deficiency
5. Medications
   a. Antidepressants: Monoamine oxidase inhibitors
   b. Antihypertensives
      (1) Calcium channel blockers
      (2) Direct vasodilators (hydralazine, minoxidil)
      (3) β-Blockers
   c. Hormones
      (1) Estrogens/progesterones
      (2) Testosterone
      (3) Corticosteroids
   d. Nonselective nonsteroidal anti-inflammatory drugs and cyclooxygenase-2 inhibitors
   e. Rosiglitazone, pioglitazone
6. Idiopathic edema
7. Refeeding edema
8. Myxedema
B. Limb edema due to a nonsystemic cause, manifested by unilateral or bilateral edema

1. Venous disease
   a. Obstruction
      (1) Deep venous thrombosis (DVT)
      (2) Lymphadenopathy
      (3) Pelvic mass
   b. Insufficiency
2. Lymphatic obstruction (lymphedema)
   a. Primary (idiopathic, often bilateral)
      (1) Congenital
      (2) Lymphedema praecox (onset in puberty) or tarda (onset > age 20)
   b. Secondary (more common, generally unilateral)
      (1) Neoplasm
      (2) Surgery (especially, following mastectomy)
      (3) Radiation therapy
      (4) Miscellaneous (tuberculosis, recurrent lymphangitis, filariasis)
C. Localized edema
1. Burns
2. Angioedema, hives
3. Trauma
4. Cellulitis, erysipelas

Mrs. V was well until a couple of months ago when she began feeling a bit more tired than usual, despite continuing to sleep well. She has had no shortness of breath or chest pain. She has noted intermittent vague abdominal pain, not related to eating, position, or bowel movements. She has been a bit constipated and feels bloated. Over the last 2 weeks, she has noted swelling in her feet and lower legs and has not been able to wear her regular shoes. As she tells you this, you note that she is wearing house slippers, and that her socks have produced a significant indentation above her ankles.

Her past medical history is notable for hypertension and diabetes, both well controlled. She had a blood transfusion during a cholecystectomy 25 years ago. Her current medications include hydrochlorothiazide, lisinopril, rosiglitazone, simvastatin, and aspirin. She has no history of heart or kidney disease, or tobacco or alcohol use.

At this point, what is the leading hypothesis, and what are the active alternatives? What other tests should be ordered?

ORGANIZING THE DIFFERENTIAL DIAGNOSIS

Even before examining Mrs. V, you can see that she has significant bilateral leg edema. Although there are some local diseases that can present with bilateral leg edema, the first step in such patients is always to look for systemic causes. While the history and physical are often not sensitive or specific enough to make a diagnosis, they are a good starting point for organizing the differential. So the first question to ask is, "Does Mrs. V have any signs or symptoms pointing to a cardiac, hepatic, or renal cause of her edema?" Mrs. V's history of a blood transfusion puts her at risk for chronic hepatitis and cirrhosis, and her vague abdominal complaints raise the possibility of ascites, more commonly seen with cirrhosis than congestive heart failure (CHF) or renal failure. She is certainly at risk for both cardiac and renal disease because of her history of hypertension and diabetes, even though she has not had such problems in the past. While most patients with heart failure complain of shortness of breath, some describe only fatigue. Medication should be considered as a cause, since rosiglitazone frequently causes edema; hypothyroidism does not cause pitting edema, and so is not likely. Finally, although it is uncommon for obstruction to cause bilateral edema, you should think about ovarian cancer causing malignant ascites and venous obstruction, either via extrinsic compression or due to associated DVT formation. Table 12–1 lists the differential diagnosis.

Always look for systemic causes of edema in patients with bilateral leg edema.

In general, Mrs. V appears fatigued. Her BP is 100/60 mm Hg, pulse is 92 bpm, and RR is 16 breaths per minute. Sclera are anicteric, jugular venous pressure is normal, and lungs are clear. On cardiac exam, she has a normal S_1 and S_2, a soft S_4, and no S_3 or murmurs. Her abdomen is slightly distended, but soft and nontender; there is a fluid wave. Her is liver is not

(continued)

Table 12–1. Diagnostic hypotheses for Mrs. V.

Diagnostic Hypotheses	Clinical Clues	Important Tests
Leading Hypothesis		
Cirrhosis	Hepatitis risk factors Ascites Spider angiomata Gynecomastia Normal or low jugular venous pressure (JVP)	Ultrasound Bilirubin Liver enzymes Prothrombin time Albumin Liver biopsy
Active Alternatives—Must Not Miss		
CHF	Cardiovascular risk factors Dyspnea Elevated JVP Crackles S_3	ECG Chest x-ray Echocardiogram
Renal disease (insufficiency or nephrotic syndrome)	Malaise Nausea Dyspnea Edema	BUN/creatinine Urinalysis
Active Alternatives—Most Common		
Medication	History	History
Other Hypotheses		
Ovarian cancer	Abdominal pain Increased abdominal girth Family history	Pelvic ultrasound, CA-125

enlarged, but the spleen is palpable. Rectal exam shows hemorrhoids and guaiac-negative stool. She has 2+ edema bilaterally.

 Is the clinical information sufficient to make a diagnosis? If not, what other information do you need?

Leading Hypothesis: Cirrhosis

Textbook Presentation

Patients with cirrhosis can be asymptomatic or have mild symptoms, such as fatigue. Some patients have the classic manifestations of portal hypertension: ascites, edema, variceal bleeding, encephalopathy, or hypersplenism.

Disease Highlights

A. Etiology

1. Long-term alcohol abuse

2. Chronic hepatitis B or C

3. Less common causes are hepatitis D, hepatitis E, hepatitis G, and cytomegalovirus

 The 2 most common causes of cirrhosis in the United States are alcoholic liver disease and chronic hepatitis C.

3. Primary biliary cirrhosis

4. Metabolic (hemochromatosis, Wilson disease, α_1-antitrypsin)

5. Cardiac

6. Drugs and toxins (isoniazid, methotrexate)

7. Autoimmune

8. Nonalcoholic fatty liver disease (NAFLD)

B. Pathophysiology of portal hypertension

1. Portal hypertension means increased portal vein pressure and an increased portal pressure gradient (the pressure difference between the portal vein and the systemic veins, such as the hepatic veins or inferior vena cava)

    a. Architectural distortion of the liver causes obstruction of blood flow through the liver with a consequent increase in portal pressure

    b. Increased intrahepatic vascular tone also contributes to increased portal pressure

    c. Increased portal blood flow also contributes to elevated portal pressure; this occurs due to splanchnic vasodilatation and sodium and water retention.

2. Consequences of portal hypertension include

    a. Formation of portosystemic collaterals (ie, varices)

    b. Increased capillary hydrostatic pressure resulting in ascites; other factors that contribute to ascites and edema formation include

        (1) Salt and water retention in response to systemic vasodilatation

        (2) Hypoalbuminemia

C. Childs-Pugh classification of cirrhosis severity predicts prognosis (Table 12–2).

Evidence-Based Diagnosis

A. Cirrhosis is a pathologic diagnosis definitively made only by examining the entire liver at autopsy or after liver transplantation.

B. The traditional gold standard is percutaneous liver biopsy, although due to sampling error, the sensitivity has been reported to be as low as 70–80%.

C. The clinical presentation is variable, making clinical diagnosis difficult.

1. Patients may have physical findings suggestive of chronic liver disease (see below), constitutional symptoms, asymptomatic liver enzyme or radiologic abnormalities, manifestations of portal hypertension (see below), or no symptoms at all. Cirrhosis is sometimes diagnosed at autopsy in patients in whom the disease never manifested.

2. Physical findings associated with chronic liver disease include

    a. Spider angiomata

    b. Palmar erythema

    c. Dupuytren contracture

    d. Gynecomastia

    e. Testicular atrophy

    f. Jaundice

    g. Ascites

    h. Peripheral edema

    i. Hepatomegaly

    j. Splenomegaly

    k. Caput medusae

    l. None of these are sensitive or specific enough to diagnose cirrhosis, although multiple findings in combination do increase the pretest probability of cirrhosis.

3. Patients who show manifestations of portal hypertension (see below) are assumed to have cirrhosis.

D. Some clinical models have been developed to predict cirrhosis *in patients with chronic hepatitis C*, although none has been extensively validated.

1. Males with platelet counts ≤ 140,000 mcL, spider angiomata, and an AST (SGOT) > 40

Table 12–2. Childs-Pugh classification.

Parameter	1 Point	2 Points	3 Points
Ascites	Absent	Slight	Moderate
Bilirubin mg/dL	≤ 2	2–3	> 3
Albumin, g/dL	> 3.5	2.8–3.5	< 2.8
INR	< 1.7	1.8–2.3	> 2.3
Encephalopathy	None	Grade 1–2	Grade 3–4

Grade A (well-compensated disease, 2-year survival 85%): 5–6 points
Grade B (significant functional compromise, 2-year survival 60%): 7–9 points
Grade C (decompensated disease, 2-year survival 35%): 10–15 points

units/L had a 99.8% probability of having cirrhosis; males and females with platelet counts > 140,000 mcL, AST < 40 units/L, and no spider angiomata had a 1.8% probability of having cirrhosis.

2. AST/ALT (SGPT) ratio ≥ 1 and globulin/albumin ratio ≥ 1 has sensitivity of 22% and specificity of 100% in diagnosing cirrhosis; platelet count ≤ 140,000 mcL and globulin/albumin ratio ≥ 1 has sensitivity of 39% and specificity of 100%; platelet count ≤ 140,000 mcL has a sensitivity of 83% and a specificity of 85%.

E. Test characteristics of ultrasound to diagnose cirrhosis are variable (LR+, 2.5–11.6; LR–, 0.13–0.73).

F. MRI has sensitivity and specificity as high as 93% and 82%, respectively.

Manifestations of Portal Hypertension

Once it has been determined that the patient probably or definitively has cirrhosis, it is important to elucidate the specific cause of the cirrhosis (see Chapter 18, Jaundice) and to determine whether the patient has manifestations of portal hypertension: variceal bleeding, ascites and its complications, hepatic encephalopathy, and hypersplenism.

1. Variceal Bleeding

See Chapter 14, GI Bleeding.

2. Ascites

Textbook Presentation

The patient complains of an inability to fasten her pants due to increasing abdominal girth, sometimes accompanied by dyspnea and edema.

Disease Highlights

A. Epidemiology

1. Ascites develops over 5 years in 30% of patients with compensated cirrhosis, defined as the absence of manifestations of portal hypertension.

2. 1-year survival rates drop significantly once ascites develops.

B. Complications of ascites

1. Respiratory compromise due to compression of lung volumes

2. Hepatorenal syndrome

a. Prevalence estimates range from 1% to 40% of cirrhotic patients

b. Median survival for patients who have acute hepatorenal syndrome is less than 2 weeks.

c. Hepatorenal syndrome is due to splanchnic vasodilation, which causes decreased systemic vascular resistance, resulting in renal arteriolar vasoconstriction, decreased renal blood flow, and a reduced glomerular filtration rate.

d. Precipitants of hepatorenal syndrome include spontaneous bacterial peritonitis (SBP), septicemia, variceal bleeding, therapeutic paracentesis, and acute alcoholic hepatitis.

e. Criteria for diagnosing hepatorenal syndrome

(1) Severe cirrhosis

(2) 24-hour creatinine clearance < 40 mL/min or creatinine > 1.5 mg/dL

(3) Absence of shock, active bacterial infection, excessive fluid loss, exposure to nephrotoxic drugs

(4) No improvement in renal function with optimization of volume status

(5) Absence of significant proteinuria or renal obstruction

f. Liver transplantation is the only effective treatment.

3. SBP

a. Prevalence of 10–30% in hospitalized cirrhotic patients, with 1-year recurrence rate of 70% and mortality rate of about 20%

b. The 3 most common isolates are *Escherichia coli, Klebsiella pneumoniae,* and pneumococci

c. Symptoms can be relatively specific (such as fever and abdominal pain) or nonspecific (such as worsening of liver or renal function).

 Consider diagnostic paracentesis in all patients with ascites.

d. Diagnosis of SBP

(1) Some experts recommend diagnostic paracentesis in all patients who have cirrhosis with ascites who are admitted to the hospital, in patients with ascites in whom signs of sepsis develop, in patients with hepatic encephalopathy, in those with renal impairment or altered GI motility, and in all ascitic patients with a GI bleed.

(2) Ascitic fluid polymorphonuclear leukocyte (PMN) count > 250/mcL confirms SBP

(3) 40% of patients have negative culture results.

Consider secondary peritonitis if more than 1 organism is cultured.

e. Treatment of SBP

(1) Recommended antibiotics include IV cefotaxime or ampicillin and sulbactam; oral ofloxacin can be used in patients with uncomplicated SBP who have not received prophylactic quinolones. (**Note:** There are not high quality randomized trials backing up these recommendations.)

(2) Patients with renal impairment should also receive albumin for volume expansion.

(3) All patients who recover from SBP should receive secondary prophylaxis with oral norfloxacin.

(4) Since 2-year survival after SBP is only about 30%, liver transplantation should be considered in patients who recover from SBP.

Evidence-Based Diagnosis

A. Physical exam: See Chapter 18, Jaundice

B. Peritoneal fluid analysis

1. Serum-ascites albumin gradient

   a. In portal hypertension, ascites occurs due to transudation, without changes in permeability that would allow albumin to leak into the ascitic fluid.

   b. Therefore, the albumin content of ascitic fluid is low relative to serum.

   c. This is in contrast to exudative types of ascites, such as ascites from infection or malignancy, in which albumin can leak into the ascitic fluid.

   d. A serum-ascites albumin gradient (serum albumin-ascitic fluid albumin) of > 1.1 mg/dL has an accuracy of 97% in distinguishing ascites due to portal hypertension from ascites with normal portal pressures (such as malignant ascites).

2. Ascitic fluid total protein

   a. Also based on the principle that ascites due to cirrhosis is transudative and should have a low protein content relative to serum

   b. Using a cut point of 2.5 mg/dL of ascitic fluid total protein to distinguish an exudate from a transudate had an accuracy of only 56%.

Serum-ascites albumin gradient is the best test for distinguishing between ascites due to portal hypertension and ascites due to other causes.

3. Encephalopathy

Textbook Presentation

The classic presentation of hepatic encephalopathy is a patient with known cirrhosis who is in a coma.

Disease Highlights

A. Present in 50–70% of patients with chronic liver disease

B. The clinical manifestations range from subtle abnormalities detectable only on neuropsychological testing to coma (Table 12–3).

C. Can be precipitated by a wide variety of insults including

1. Increased ammonia production due to

   a. Excess dietary protein

   b. Constipation

   c. GI bleeding

   d. Infection

   e. Azotemia

   f. Hypokalemia

   g. Systemic alkalosis

2. Reduced metabolism of toxins because of hepatic hypoxia due to

   a. Dehydration

   b. Arterial hypotension

   c. Anemia

3. Increased central nervous depressant effect with use of benzodiazepines or other psychoactive drugs

4. Reduced metabolism of toxins because diversion of portal blood, due to surgical or transhepatic shunts

Table 12–3. Grading system for hepatic encephalopathy.

Grade	Level of Consciousness	Clinical Symptoms	Neurologic Signs	EEG Abnormalities
0	Normal	None	None	None
Subclinical	Normal	Normal	Abnormal neuropsychiatric testing	None
1	Sleep-wake reversal, restlessness	Forgetfulness, agitation, irritability, mild confusion	Tremor, apraxia, incoordination	Present
2	Lethargy, slow responses	Disorientation, amnesia, inappropriate behavior	Asterixis, dysarthria, ataxia, hypoactive reflexes	Present
3	Somnolence, confusion	Disorientation, aggressive behavior	Asterixis, hyperactive reflexes, positive Babinski sign, muscle rigidity	Present
4	Coma	Unresponsive	Decerebration	Present

 Always look for the underlying cause of worsening hepatic encephalopathy.

Evidence-Based Diagnosis

A. There is some correlation between the degree of elevation of ammonia (either arterial or venous) and the severity of the encephalopathy, but the ammonia level cannot be used to determine the presence or absence of hepatic encephalopathy.

B. Diagnosis is based on history and exclusion of other causes of encephalopathy in a patient with significant liver dysfunction.

4. Hypersplenism

Textbook Presentation

Anemia, thrombocytopenia, or both are found on routine blood testing in a patient with cirrhosis.

Disease Highlights

A. Splenomegaly is found in 36–92% of patients with cirrhosis; 11–55% have the clinical syndrome of hypersplenism.

B. There is a rough correlation between spleen size and degree of decrease in blood cells.

C. Blood cell abnormalities in liver disease

1. Anemia is due to increased destruction in the spleen as well as iron or folate deficiency; there is also reduced erythropoietin production.

2. Thrombocytopenia is due to platelet sequestration in the spleen, impaired bone marrow production, and decreased platelet survival.

3. Leukopenia is due to sequestration in the spleen and is rare compared with thrombocytopenia (1 series found 64% of cirrhotic patients had thrombocytopenia, but only 5% had leukopenia).

Evidence-Based Diagnosis

A. Hypersplenism is a clinical syndrome without a specific set of diagnostic criteria.

B. Hypersplenism is manifested by splenomegaly and a significant reduction in 1 or more cellular elements of the blood, in the presence of normal or hypercellular bone marrow.

MAKING A DIAGNOSIS

Initial laboratory test results follow: WBC, 9,700/mcL; Hgb, 10.5 g/dL; Hct, 31%; MCV, 86 mcm³; platelet, 123,000 mcL; electrolytes normal; BUN, 8 mg/dL; creatinine, 0.4 mg/dL; glucose, 97 mg/dL; albumin, 2.1 g/dL; alkaline phosphatase, 95 units/L; total bilirubin, 1.2 mg/dL; ALT, 102 units/L; AST, 66 units/L; PT/PTT normal; urinalysis, 2+ protein with no cells or casts.

Have you crossed a diagnostic threshold for the leading hypothesis, cirrhosis and portal hypertension? Have you ruled out the active alternatives? Do other tests need to be done to exclude the alternative diagnoses?

Mrs. V's physical exam suggests that she has splenomegaly, ascites, and edema, without pulmonary findings or an elevated jugular venous pressure, making CHF unlikely. Her laboratory results are notable for elevation of transaminases and hypoalbuminemia—all consistent with chronic liver disease. However, the findings of proteinuria and hypoalbuminemia are also consistent with nephrotic syndrome.

Alternative Diagnosis: Nephrotic Syndrome

Textbook Presentation

Patients with nephrotic syndrome classically have edema (often periorbital), hypertension, hypoalbuminemia, hyperlipidemia, and at least 3.5 g/d of proteinuria.

Disease Highlights

A. Etiology
  1. Occurs when the glomerulus loses the ability to prevent filtration of protein
  2. Diabetic nephropathy is the most common cause.
  3. In adults, the most common primary glomerular disease is membranous glomerulonephritis (40%), followed by minimal change glomerulopathy (20%); focal segmental glomerulosclerosis and membranoproliferative glomerulonephritis account for about 15% and 7% of cases respectively.
  4. Nephrotic syndrome can be associated with chronic hepatitis B or C.

 Membranous and other glomerulopathies can be a manifestation, or even a presenting symptom, of cancer.

  5. Myeloma and amyloid are other causes of nephrotic range proteinuria.

B. Clinical consequences
  1. Primary sodium retention by the kidney causes edema and hypertension.
  2. Albumin excretion leads to hypoalbuminemia.
  3. Alterations in lipoprotein production and catabolism lead to elevations of low-density lipoprotein and sometimes triglycerides.
  4. Immunoglobulin excretion causes increased susceptibility to infection.
  5. Thromboembolic complications
    a. Due to increased procoagulatory factors and fibrinogen, altered fibrinolytic system, urinary loss of antithrombin III, and increased platelet activity
    b. Venous thromboses (eg, renal vein thrombosis, pulmonary embolism, DVT) occur in up to 50% of patients with nephrotic syndrome.
      (1) Risk factors include serum albumin < 2.5 mg/dL, protein excretion > 10 g/24 hrs, high fibrinogen levels, and antithrombin III levels < 75% of normal.
      (2) The role of prophylactic anticoagulation is unclear, but it should be considered in high-risk patients.
    c. Arterial thrombosis is less common, but an increased risk of MI has been found.

Evidence-Based Diagnosis

A. Nephrotic syndrome is defined by the presence of urinary protein excretion of at least 3.5 g/24 hours.
B. Serum and urine electrophoreses should be done to rule out underlying myeloma or amyloid.
C. Renal biopsy is necessary to establish the specific etiology.

Treatment

A. Loop diuretics are used to treat the edema; high doses are often needed due to the primary sodium retention by the kidney.
B. ACE inhibitors reduce proteinuria in both hypertensive and normotensive patients.
  1. The antiproteinuric effect becomes maximal in 28 days.
  2. The effect can be increased by a low-salt diet, diuretic treatment, or both.
C. Corticosteroids and other immunosuppressives are used in selected patients.

CASE RESOLUTION

Mrs. V's hepatitis C antibody is positive, with negative hepatitis B serologies. Her total cholesterol is 145 mg/dL, and her 24-hour urinary protein excretion is 1.4 g. An abdominal CT scan demonstrates a small, nodular liver; splenomegaly; and ascites. You schedule an esophagogastroduodenoscopy to screen for varices, start spironolactone because of the discomfort she is having from the edema, and refer her to a hepatologist.

Treatment of Cirrhosis

The treatment of cirrhosis depends on the underlying cause. Treatments for selected causes of cirrhosis are discussed in Chapter 18, Jaundice.

Treatment of Manifestations of Portal Hypertension

1. Variceal Bleeding

See Chapter 14, GI Bleeding.

2. Ascites

A. Sodium and water restriction (sodium intake < 2 g/d) is commonly recommended, but there are no clinical trials showing that they lead to improved outcomes.

B. Spironolactone is the diuretic of choice to treat the aldosterone driven salt and water retention seen in cirrhosis.
   1. 75% of patients respond
   2. Furosemide or other loop diuretics can be added in patients who do not respond to spironolactone alone; 90% of patients respond to sodium restricted diets, spironolactone, and loop diuretics.
   3. In order to avoid hypovolemia and renal impairment, the rate of weight loss should not exceed 0.5 kg/d in the absence of peripheral edema or 1 kg/d in the presences of edema.

Aspirin and nonsteroidal anti-inflammatory drugs blunt the natriuretic effect of diuretics and should be avoided in patients with ascites.

C. Large volume paracentesis with volume expansion (dextran or albumin) for patients unresponsive to diuretics

D. Transvenous intrahepatic portosystemic shunts (TIPS)
   1. Creates a shunt between the high-pressure portal vein and the low-pressure hepatic vein, leading to improved hemodynamics and a decrease in ascites
   2. Complications include bleeding, shunt stenosis or thrombosis, and encephalopathy in 30% of patients.

E. Liver transplantation

F. When should ascites be treated with measures beyond sodium restriction?
   1. Not in grade 1 ascites (detectable only by ultrasound)
   2. Grade 2 (moderate) and grade 3 (severe) ascites are generally treated due to patient discomfort and respiratory compromise.
      a. Grade 2 should be treated with diuretics.
      b. Grade 3 should be treated with paracentesis, followed by diuretics.
   3. Refractory ascites (ascites not responsive to maximal tolerated medical therapy) should be treated with repeated paracentesis or TIPS, or both.

3. Encephalopathy

A. Treatment focuses on reduction of intestinal production of ammonia.

B. Lactulose removes both dietary and endogenous sources of ammonia through its cathartic action; it also lowers pH, which reduces the population of urease-producing bacteria.
   1. Efficacy shown in randomized trials
   2. Daily dose should be titrated to result in 2–4 soft stools/d.
   3. Complications include hypovolemia and hypernatremia.

C. Neomycin reduces the population of urease-producing bacteria.
   1. Efficacy is equivalent to lactulose, but potential ototoxicity and nephrotoxicity precludes long-term use.
   2. May have an additive effect when given with lactulose.

4. Hypersplenism

A. Treatment is usually not necessary.

B. Splenectomy or partial splenic embolization is sometimes done for severe thrombocytopenia with bleeding complications.

C. Granulocyte-macrophage colony-stimulating factor (GM-CSF) and erythropoietin are sometimes used.

D. TIPS does not correct thrombocytopenia.

CHIEF COMPLAINT

PATIENT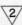

Mrs. E is a 62-year-old woman with a long history of hypertension that is well controlled with hydrochlorothiazide, atenolol, and amlodipine. She comes in today with a new complaint of swelling in her legs and feet for several weeks. It is generally most noticeable late in the day and is often absent when she first gets up in the morning. She has no history of liver or kidney disease or alcohol use. She has no chest pain and no shortness of breath, although notes she occasionally finds it tiring to climb stairs. She smoked a few cigarettes a day for 20 years, but quit 20 years ago.

Her physical exam is notable for clear lungs, an S_4 with no S_3 or murmurs, and a normal abdomen. Her legs show 1+ edema to the knees bilaterally. She has a longstanding goiter that is unchanged from previous exams. It is difficult to identify her jugular venous pressure due to the shape of her neck.

 At this point, what is the leading hypothesis, and what are the active alternatives? What other tests should be ordered?

ORGANIZING THE DIFFERENTIAL

Once again, given the finding of bilateral edema, the first step is to look for systemic causes, focusing first on cardiac, hepatic, and renal causes. Mrs. E's longstanding history of hypertension raises the possibility of diastolic dysfunction, and the lack of physical exam findings does not rule this out. There are no clinical clues to suggest liver or kidney disease, but these are easy to test for and should always be ruled out. Amlodipine commonly causes edema, but she has taken it for years without symptoms. "Dependent edema," edema that is worsened by standing and improves or resolves with leg elevation, is consistent with, but not specific for, venous insufficiency. A final consideration would be pulmonary hypertension. Patients with pulmonary hypertension commonly complain of dyspnea in addition to edema; however, she has no diseases associated with pulmonary hypertension, and primary pulmonary hypertension is rare. Table 12–4 lists the differential diagnosis.

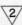

Initial laboratory test results include BUN, 15 mg/dL; creatinine, 0.9 mg/dL; urinalysis negative for protein; normal liver enzymes, albumin, and prothrombin time.

The ECG and chest x-ray are normal. An echocardiogram shows normal left ventricle size and function, elevated pulmonary pressures consistent with moderate pulmonary hypertension (estimated mean PAP 40 mm Hg), mild tricuspid regurgitation, and normal right ventricle size and function.

Is the clinical information sufficient to make a diagnosis? If not, what other information do you need?

There is no evidence of renal disease, liver disease, or diastolic dysfunction. However, the echocardiogram shows the somewhat unexpected finding of pulmonary hypertension. This necessitates revising the original set of diagnostic hypotheses: the leading hypothesis is now pulmonary hypertension, and venous insufficiency is the remaining active alternative.

Leading Hypothesis: Pulmonary Hypertension

Textbook Presentation

Patients commonly complain of longstanding dyspnea, or sometimes exercise-induced weakness or fatigue; syncope occurs in 33% of patients. Edema occurs later in the course of the disease, when right ventricular dysfunction is present. Physical exam findings suggestive of pulmonary hypertension include an accentuated pulmonary component of S_2, sustained left lower parasternal movement, an early systolic click, increased jugular a and v waves, tricuspid regurgitation murmur, hepatojugular reflux, pulsatile liver, elevated jugular venous pressure, and edema.

Disease Highlights

A. Definition

1. The normal mean pulmonary artery pressure (PAP) is 12 mm Hg.

2. Pulmonary hypertension is defined as a mean PAP of at least 25 mm Hg at rest or 30 mm Hg with exercise; severe pulmonary hypertension is defined as a mean PAP of at least 50 mm Hg.

Table 12–4. Diagnostic hypotheses for Mrs. E.

Diagnostic Hypotheses	Clinical Clues	Important Tests
Leading Hypothesis		
Diastolic dysfunction	History of hypertension, dyspnea, edema Elevated jugular venous pressure (JVP) S_3	Echocardiogram
Active Alternatives—Most Common		
Venous insufficiency	Dependent edema Varicose veins Typical skin changes (see description below)	Physical exam Duplex ultrasound
Active Alternatives—Must Not Miss		
Renal and liver disease	See Diagnostic hypotheses for Mrs. V	See Diagnostic hypotheses for Mrs. V
Other Hypotheses		
Pulmonary hypertension	Dyspnea, often longstanding Edema Syncope	Echocardiogram Right-heart catheterization

B. Clinical classification, using a pathophysiologic framework

1. Pulmonary arterial hypertension
   a. Primary pulmonary hypertension (familial or sporadic)
   b. Related to
      (1) Collagen vascular disease
      (2) Congenital shunts
      (3) Portal hypertension
      (4) HIV infection
      (5) Drugs or toxins (eg, appetite suppressants)

2. Pulmonary venous hypertension is caused by
   a. Left-sided atrial or ventricular heart disease or valvular heart disease
   b. Extrinsic compression of central pulmonary veins (adenopathy, tumors, fibrosing mediastinitis)
   c. Pulmonary veno-occlusive disease

3. Pulmonary hypertension associated with disorders of the respiratory system or hypoxemia
   a. Chronic obstructive pulmonary disease
   b. Interstitial lung disease
   c. Sleep disordered breathing

4. Pulmonary hypertension due to chronic thromboembolic disease
   a. Pulmonary embolism
   b. In situ thrombosis
   c. Sickle cell disease

5. Pulmonary hypertension due to disorders directly affecting the pulmonary vasculature
   a. Schistosomiasis
   b. Sarcoidosis

Evidence-Based Diagnosis

A. Physical exam

1. Sustained left lower parasternal movement for detecting a mean PAP > 50 mm Hg: sensitivity, 71%; specificity, 80%; LR+, 3.6; LR−, 0.4

2. A palpable P_2 for detecting a mean PAP > 50 mm Hg (studied in patients with mitral stenosis): sensitivity, 96%; specificity, 73%; LR+, 3.6; LR−, 0.05

3. A loud P_2 is neither sensitive nor specific for the diagnosis of pulmonary hypertension.

B. ECG

1. Expected findings include right axis deviation, right ventricular hypertrophy, and P-pulmonale pattern (right atrial enlargement).

2. Not sensitive or specific enough to diagnosis pulmonary hypertension

   a. Sensitivity, 51%; specificity, 86%

   b. LR+, 3.6; LR−, 0.56

C. Chest film

   1. Expected findings include enlargement of pulmonary arteries and right ventricular enlargement.

   2. Not sensitive or specific enough to diagnose pulmonary hypertension (sensitivity, 46%; specificity, 63%)

D. Transthoracic echocardiogram

   1. Most common noninvasive way to estimate pulmonary pressure

   2. Sensitivity ranges from 78% to 85% but can be as high as 97% in selected populations with very severe disease.

   3. Specificity ranges from 55% to 75%.

E. Right heart catheterization is the gold standard for diagnosing pulmonary hypertension.

F. See Figure 12–2 for a diagnostic approach to pulmonary hypertension.

Treatment

A. Depends on underlying etiology

B. Correct underlying cause when possible

   1. For obstructive sleep apnea, administer continuous positive airway pressure.

   2. For chronic thromboembolism, begin anticoagulation and consider thromboendarterectomy.

   3. For valvular disease, replace the valve.

   4. For congenital heart disease, repair surgically.

   5. For left ventricular dysfunction, optimize medical regimen.

C. Oxygen therapy for patients with hypoxemia (PO_2 < 55 mm Hg at rest, oxygen saturation < 85% with exercise)

D. Epoprostenol (prostacyclin) for patients with primary pulmonary hypertension and selected other patients

E. Bosentan and sildenafil are being studied in patients with primary pulmonary hypertension.

F. The role of calcium channel blockers is unclear.

G. Diuretics should be used cautiously to control edema; patients with right ventricular dysfunction need relatively high filling pressures to maintain systemic BP.

H. Anticoagulation should be given to patients with chronic thromboemboli.

MAKING A DIAGNOSIS

Mrs. E has a normal physical exam, ECG, and chest x-ray, normal right ventricular function on echocardiogram, and the isolated finding of moderately elevated PAP seen on an echocardiogram. The echocardiogram estimate of PAP alone is not specific enough to make the diagnosis of pulmonary hypertension, and Mrs. E has no other findings supporting the diagnosis of pulmonary hypertension. Furthermore, Mrs. E's dyspnea is minimal, suggesting that she has neither significant pulmonary hypertension nor pulmonary disease.

You explain the puzzling finding to Mrs. E. She does not want to undergo a right heart catheterization to verify the PAP. She reports that she is able to walk a mile every morning without shortness of breath, and that her edema is most noticeable when she has been on her feet for a long time.

Have you crossed a diagnostic threshold for the leading hypothesis, pulmonary hypertension? Have you ruled out the active alternatives? Do other tests need to be done to exclude the alternative diagnoses?

Alternative Diagnosis: Venous Insufficiency

Textbook Presentation

Venous insufficiency can be asymptomatic or manifested just by small reticular veins. In more severe cases, the patient has large varicose veins and skin changes ranging from edema to fibrosing panniculitis to ulceration. Symptoms include leg fullness or heaviness, aching leg pain, and nocturnal leg cramps.

Disease Highlights

A. Anatomy

   1. The superficial saphenous veins join the deep system at the knee (popliteal vein) and the groin (femoral vein).

   2. Perforating veins directly connect the saphenous veins and the deep veins at various points along their parallel courses.

B. Pathophysiology and epidemiology

1. Venous insufficiency is due to elevated venous pressures from venous valvular incompetence, venous obstruction, or a combination of both.

2. Varicose veins are found in 25–33% of women and 10–20% of men.

3. Prevalence of skin changes is 3–11%; prevalence of skin ulcers is 0.3–1%.

4. Risk factors for venous insufficiency include advancing age, obesity, a history of phlebitis or venous thrombosis, and serious leg trauma.

5. Postthrombotic syndrome (venous insufficiency after a DVT) occurs in 35–69% of patients at 3 years and in 49–100% of patients at 5–10 years; incidence is reduced to 8% if patients are treated with adequate anticoagulation, early mobilization, and long-term use of compression stockings.

C. Classification

1. Class 1: telangiectasias or reticular veins (nonpalpable subdermal veins up to 4 mm in diameter)

2. Class 2: varicose veins (palpable, subcutaneous veins > 4 mm in diameter)

3. Class 3: edema

   a. Initially present just at the end of day but can become persistent and massive

   b. Can be unilateral initially

   c. Often begins around medial malleolus

4. Class 4: skin changes

   a. Pigmentation due to breakdown of extravasated RBCs

   b. Stasis dermatitis: itching, weeping, scaling, erosions, and crusting

   c. Lipodermatosclerosis or fibrosing panniculitis

      (1) Induration initially at medial ankle, spreading circumferentially round the entire leg, up to mid calf

      (2) The skin is heavily pigmented and fixed to subcutaneous tissues, with brawny edema above the fibrosis and in the foot below

      (3) High risk for cellulitis

5. Classes 5 and 6: healed or nonhealed ulcers

   a. Usually low on the medial ankle or along the path of the long or short saphenous vein

   b. Never above the knee or on the forefoot

   c. Chronic and recurrent, often lasting for months or even years

Evidence-Based Diagnosis

A. Diagnosis is often made based on the appearance of the leg.

B. Venography is the gold standard.

C. Duplex ultrasonography is the best noninvasive test.

1. Should be done if the diagnosis is in doubt (especially to rule out DVT), in patients with atypical symptoms or presentations, or if surgery is being considered

2. For diagnosing valvular incompetence, the sensitivity is 84%, specificity is 88%, LR+ = 7, and LR− = 0.18.

3. For diagnosing severe venous insufficiency, the sensitivity is 77%, specificity is 85%, LR+ = 5.1, and LR− = 0.26.

D. Because many patients have both arterial and venous insufficiency, concurrent arterial disease must be ruled out with the ankle brachial index (ABI).

1. In 1 study, 21% of patients with venous insufficiency had concomitant arterial insufficiency.

2. Use Doppler ultrasonography to measure systolic BP in brachial, posterior tibial, and dorsalis pedis arteries, and then divide the highest foot or ankle pressure by the brachial pressure.

   a. Normal is > 1.0

   b. ABI < 0.9 has 95% sensitivity for detecting peripheral vascular disease (PVD).

   c. ABI of 0.5–0.89 suggests moderate PVD.

   d. ABI < 0.5 suggests severe PVD.

CASE RESOLUTION

2

You decide that Mrs. E's symptoms are more consistent with venous insufficiency than with pulmonary hypertension. Duplex ultrasonographic scans confirm valvular incompetence, and you recommend that Mrs. E wear compression stockings. She returns in 3 months reporting that she has no edema when she wears the stockings, and that she continues to walk 1 mile daily without any dyspnea.

Treatment of Venous Insufficiency

A. Compression stockings are the most important treatment modality.

1. Have been shown to reduce risk of postthrombotic syndrome, to accelerate ulcer healing, and to prevent recurrent ulceration

2. Classified into several grades, based on degree of compression at the ankle

   a. 20–30 mm Hg: for patients with varicose veins, edema, leg fatigue

   b. 30–40 mm Hg: for patients with severe varicosities or moderate disease

   c. 40–50 mm Hg or > 60 mm Hg: for patients with severe disease or ulceration, or both

3. Knee high stockings are better tolerated than thigh high stockings.

4. Compliance often poor due to skin irritation, discomfort, and difficulty putting on the stockings.

 Compression stockings should not be used in patients with PVD or with invasive infection at an ulcer site.

5. Ulcers should be covered with a dressing before putting on the compression device.

6. Alternative ways to provide compression include elastic wraps and intermittent pneumatic compression pumps.

B. Diuretics are ineffective for the edema unless given with compression therapy.

C. Treatment of venous insufficiency ulcers

1. Occlusive dressing

2. Leg elevation and compression

3. Aspirin, 325 mg daily, might accelerate healing.

4. Pentoxifylline might accelerate healing.

5. Topical antibiotics have no role.

6. Systemic antibiotics indicated only if cellulitis or other invasive infection is present.

D. Role of surgery is unclear.

CHIEF COMPLAINT

PATIENT 3

Mrs. K is a 64-year-old woman who had a right mastectomy 2 years ago for breast cancer. She was treated with adjuvant radiation therapy and has been taking tamoxifen since completing the radiation. She has had no evidence of recurrent disease but has had some right arm swelling for at least 18 months. She comes to see you now because 2 days ago the swelling of her right arm worsened, with associated pain and redness. This morning her temperature was 37.9 °C.

 At this point, what is the leading hypothesis, and what are the active alternatives? What other tests should be ordered?

ORGANIZING THE DIFFERENTIAL

Mrs. K has chronic lymphedema due to disruption of her lymphatic drainage by her previous surgery and radiation therapy. Patients with lymphatic disruption and lymphedema are at high risk for skin and subcutaneous infections. Although pathophysiologically, the edema found in cellulitis is due to a localized increase in capillary permeability due to inflammation, in patients with underlying limb abnormalities, the edema can be more diffuse. The other primary consideration in any patient with unilateral limb swelling is DVT. Mrs. K has several risk factors for this, including history of cancer, possible venous scarring secondary to radiation, and use of tamoxifen (a drug associated with a relative risk for DVT of about 3). Table 12–5 lists the differential diagnosis.

Always think about DVT in a patient with unilateral limb swelling.

Table 12–5. Diagnostic hypotheses for Mrs. K.

Diagnostic Hypotheses	Clinical Clues	Important Tests
Leading Hypothesis		
Cellulitis	Edema Erythema Pain Fever Entry site for infection Underlying venous insufficiency or lymphedema	WBC count
Active Alternative—Must Not Miss		
Upper extremity DVT	Unilateral arm or neck swelling Feeling of fullness or heaviness DVT risk factors (especially indwelling IV catheter)	Duplex ultrasound CT MRA Venography

On physical exam, Mrs. K is clearly uncomfortable. Her temperature is 38.3 °C, pulse 102 bpm, RR 16 breaths per minute, and BP 125/80 mm Hg. Her right upper arm and chest are bright red, hot, and tender. The border of the erythema is sharply demarcated, and the area of erythema feels indurated. She has eczema of all of her fingers, with multiple areas of cracked skin.

Is the clinical information sufficient to make a diagnosis? If not, what other information do you need?

Leading Hypothesis: Cellulitis & Erysipelas

Textbook Presentation
A painful, red, hot, and swollen limb develops acutely in a patient with underlying venous or lymphatic disease.

Disease Highlights
A. Definitions
   1. Cellulitis is an infection of the skin that extends into the subcutaneous tissue.
   2. Erysipelas is a type of cellulitis limited to the dermis and hypodermis.

B. Cellulitis highlights
   1. Risk factors for development of cellulitis
      a. Lymphedema
      b. Breast cancer treatment
         (1) Cellulitis developed in 5.5% of women in 42 months of observation after mastectomy and axillary node dissection
         (2) Cellulitis of the breast is seen after lumpectomy.
      c. Entry site for infection (eg, leg ulcer, trauma, tinea pedis, eczema)
      d. Venous insufficiency
      e. Leg edema
      f. Obesity
   2. Clinical presentation
      a. Presence of systemic symptoms (eg, fever, chills, myalgias) is variable.
      b. Physical findings
         (1) Nonpalpable, confluent erythema with vague margins
         (2) Generalized swelling
         (3) Warmth and tenderness of involved skin
         (4) Tender regional adenopathy sometimes found
         (5) Lymphangitis and abscess formation sometimes seen
         (6) In women who have been treated for breast cancer, the humeral area of the ipsilateral extremity is most often involved, with extension to the shoulder and forearm.

(7) In breast cellulitis, the infection starts at the lumpectomy site and can extend to the remainder of the breast, the anterior shoulder, back, and ipsilateral upper extremity.

3. Microbiology

    a. β-Hemolytic streptococci (groups A, B, C, and G) are the most common organisms.

    b. *Staphylococcus aureus* is the other most common organism.

    c. Gram-negative organisms or anaerobes seen only in immunocompromised patients or diabetic patients

C. Erysipelas highlights

    1. Risk factors for development of erysipelas

        a. Similar to those for cellulitis

        b. Lymphedema and portal of entry (primarily tinea pedis) are the 2 strongest risk factors in 1 study.

Always treat tinea pedis in a patient with cellulitis, erysipelas, or risk factors for developing those infections.

    2. Clinical presentation

        a. Sudden onset of fever (85% of patients), erythema, edema, and pain

        b. Physical findings

            (1) Palpable plaque of erythema that extends by 2–10 cm/d

            (2) Sharply demarcated border

            (3) Leg is the most common site (90%), then the arm (5%), and then the face (2.5%).

            (4) Regional adenopathy and lymphangitis sometimes seen

        c. Recurrence rate of 10% at 6 months and 30% at 3 years is usually due to untreated local factors.

    3. Microbiology

        a. Streptococci are the causative organisms in 90% of cases.

        b. *S aureus* is also found in 10% of cases, although it is unclear whether it is contributing to the infection or just colonizing.

Evidence-Based Diagnosis

A. Both cellulitis and erysipelas are clinical diagnoses.

B. Blood cultures are positive in 2–5% of patients.

C. Skin biopsy cultures were positive in 10% of patients in 1 study.

D. Aspiration of the leading edge of erythema is sometimes done, but the yield is low.

E. Toe web cultures are sometimes helpful in patients with tinea pedis.

Cultures are rarely helpful in cellulitis or erysipelas.

MAKING A DIAGNOSIS

Initial laboratory tests include the following: WBC 11,700/mcL, 83% PMNs, 10% basophils, 7% lymphocytes; Hgb, 13.5 g/dL; glucose, 88 mg/dL; creatinine, 0.8 mg/dL.

Have you crossed a diagnostic threshold for the leading hypothesis, cellulitis? Have you ruled out the active alternatives? Do other tests need to be done to exclude the alternative diagnoses?

Alternative Diagnosis: Upper Extremity DVT (UEDVT)

Textbook Presentation

Patients can be asymptomatic, but generally arm, shoulder, or neck discomfort or fullness as well as arm swelling are the presenting symptoms.

Disease Highlights

A. Classification

    1. Primary UEDVT (20% of cases)

        a. Idiopathic

        b. Effort thrombosis, also known as Paget-Schroetter syndrome

            (1) Occurs in young men after strenuous exercise, which causes microtrauma to the veins

            (2) May or may not find compression by hypertrophied muscles or a cervical rib

2. Secondary UEDVT (80% of cases)

   a. Indwelling central venous catheter–associated UEDVT (> 50% of cases)

     (1) UEDVT occurs more often with large catheters than with smaller ones.

     (2) Risk increases with duration of catheter use.

     (3) Higher risk with polyvinyl chloride-coated catheters than with silicone ones.

   b. Malignancy (up to 37%)

   c. Hypercoagulable states

   d. Other miscellaneous causes (surgery, infection, immobility, concurrent lower extremity DVT)

B. Sites

   1. Subclavian in 18–69% of cases

   2. Axillary in 5–42% of cases

   3. Internal jugular in 8–29% of cases

   4. Brachial in 4–13% of cases

   5. Multiple veins are often involved, but bilateral UEDVT is rare.

C. Clinical features

   1. Pain is present in 68% of patients.

   2. Edema is present in 98% of patients in some series, but patients with catheter-related UEDVT often do not have edema.

   3. Patients may note numbness, heaviness, paresthesias, pruritus, and coldness.

   4. Dilated cutaneous veins sometimes visible.

D. Complications

   1. Pulmonary embolism occurs in up to 36% of cases and is more often seen with secondary UEDVT, especially catheter-related.

UEDVT can cause pulmonary embolism.

   2. Postthrombotic syndrome is seen in up to 90% of patients.

Evidence-Based Diagnosis

A. Venography is the gold standard.

B. Duplex ultrasonography is the most commonly used noninvasive test.

   1. Disadvantages include a blind spot caused by the clavicle and difficulties interpreting the study if there are collateral veins.

2. Sensitivity ranges from 56% to 100%, and specificity from 94% to 100%

3. Magnetic resonance angiography and CT are sometimes done; sensitivity and specificity are unknown.

Treatment

A. Anticoagulation with heparin, followed by at least 3 months of warfarin.

B. Thrombolysis with or without stent placement is sometimes done, especially in patients who require permanent indwelling catheters.

CASE RESOLUTION

Mrs. K's presentation of a sharply demarcated, erythematous plaque, fever, and leukocytosis is diagnostic of erysipelas. The portal of entry is the eczematous, cracked skin on her hands. Although she has some risk factors for UEDVT, it is not necessary to test for it at this point. Because of the extent of infection, Mrs. K is admitted to the hospital and treated with IV cefazolin. One of 2 blood cultures grows group A β-hemolytic streptococci. She improves rapidly and is switched to oral penicillin and is discharged.

Treatment of Cellulitis & Erysipelas

A. Cellulitis

   1. Initial therapy is generally empiric.

   2. Must cover staphylococcus and streptococcus

     a. Cefazolin or nafcillin are common initial choices.

     b. Clindamycin, macrolides, or fluoroquinolones (levofloxacin, gatifloxacin, moxifloxacin) can be used in patients who are allergic to penicillin.

     c. Vancomycin should be used if methicillin-resistant staphylococcus is suspected.

   3. Should treat for 10–14 days

B. Erysipelas

   1. Penicillin G can be used for erysipelas.

   2. If the patient is allergic to penicillin, other options listed above can be used.

C. Uncomplicated, slowly progressive infection in a well-appearing patient can be treated with oral antibiotics if

 1. The patient has no GI upset

 2. The limb can be elevated

 3. Serial exams are feasible

D. Another option for patients who do not need admission is 1 dose of a long-acting IV antibiotic (such as ceftriaxone), followed by oral therapy.

E. Patients who appear ill, who have rapidly progressive infection, or who might not be able to follow treatment instructions should be admitted for IV antibiotics.

F. Obtain infectious disease and surgical consultations for patients with rapidly progressive infections, especially if progression occurs while on appropriate antibiotics.

Diagnostic Approach: Suspected Pulmonary Hypertension

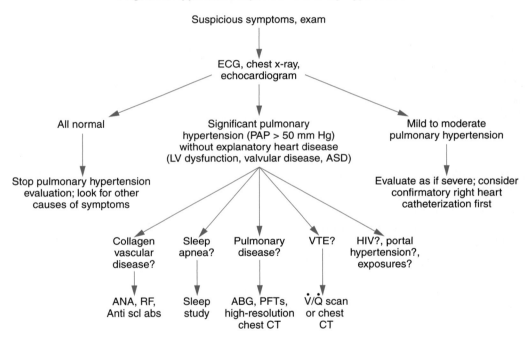

PAP, pulmonary artery pressure; LV, left ventricular; ASD, atrial septal defect; ANA, antinuclear antibodies; RF, rheumatoid factor; PFTs, pulmonary function tests; V̇/Q̇, ventilation-perfusion.

I have a patient with fatigue. How do I determine the cause?

CHIEF COMPLAINT

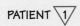

PATIENT 1

Mrs. M is a 42-year-old woman who has had fatigue for the past 6 months.

What is the differential diagnosis of fatigue? How would you frame the differential?

CONSTRUCTING A DIFFERENTIAL DIAGNOSIS

Before considering the differential diagnosis, it is important to understand what the patient means by fatigue, which is conventionally defined as a sensation of exhaustion after usual activities, or a feeling of insufficient energy to begin usual activities. Most people consider the terms fatigue, tiredness, and lack of energy synonymous. However, patients sometimes use these terms when they are actually experiencing other symptoms, especially excessive sleepiness, weakness, or dyspnea on exertion.

Always ask patients what they mean when they report fatigue. Always ask directly about weakness, excessive sleepiness, and dyspnea.

Acute fatigue is common in conjunction with a variety of acute illnesses, ranging from uncomplicated viral infections to exacerbations of congestive heart failure. Fatigue is also a prominent symptom in some chronic diseases, such as multiple sclerosis and cancer. This chapter will not discuss fatigue in such patients but will focus on evaluating the symptom of fatigue lasting weeks to months in patients without already diagnosed conditions known to cause fatigue.

The differential diagnosis of fatigue is extremely broad and best organized with an organ/system approach.

A. Psychiatric
   1. Depression
   2. Anxiety
   3. Somatization disorder
   4. Substance abuse
B. Sleep disorders
   1. Insomnia
   2. Obstructive sleep apnea
   3. Periodic leg movements
   4. Narcolepsy
C. Endocrine
   1. Thyroid disease
   2. Diabetes
   3. Hypoadrenalism
D. Medications (Table 13–1)
E. Hematologic or oncologic
   1. Anemia
   2. Cancer
F. Renal: renal failure
G. GI: liver disease
H. Cardiovascular: chronic heart disease
I. Pulmonary: chronic lung disease
J. Neuromuscular: myositis, multiple sclerosis
K. Infectious: chronic infections
L. Rheumatologic: autoimmune diseases
M. Fatigue of unknown etiology
   1. Chronic fatigue syndrome
   2. Idiopathic chronic fatigue: fatigue for which no medical, psychiatric, or sleep pattern explanation can be found.

Table 13–1. Medications that affect sleep.

Medications that cause insomnia	Antihypertensives: Clonidine, methyldopa, reserpine, propranolol, atenolol Anticholinergics: Ipratropium CNS stimulants: Methylphenidate Hormones: Oral contraceptives, thyroid hormone, corticosteroids, progesterone Sympathomimetic amines: Albuterol, theophylline, phenylpropanolamine, pseudoephedrine Antineoplastics: Leuprolide, goserelin, pentostatin, interferon alfa Miscellaneous: Phenytoin, nicotine, levodopa, quinidine, caffeine, alcohol
Medications that cause drowsiness	Tricyclic antidepressants: Amitriptyline, imipramine Narcotics Benzodiazepines Nonsteroidal anti-inflammatory drugs Anticonvulsants: Gabapentin Alcohol

 The most common causes of fatigue are psychiatric disorders, sleep disorders, and medication side effects.

Mrs. M reports that she is tired all the time, beginning first thing in the morning and lasting all day. She also reports frontal headaches several times per week, intermittent lower abdominal pain relieved by bowel movements, and low back pain. She does not complain of any trouble sleeping.

Her past medical history is notable for menorrhagia and iron deficiency anemia when she was in her 20s and is otherwise unremarkable. Currently, her menses occur every 30 days, with bleeding for 3–4 days. Her family history is notable for thyroid disease in her mother and breast cancer in her paternal grandmother.

She takes no medications, does not smoke, and does not drink alcohol. She has never used illicit drugs. She works as a teacher, and her husband is a security guard. They have 2 children, ages 9 and 12.

 At this point, what is the leading hypothesis, and what are the active alternatives? What other tests should be ordered?

ORGANIZING THE DIFFERENTIAL DIAGNOSIS

A specific causative medical disease that explains fatigue is found in less than 10% of patients who seek medical attention from their primary care physician. Up to 75% of patients with fatigue have psychiatric symptoms. Sleep disorders are also common in patients with fatigue, and in one referral clinic, 80% of patients with fatigue had sleep disorders. Patients with several somatic complaints, such as Mrs. M, are particularly likely to have psychiatric causes for fatigue, as are patients who feel tired constantly. Because sleep disorders are so common, either in association with psychiatric disorders or alone, they are always an active alternative in patients with fatigue. Patients often do not spontaneously describe sleep disturbances and psychiatric symptoms, so it is important to ask about them directly.

 All patients with fatigue need a detailed psychosocial and sleep pattern history.

Although most patients with fatigue do *not* have anemia, hypothyroidism, or diabetes, they are important and treatable, and so are generally considered "must not miss" diagnoses. Anemia and hypothyroidism are somewhat likely in Mrs. M because of her previous history of anemia and her family history of thyroid disease. Finally, on occasion, fatigue may be the presenting symptom in patients with surprisingly severe cardiac, pulmonary, renal, or liver disease. Table 13–2 lists the differential diagnosis.

Table 13–2. Diagnostic hypotheses for Mrs. M.

Diagnostic Hypotheses	Clinical Clues	Important Tests
Leading Hypotheses		
Depression	History of loss Prior depression Postpartum state Family history > 6 somatic symptoms Positive depression screen	History
Anxiety	Multiple somatic symptoms Anxiety Panic attacks	History
Active Alternative—Most Common		
Sleep disorders	Fatigue Excessive daytime sleepiness	History
Active Alternatives—Must Not Miss		
Anemia	Fatigue Dyspnea Symptoms of blood loss	CBC
Hypothyroidism	Fatigue Constipation Cold intolerance	TSH
Diabetes	Family history Obesity Hypertension Ethnic group Polyuria Polydipsia	Fasting plasma glucose
Other Hypotheses		
Advanced renal disease	Fatigue Anorexia Nausea Edema	BUN, creatinine
Advanced liver disease	Fatigue Anorexia Nausea Edema	AST ALT Bilirubin
Advanced cardiac disease	Dyspnea Orthopnea Paroxysmal nocturnal dyspnea Edema	ECG Echocardiogram Stress test
Advanced pulmonary disease	Dyspnea Cachexia	Pulmonary exam Pulmonary function tests Chest x-ray

Despite the rarity of positive results, most patients with fatigue need basic laboratory testing consisting of a blood count, chemistry panel, and TSH.

Mrs. M does not lack interest in her usual activities or feel depressed. She has not lost or gained weight. She worries about money and her family but has never had a panic attack and does not consider herself excessively nervous or anxious.

On physical exam, she appears healthy and her affect is normal. HEENT exam is normal. There is no thyromegaly or adenopathy. Lungs are clear. There are no breast masses. Cardiac and abdominal exams are normal, and there is no edema. Her CBC, glucose, BUN, creatinine, liver function tests, and TSH are all normal.

 Is the clinical information sufficient to make a diagnosis? If not, what other information do you need?

Leading Hypotheses: Depression & Anxiety

See Chapter 22, Unintentional Weight Loss.

MAKING A DIAGNOSIS

Mrs. M does not meet DSM criteria for anxiety or depression. It is therefore necessary to consider the alternative diagnoses.

Mrs. M works as a teacher, rising at 6 AM, leaving her house at 7 AM, and returning home about 5 PM. She then prepares dinner for her family, helps her 2 children with their homework, and grades papers until 9:30 PM. She watches a little television, and then goes to sleep about 10:00 PM. Her husband works from 3 PM to 11 PM, and she often wakes up when he gets home at midnight. He needs some time to "wind down" before he goes to sleep, so they often talk and watch TV in bed for an hour or so. She usually then falls asleep immediately but occasionally

has to watch another hour of TV before she can get back to sleep. Considering the additional history, the leading hypothesis is now sleep disorders.

 Is the clinical information sufficient to make a diagnosis? If not, what other information do you need?

Revised Leading Hypothesis: Sleep Disorders

Textbook Presentation

Patients with sleep disorders can present with a variety of symptoms, including insomnia, excessive daytime sleepiness, or disturbed behavior during sleep.

Disease Highlights

A. International Classification of Sleep Disorders (abridged)

  1. Dyssomnias produce either excessive sleepiness or insomnia, which is defined as difficulty initiating or maintaining sleep or nonrestorative sleep.

    a. Intrinsic sleep disorders

      (1) Narcolepsy

      (2) Obstructive sleep apnea

      (3) Central sleep apnea

      (4) Periodic limb movement disorder (PLMD)

    b. Extrinsic sleep disorders

      (1) Psychophysiologic insomnia (insomnia not due to another disorder; lasts for at least 1 month and causes functional impairment)

      (2) Inadequate sleep hygiene

      (3) Adjustment sleep disorder

      (4) Related to stimulant, alcohol, or hypnotic medication use

    c. Circadian rhythm sleep disorders

      (1) Jet lag

      (2) Shift work sleep disorder

      (3) Irregular sleep-wake pattern (going to sleep and waking up at different times each day)

      (4) Delayed or advanced sleep phase syndrome

(a) When the major sleep episode is delayed in relation to the desired clock time, the person cannot fall asleep until very late and then cannot get up at the required time in the morning.

(b) When the major sleep episode is advanced, the person is unacceptably sleepy in the evening and then wakes up much earlier than desired.

2. Parasomnias

   a. Undesirable physical phenomena that disrupt normal sleep

   b. Examples include sleepwalking, sleep terrors, nightmares, bruxism

3. Sleep disorders associated with mental, neurologic, or other medical disorders

   a. Psychiatric disorders with sleep disturbances such as psychoses and mood disorders

   b. Neurologic disorders with sleep disturbances such as dementia and epilepsy

   c. Medical diseases with sleep disturbances such as chronic obstructive pulmonary disease, reflux, fibromyalgia

B. Common sleep disorders

1. Obstructive sleep apnea

   a. Recurrent episodes of partial (hypopnea) or complete (apnea) upper airway obstruction resulting in oxygen desaturation and arousals from sleep.

   b. Present in up to 24% of men and 9% of women

   c. Severity assessed by 2 measures

      (1) Patient description of daytime sleepiness: mild, moderate, severe

      (2) Apnea/hypopnea index (AHI)

         (a) Mild = 5–15 events/hour

         (b) Moderate = 15–30 events/hour

         (c) Severe = greater than 30 events/hour

         (d) Predisposing factors include obesity, male gender, large neck girth, craniofacial abnormalities, increased pharyngeal soft tissue, nasal obstruction, hypothyroidism, family history.

         (e) Treatment modalities include weight loss, uvulopalatopharyngoplasty, continuous positive airway pressure (CPAP), tracheostomy

2. Central sleep apnea

   a. Recurrent apneic episodes in the absence of upper airway obstruction

   b. Accounts for 5% of sleep apnea

   c. Can be idiopathic or associated with congestive heart failure, restrictive lung disease, or obesity

   d. Treatment options include CPAP, diaphragmatic pacing, acetazolamide, theophylline

3. PLMD

   a. Periodic episodes of repetitive and stereotyped limb movements occurring during sleep, generally consisting of big toe extension in combination with partial flexion of the ankle, knee, and hip

   b. Rare in persons younger than 30 years; found in 5% of persons aged 30–50, and in 44% of persons older than 65 years

   c. Primary cause of insomnia in 17% of patients

   d. Most patients with PLMD do not have restless legs syndrome (disagreeable leg sensations causing an irresistible urge to move the legs), but 80% of patients with restless legs syndrome have PLMD

   e. Can be unmasked after successful treatment of obstructive sleep apnea

   f. Effective medications include carbidopa-levodopa, other dopamine agonists, and clonazepam

4. Narcolepsy

   a. Recurrent and uncontrollable lapses into daytime sleep, sometimes with emotion-induced sudden bilateral loss of postural muscle tone (cataplexy)

   b. Prevalence of 0.05%, with peak age of onset ranging from 15 to 25 years

   c. Treatment modalities include lifestyle adjustment, such as avoidance of alcohol, and use of stimulant medications

5. Alcohol-related sleep disorders

   a. Alcohol consumed 30–60 minutes before bedtime results in reduced sleep latency (falling asleep faster).

   b. However, during the second half of the night there is disruption of sleep continuity, due to a "rebound" effect after the alcohol is fully metabolized.

   c. Tolerance to both the sedative and disruptive effects of alcohol occurs within 3 nights.

6. Psychophysiologic insomnia

   a. Chronic sleep disturbance *not* due to an intrinsic sleep disorder; psychiatric, neurologic, medical condition; or medication

b. Leads to fatigue, irritability, impaired memory, and decreased concentration

c. Often due to a combination of tension and learned sleep-preventing associations

Evidence-Based Diagnosis

A. History and physical exam

1. The complaint of sleepiness has traditionally been thought to suggest the diagnosis of an intrinsic sleep disorder.

2. One study of patients with obstructive sleep apnea showed that patients more often reported fatigue, tiredness, or lack of energy than sleepiness.

   a. When patients were asked to choose 1 of these symptoms, they chose lack of energy most often.

   b. Severity of sleep apnea did not correlate with choice of symptom terminology.

3. Since no 1 historical or physical exam finding can reliably predict obstructive sleep apnea, several clinical decision rules have been developed.

   a. A model including neck circumference, hypertension, habitual snoring, and bed partner reports had an LR− = 0.25 and an LR+ = 5.17 for predicting an AHI of at least 10 events/hour

   b. Another model found that presence of an overbite, an abnormal pharyngeal grade, and cricomental distance ≤ 1.5 cm had an LR+ = 10 and an LR− = 0.62; a cricomental distance > 1.5 cm had a negative predictive value of 100% (Figure 13–1).

B. Polysomnography

1. Records electroencephalogram, electromyelogram, ECG, heart rate, respiratory effort, airflow, and oxygen saturation during sleep

2. Gold standard for diagnosis of obstructive and sleep apnea

3. Often used to diagnose PLMD

C. Multiple sleep latency test (MSLT)

1. Used to determine whether abnormal daytime sleepiness is present

2. Consists of 4–5 "nap opportunities" at 2-hour intervals throughout a day, with sleep latency defined as the elapsed time from lights being turned off to the onset of sleep

3. Greater than 70% of patients with narcolepsy have a mean MSLT sleep latency of < 5 minutes

4. 2 or more episodes of REM sleep on MSLT testing is 80% sensitive for the diagnosis of narcolepsy.

 Have you crossed the diagnostic threshold for the leading hypothesis, sleep disorder? Have you ruled out the active alternatives? Do other tests need to be done to exclude the alternative diagnoses?

It is clear that Mrs. M has psychophysiologic insomnia. Further evaluation is not necessary.

CASE RESOLUTION

Mrs. M is reassured that her laboratory tests are normal. She realizes that she often gets 6 hours of sleep or less a night. After listening to you explain the principles of sleep hygiene, she decides to talk with her husband about ways they could spend time together without interrupting her sleep so often.

When she returns 6 months later, she reports that she is still tired because she values the time she spends with her husband at night. However, she now asks him to sleep in the guest room when she feels exceptionally fatigued, so she can have a few nights of uninterrupted sleep. She has also found that a 15-minute nap at lunchtime helps.

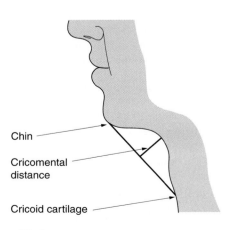

Chin

Cricomental distance

Cricoid cartilage

Figure 13–1. Cricomental distance.

Treatment of Psychophysiologic Insomnia

A. Behavioral therapy

1. Stimulus control therapy

   a. Also known as sleep hygiene

   b. Based on premise that insomnia is a conditioned response to temporal and environmental cues

   c. Has been shown to be effective for sleep onset and maintenance

   d. Principles of sleep hygiene

      (1) Go to bed only when sleepy.

      (2) Use the bedroom only for sleep and sex, not reading, watching television, eating, or working.

      (3) If unable to sleep after 20 minutes in bed, get out of bed, go into another room, read or listen to quiet music, and then return to bed when sleepy.

      (4) Maintain a consistent sleep-wake schedule; go to bed and get up at the same time each day.

      (5) Avoid daytime napping; if napping is necessary, limit the nap to less than 30 minutes and take the nap no later than the early afternoon.

      (6) Avoid caffeine, alcohol, and other stimulants (such as decongestants).

      (7) Exercise regularly, but not in the late evening.

2. Relaxation therapy

   a. Methods include progressive muscle relaxation, biofeedback to reduce somatic arousal, imagery training, meditation

   b. Useful for both sleep onset and maintenance

   c. Often requires practice with a trained professional

3. Sleep restriction therapy

   a. Decreases the amount of time spent in bed in order to increase the percentage of time in bed spent sleeping

   b. Usually keep waking time constant and make bedtime later, with progressive moving up of bedtime as sleep improves

   c. Effective for sleep onset and maintenance

B. Cognitive therapy involves identifying dysfunctional beliefs about sleep and then substituting more functional attitudes that can reduce anxiety.

C. Combination therapy: combining cognitive and behavior therapy has been shown to be superior to relaxation therapy alone.

D. Pharmacotherapy

1. Data comparing pharmacotherapy with behavioral and cognitive therapy are limited.

   a. Overall, treatment effects are similar.

   b. Perhaps more rapid improvement with pharmacotherapy

   c. Perhaps more sustained improvement with behavioral therapy

2. There is little or no information about the use of any medication for more than a few weeks.

3. Basic principles for using pharmacotherapy to treat chronic insomnia

   a. Use agents with shorter half-lives to minimize daytime sedation

   b. Use the lowest effective dose

   c. Try to dose intermittently, such as 2–4 times per week, rather than daily.

   d. Try to limit daily use to a maximum of 3–4 weeks.

   e. Discontinue medication gradually.

   f. Monitor for rebound insomnia when medications are stopped.

4. Categories of medications (Table 13–3)

   a. Benzodiazepines

      (1) Effective in initiating and maintaining sleep

      (2) Efficacy decreases with duration of administration, with tolerance developing after about 3 weeks of daily administration

      (3) Can develop rebound insomnia or withdrawal symptoms when stopped

      (4) Should use only short-acting benzodiazepines for insomnia, since daytime drowsiness, cognitive impairment, and potential for delirium are all greater with longer-acting drugs (but can still occur with short-acting drugs)

   b. Benzodiazepine receptor agonists

      (1) Nonbenzodiazepine compounds that bind to only 1 type of benzodiazepine receptor

      (2) Both zolpidem and zaleplon are effective in initiating sleep; zolpidem is possibly more effective in maintaining sleep.

Table 13–3. Medications used to treat insomnia.

Medication	Dose Range (mg)	Elimination Half-life (h)
Benzodiazepines		
Triazolam	0.125–0.25	1.5–5.5
Temazepam	15–30	3.5–18
Estazolam	1–2	10–24
Lorazepam	0.5–4	8–24
Clonazepam	0.5–2	19–60
Benzodiazepine receptor agonists		
Zaleplon	5–10	1
Zolpidem	5–10	2.5
Miscellaneous		
Diphenhydramine	25–50 mg	2.4–9.3
Trazodone	25–100	5–9

(3) Because of its extremely short half-life, zaleplon can be taken during the night.

(4) No tolerance, dependence, or rebound insomnia

(5) Little or no daytime drowsiness

(6) No evidence of cognitive impairment with zaleplon; zolpidem may cause mild impairment

c. Antihistamines

(1) Should not be used as sleeping aids due to minimal effectiveness and impairment of sleep quality

(2) Daytime drowsiness is common

(3) Commonly cause delirium in elderly patients

d. Antidepressants

(1) Trazodone is frequently used for sleep, although there is no supporting evidence.

(2) Low-dose tricyclic antidepressants, such as amitriptyline, are sometimes used.

(a) Elimination half-lives are long, leading to daytime sedation.

(b) Potential for anticholinergic side effects, even at low doses

I have a patient with GI bleeding. How do I determine the cause?

CHIEF COMPLAINT

PATIENT $\boxed{1}$

Mr. T is a 66-year-old man who arrives at the emergency department with bloody stools and dizziness that started 2 hours ago.

What is the differential diagnosis of GI bleeding. How would you frame the differential?

CONSTRUCTING A DIFFERENTIAL DIAGNOSIS

The approach to GI bleeding is similar to the approach to other imminently life-threatening illnesses. Patient stabilization, specifically, hemodynamic stabilization is the first step in management. In a patient with GI bleeding, management precedes diagnosis, usually made by colonoscopy or esophagogastroduodenoscopy (EGD).

Initial management takes a very regimented course. The patient must be hemodynamically stabilized, preparation must be made in case of further bleeding, and initial diagnostic tests must be completed.

A. Hemodynamic stabilization

   1. Clinically assess volume status.

      a. Signs of shock may be seen with 30–40% volume depletion.

      b. Orthostasis can be seen with 20–25% volume depletion.

      c. Tachycardia may be present with 15% volume depletion.

   2. Calculate necessary replacement (weight in kg × 0.6 (lean body weight made up of water) × % volume depletion).

   3. Replace fluid losses initially with normal saline or Ringers solution.

   4. Administer typed (or O–) blood if there has been a large degree of blood loss.

B. Preparation for further bleeding

   1. All patients should have their blood typed and be cross-matched for at least 2 units.

   2. Patients may initially have normal hematocrits (Hcts) that drop only with fluid replacement.

It is common for a patient with a significant GI bleed to have a normal hematocrits at presentation.

   3. Remember that the physical exam is insensitive for anemia (see Chapter 4, Anemia).

   4. Two large bore IVs

      a. IVs should be 16 gauge or greater.

      b. Flow = $\Delta P \, (\pi r^4 / 8\mu L)$ where ΔP is the pressure differential, r is the radius of the IV, μ is the viscosity of the fluid, and L is the length of the IV.

      c. Flow can therefore be maximized by

         (1) Increasing the pressure behind the fluid being infused (squeezing the bag).

         (2) Decreasing the length of the IV.

         (3) Increasing the gauge of the IV (the most effective as the flow goes up by the fourth power of any increase).

      d. Large gauge IVs (16 and larger) are much more effective than central lines for volume resuscitation.

Always make sure your patient has 2 usable large bore IVs, so you do not have to worry about IV access should life-threatening bleeding develop.

e. In large bleeds, a Foley catheter can help monitor fluid status.

C. Initial diagnostic tests

1. CBC and platelet count

2. Chem-7

3. Liver function tests (LFTs) (Abnormal LFTs raise the risk of underlying severe liver disease and thus coagulopathy and varices.)

4. Prothrombin time and partial thromboplastin time

5. Upright chest x-ray

a. Can diagnose perforated viscus

b. May provide clues to other diagnoses

6. Nasogastric (NG) tube placement helps assess source and acuity of blood loss.

The differential diagnosis of GI bleeding is based on an anatomic framework. Upper GI bleeds originate proximal to the ligament of Treitz, while lower GI bleeds are distal and primarily colonic. The causes of upper and lower GI bleeding are arranged in the approximate order of frequency. Bleeding from a small bowel source is uncommon. The last category is anorectal bleeding. These are generally smaller bleeds with limited potential to cause hemodynamic instability.

A. Upper GI bleeds

1. Common

a. Peptic ulcer disease

b. Gastritis

c. Varices

2. Less common

a. Angiodysplasia

b. Mallory-Weiss tear

c. Malignancy

d. Esophagitis

e. Dieulafoy lesion

B. Lower GI bleeds

1. Common

a. Diverticulosis

b. Malignancy or polyp

c. Colitis

(1) Inflammatory

(2) Infectious

(3) Ischemic

d. Angiodysplasia

2. Less common small bowel sources

a. Angiodysplasia

b. Ulcers

c. Malignancy

d. Crohn disease

e. Meckel diverticulum

C. Anorectal bleeding

1. Hemorrhoids

2. Anal fissures

Mr. T was well until this morning. Abdominal cramping developed while he was eating breakfast. He did not have nausea. He went to the bathroom and passed a large bowel movement of stool mixed with blood. Afterward, he felt better and went to lie down. About 30 minutes later, he had the same sensation and this time passed what he described as "about a pint" of bright red blood. While getting up from the toilet, he became dizzy and had to sit on the bathroom floor for 15 minutes before he could crawl to the phone to dial 911.

At this point, what is the leading hypothesis, and what are the active alternatives? What other tests should be ordered?

ORGANIZING THE DIFFERENTIAL DIAGNOSIS

The lack of nausea, vomiting, or abdominal pain, and the presence of bright red blood per rectum make a lower GI source most likely. Cramping is often seen with GI bleeds, caused by blood passing through the bowel. The volume of blood makes hemorrhoids or fissures unlikely, so bleeding from diverticuli, colitis, malignancy, or angiodysplasia have to be considered most likely. Whether he has had recent change in bowel habits, weight loss, or previous bloody stools is unknown; all these factors would heighten suspicion for colitis or malignancy. Upper sources of bleeding must also be considered. A brisk bleed from an upper source can present with bright red blood per rectum. Assuming there is no history of liver disease, peptic ulcer disease and gastritis would be the most likely causes. Table 14–1 lists the differential diagnosis.

Table 14–1. Diagnostic hypotheses for Mr. T.

Diagnostic Hypotheses	Clinical Clues	Important Tests
Leading Hypothesis		
Diverticular bleed	Brisk self-limited bleeds History of diverticuli	Colonoscopy
Active Alternative		
Angiodysplasia	Brisk lower GI bleeds More common with end-stage renal disease	Colonoscopy or small bowel endoscopy
Other Alternative		
Peptic ulcer disease	Epigastric pain improved or worsened with eating	EGD
Active Alternative—Must Not Miss		
Colon cancer	History of anemia or changing bowel habits	Colonoscopy

Blood is cathartic to the bowel. A brisk bleed from an upper source can present with bright red blood per rectum.

Mr. T reports no recent illness or change in bowel habits. He reports no family history of colon cancer, and he has never had a colonoscopy. He has a fifty-pack year smoking and quit about 6 years ago. He reports drinking 2–4 beers each night.

On physical exam, Mr. T looks somewhat anxious but is otherwise well. While sitting, his BP is 120/92 mm Hg and his pulse is 100 bpm. While standing, his BP is 100/80 mm Hg and his pulse his 122 bpm. His temperature is 37.0 °C and his RR is 16 breaths per minute. There is no conjunctival pallor. Lungs and heart exams are normal. There are hyperactive bowel sounds but the abdomen is soft, nontender, and with no organomegaly. Rectal exam reveals bright red blood.

Is the clinical information sufficient to make a diagnosis? If not, what other information do you need?

Leading Hypothesis: Diverticular Bleed

Textbook Presentation
The typical presentation is an episode of bright red blood per rectum in an older patient. There is abdominal cramping but no real pain. A history of previously diagnosed diverticuli (on a screening colonoscopy, for instance) and possibly a previous, self-limited hemorrhage is often present.

Disease Highlights
A. Most common cause of lower GI bleeding
   1. Prevalence of causes of GI bleeding varies from study to study.
   2. One large review gave the following data:
      a. Diverticulosis: 33%
      b. Colonic malignancy or polyp: 19%
      c. Inflammatory bowel disease (IBD) or ulcers: 18%
      d. Angiodysplasia: 8%
      e. Anorectal cause: 4%
B. The risk of diverticular hemorrhage in a patient with diverticuli is not known but is estimated to be 3–15%.
C. Although diverticuli are most commonly left sided, right-sided lesions seem to cause the heaviest bleeds.

D. Bleeding occurs as a vessel is stretched over the dome of a diverticulum. Luminal trauma likely leads to bleeding from the weakened vessel.

E. Spontaneous cessation and only moderate blood loss is the rule, but recurrence is common.

   1. ≅ 75% of patients experience spontaneous cessation of hemorrhage.

   2. Nearly all patients require less than 4 units of packed RBCs.

   3. ≅ 40% of patients will have recurrent bleeding.

F. Diverticular hemorrhage carries a poor short-term prognosis.

   1. In general, lower GI bleeding carries a better overall prognosis than upper GI bleeding with about half the mortality rate.

   2. Mortality rates for diverticular hemorrhage are higher (11% at 1 year and 20% at 4 years) although the cause of death is rarely related to the GI hemorrhage.

 Although diverticular hemorrhage seldom causes death, it is a marker for a poor, short-term prognosis.

Evidence-Based Diagnosis

The first step in making the diagnosis of any GI bleed is to determine whether the source of the bleeding is the upper or lower tract.

A. History

   1. Certain historical features may point to a specific diagnosis (Table 14–2).

      a. These features should be sought in every patient with GI bleeding.

      b. They are only suggestive, however, and by no means diagnostic.

   2. A physician's assessment of the appearance of stool is somewhat predictive of the site of bleeding (Table 14–3).

   3. Certain features suggest upper GI bleeds

      a. Nausea and vomiting

      b. Hematemesis or coffee-ground emesis

      c. Melena

      d. An elevated BUN/creatinine ratio has traditionally been considered suggestive of an upper GI bleed, but test characteristics suggest it is only minimally useful.

         (1) Test characteristics of BUN/creatinine ratio ≤ 33 for the diagnosis of lower GI bleeding are 96% sensitivity, 17% specificity, LR+ = 1.16, and LR− = 0.24.

   4. Lower GI bleeds

      a. Hematochezia generally suggests a lower GI source of bleeding.

      b. 10–15% of patients with hematochezia have an upper GI source. These patients are more likely to be older and to have duodenal ulcers.

Table 14–2. Historical features in the diagnosis of GI bleeding.

Historical Feature	Suggested Diagnosis
NSAID use	Peptic ulcer disease
Severe vascular disease	Ischemic colitis
Pelvic radiation	Radiation colitis
Febrile illness	Infectious colitis
Aortic graft	Aortoenteric fistula (duodenal most common)
Liver disease or alcohol history	Esophageal varices
Retching preceding hematemesis	Mallory-Weiss tear
Recent colonic polypectomy	Post polypectomy bleeding
Severe constipation	Stercoral ulcer

NSAID, nonsteroidal anti-inflammatory drug.

Table 14–3. Test characteristics of physician assessment of stool appearance.

Physician Descriptor and Corresponding Bleeding Site	Sensitivity	Specificity	LR+	LR–
Bright red blood for lower GI bleeding	46%	90%	4.6	0.6
Black stool for upper GI bleeding	71%	88%	5.92	0.33

Adapted from Zuckerman GR, Trellis DR, Sherman TM, Clouse RE. An objective measure of stool color for differentiating upper from lower gastrointestinal bleeding. *Dig Dis Sci.* 1995;40:1614–1621 with kind permission from Springer Science and Business Media.

5. Patients, as well as nurses and doctors, overestimate blood volume when seeing blood in a toilet.

B. Physical exam

1. Aids in the localization of GI bleeding by identifying related diseases.

   a. Look for stigmata of chronic liver disease, cancer-related cachexia, or extraintestinal manifestations of IBD.

   b. Patients who are volume depleted, orthostatic, or hypotensive are about twice as likely to have an upper GI bleed than a lower GI bleed.

2. An NG tube is a minimally invasive way to assess the acuity of bleeding and to help localize its source.

   a. An NG tube should always be placed unless there is a really obvious lower GI source.

   b. After placement, the contents of the stomach are withdrawn, and the tube is flushed until the return is clear.

   c. A bloody return is essentially diagnostic of an upper GI bleed (LR+ = 7.7).

   d. A negative lavage does not exclude an upper GI source.

   e. Although it is usually taught that a negative return (in which there is bilious material) rules out *active* upper GI bleeding, some studies question this.

   f. The test characteristics for NG aspiration diagnosing an actively bleeding upper GI source are

     (1) Sensitivity, 79%; specificity, 55%

     (2) LR+, 1.76; LR–, 0.38

 A positive NG diagnoses upper GI bleeding, although not necessarily active bleeding. It does predict a worse overall prognosis.

C. Endoscopy

1. EGD is usually recommended as the first procedure unless there is a clearly negative NG tube aspirate. This recommendation is based partly on the higher potential for severe blood loss from upper GI bleeds.

2. Colonoscopy

   a. The diagnosis of diverticular hemorrhage is usually made on colonoscopy.

   b. It is important to realize that this diagnosis is usually presumptive (87% of the time in some studies) based on seeing diverticuli and blood in that region of the colon.

   c. Less commonly, a definitive diagnosis is made when active bleeding or stigmata of recent bleeding in a diverticulum is seen.

D. Tagged RBC scan

1. Tc 99m-labeled RBC scans are most commonly used.

2. Can detect bleeds as slow as 0.1 mL/min.

3. Most commonly used for detecting the source of bleeding in patients with persistent bleeding and normal endoscopy.

4. Test characteristics are not very good.

   a. Scans detect bleeding in about half of patients (sensitivity ≅ 45%).

   b. The specificity of bleeding scans is unknown and their ability to accurately localize bleeds is only moderate, succeeding 78% of the time.

   c. Scans that turn positive early are most helpful in localizing bleeds (≅ 95%).

E. Angiography

1. Requires bleeding at a rate of about 0.5 mL/min to detect active bleeding.

2. Sensitivity is about 50% but depends greatly on selection of patients.

3. In diverticular bleeding, angiography is very useful at localizing the site of bleeding before surgery.

MAKING A DIAGNOSIS

Mr. T was given 1 L of normal saline. While in the emergency department, he again passed a large amount of blood.

Initial lab tests are normal. Important values are BUN, 12 mg/dL; creatinine, 1.1 mg/dL; Hgb, 13.9 g/dL; Hct, 39%. NG tube lavage did not reveal any blood, but there was no bilious return.

Have you crossed a diagnostic threshold for the leading hypothesis, diverticular bleed? Have you ruled out the active alternatives? Do other tests need to be done to exclude the alternative diagnoses?

Mr. T weighs 75 kg. His orthostasis suggests 20% volume depletion. Given this weight, his fluid deficit is about 9 L (75 kg × 20% volume depletion × 60%). Assuming this deficit is all from the GI bleed, it is very likely that his Hct will fall once he is hydrated.

His history, normal BUN/creatinine ratio, and clear NG tube lavage are suggestive of a lower GI bleed. Following stabilization, initial endoscopy with either colonoscopy or EGD would be reasonable.

Alternative Diagnosis: Angiodysplasia

Textbook Presentation

Bleeding from angiodysplasia can look like any other cause of lower GI bleeding. It is seen almost exclusively in older adults and can present with anything from hematochezia to occult blood loss. In general, hemorrhage from angiodysplasia tends to be less brisk than that from diverticuli.

Disease Highlights

A. Angiodysplasia, also called arteriovenous malformations, are dilated submucosal veins that are most commonly seen in the right colon of adults over age 60.

B. Present in < 5% of patients over 60.

C. Well over 50% of patients with angiodysplasias do not bleed.

D. Angiodysplasia has historically been associated with various other diseases (eg, aortic stenosis and cirrhosis).

1. These relationships have not been proved.

2. Angiodysplasia is a common cause of bleeding in patients with end-stage renal disease.

Evidence-Based Diagnosis

A. Similar to the diagnosis of diverticular hemorrhage, colonoscopy, tagged RBC scan, and angiography are all used.

B. Colonoscopy is the most common tool. It allows good visualization of the cecum, which is the site of most angiodysplasias.

C. Angiography can provide evidence of a diagnosis even without active bleeding if suspicious vascular patterns are seen.

D. As in diverticular hemorrhage, the diagnosis is often presumptive, made on the basis of visualizing non-bleeding angiodysplasia in a patient with GI bleeding.

Treatment

A. Both acute and chronic bleeding is generally treated endoscopically with thermal or laser ablation. This method can be repeated for recurrent bleeding.

B. Angiographic intervention, with vasoconstrictor agents or embolization, is rarely used.

C. Surgical management (right hemicolectomy) is sometimes required for frequent, recurrent bleeding.

D. Hormonal therapy with estrogen has been used to prevent recurrent bleeding in angiodysplasia, but a recent study suggests that this is not very effective.

Alternative Diagnosis: Colon Cancer

Textbook Presentation

A typical presentation is iron deficiency anemia, weight loss, cachexia, and constipation in a middle-aged patient. Physical exam may reveal anemia and fullness in the left lower quadrant.

Disease Highlights

A. The most common presenting symptoms in patients with colon cancer are listed below. It should be noted that these data are from 1991. Colon cancer screening has become more widespread since this time, presumably reducing the proportion of cases that present with acute GI bleeding.

1. Acute GI bleeding: 34%

2. Abdominal pain: 22%

3. Screening: 12%

4. Anemia: 11%

5. Large bowel obstruction: 4%

B. Unlike colon cancer, colonic polyps are an unlikely cause of acute bleeding. Colonic polyps are most likely to bleed when they are removed. GI bleeding after polypectomy is not uncommon, occurring after about 1 in 200 procedures.

Evidence-Based Diagnosis

A. Colon cancer and colonic polyps are diagnosed either by barium enema, colonoscopy, or virtual colonoscopy. All tests effectively detect large tumors but test characteristics vary for adenomas of around 1 cm.

    1. Colonoscopy is generally considered the gold standard. Sensitivity is about 95% overall and is close to 100% for polyps > 1 cm but lower for cecal polyps.

    2. Barium enema: sensitivity $\cong$ 50%

    3. Virtual colonoscopy

        a. In virtual colonoscopy, data from CT scans are used to generate displays of the interior of the colon.

        b. Studies have reported sensitivities for detecting polyps > 1 cm ranging from 55% to 95%.

        c. In a study using the most advanced techniques, virtual colonoscopy actually outperformed traditional colonoscopy in finding large polyps.

B. Definitive diagnosis is made by obtaining a biopsy specimen, usually endoscopically.

Treatment

Surgical excision is the mainstay of treatment for colon cancer with chemotherapy indicated for those patients with more advanced disease.

CASE RESOLUTION

Following the episode of bleeding in the emergency department, Mr. T was given 1 liter of normal saline. His initial Hct was 38%; 6 hours later, it was 30% and he was given 2 units of packed RBCs. Given the clinical suspicion of a lower GI bleed, colonoscopy was done about 6 hours after admission. There were multiple left-sided diverticuli and a right-sided diverticulum with a nonbleeding visible vessel. A diagnosis of a diverticular bleed was made.

Following the 2 units of packed RBCs and 3 L of normal saline, Mr. T was clinically euvolemic and his Hct stabilized at 31%. He remained in the hospital for about 48 hours during which there was no recurrent bleeding and his Hct remained stable.

This is one of the rare cases when the diagnosis of a diverticular hemorrhage can be made with certainty. The patient required only 2 units of blood and the bleeding stopped spontaneously.

Treatment of Diverticular Hemorrhage

A. Management of blood loss

    1. All GI bleeds call for similar treatment of a patient who has lost, or has the potential to lose, a significant amount of blood.

    2. Monitoring

        a. Clinically: Is there recurrent bleeding, increasing tachycardia, or orthostasis?

        b. Laboratory: Is the Hct falling?

            (1) Typically, patients have a CBC checked every 6 hours until stability has been achieved.

            (2) Intensity of monitoring varies with risk of rebleeding.

    3. Transfusion

        a. Transfusion is generally initiated when Hct < 20% or < 25% in patients with cardiopulmonary disease.

        b. In the setting of acute hemorrhage, transfusion needs to be used more liberally in order to address the expected falls in blood counts.

        c. Transfusion is recommended for blood loss of > 30% ($\cong$ 1 L).

        d. Alternatively, it is recommended when the Hct is $\cong$ 24% in a patient who is actively bleeding or when Hct is $\cong$ 30% in a patient with cardiopulmonary disease who is actively bleeding.

        e. In general, there should be a low threshold for giving a transfusion to a patient who is orthostatic and actively bleeding.

B. Management of diverticular hemorrhage

    1. Treatment is seldom necessary because most diverticular hemorrhages stop spontaneously.

    2. Endoscopic treatment, primarily thermocoagulation or sclerotherapy, is occasionally used.

3. Angiographic intervention, with vasoconstrictor agents or embolization, is rarely used. Occasionally, local vasopressin infusion may be a temporizing measure.

C. Colectomy

1. Ultimate therapy for diverticular bleeding is to remove the part of the colon containing the diverticuli.

2. Recommended for either persistent, large bleeds (over 4 units in 24 hours or 10 units during the course of a single bleed) or for frequent recurrences.

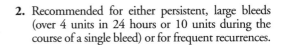 The diagnosis of diverticular hemorrhage is often presumptive. Localization of the bleeding site before surgery must be as definitive as possible.

CHIEF COMPLAINT

PATIENT 2

Mr. M is a 39-year-old man who arrives at the emergency department after vomiting blood. He reports waking the morning of admission with an "upset stomach." He initially attributed this to a hangover. After about an hour he vomited "a gallon of blood" with no other stomach contents. Almost immediately afterward, he had another episode and called 911.

 At this point, what is the leading hypothesis, and what are the active alternatives? What other tests should be ordered?

ORGANIZING THE DIFFERENTIAL DIAGNOSIS

Mr. M is having an upper GI bleed. The hematemesis localizes the source of the bleeding to above the ligament of Treitz. Peptic ulcer disease and gastritis are the most common causes of upper GI bleeding. Although not always present, preceding symptoms of abdominal distress are common with peptic ulcer disease and gastritis. Esophageal varices should be considered in the differential diagnosis given the patient's alcohol history. The severity of the patient's alcohol use is still unknown, so we do not know whether he is at risk for portal hypertension. A Mallory-Weiss tear is also possible, but the patient would report vomiting before the onset of bleeding. Table 14–4 lists the differential diagnosis.

2

On further history, the patient reports no previous episodes of GI bleeding. He reports occa-

sional stomach upset, usually following drinking binges. He denies NSAID use. Mr. M says that he has been drinking heavily since his late teens. He reports drinking at least a fifth of hard liquor and a 6-pack of beer daily for the last 20 years. He reports that he has not seen a doctor since his pediatrician.

On physical exam, Mr. M is anxious and appears tired. He smells of alcohol. While sitting, his BP is 140/80 mm Hg and his pulse is 100 bpm. While standing, his BP is 100/80 mm Hg and his pulse is 130 bpm. His temperature is 37.0 °C and RR is 16 breaths per minute. Sclera are slightly icteric. Lungs are clear and heart is tachycardic but regular. Abdomen is soft without hepatomegaly. There is no ascites but the spleen is palpable about 2 cm below the costal margin.

Given the alcohol history, scleral icterus, and splenomegaly, a hemorrhage from esophageal varices needs to move above peptic ulcer disease on the differential diagnosis.

 Is the clinical information sufficient to make a diagnosis? If not, what other information do you need?

Leading Hypothesis: Esophageal Variceal Hemorrhage

Textbook Presentation

A patient with known cirrhosis presents with heavy upper GI bleeding (hematemesis or melena). There are stigmata of chronic liver disease and frequently history of previous hemorrhages. Laboratory data demonstrate LFTs consistent with cirrhosis and thrombocytopenia.

Table 14–4. Diagnostic hypotheses for Mr. M.

Diagnostic Hypotheses	Clinical Clues	Important Tests
Leading Hypothesis		
Peptic ulcer disease	Abdominal pain NSAID use Relationship to eating	EGD
Active Alternative		
Gastritis	Often asymptomatic prior to hemorrhage	EGD
Active Alternative—Must Not Miss		
Esophageal varices	History of portal hypertension, usually due to cirrhosis Stigmata of chronic liver disease	EGD
Other Alternative		
Mallory-Weiss tear	Hematemesis preceded by vomiting, especially with retching	EGD

Disease Highlights

A. Esophageal varices are portosystemic collaterals that dilate when portal pressures exceed 12 mm Hg.

B. Although varices are the second most common cause of GI bleeding, they account for 80–90% of GI bleeds in patients with cirrhosis.

C. Gastroesophageal varices are present in about 50% of patients with cirrhosis.

   1. The prevalence of varices depends on the severity of the cirrhosis.

   2. The Child-Turcotte-Pugh system classifies patients based on the severity of their cirrhosis. The system takes into account the presence of encephalopathy, ascites, hyperbilirubinemia, hypoalbuminemia, and clotting deficiencies (Table 14–5).

   3. 40% of patients with Child A disease have varices, while 85% of patients with Child C disease have varices.

D. Approximately 33% of patients with varices will experience hemorrhage.

E. Varices may develop from cirrhosis of any cause.

F. Varices carry the worst prognosis of GI bleeds.

   1. Nearly 33% of patients die at the time of their first variceal hemorrhage.

   2. Up to 70% of survivors have recurrent bleeding in the first year.

   3. A variceal bleed carries a 32–80% 1-year mortality.

 Esophageal varices are by far the most lethal type of GI bleeding.

Evidence-Based Diagnosis

A. Of all causes of GI bleeding, varices are probably the easiest to predict. One study has the sensitivity and specificity of physicians predicting variceal hemorrhage at 82% and 96% respectively, much better than for other diagnoses.

B. The gold standard for the diagnosis of varices is endoscopy.

MAKING A DIAGNOSIS

NG tube lavage in the emergency department revealed bright red blood that did not clear with flushing. The patient was admitted to the ICU and received 1 L of normal saline and 2 units of O– packed RBCs. A Foley catheter was placed for close monitoring of volume status. After another large episode of hematemesis, Mr. M was intubated for airway protection. IV octreotide was begun, and the GI service was called to perform urgent endoscopy.

Table 14–5. Child-Turcotte-Pugh classification.

Parameter	1 Point	2 Points	3 Points
Ascites	Absent	Slight	Moderate
Bilirubin mg/dL	≤ 2	2–3	> 3
Albumin, g/dL	> 3.5	2.8–3.5	< 2.8
INR	< 1.7	1.8–2.3	> 2.3
Encephalopathy	None	Grade 1–2	Grade 3–4

Grade A (well-compensated disease, 2-year survival 85%): 5–6 points
Grade B (significant functional compromise, 2-year survival 60%): 7–9 points
Grade C (decompensated disease, 2-year survival 35%): 10–15 points

 Have you crossed a diagnostic threshold for the leading hypothesis, variceal hemorrhage? Have you ruled out the active alternatives? Do other tests need to be done to exclude the alternative diagnoses?

The patient is having a large upper GI bleed and is clearly actively bleeding. Initial management is aimed at hemodynamic stabilization. The decision to place the patient in the ICU was based on his hemodynamic instability, active bleeding, and need for close monitoring. Given the alcohol history, the volume of the bleed, and the lack of previous abdominal symptoms, esophageal varices is highest on the differential diagnosis, and empiric therapy has begun with octreotide. Peptic ulcer disease is the most common cause of upper GI bleeding, and we do not yet know whether this patient has cirrhosis. Dieulafoy lesions can also cause large upper GI bleeds.

Alternative Diagnosis: Peptic Ulcer Disease

The details of peptic ulcer disease are given in Chapter 22, Unintentional Weight Loss. This section will only deal with hemorrhage from peptic ulcers.

Textbook Presentation

The classic presentation is chronic dyspepsia, long-term use of nonsteroidal anti-inflammatory drugs (NSAIDs), or *Helicobacter pylori* infection in a middle-aged person who has an episode of hematemesis or melena, or both.

Disease Highlights

A. Most common cause of GI bleeds.

  1. Upper GI bleeds are 4–8 times more common than lower GI bleeds.

  2. Peptic ulcer disease accounts for at least 50% of upper GI bleeds.

B. Bleeding occurs when an ulcer erodes into a vessel in the stomach or duodenal wall.

C. About 50% of patients with bleeding or perforation have had no previous symptoms.

D. Causative factors are long-term use of NSAIDs, *H pylori* infection, or stress from critical illness.

E. Similar to diverticuli, most cases are self-limited (≅ 80%).

Evidence-Based Diagnosis

A. Except in rare cases, all patients with GI bleeding in whom an ulcer is suspected undergo endoscopy. Endoscopy is useful from diagnostic, prognostic, and therapeutic standpoints.

B. Endoscopy has a 92% sensitivity for ulcers and allows for exclusion of malignancy as a cause of the ulcer.

C. Endoscopy is also useful because it gives information about a patient's risk of recurrent bleeding and thus enables discharge planning. Table 14–6 gives approximate rates for recurrent bleeding by endoscopic finding.

D. Other endoscopic findings associated with high-risk are ulcer size > 2 cm and arterial bleeding.

E. Clinical factors such as transfusion requirements, age, comorbid conditions, and hemodynamic stability must also be taken into account.

Table 14–6. Approximate rates for recurrent bleeding by endoscopic finding.

Lesion	Rebleeding Rate
Actively oozing vessel	55%
Nonbleeding visible vessel	45%
Adherent clot	15–35%
Clean based ulcer	5%

Treatment

A. Hemodynamic stabilization

B. Endoscopy

   1. Early endoscopy achieves hemostasis in > 94% of patients and decreases length of hospital stay.

   2. There are many different modes of controlling bleeding endoscopically, including thermocoagulation, sclerotherapy, and laser therapy.

   3. Repeat endoscopy is effective in the 15–20% of patients who have a recurrence of bleeding.

C. Medication

   1. IV H_2-blockers are commonly used in the United States, although they are probably only slightly effective in treating gastric ulcers.

   2. One well-done study has shown that compared with placebo, IV omeprazole is effective in treating patients with ulcers who are actively bleeding.

     a. Relative risk reduction (RRR) of 70% with a number needed to treat (NNT) of 8.

     b. There was a trend toward decreased mortality in the omeprazole group.

     D. Although surgical therapy is less frequently necessary than it once was, it does still play a role for patients whose severe bleeding cannot be controlled endoscopically.

Alternative Diagnosis: Mallory-Weiss Tear

Textbook Presentation

Mallory-Weiss tear is typically seen in patients with vomiting of any cause who acutely develop hematemesis.

Disease Highlights

A. Mallory-Weiss tears are mucosal tears at the gastroesophageal junction.

B. It is a common misconception that Mallory-Weiss tears always follow retching when in fact a history of retching preceding hematemesis is present in about 33% of cases.

Evidence-Based Diagnosis

Diagnosis is routinely made on upper endoscopy.

Treatment

Mallory-Weiss tears seldom require specific treatment. Rebleeding is quite rare.

CASE RESOLUTION

Emergency endoscopy was performed in the ICU. Mr. M was found to have large esophageal and gastric varices. A clear bleeding source was found and treated with sclerotherapy. Although there was no clinically significant rebleeding, other complications developed. He remained intubated for 5 days for presumed aspiration pneumonia, and his recovery was delayed by alcohol withdrawal and mild encephalopathy.

During the hospitalization he was found to have Child-Turcotte-Pugh grade B cirrhosis. At the time of discharge, he was taking propranolol, isosorbide mononitrate and lactulose. Follow-up in an outpatient alcohol program and the hepatology practice was scheduled. He did not come to any follow-up visits.

Mr. M's emergent endoscopy was indicated by the severity of the bleeding. His bleeding was controlled with a combination of medical and endoscopic management. The complicated hospital course is not surprising given the comorbid conditions frequently present in patients with varices. Mr. M had advanced cirrhosis and alcohol dependence.

Treatment of Esophageal Varices

A. Prophylactic treatment

   1. Because variceal bleeding carries such a high mortality, the goal is to predict bleeding and treat prophylactically.

   2. All patients with cirrhosis should undergo screening endoscopy every other year.

     a. Patients without splenomegaly or thrombocytopenia are at the lowest risk for having varices ($\cong$ 4%). Endoscopy may be delayed in these patients.

   b. Patients who continue to drink, have poor liver function, and have various endoscopic markers have the highest chance of bleeding.

3. Once diagnosed, β-blockers (usually propranolol or nadolol) and nitrates are prescribed to decrease portal pressures.

   a. Nitrates reduce portal pressure but are inferior to β-blockers in reducing rate of first bleed.

   b. Shunt procedures reduce bleeding rates at the cost of more frequent encephalopathy and higher mortality rates.

   c. Sclerotherapy of varices is not effective as primary prevention.

4. Patients with the highest risk of bleeding or those who are intolerant of β-blockers should undergo band ligation of the varices.

5. Liver transplantation is the definitive therapy.

B. Treatment of acute hemorrhage

1. Even more than other GI bleeds, achievement of hemodynamic stability in variceal bleeds is of primary importance because the hemorrhage is potentially massive.

2. Transfuse to a target Hct of 25–30%; overexpansion of blood volume increases portal pressure and the risk of rebleeding.

3. IV octreotide should be given as soon as variceal hemorrhage is suspected. It achieves cessation of variceal bleeding in about 80% of patients.

4. Endoscopic banding and sclerotherapy are done initially and if bleeding persists.

5. Other therapies include balloon tamponade of varices and transvenous intrahepatic portosystemic shunting (TIPS).

6. Surgical intervention is seldom called for as the mortality is extremely high.

7. Cirrhotic patients with upper GI bleeding are at high risk for bacterial infections. Administration of norfloxacin for 7 days has been shown to decrease both the rate of bacterial infections and mortality.

CHIEF COMPLAINT

PATIENT 3

Ms. S is a 35-year-old woman who comes to the outpatient clinic for an initial visit. She is well and is without complaints. On review of systems, she notes that she occasionally passes bright red blood per rectum. This has happened about 4 times over the past 5 years. It is never associated with pain. She sometimes sees the blood on the toilet paper and sometimes in the bowl.

At this point, what is the leading hypothesis, and what are the active alternatives? What other tests should be ordered?

ORGANIZING THE DIFFERENTIAL DIAGNOSIS

Ms. S has recurrent, lower GI bleeding that has occurred intermittently over a number of years without obvious negative health effects. This type of bleeding can be categorized as benign sounding anorectal bleeding. It is bleeding in a young patient without "red flags" for serious disease such as anemia, change in bowel habits, weight loss, or diarrhea. Between 10% and 20% of the population will have this type of bleeding. The goal is to diagnose these patients appropriately without missing occasional serious lesions and without subjecting excessive numbers of patients to unpleasant evaluation.

The differential diagnosis has to include hemorrhoidal bleeding and bleeding from anal fissures. Anal fissures are usually painful so hemorrhoids are probably the more likely diagnosis. IBD, especially ulcerative colitis, could cause similar symptoms, although because of the intermittent nature in this case, IBD would be surprising. You need to know more about the patient's bowel habits. Diverticuli and colonic angiodysplasia could account for the patient's symptoms but would be very unusual in a patient this age. Colon or rectal cancer are also rare in this age group but should be considered. Table 14–7 lists the differential diagnosis.

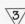 3

On further history Ms. S reports no recent change in bowel habits, no weight loss, and says she feels well. She does report that although the bleeding has never been associated with pain, it is sometimes associated with constipation. She has never used any treatment.

Table 14–7. Diagnostic hypothesis for Ms. S.

Diagnostic Hypotheses	Clinical Clues	Important Tests
Leading Hypothesis		
Hemorrhoids	Painful or painless bright red blood per rectum	Anoscopy
Active Alternative—Most Common		
Anal fissures	Bright red blood per rectum, often associated with severe pain	External inspection and anoscopy
Active Alternative—Must Not Miss		
Ulcerative colitis	Usually associated with diarrhea	Colonoscopy
Colon cancer	History of anemia or changing bowel habits	Colonoscopy

 Is the clinical information sufficient to make a diagnosis? If not, what other information do you need?

Leading Hypothesis: Hemorrhoidal Bleeding

Textbook Presentation

Hemorrhoidal bleeding typically presents with severe rectal pain and bleeding. The pain is worst with bowel movements, straining, or sitting. Occasionally, hemorrhoids can present with painless bleeding.

Disease Highlights

A. Hemorrhoids are generally classified as internal or external.

  1. External hemorrhoids

   a. Occur below the dentate line.

   b. Present either as painless bleeding; engorged, painful, swollen perianal tissue; or as thrombosed hemorrhoids. Thrombosed hemorrhoids are purple and extremely painful and may also bleed.

  2. Internal hemorrhoids

   a. Occur above the dentate line.

   b. Symptoms can be a feeling of internal fullness, painless bleeding, or prolapse. Prolapse is usually painful and sometimes associated with bleeding.

B. Both internal and external hemorrhoids will be most symptomatic with sitting, straining, and constipation.

 A physician should always verify a patient's self-diagnosis of hemorrhoids. Many patients refer to all perianal symptoms as hemorrhoids.

Evidence-Based Diagnosis

A. Hemorrhoidal bleeding is diagnosed by direct observation.

  1. This may be accomplished visually in patients with external hemorrhoids.

  2. Patients with internal hemorrhoids require anoscopy to see hemorrhoids.

B. An important question is "When does benign sounding anorectal bleeding need a more extensive evaluation than an anal exam with or without anoscopy?"

  1. One study looked at 201 patients who had the complaint of rectal bleeding elicited on a review of symptoms.

   a. 24% of these patients were found to have serious disease. The diseases were polyps in 13%, colon cancer in 6.5%, and IBD in 4% of patients.

   b. Factors associated with risk of serious disease were age, short duration of bleeding, and blood mixed with stool.

   c. No cancers were found in patients younger than 50.

   d. 6 of the 37 patients who had a clear source of anorectal bleeding (fissures or hemorrhoids) also had polyps or cancer.

2. Another study found only 10 polyps among 314 patients under 40 with rectal bleeding compared with 27 polyps and 1 case of cancer among 256 patients between the ages of 40 and 50.

C. In general, if a young patient with rectal bleeding does not have a clear anorectal source or if the bleeding continues despite treatment of the anorectal source, a more complete evaluation (with colonoscopy) should be done. Patients over 40 should always be evaluated.

 Although serious disease is rare among young people with rectal bleeding, it does occur.

MAKING A DIAGNOSIS

 Ms. S has a normal general physical exam. External anal exam and digital rectal exam are normal. Anoscopy reveals 1 large, nonbleeding internal hemorrhoid.

 Have you crossed a diagnostic threshold for the leading hypothesis, hemorrhoidal bleeding? Have you ruled out the active alternatives? Do other tests need to be done to exclude the alternative diagnoses?

The patient has an internal hemorrhoid on exam. This is almost certainly, but not definitely, the cause of her bleeding. Because she is currently asymptomatic, it would be reasonable to postpone further work-up for now.

Alternative Diagnosis: Anal Fissures

Textbook Presentation

Patients typically have severe rectal pain with bowel movements and bright red blood on the toilet paper. On physical exam, a fissure can be found at the midline, posterior to the anal opening.

Disease Highlights

A. Anal fissures occur secondary to trauma to the mucosa of the anal canal, most commonly by hard stool.

B. Fissures usually present as acute onset, painful defecation, usually with bleeding.

C. Fissures can become chronic.

   1. Pain causes anal sphincter spasm that, in turn, causes recurrent trauma.

   2. Chronic fissures can be associated with sentinel piles.

D. Fissures are present at the midline.

   1. Fissures are usually posterior in men and can be posterior or anterior in women.

   2. Other diagnoses, such as Crohn disease or sexually transmitted diseases, should be considered when fissures are lateral to the anal opening.

Evidence-Based Diagnosis

A. Fissures are diagnosed by direct observation.

B. Physical exam is sometimes difficult since patients are often in such acute pain.

Treatment

A. In most cases, general supportive recommendations outlined below for the treatment of hemorrhoids will cause relief of symptoms in days to weeks.

B. More chronic fissures often need therapy to relax the anal sphincter.

   1. Topical nitrates and injected botulinum toxin are effective.

   2. Surgical sphincterotomy is almost always effective but carries a small risk of permanent fecal incontinence.

CASE RESOLUTION

 One year later Ms. S returns to the clinic with recurrent bleeding. Anoscopy revealed a bleeding internal hemorrhoid. Symptoms resolve with supportive care, but bleeding recurs 1 month later. Colonoscopy is performed and reveals only internal hemorrhoids. The patient declines definitive therapy and continues to experience rare episodes of hemorrhoidal bleeding.

The patient's history of recurrent bleeding is quite common. Many patients with hemorrhoids will have occasional flares. The decision to perform colonoscopy was a difficult one. Although her young age and presence of an abnormality on anoscopy makes serious disease unlikely, evaluation of any patient with recurrent rectal bleeding is appropriate.

Treatment of Hemorrhoids

A. Most hemorrhoids and anal fissures can be treated conservatively with general recommendations for perianal well being.

1. Sitz baths to relax anal sphincter.

2. Analgesia with acetaminophen, topical creams or short-term topical corticosteroids. A doughnut cushion is sometimes helpful for prolonged sitting.

3. Soften stool with increased fluid intake, a high-fiber diet, and docusate sodium.

4. Avoid anything that may lead to constipation.

5. Avoid prolonged sitting, especially on the toilet.

B. Internal hemorrhoids that prolapse or continue to bleed usually require surgical removal.

C. Thrombosed, irreducible internal hemorrhoids and thrombosed external hemorrhoids require rapid surgical treatment.

REVIEW OF OTHER IMPORTANT DISEASES

Occult GI Bleeding

Textbook Presentation

Occult GI bleeding presents in 1 of 2 ways: either in a patient with newly discovered iron deficiency anemia or in a patient with positive fecal occult blood tests.

Disease Highlights

A. Generally a disease of older patients; average age in most studies is the early 60s.

B. Upper GI lesions cause occult GI bleeding slightly more commonly than lower GI lesions.

C. Common upper and lower GI tract diseases account for most causes of occult GI bleeding.

1. Upper

   a. Esophagitis

   b. Peptic ulcer disease

   c. Gastritis or duodenitis

   d. Angiodysplasia

   e. Gastric cancer

2. Lower

   a. Colonic adenomas

   b. Colonic carcinoma

   c. Colitis

   d. Angiodysplasia

D. Chronic aspirin, NSAID, or alcohol use is found in about 40% of patients with an upper GI tract lesion.

E. A small percentage of patients, $\cong 5\%$, have lesions of both the upper and lower GI tract.

Evidence-Based Diagnosis

A. All patients with occult GI bleeding need evaluation of the GI tract.

B. All patients with iron deficiency anemia need to have cause of the iron deficiency identified.

1. Iron deficiency is usually due to chronic blood loss. Very rarely it is due to poor iron intake or iron malabsorption.

2. Menstrual and GI blood loss are the most common sources.

3. All men, all women without menorrhagia, and all women over 50 (even those with menorrhagia) need to have an evaluation of the GI tract.

4. Women under age 50 with menorrhagia do not necessarily need further GI evaluation, unless they have GI symptoms or a family history of early colon cancer. That said, there should be a low threshold for evaluation of the GI tract.

5. Women under age 50 with menorrhagia need to be asked about minimal GI symptoms. Celiac sprue causes iron deficiency through malabsorption, and the symptoms can be easily attributed to irritable bowel syndrome.

 Always determine the source of blood loss in occult GI bleeding and iron deficiency anemia.

C. Evaluation of the GI tract in patients with occult GI bleeding should be done as follows:

1. If the patient is older than 50 years or has a family history of colon cancer, evaluation should begin with colonoscopy.

2. If there are symptoms of upper GI disease, evaluation should begin with an EGD.

3. If neither of the above is true, evaluation should begin with colonoscopy.

4. If the first test is unrevealing, the other test should be done.

5. Evaluation should end after the first positive test.

6. If no diagnosis is made after both EGD and colonoscopy, the patient should be treated with iron supplements for 6 months. If anemia recurs, the patient should be treated as though he or she has obscure GI bleeding (see below). A

definite source of bleeding is not found in 30–50% of patients after initial evaluation with upper and lower endoscopy.

7. If iron deficiency anemia or occult bleeding does not recur following iron supplementation, no further evaluation is necessary.

Obscure GI Bleeding

Textbook Presentation

Obscure GI bleeding refers to GI bleeding with normal upper and lower endoscopy. Included in the diagnosis are patients with occult bleeding, as discussed above, who have normal endoscopy but persistent bleeding. The usual presentation is acute GI bleeding in a patient in whom initial evaluation is unrevealing.

Disease Highlights

A. Obscure GI bleeding either comes from an upper GI or colonic source missed on the initial evaluation or from a small bowel source.

B. Small bowel bleeding is rare, accounting for < 5% of patients with GI bleeding.

C. About 50% of the patients with obscure GI bleeding have an upper or colonic source. Peptic ulcer disease or ulcers within hiatal hernias are the most common diagnosis.

D. In patients with a small bowel source, angiodysplasia is the most common diagnosis followed by ulcers, malignancy (accounting for about 10% of small bowel bleeding), Crohn disease, and Meckel diverticula, among others.

Evidence-Based Diagnosis

A. A directed history may provide clues to the source of obscure GI bleeding. Ask about use of medications that can cause mucosal damage (eg, NSAIDs, bisphosphonates) as well as a history of diseases that predispose patients to GI bleeding (HIV, neurofibromatosis).

B. In patients who are actively bleeding, the first step in evaluation is usually a tagged RBC scan. (See discussion above under diverticular hemorrhage).

C. When tagged RBC scanning is negative, various means of imaging the small bowel are used.

1. Enteroscopy is usually the next procedure recommended.

   a. In enteroscopy, a long endoscope (often a colonoscope) is passed orally.

   b. Access 40–60 cm into the jejunum is common.

   c. Diagnostic yields of 40–75% have been reported.

   d. In rare cases, endoscopy of the small bowel can be done at the time of exploratory laparotomy. This yields diagnoses 70–90% of the time but the invasive nature limits its usefulness.

2. Enteroclysis is another alternative.

   a. In enteroclysis, a tube is placed in the duodenum. Barium is then instilled into the bowel allowing for images similar to double contrast barium enema.

   b. Can be combined with enteroscopy.

   c. Diagnostic yields about twice that with traditional small bowel follow-through (10% vs 5%).

3. Meckel diverticulum scan uses a nuclear tracer that binds to parietal cells.

   a. Sensitivity is between 75% and 100%.

   b. Diagnosis only really considered when obscure bleeding occurs in a patient younger than 30.

4. Video capsule endoscopy appears to be the most effective of all means of imaging the small bowel.

   a. After being swallowed, the capsule transmits 2 images per second to a receiving device worn by the patient.

   b. Initial data suggest diagnostic yields of 40–80%, potentially higher than any of the procedures above.

   c. Video capsule endoscopy is likely to become the procedure of choice following repeat endoscopy in patients with obscure bleeding.

Treatment

The treatment of obscure bleeding varies by the cause of bleeding.

I have a patient with headache. How do I determine the cause?

CHIEF COMPLAINT

PATIENT

Mr. M is a 34-year-old man who comes to an outpatient practice complaining of intermittent headaches.

What is the differential diagnosis of headache? How would you frame the differential?

CONSTRUCTING A DIFFERENTIAL DIAGNOSIS

Headache is one of the most common physical complaints. Because less than 1% of all headaches are life-threatening, the challenge is to reassure and treat patients with benign headaches appropriately while finding the rare, life-threatening headache without excessive evaluation.

Headaches are often classified as primary or secondary. Primary headaches are syndromes unto themselves rather than signs of other diseases. Although potentially disabling, they are reliably not life-threatening. Secondary headaches are symptoms of other illnesses. Unlike primary headaches, secondary headaches are potentially dangerous.

The distinction of primary and secondary headaches is useful diagnostically. Primary headaches are diagnosed clinically, sometimes using diagnostic criteria. Traditional diagnostic studies cannot verify the diagnosis. Secondary headaches often can be definitively diagnosed by recognizing the underlying disease.

Clinically, primary and secondary headaches can be difficult to distinguish. The single most important question when developing a differential diagnosis for a headache is, "Is this headache new or old?" Chronic headaches tend to be primary, while new-onset headaches are usually secondary. This distinction is not perfect. There are some chronic headaches that are secondary headaches and even classic, primary headaches (such as migraines) can present as a new headache. The differentiation of old versus new also depends on how rapidly a patient brings his or her symptoms to medical attention. This being said, the following breakdown provides a clinically useful way of organizing headaches.

A. Old headaches
   1. Primary
      a. Tension headaches
      b. Migraine headaches
      c. Cluster headaches
   2. Secondary
      a. Cervical degenerative joint disease
      b. Temporomandibular joint syndrome
      c. Headaches associated with substances or their withdrawal
         (1) Caffeine
         (2) Nitrates
         (3) Analgesics
         (4) Ergotamine
B. New headaches
   1. Primary
      a. Benign cough headache
      b. Benign exertional headache
      c. Headache associated with sexual activity
      d. Benign thunderclap headache
   2. Secondary
      a. Infectious
         (1) Upper respiratory tract infection
         (2) Sinusitis
         (3) Meningitis

b. Vascular

    (1) Temporal arteritis

    (2) Subarachnoid hemorrhage (SAH)

    (3) Parenchymal hemorrhage

    (4) Malignant hypertension

    (5) Cavernous sinus thrombosis

c. Space occupying lesions

    (1) Brain tumors

    (2) Subdural hematoma

d. Medical morning headaches

    (1) Sleep disturbance

    (2) Night-time hypoglycemia

Mr. M reports similar headaches for 10 years. He comes in now because while they used to occur 2–3 times a year, they have become more frequent, occurring 3–4 times a month. The headaches are so severe that he is unable to work while experiencing one. He describes them as a throbbing pain behind his right eye. (When describing the headache, he places the base of his hand over his eye with his fingers wrapping over his forehead.) The headaches are often associated with nausea and, in the last few months, he has occasionally vomited with them.

At this point, what is the leading hypothesis, and what are the active alternatives? What other tests should be ordered?

ORGANIZING THE DIFFERENTIAL DIAGNOSIS

Although Mr. M's headaches are terribly severe, they have to be classified as old headaches since they have been occurring for years. This fact is reassuring, meaning that his headaches are most likely a primary headache. In a young healthy person with chronic headaches, migraines and tension headaches are most likely. Given the severity of the headaches, migraines are more likely than tension headaches. Given the severe, throbbing nature of the headaches, a vascular cause should at least be considered. An intracranial aneurysm could cause similar symptoms, but the chronicity makes this less likely. Table 15–1 lists the differential diagnosis.

Severity is less important than quality in distinguishing a new headache from an old headache. A severe headache that is identical in quality to chronic headaches is less worrisome than a mild headache that is dissimilar to any previous headache.

Table 15–1. Diagnostic hypotheses for Mr. M.

Diagnostic Hypotheses	Clinical Clues	Important Tests
Leading Hypothesis		
Migraine headache	Moderate to severe, unilateral throbbing headache, sometimes associated with aura	Diagnostic criteria and exclusion of secondary headaches
Active Alternative—Most Common		
Tension headache	Chronic, pressure-type headache of mild to moderate intensity	Diagnostic criteria and exclusion of secondary headaches
Active Alternative—Must Not Miss		
Intracranial aneurysm	Acute or subacute headache Headache features are nonspecific	CT scan MR angiography or traditional angiography

Mr. M has used ibuprofen in the past with good response, but this is no longer working well. His past history is remarkable only for severe car-sickness as a child.

Is the clinical information sufficient to make a diagnosis? If not, what other information do you need?

Leading Hypothesis: Migraine Headaches

Textbook Presentation

Migraines most often first present in women in their teens or 20s. The headaches are unilateral and throbbing and are severe enough to make it impossible to do work during an attack. They are occasionally preceded by about 20 minutes of flickering lights in a visual field. Patients usually find it necessary to lie in a dark, quiet room.

Disease Highlights

A. The description of migraine headaches adopted by the International Headache Society (IHS) is, "Idiopathic, recurring headache disorder manifesting in attacks lasting 4–72 hours. Typical characteristics of headache are unilateral location, pulsating quality, moderate or severe intensity, aggravation by routine physical activity and association with nausea, photophobia, and phonophobia."

B. Migraine headaches are a chronic headache syndrome caused by a neurovascular disorder. Neural events lead to intracranial vasodilatation.

C. They may begin at any age but most commonly begin during adolescence.

D. They are 2–3 times more common in women than men.

E. Auras frequently accompany migraines.

   1. Somewhere between 33% and 75% of patients with migraines have auras. Of all people with migraine,
      a. 18% always have auras
      b. 13% sometimes have auras
      c. 8% have auras without headaches.
   2. Auras are usually visual, precede the headache, and last for about 20 minutes.

3. Descriptions of auras
   a. Frequently, patients will initially describe a blind spot.
   b. Auras usually involve 1 portion of the visual field.
   c. Auras may vary. The frequency of some types of aura is given in Table 15–2.
   d. Scintillating scotoma often occur. These are often described as flashing lights, spots of light, zigzag lines, or squiggles.

Evidence-Based Diagnosis

A. Migraine headaches are the most severe of all the recurrent headache syndromes.

   1. They should be considered in any patient presenting to a physician with the chief complaint of headaches.
   2. Of initial visits for headaches in the primary care setting, 90% meet criteria for migraines.

The diagnosis of migraine headache should be seriously considered in any patient who has recurrent headaches that cause disability.

Table 15–2. Qualities of migraine auras.

Types of Aura	Prevalence
Zigzags	56%
Stars or flashes	83%
Scotoma	40%
Hemianopsia	7%
Sensory aura	20%
Aphasia	11%
Motor aura	4%
Duration of Aura	**Prevalence**
< 30 minutes	70%
30–60 minutes	18%
> 60 minutes	7%

B. As with other primary headaches, diagnosis is guided by the IHS's diagnostic criteria rather than by diagnostic tests.

C. The criteria for migraines are divided into migraines with and without aura.

  1. Migraine without aura

    a. A patient must have at least 5 attacks that last 4–72 hours

    b. The headache must have 2 of the following qualities:

      (1) Unilateral pain

      (2) Pulsating pain

      (3) Moderate to severe (must limit activity)

      (4) Aggravated by movement

    c. And have 1 of the following associated symptoms:

      (1) Nausea and vomiting

      (2) Photophobia or phonophobia

  2. Migraine with aura

    a. Definition: "Idiopathic, recurring headache disorder manifesting in attacks of neurological symptoms unequivocally localizable to cerebral cortex or brainstem, usually gradually developed over 5–20 minutes and usually lasting less than 60 minutes. Headache, nausea and/or photophobia usually follow neurological aura symptoms directly or after a free interval of less than an hour. The headache usually lasts 4–72 hours but may be absent."

    b. A patient must have at least 2 attacks.

    c. 3 of the following must be present:

      (1) 1 or more reversible aura symptoms referable to the cortex or brainstem

      (2) The aura must develop gradually over 4 minutes or more.

      (3) The aura must resolve after 60 minutes.

      (4) Headache either begins at the same time as the aura or follows within 60 minutes.

D. It is important to remember that diagnostic criteria, although helpful, need to be used carefully when applied to an individual patient. A patient who clearly has the disease in question may not perfectly fit the criteria. Consider these data about some of classic migraine symptoms:

  1. 50% of patients with migraines have nonpulsatile headaches.

  2. 40% have bilateral headaches.

 Diagnostic criteria are more helpful for research than patient care. They should be used cautiously with individual patients.

E. Other less common types of migraine occur.

  1. These include headaches with aura lasting longer than 60 minutes and migraine aura without a headache.

  2. These syndromes are difficult to diagnose and require exclusion of other diseases (such as cerebrovascular accident, transient ischemic attack, or retinal detachment) that could cause similar symptoms.

F. Besides the diagnostic criteria, there are many other aspects of the history that are suggestive of migraine headaches.

  1. An excellent recent review provided test characteristics for various headache qualities in distinguishing migraines from tension headaches.

  2. Table 15–3 shows those characteristics that have at least a moderate effect on posttest probability.

 Nausea is helpful in differentiating migraines from tension headaches. The LR+ is over 20.

  3. Interestingly, some commonly considered characteristics such as headache duration and relationship of headache to stress, weather, menses, fatigue, and odors were not helpful in making the diagnosis of migraines.

  4. Presence of a family history was helpful in making the diagnosis with an LR+ of 5.0.

  5. Patients with migraines are also more likely to have had vomiting attacks as children and to have suffered from motion sickness.

G. Given the severity of migraine, a common issue is when does a patient with a probable migraine need neuroimaging?

  1. The following are predictors of abnormal neuroimaging and are generally agreed upon indications for imaging.

    a. Abnormal neurologic exam

    b. Neurologic symptoms that are atypical for aura, especially dizziness, lack of coordination, numbness or tingling, or worsening of headache with Valsalva maneuver

    c. Increasing frequency of headaches.

    d. Headaches that awaken patients from sleep.

    e. New headaches in patients over 50.

Table 15–3. Characteristics for symptoms of migraine.

Criteria	Sensitivity (%)	Specificity (%)	LR+	LR−
Nausea	82	96	23.2	0.19
Photophobia	79	87	6.0	0.24
Phonophobia	5.2	3.7	5.2	0.38
Exacerbated by physical activity	81	78	3.7	0.24
Unilateral	66	78	3.1	0.43
Throbbing	76	77	3.3	0.32
Precipitated by chocolate	22	95	4.6	0.82
Precipitated by cheese	38	92	4.9	0.68

Adapted from Smetana GW. The diagnostic value of historical features in primary headache syndromes: A comprehensive review. *Arch Intern Med.* 2000;160:2729–2737. Copyrighted © 2000. American Medical Association. All rights reserved.

2. More generally, and in addition to those above, other indications for imaging in persons with headaches are:
   a. Change in headache quality or pattern
   b. First headache, worst headache, or abrupt-onset headache
   c. New headache in patients with cancer, immunosuppression, or pregnancy
   d. Headache associated with loss of consciousness
   e. Headache triggered by exertion

MAKING A DIAGNOSIS

Mr. M's physical exam, including a detailed neurologic exam is completely normal.

Mr. M's headaches fulfill the criteria for migraine headaches. The severity and personal history of motion sickness provide other clues. The increasing frequency and severity of the headaches is somewhat worrisome, and neurologic imaging would be reasonable.

Have you crossed a diagnostic threshold for the leading hypothesis, migraine headaches? Have you ruled out the active alternatives? Do other tests need to be done to exclude the alternative diagnoses?

Alternative Diagnosis: Tension Headaches

Textbook Presentation

Tension headaches are the most common type of headache. They generally occur a few times each month and are described as bilateral and squeezing. They are usually relieved with over-the-counter analgesics and are seldom severe enough to cause real disability.

Disease Highlights

A. The IHS definition of episodic tension type headache is, "Recurrent episodes of H/A lasting minutes to days. The pain is typically pressing/tightening in quality, of mild or moderate intensity, bilateral in location and does not worsen with routine physical activity. Nausea is absent, but photophobia or phonophobia may be present."

B. Most common type of headache, it is 1 of the only conditions discussed in this book that is more likely to be present than not, the 1-year prevalence of tension headaches is 63% in men and 86% in women.

C. The IHS criteria differentiate headaches as episodic or chronic and with or without associated tenderness of pericranial muscles.

D. The pathophysiology of tension headaches is still a topic of debate.

   1. Episodic tension headaches are likely related to tenderness and spasm in the pericranial muscles while chronic tension headaches are related to changes in the CNS caused by the chronic pain of tension headaches.

2. There is evidence to suggest that people who suffer from more frequent tension headaches have higher levels of perceived stress and lower pain thresholds than those without headaches.

E. Tension headaches can be troublesome but are seldom disabling.

Evidence-Based Diagnosis

A. Because tension headaches are the most common form of headaches, they are the default diagnosis in almost every patient with a mild to moderate headache syndrome.

B. A detailed history and physical exam is required to exclude other headache syndromes that require specific treatment.

C. Special attention should be given to excluding migraines.

D. The IHS diagnostic criteria for episodic tension headaches are:

1. At least 10 previous headaches

2. Duration of 30 minutes to 7 days

3. 2 of the following

   a. Pressing or tightening (nonpulsating) quality

   b. Mild to moderate in severity (inhibits but does not prevent activity)

   c. Bilateral

   d. Not aggravated by routine activity

4. No nausea or vomiting

5. Photophobia or phonophobia may be present, but not both

E. Chronic tension type headaches often develop from the more common episodic headaches. These are similar in quality but occur at least 15 days of the month.

Treatment

A. Episodic tension headaches

1. Usually treated by patients without the input of a physician.

2. Simple analgesics (acetaminophen or nonsteroidal anti-inflammatory drugs [NSAIDs]) are the basis of most treatment.

3. For more severe headaches combinations that include caffeine or codeine can be used.

4. In patients with frequent, but still episodic tension headaches, efforts at stress reduction are helpful.

B. Chronic tension headaches

1. These are often quite difficult to treat.

2. The first intervention should almost always be "detoxification" from the patient's regimen of pain medications.

   a. Chronic use of many headache medications has the potential to cause or exacerbate chronic tension headaches.

   b. The most common culprit medications are ergotamine, NSAIDs, caffeine, and narcotics.

   c. Detoxification can be difficult and occasionally requires hospitalization.

 The first step in managing chronic tension headaches is the withdrawal of all previously used headache medications.

3. Once all previous medications have been withdrawn, tricyclic antidepressants (TCAs) and stress management, either alone or in combination, are effective.

   a. TCAs work faster than stress management.

   b. Even a combination of both TCAs and stress management only reduce headache frequency and severity by about 50%.

Alternative Diagnosis: Headache due to Unruptured CNS Aneurysm

Textbook Presentation

The classic presentation of a headache caused by a CNS aneurysm is a unilateral and throbbing headache that is new in a middle-aged patient.

Disease Highlights

A. CNS aneurysm may present in 3 ways

1. Asymptomatic detection: This commonly occurs when a patient has a ruptured aneurysm and another, nonruptured aneurysm is found during the evaluation.

2. Acute rupture or acute expansion (discussed later in the chapter)

3. Chronic headache

B. The studies of the chronic headaches caused by unruptured aneurysms are, by their nature, somewhat flawed since they must be retrospective.

Evidence-Based Diagnosis

A. The headaches of unruptured aneurysms are non-specific.

1. One study looked retrospectively at the symptoms of 111 patients referred for therapy of unruptured aneurysms; 54 of the patients had symptoms referable to the aneurysm at the time of diagnosis.

2. Of the 54 patients with symptoms, 35 (65%) had chronic symptoms.

3. In 18 of these 35 patients, the chronic symptom was headache without other neurologic sign.

4. Patient's headaches were divided equally between unilateral and bilateral.

B. Neuroimaging

1. CT and magnetic resonance angiography (MRA) are very sensitive means of detecting CNS aneurysms.

   a. Sensitivity for aneurysms > 1 cm in diameter is probably 100%.

   b. Sensitivity for all aneurysms is lower (62% for CT and 45% for MRI).

      (1) Aneurysms < 1 cm can, rarely, cause symptoms. These symptoms may include chronic headaches.

      (2) Repair of aneurysms < 1 cm in a patient who has not had a previous rupture is generally not recommended since the rupture rates are so low.

2. Traditional angiography

   a. Considered the gold standard for diagnosis

   b. Usually required prior to repair

   c. There are case reports of small aneurysms being missed on traditional angiography and being seen on CT and MRA.

Treatment

A. The treatment of CNS aneurysms can be accomplished with neurosurgical or endovascular procedures.

B. Management decisions are difficult in a patient with a small aneurysm and a suspicious headache because there is no definitive way to know whether the aneurysm is causing the headache prior to surgery.

CASE RESOLUTION

Because the quality of Mr. M's headaches had not changed at all, the decision was made not to image his brain. He was given long-acting propranolol at 80 mg/d and prescribed oral sumatriptan to be used as needed. At a 1-month follow-up, the patient reported only a single mild headache for which he used ibuprofen.

The decision to forgo imaging was difficult. Although the likelihood of finding another cause of headaches was small, the patient's headaches had changed. His complete response to migraine prophylaxis is diagnostic.

Treatment of Migraines

A. Treatment of migraines is either abortive or prophylactic.

B. Abortive therapy

1. Abortive therapy should be used at the very first sign of a migraine. Patients should be advised not to wait until they "are sure it is a migraine."

2. Effective drugs are outlined in Table 15–4 with the individual considerations mainly from the consensus comments from the US Headache Consortium.

C. Prophylactic therapy

1. Prophylactic therapy is instituted when patient and doctor agree that the migraines are frequent enough, severe enough, or persistent enough to warrant regular medications.

2. Prophylactic therapy does not need to be used every day. It can be used only around the times that migraines predictably occur (such as perimenstrually).

3. The most effective medications are:

   a. β-Blockers

      (1) Propranolol

      (2) Timolol

   b. Divalproex

   c. Amitriptyline

Table 15–4. Recommended treatments for migraine.

Drug	Considerations
NSAIDs	First-line therapy; may be used with antiemetics
Acetaminophen plus aspirin plus caffeine	Another first-line therapy; may also be used with antiemetics
Triptans (SQ, PO, IN)	For moderate to severe migraines
Dihydroergotamine (SQ, IV, IM, IN)	For moderate to severe migraines; may be used with antiemetics
Antiemetics (prochlorperazine maleate or metoclopramide)	Used as adjuncts as above
Opiates	For moderate to severe migraine—rescue therapy Limit use due to risk of rebound and medication overuse
Corticosteroids	Rescue therapy for intractable migraines
Butalbital plus aspirin plus caffeine	Occasional use for moderate and severe migraines
Acetaminophen, dichloralphenazone, and isometheptene	Occasional use for mild to moderate migraines

NSAIDs, nonsteroidal anti-inflammatory drugs; SQ, subcutaneous; PO, oral; IN, intranasal; IV, intravenous; IM, intramuscular.

CHIEF COMPLAINT

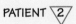

PATIENT 2

Mrs. L is a 65-year-old woman who comes to an outpatient clinic complaining of headaches. She reports waking up almost every morning with a moderate to severe, bitemporal headache. She reports never having headaches of any consequence in the past but has been quite troubled for the last 2 months.

 At this point, what is the leading hypothesis, and what are the active alternatives? What other tests should be ordered?

ORGANIZING THE DIFFERENTIAL DIAGNOSIS

Mrs. L's headaches are of concern because she is older and the headaches are new. Both these features raise the likelihood that the headaches are secondary and, therefore, potentially dangerous. Morning headaches are classically associated with brain tumors. Edema forms around the CNS lesion while the patient is supine at night leading to headaches from increased intracranial pressure in the morning. Further history is needed, as brain tumors are most likely in patients with other types of cancer.

Morning headaches are also a fairly common symptom of many habits, diseases, and exposures. Headaches associated with substances or their withdrawals are a common cause of morning headaches. Alcohol, caffeine, and carbon monoxide are probably the most common. Other common causes of morning headaches can be grouped as "medical morning headaches." These are headaches caused by diseases that are active at night or that disturb sleep. Nighttime hypoglycemia and obstructive sleep apnea (OSA) are common causes of headaches in this category. Tension headaches should always be in the differential of headaches and may, on occasion, cause morning headaches.

The presence of a new, bitemporal headache in an older patient should raise the possibility of temporal arteritis. Although these headaches are not classically morning headaches, they should still be considered. Temporal arteritis will be discussed later in the chapter. Table 15–5 lists the differential diagnosis.

 Even more than with most headaches, an extensive history is necessary in a patient with morning headaches.

Table 15–5. Diagnostic hypotheses for Mrs. L.

Diagnostic Hypotheses	Clinical Clues	Important Tests
Leading Hypothesis		
Brain tumor	History of malignancy Focal neurologic deficit	CNS imaging
Active Alternative		
Substance exposure or withdrawal	*Caffeine:* Worst when sleeping late, often worst on vacations or weekends *Alcohol:* Occurs following intoxication *Carbon monoxide poisoning:* Headache that occurs in an exposed cohort and resolves upon leaving site of exposure	Response to caffeine. Relation only to alcohol use. Carboxyhemoglobin levels.
Medical morning headaches	*Nighttime hypoglycemia:* Most common in diabetics with recent medication or diet changes. *Obstructive sleep apnea:* Obesity and daytime somnolence	2 AM finger stick. Polysomnogram
Tension headaches	Chronic, pressure-type headache of mild to moderate intensity	Diagnostic criteria and exclusion of secondary headaches

Mrs. L reports otherwise feeling well. She says the headaches occur nearly every morning, irrespective of day of the week or whether she has slept at home or at her weekend house. She denies neurologic symptoms such as focal numbness, weakness, or visual disturbances. She denies snoring or excessive daytime somnolence. She read on an Internet site that new-onset, morning headaches are classic for brain tumors, and she is very nervous.

Her medical history is notable only for non-insulin-dependent diabetes mellitus, which has always been under good control. She reports no recent change in her diet, weight, or medication.

Medications are 325 mg/d of aspirin, 10 mg/d orally of atorvastatin, and 5 mg of oral glyburide taken twice daily.

Many patients seeking care for a headache believe they have a brain tumor. It is important to recognize this—a little definitive reassurance can go a long way.

Is the clinical information sufficient to make a diagnosis? If not, what other information do you need?

Leading Hypothesis: Intracranial Neoplasms

Textbook Presentation

Brain tumors classically present with progressive morning headaches associated with focal neurologic deficits.

Disease Highlights

A. Brain tumors are classified as metastatic, primary extra-axial, and primary intra-axial.

B. The relative frequency of types of tumors within each type are listed below:

1. Metastatic
   a. Lung, 37%
   b. Breast, 19%
   c. Melanoma, 16%
2. Primary extra-axial
   a. Meningioma, 80%
   b. Acoustic neuroma, 10%
   c. Pituitary adenoma, 7%

3. Primary intra-axial

    a. Glioblastoma, 47%

    b. Astrocytoma, 39%

C. Metastatic tumors are about 7 times more common than primary tumors. Thus, a patient with known malignancy and new headaches should undergo imaging.

D. Intracranial neoplasms generally present with focal signs, including seizure, or signs of increased intracranial pressure such as headache.

E. Although the presenting symptoms vary with type of tumor, the most common symptoms are:

    1. Headache (about 50% of the time)

    2. Seizure

    3. Hemiparesis

    4. Change in mental status

Evidence-Based Diagnosis

A. History

    1. The history of a patient's headache is not particularly helpful in making a diagnosis of intracranial neoplasms.

    2. One very good report retrospectively studied 111 patients with brain tumors. The symptoms were nonspecific.

        a. Only 48% of patients had headaches.

        b. Only 17% had classic brain tumor headache (defined as severe, worse in the morning and associated with nausea and vomiting).

        c. 77% of patients met the criteria for tension headaches.

        d. 9% of patients had migraine-like headaches.

        e. The most common qualities were

            (1) Intermittent, 62%

            (2) Frontal, 68%

            (3) Bilateral, 72%

 Brain tumor headaches are nonspecific. A patient with a new headache and a preexisting cancer that could potentially metastasize to the CNS should undergo imaging.

B. Neuroimaging

    1. CT

        a. A reasonable choice for screening patients in whom there is a low suspicion.

        b. The sensitivity of a contrast-enhanced CT for intracranial neoplasm is around 90%.

    2. MRI with contrast is the procedure of choice for imaging brain tumors. The sensitivity of MRI is nearly 100% and the detail provided often suggests a likely pathology.

Treatment

A. The treatment of brain tumors depends on the pathology.

B. Importantly, patients with signs of increased intracranial pressure or seizure should be hospitalized immediately enabling both rapid diagnosis and treatment.

MAKING A DIAGNOSIS

 Mrs. L's physical exam, including a detailed neurologic exam, is normal. Laboratory tests done on the day of the visit revealed a normal CBC, normal chem-7, and a glycosylated Hgb of 5.9% (down from 7% 3 months earlier). A noncontrast head CT done on the day of the visit was normal. The patient was asked to set her alarm and check a finger-stick glucose at 2 AM. Her reading was 42 mg/dL.

 Have you crossed a diagnostic threshold for the leading hypothesis, intracranial neoplasms? Have you ruled out the active alternatives? Do other tests need to be done to exclude the alternative diagnoses?

Given that intracranial neoplasms are relatively rare in patients without preexisting cancers and the presence of morning headaches is a nonspecific finding, it is unlikely that the patient has a brain tumor. The noncontrast head CT was probably a reasonable test to do. It essentially rules out a tumor and, given the patient's concern, it was an effective method of calming her.

After the negative CT and unrevealing laboratory test results, attention must be turned to possible exposures or the "medical morning headaches." The patient's marked drop in her glycosylated Hgb and early morning hypoglycemia are suggestive of a diagnosis.

Alternative Diagnosis: Medical Morning Headaches

Textbook Presentation

Various diseases can cause headaches that occur predominantly in the morning. The headaches are generally worst upon awakening and then improve as the day progresses. Classically, the more common symptoms of the underlying disease (daytime hypoglycemia with overly controlled diabetes mellitus or daytime somnolence with OSA) are present.

Disease Highlights

A. The most rigorously defined morning headaches are those caused by disturbed sleep. The sleep disturbance can be of almost any etiology.

    1. Primary sleep disturbance

      a. OSA

      b. Periodic leg movement of sleep (PLMS)

    2. Abnormal sleep duration

      a. Excessive sleep

      b. Interrupted sleep

      c. Sleep deprivation

    3. Secondary to another disease

      a. Chronic pain

      b. Depression

B. Hypoglycemia that occurs while asleep or awake can cause headaches.

Evidence-Based Diagnosis

A. The diagnosis of a medical morning headaches depends on recognition of the underlying disease, its treatment, and the response of the presenting headache.

B. Recognition of the OSA and nighttime hypoglycemia can be difficult since clinical clues are nonspecific.

    1. Nighttime hypoglycemia should be considered

in any patient with diabetes and morning headaches. Abnormal nocturnal glucose readings are diagnostic.

2. Clinical predictors of OSA are poor (Table 15–6). Polysomnography is diagnostic and will also provide information about PLMS and, sometimes, insomnia related to chronic pain.

 A sleep study is a reasonable diagnostic test in a patient with morning headaches and no readily apparent cause.

Alternative Diagnosis: Headaches Associated with Substances or Their Withdrawal

Textbook Presentation

The IHS defines this type of headache as "a new form of headache (including migraine, tension-type headache or cluster headache) in close temporal relation to substance use or substance withdrawal."

Disease Highlights

A. Many substances can cause headaches acutely, with chronic use, or after their withdrawal.

    1. Acute exposure

      a. Nitrites ("hot dog headache")

      b. MSG ("Chinese restaurant syndrome")

      c. Carbon monoxide

Table 15–6. Test characteristics for clinical predictors of obstructive sleep apnea.

Criteria	Sensitivity	Specificity	LR+	LR−
Snoring	94%	12%	1.07	0.5
Nocturnal choking	25%	85%	1.67	0.88
Daytime somnolence	23%	84%	1.44	0.92
Apneic events	78%	45%	1.45	0.49
Abnormal pharyngeal exam	51%	78%	2.32	0.63
Expert impression	52%	70%	1.73	0.69
BMI > 29	55%	65%	1.57	0.69
Observed apnea + involuntary falling asleep	69%	70%	2.3	0.44
Observed apnea + involuntary falling asleep + BMI > 29	41%	88%	3.42	0.67

BMI, body mass index.

2. Chronic exposure (analgesics)

3. Withdrawal from acute exposure (alcohol)

4. Withdrawal from chronic exposure

    a. Caffeine

    b. Narcotics

B. Of these headaches, caffeine withdrawal, hangovers, and carbon monoxide poisoning are probably the most common causes of morning headaches.

Evidence-Based Diagnosis

A. Caffeine withdrawal headaches

    1. The IHS criteria require that:

        a. Patients drink caffeine daily and > 15 g/month.

        b. The headaches occur within 24 hours of the last caffeine intake.

        c. 100 mg of caffeine cures the headache within 1 hour.

    2. An average cup of coffee contains about 100 mg of caffeine.

    3. The average adult American ingests approximately 280 mg of caffeine each day.

    4. The requirement of > 15 g/month may be excessive.

    5. Caffeine withdrawal should be suspected if headaches seem to occur when coffee intake changes, such as on weekends and during vacations.

Caffeine withdrawal should be considered when headaches occur when patients sleep later than usual or occur mainly on weekends or vacations.

B. Carbon monoxide poisoning

    1. Presentation runs the spectrum from mild headache to headache with nausea, vomiting, and anxiety to cardiovascular collapse.

    2. Various aspects of a patient's history increase suspicion of this diagnosis.

        a. A patient's headache only occurs in a single location and resolves when the patient is removed from this setting.

        b. Multiple family members or roommates have similar symptoms.

        c. Carbon monoxide poisoning is most common in the winter.

    3. An elevated carboxyhemoglobin level makes the diagnosis. ABG measurement and pulse oximetry do not detect carbon monoxide poisoning.

Because carbon monoxide poisoning is potentially life-threatening, the diagnosis should be considered whenever a patient has a potentially consistent history.

Treatment

A. Treatment of headaches associated with substances or their withdrawal depends on the substance.

B. Patients with headaches from carbon monoxide poisoning should be removed from their house while the source is repaired.

C. Patients with caffeine withdrawal headaches should either be weaned off caffeine or counseled on the need to continue regular use (an option generally preferred by medical students).

CASE RESOLUTION

A tentative diagnosis of morning headaches due to nocturnal hypoglycemia was made. The patient was advised not to take the evening dose of glyburide; her headaches resolved the next day. At her next visit, the patient's medications were inspected. The label on the bottle was correct, but inspection of the pills revealed that 10 mg pills had been mistakenly dispensed, doubling her dose.

Adverse effects of medications are common. Although most commonly intrinsic to the medication, they can also be related to inappropriate prescribing or incorrect dispensing.

Treatment of Medical Morning Headaches

The treatment of medical morning headaches depends on the cause.

A. Nighttime hypoglycemia: improved management of diabetes

B. OSA: Continuous positive airway pressure

C. PLMS: Carbidopa and levodopa

D. Pain syndromes: Improved pain control

CHIEF COMPLAINT

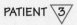

PATIENT 3

Mr. J is a 27-year-old man who arrives at his primary care physician's office complaining of a headache. He has a long history of mild tension-type headaches managed with acetaminophen. Three days ago, a severe headache suddenly developed while he was weight lifting. He describes this headache as the "worst headache of his life." The headache slowly resolved over about 2 hours. He is now feeling completely well. He has been afraid to exercise since this headache.

At this point, what is the leading hypothesis, and what are the active alternatives? What other tests should be ordered?

ORGANIZING THE DIFFERENTIAL DIAGNOSIS

Both the acuity and severity of this headache are worrisome. The onset during exercise is also concerning. This type of headache, one that begins at its peak intensity, is referred to as a thunderclap headache.

SAH is the leading hypothesis and must not miss diagnosis for this type of headache. His designation of the headache as the "worst headache of his life" is classic for SAH, although the resolution of the pain is not typical. Other headaches can present in similar fashion. Benign thunderclap headaches are clinically indistinguishable from SAH. Headaches due to cough, exertion, and sexual activity are primary headache syndromes that may mimic SAH. A parenchymal hemorrhage is possible but unlikely given the patient's age and absence of a history of hypertension.

There are some rare diseases that can occasionally present with a thunderclap headache; these include cerebral venous sinus thrombosis, pituitary apoplexy, carotid dissection, and spontaneous intracranial hypotension from cerebrospinal fluid (CSF) leaks. Table 15–7 lists the differential diagnosis.

Assume that a thunderclap headache is caused by a SAH until proven otherwise.

3

Mr. J's past medical history is notable only for mild asthma for which he uses albuterol as needed.

On physical exam, he appears well and not in any distress. His vital signs are temperature, 36.9 °C; pulse, 82 bpm; BP, 112/82 mm Hg; RR, 14 breaths per minute. His neck is supple and detailed neurologic exam is also normal.

Is the clinical information sufficient to make a diagnosis? If not, what other information do you need?

Table 15–7. Diagnostic hypotheses for Mr. J.

Diagnostic Hypotheses	Clinical Clues	Important Tests
Leading Hypothesis		
Subarachnoid hemorrhage (SAH)	"Worst headache of life" Acute onset	Noncontrast head CT scan Lumbar puncture
Active Alternative		
Cough, exertional and sexual headaches	Acute headaches associated with cough, exertion, or sexual activity	History CNS imaging
Benign thunderclap headaches	Indistinguishable from SAH	Noncontrast head CT scan Lumbar puncture
Intracerebral hemorrhage	Headache with focal neurologic signs	Noncontrast head CT scan

Leading Hypothesis: SAH

Textbook Presentation

A middle-aged patient describes the pain as the worst headache of his or her life. Soon after the headache begins, the patient experiences vomiting and then focal neurologic symptoms. On physical exam, focal neurologic signs are present as is meningismus. Soon after presentation the patient loses consciousness.

Disease Highlights

A. SAH is primarily caused by rupture of a saccular aneurysm in the circle of Willis ($\cong$ 80%).

B. Aneurysms are present in about 4% of the population.

C. Largest aneurysms (> 1 cm) rupture at a rate of about 0.5%/year.

D. The vast majority of ruptures occur in persons 40–65 years old.

E. SAH carries a mortality of about 50%.

F. It is generally accepted that anywhere from 10–50% of patients will have a warning or sentinel headache in the weeks preceding the SAH.

   1. Likely caused by expansion or a small leak from an aneurysm.

   2. This headache is usually the same sort of abrupt onset (thunderclap) headache as SAH but resolves within 24 hours.

   3. About 50% of patients with warning headaches actually seek medical care at the time of their headache.

Evidence-Based Diagnosis

A. Pretest probability

   1. SAH accounts for 1–4% of headaches presenting to the emergency department.

   2. Among headaches presenting to the emergency department, SAH accounts for

      a. 12% of patients with the "worst headache of my life"

      b. 25% of patients with the "worst headache of my life" and neurologic findings

   3. The prevalence of the various possible symptoms of SAH vary from study to study. Some of the more common symptoms are listed below (with prevalence figures from 1 large review).

      a. Headache, 90%

      b. Stiff neck, 74%

      c. Change in mental status, 60%

      d. Stupor or coma, 27%

B. Diagnostic tests

   1. The initial diagnostic test is a noncontrast head CT. The sensitivity of this test varies with the time since the onset of symptoms.

      a. First 12 hours, 97%

      b. 12–24 hours, 93%

      c. Falls to as low as 80% after 2 weeks.

   2. Next to angiography, CSF exam for RBC and xanthochromia from deteriorating RBCs is the most accurate diagnostic method.

      a. RBCs are seen immediately in the CSF in 100% of patients. The specificity, however, can be limited by traumatic lumbar punctures.

      b. Sensitivity of RBCs begins to fall after about 24 hours.

      c. Spectrophotometric % detection of xanthochromia is 100% specific for SAH and reaches nearly 100% sensitivity by 24 hours.

      d. The sensitivity of xanthochromia remains at 100% for over 1 week.

   3. In all patients with documented SAH, angiography is performed to assist in surgical planning. Angiography might also be done for patients in whom the diagnosis is unclear even after lumbar puncture.

C. Importance of correct diagnosis

   1. About 25% of patients with SAH are initially misdiagnosed.

   2. Patients with less severe clinical presentations are most commonly misdiagnosed.

   3. Patients who are initially misdiagnosed are only about half as likely to have a good or excellent outcome.

 All patients in whom SAH is suspected should undergo a noncontrast head CT. Lumbar puncture should be done in a patient with a normal head CT and even only minimal suspicion of a SAH.

Treatment

A. Medical

   1. The primary treatment of SAH is neurosurgical.

   2. Medical therapy includes

      a. Pain control

      b. Reduction of cerebral vasospasm with nimodipine

      c. Judicious treatment of hypertension since lowering the BP too much in the setting of cerebral vasospasm potentially increases the risk of ischemic injury.

B. Surgical

1. Following angiography, the culprit aneurysm is repaired.

   a. This is usually done with surgical clipping.

   b. Intravascular devices can be used in selected patients.

2. Surgery for aneurysms is most successful when performed either before or after vasospasm has occurred.

MAKING A DIAGNOSIS

The patient had a thunderclap headache that he describes as the worst headache of his life, which mandates urgent evaluation.

Mr. J is referred from clinic for a noncontrast head CT. The results are normal.

Have you crossed a diagnostic threshold for the leading hypothesis, SAH? Have you ruled out the active alternatives? Do other tests need to be done to exclude the alternative diagnoses?

Alternative Diagnoses: Benign Cough Headache, Benign Exertional Headache, and Headache Associated with Sexual Activity

Textbook Presentation

These headaches are precipitated by cough, exertion (usually involving the Valsalva maneuver), and sexual activity (peaking at orgasm). They may mimic SAH.

Disease Highlights

A. Cough headaches

1. Most common in men (~ 3:1)

2. More common in older patients (mean age, 67)

3. Last < 1 minute

B. Exertional headaches

1. Most common in men (~ 90%)

2. Occurs in young people (mean age, 24)

3. Often bilateral and throbbing

4. Sometimes related to migraines (some patients may induce migraines with physical activity)

5. Lasts from 5 minutes to 24 hours

C. Sexual headaches

1. Also most common in men (~ 85%)

2. Mean age, 41

3. Lasts less than 3 hours

4. Can occur as 3 types

   a. Dull type: dull headache worsening with sexual excitement

   b. Explosive type: SAH-like headache occurring at orgasm

   c. Postural type: postural headache developing after coitus

Evidence-Based Diagnosis

A. Although these headaches may be indistinguishable from more concerning headaches, the clinical presentation can sometimes help identify the diagnosis.

B. They should be considered when the headache starts with cough, sexual activity, or exercise.

C. One review suggested other distinguishing features.

1. Cough headaches

   a. Either represented the primary headache syndrome or symptoms of a Chiari type I malformation

   b. Those headaches lasting > 30 minutes were usually secondary to a Chiari type I malformation.

   c. Patients with Chiari type I malformations were younger than those with primary cough headaches (mean age, 39 vs. 67)

2. Sexual headaches

   a. Almost always (93%) benign

   b. The only sexual headache not part of the primary syndrome was a SAH.

   c. Patients with benign sexual headaches tended to have multiple episodes of the headache.

3. Exertional headaches

   a. Either represented the primary headache syndrome or secondary headache including SAH and brain tumor.

   b. The primary and secondary headaches were generally indistinguishable.

Exertional headaches are clinically indistinguishable from SAH.

Alternative Diagnosis: Benign Thunderclap Headache

Textbook Presentation

Benign thunderclap headaches present in a way indistinguishable from SAH. The diagnosis is made after normal results are obtained on CT scan and lumbar puncture. These headaches occasionally recur.

Disease Highlights

A. Primary headache syndrome likely related to diffuse segmental cerebral vasospasm.

B. Clinically indistinguishable from SAH but lacks any associated neurologic symptoms or signs.

C. Headaches frequently recur over 1–2 weeks and then intermittently over years.

D. In the best study of these headaches:

   1. SAH developed in none of the 71 patients studied.

   2. 51 (72%) of the patients had their headaches unrelated to cough, sexual activity, or exertion.

   3. 17% of the patients had recurrent, similar headaches.

Evidence-Based Diagnosis

A. Benign thunderclap headaches are diagnosed when there is a suspicious clinical presentation and SAH is ruled out.

B. Given the poor prognosis of SAH, CT scan and lumbar puncture should be performed in all patients prior to the diagnosis.

 Because benign thunderclap headaches are clinically indistinguishable from SAH, they can only be diagnosed after SAH has been ruled out.

Treatment

A. Treatment is challenging because these headaches are short-lived and very intermittent.

B. As-needed analgesics are probably the only reasonable therapy.

Alternative Diagnosis: Intracerebral Hemorrhage

Textbook Presentation

Intracerebral hemorrhage generally presents in older, hypertensive patients with acute-onset headache and focal neurologic symptoms and signs.

Disease Highlights

A. Intracerebral hemorrhage accounts for about 10% of strokes, being less common than embolic and thrombotic strokes.

B. Hypertension is the most important cause, followed by amyloid angiopathy, saccular aneurysm rupture, and arteriovenous malformation rupture.

C. Among patients with hypertension, Asians and blacks have the highest risk of hemorrhagic cerebrovascular accidents.

D. The incidence of hypertension-related intracerebral hemorrhage has declined with better control of hypertension.

E. In young patients without hypertension, arteriovenous malformation, aneurysm rupture, and drug use should be considered.

F. Arteriovenous malformations are present in 0.01% to 0.05% of the population and usually present in persons between the ages of 20 and 40 years.

   1. Presentation may be with hemorrhage, seizure, or headache.

   2. About 50% of patients with arteriovenous malformation will experience bleeding. Patients with hypertension or a previous hemorrhage have the highest rate of bleeding.

Evidence-Based Diagnosis

A. Patients with intracerebral hemorrhage usually have headache and focal neurologic signs.

B. A thunderclap-type headache is the presenting sign in nearly 60% of patients.

C. Vomiting is present in about 50% of patients, and seizures are present in about 10%.

D. Noncontrast CT scan is the test of choice with a sensitivity of nearly 100%.

Treatment

See the Treatment section under Cerebellar Hemorrhage in Chapter 10, Dizziness.

CASE RESOLUTION

Given the acute-onset during exercise, the normal neurologic exam, and the lack of symptoms during the intervening 3 days, the patient was thought to have primary exertional headache. A sentinel headache, preceding an SAH, however,

(continued)

was thought a possible alternative. Given this, the patient underwent lumbar puncture that revealed no RBCs and no xanthochromia. He subsequently experienced a similar headache 2 weeks later with exercise. He was then treated with preexercise propranolol with good response.

The evaluation of this patient was reasonable. Although he was feeling well at the time of the visit, the test threshold for SAH needs to be very low given the severity of disease. SAH tends to be misdiagnosed in patients with the mildest symptoms. This is because the physician's suspicion is lowest in these patients and probably because the CT scan may be least sensitive in people with presumably small hemorrhages. Physicians need a higher suspicion in these patients because they could have the best outcomes.

With a normal CT scan and a negative lumbar puncture, the diagnosis becomes either benign thunderclap headache or benign exertional headache. The difference is likely semantic, but the headache's onset and recurrence during exercise makes benign exertional headache the diagnosis. Intracerebral bleed from an arteriovenous malformation was a possibility but was ruled out with the normal CT scan.

Treatment of Benign Cough Headache, Benign Exertional Headache, & Headache Associated with Sexual Activity

A. Cough headaches are effectively treated with cough suppression and NSAIDs.

B. Exertional headaches are treated by avoiding strenuous activity, especially in hot weather or at high altitudes or by using preexertion ergotamine, β-blockers, or NSAIDs.

C. Sexual headaches are effectively treated with prophylactic β-blockers.

CHIEF COMPLAINT

PATIENT 4

Mrs. T is an 80-year-old woman who comes to your office complaining of headaches for the past 3 months. She reports always having had mild headaches that never troubled her enough to see a doctor. This headache has been persistent, bilateral, band-like, and throbbing.

At her present visit, she reports no visual changes, no recent head trauma, and no neurologic deficits. She does report fatigue and says that she has lost about 15 lbs over the last month.

Her past medical history is notable for hypertension for which she takes hydrochlorothiazide and a breast mass noted 2 years before. The mass was thought to be low suspicion for malignancy and the patient declined work-up.

 At this point, what is the leading hypothesis, and what are the active alternatives? What other tests should be ordered?

ORGANIZING THE DIFFERENTIAL DIAGNOSIS

This presentation is of concern because the patient is elderly and she has a new headache. The differential diagnosis must therefore include "new headaches" which could be persistent and progressive. The persistence of the headache probably excludes diagnoses such as intracerebral hemorrhage or infections.

Temporal arteritis and malignancy are both possible given the patient's age and subacute presentation. The throbbing nature of the pain and weight loss could certainly be consistent with either of these types of headache. The history of a breast mass has to make metastatic disease a real consideration. Subdural hematoma is possible, although the lack of a history of head trauma makes this less likely. Although the diagnosis should be given with extreme caution in an elderly person with new headaches, the persistent band-like description raises the possibility of tension headaches. Table 15–8 lists the differential diagnosis.

 4

Soon after the headache began (3 months prior to her current presentation), she went to

Table 15–8. Diagnostic hypotheses for Mrs. T.

Diagnostic Hypotheses	Clinical Clues	Important Tests
Leading Hypothesis		
Temporal arteritis	Throbbing headache Symptoms of polymyalgia rheumatica Temporal artery abnormalities	ESR Temporal artery biopsy
Active Alternative—Most Common		
Tension headache	Chronic, pressure-type headache of mild to moderate intensity	Diagnostic criteria and exclusion of secondary headaches
Active Alternative		
Brain tumor	History of malignancy Focal neurologic deficit	CNS imaging
Other Alternative		
Subdural hematoma	Elderly patients with a history of falls	Noncontrast head CT scan

an emergency department and cervical osteoarthritis was diagnosed. She was given ibuprofen, muscle relaxants, and a referral to a rheumatologist. She saw the rheumatologist about 2 weeks later. An ESR done at that visit was 56 mm/h.

 Is the clinical information sufficient to make a diagnosis? If not, what other information do you need?

Leading Hypothesis: Temporal Arteritis

Textbook Presentation

Temporal arteritis classically presents in white women over age 50 as a bilateral, throbbing headache. Jaw pain and fatigue (jaw claudication) may be present. There may be a history of polymyalgia rheumatica or consistent symptoms and the physical exam can reveal beading and tenderness of the temporal arteries. The erythrocyte sedimentation rate (ESR) is usually elevated.

Disease Highlights

A. Temporal (or giant cell) arteritis is a vasculitis of large- and medium-sized arteries.

B. Primarily involves the vessels of the aortic arch, particularly the external carotid.

C. Affects persons over age 50, women more commonly than men.

D. Although the most common presentation is with a new headache, temporal arteritis can present with nonspecific manifestations of a chronic inflammatory disorder.

1. Fever
2. Anemia
3. Fatigue
4. Weight loss
5. Elevated ESR or C-reactive protein

E. It can also present with specific complications of the disease.

1. Jaw claudication
2. Blindness

F. Related to polymyalgia rheumatica

1. 15% of patients with polymyalgia rheumatica have temporal arteritis
2. 60% of patients with temporal arteritis have polymyalgia rheumatica

G. Rapid diagnosis and treatment are critical to prevent vasculitis-associated thrombosis in the effected vessels. Ophthalmic artery involvement can lead to sudden blindness.

Evidence-Based Diagnosis

A. Clinical findings

1. The clinical signs and symptoms of temporal arteritis are not highly predictive.
2. One recent review presented test characteristics for many of the commonly sited findings. These are outlined in Table 15–9.

Table 15–9. LRs for signs and symptoms of temporal arteritis.

Symptom or Sign	LR+	LR–
Jaw claudication	4.2	0.72
Diplopia	3.4	0.95
Beaded temporal artery	4.6	0.93
Enlarged temporal artery	4.3	0.67
Loss of temporal pulse	2.7	0.71
Temporal artery tenderness	2.6	0.82
Any temporal artery abnormality	2.0	0.53
Synovitis	0.41	1.1

Adapted from Smetana GW, Shmerling RH. Does this patient have temporal arteritis? *JAMA.* 2002;287:92–101. Copyrighted © 2002. American Medical Association. All rights reserved.

3. Reflecting the poor performance of these clinical predictors, only about 40% of patients referred for temporal artery biopsy have the disease.

 Because the clinical signs and symptoms of temporal arteritis are not highly predictive, temporal artery biopsy should be used in any patient in whom the clinical suspicion is moderate or high.

B. ESR has been used to "rule out" temporal arteritis.
   1. The sensitivity of an abnormal ESR is 96%.
   2. The test characteristics of the ESR at various cut points are shown below. (A normal ESR is usually considered to be < age/2 in men and age + 10/2 in women.)
      a. Abnormal: LR+, 1.1; LR–, 0.2
      b. ESR > 50 mm/h: LR+, 1.2; LR–, 0.35
      c. ESR > 100 mm/h: LR+, 1.9; LR–, 0.8
C. Temporal artery ultrasound
   1. Ultrasound has been used as a diagnostic tool
   2. Inflamed arteries have a hypoechoic halo around the lumen.
   3. Most studies have found this finding to be insensitive and not specific enough to avoid biopsy.
D. Temporal artery biopsy
   1. Considered the gold standard for diagnosing temporal arteritis.

2. Given the difficulty of clinically diagnosing temporal arteritis and the common side effects of the treatment, temporal artery biopsy is always recommended to establish the diagnosis of temporal arteritis.
3. Although biopsy should be done as quickly as possible once the disease is suspected, a short delay after beginning treatment ($\cong$ 7 days) probably does not effect the results.
4. Biopsy of palpably abnormal artery is the most accurate. If the artery is palpably normal, longer and bilateral biopsies are useful.
5. There are cases of biopsy-negative temporal arteritis. One much quoted study gave the following test characteristics for temporal artery biopsy.
   a. Sensitivity, 85%; specificity, 100%
   b. LR+, ∞; LR–, 0.15

 Even in the setting of a negative temporal artery biopsy, a patient with very high suspicion for temporal arteritis should be monitored closely or treated.

MAKING A DIAGNOSIS

 Physical exam is notable for vital signs of temperature, 37.1 °C; BP, 130/82 mm Hg; pulse, 72 bpm; RR, 10 breaths per minute. Head and neck exam revealed bilateral cataracts with some prominence of the temporal arteries. Heart, lung, and abdominal exams were normal. Breast exam revealed a 2 × 3 cm mass in the left breast that was soft and freely mobile, which seemed unchanged from a description in the patient's chart from 2 years earlier. Extremity exam was notable for bruises over her left elbow and shoulder from a fall. Neurologic exam is fully intact.

 Have you crossed a diagnostic threshold for the leading hypothesis, temporal arteritis? Have you ruled out the active alternatives? Do other tests need to be done to exclude the alternative diagnoses?

Temporal arteritis certainly remains high on the differential diagnosis. Her headache and physical exam are both suspicious. Assuming a pretest probability of 40% (the usual percentage of positive biopsies among people in whom temporal arteritis is suspected), the prominence of her temporal arteries (LR+ = 2) increases the likelihood of the diagnosis to 57%.

Both her history of falls and the breast mass (although likely benign) keep subdural hematoma and brain metastasis in the differential diagnosis.

Alternative Diagnosis: Subdural Hematoma

Textbook Presentation

Subdural hematoma is usually seen in older patients with a history of falls and neurologic deterioration. The classic triad of symptoms of chronic subdural hematoma is headache, somnolence, and change in mental status.

Disease Highlights

A. Subdural hematomas may be acute (within 24 hours of injury), subacute (1–14 days after injury), or chronic.

B. Acute and subacute subdural hematomas generally pose little diagnostic problem. They usually produce evolving, focal neurologic deficits.

C. Chronic subdural hematomas can present with subtle symptoms, weeks to months after trauma and can pose a real diagnostic challenge.

D. Chronic subdural hematoma is a disease seen in the elderly and others with cerebral atrophy who can accommodate a slowly expanding mass of blood in the subdural space.

Evidence-Based Diagnosis

A. History and physical exam

1. Diagnosis requires a high index of suspicion.

2. Below are the frequencies of the presenting symptoms of 43 patients, mean age 83, with subdural hematomas:

   a. Falls, 74%

   b. Progressive neurologic deficit, 70%

   c. Head trauma, 37%

   d. Transient neurologic deficit, 21%

   e. Seizure, 6%

   f. Headache, 6%

3. The absence of a trauma history should not be

particularly reassuring as this history is often hard to establish.

 The most common presenting symptom of chronic subdural hematoma is a history of falls. A high index of suspicion should be present for subdural hematoma in any elderly patient with a history of falls and subacute neurologic deficits.

B. Neuroimaging

1. CT scan and MRI are both effective means of diagnosing chronic subdural hematoma.

2. Caution should be used with noncontrast head CT scan because the blood in a chronic subdural hematoma can sometimes be isodense with cortical tissue.

Treatment

Unless a chronic subdural hematoma is small and causing no symptoms, the treatment is surgical drainage.

CASE RESOLUTION

Laboratory tests are done, and the patient is sent for a precontrast and postcontrast head CT scan. The patient's test results follow: Hgb, 9.0 g/dL (11.7 g/dL 1 month earlier); Hct, 28.1% (36.6% 1 month earlier); ESR, 125 mm/h. The head CT was normal other than cerebral atrophy expected for the patient's age.

Mrs. T was given 60 mg of prednisone daily and referred for a temporal artery biopsy. This was done 3 days later and was diagnostic for temporal arteritis. Her headache improved after 1 week of therapy. Over the next 2 years, multiple attempts at weaning corticosteroids failed, and the patient continues to take 15 mg of prednisone. While taking prednisone, a spinal compression fracture, acne, diabetes mellitus, and difficult-to-control hypertension develop.

The elevated ESR made the diagnosis of temporal arteritis likely but by no means certain. Taking the pretest probability of 57%, as it stood after the physical exam, an ESR > 100 mm/h raises the probability to 72%. This is probably not high enough to accept the side effects of long-term prednisone therapy without a more definitive diagnosis.

Treatment of Temporal Arteritis

A. The treatment of temporal arteritis is corticosteroids.

B. Corticosteroids should be started immediately in a patient in whom temporal arteritis is suspected.

C. Corticosteroids can be tapered slowly once there has been clinical remission as long as the inflammatory markers (ESR, C-reactive protein) remain depressed.

D. Methotrexate might be an option in patients who do not tolerate corticosteroid withdrawal as a steroid-sparing agent.

REVIEW OF OTHER IMPORTANT DISEASES

Meningitis

Textbook Presentation

Classically, meningitis presents with the acute onset of the triad of headache, fever, and a stiff neck. Meningitis may occur in the setting of a cluster of cases.

Disease Highlights

A. The presentation of fever and headache is common and can be worrisome, potentially caused by anything from influenza to meningitis. The differential includes:
   1. Viral infections and almost any other febrile illness
   2. Meningitis (bacterial, fungal, viral, or parasitic)
   3. Encephalitis
   4. Sinusitis
   5. CNS abscess
   6. Septic cavernous sinus thrombosis

B. Although certainly not the most common cause of fever and headache, meningitis is a relatively common, potentially life-threatening illness.

C. Viral causes are 3–4 times more common than bacterial causes and have a generally favorable prognosis.

D. Bacterial meningitis must be treated as a medical emergency.

E. Mortality rates vary by organism but community-acquired bacterial meningitis has a mortality rate of about 25%.

F. Mortality rates are higher for nosocomial infections.

G. The most common organisms are listed in Table 15–10.

Evidence-Based Diagnosis

A. The prevalence of various exam features in patients with meningitis comes from 1 hospital's review of 27 years of meningitis cases.
   1. 100% of patients had fever, stiff neck, or mental status changes
      a. 95% had fever > 37.8 °C
      b. 88% had stiff neck
      c. 66% had all 3 signs
   2. 11% had rash (67% of these cases were infected with *Neisseria meningitidis*)
   3. 28% had focal neurologic findings
   4. 44% of those who had imaging done had an abnormal CT scan

B. About 50% of patients with meningitis present with headache.

C. Patients with suppressed immune systems and the elderly are less likely to have a stiff neck.
   1. Two of the most commonly used meningeal signs are Kernig (the inability to extend the knee with a flexed hip) and Brudzinski (the demonstration of flexion of both the knees and hips upon forced flexion of the neck).
   2. These signs are present in only about 60% of patients with meningitis.

D. Lumbar puncture
   1. Lumbar puncture is the only means of making a definitive diagnosis.
   2. The CSF in acute bacterial meningitis will demonstrate WBCs with neutrophil predominance, low glucose, and high protein.

E. Patients with contraindications to lumbar puncture
   1. Frequently the question of contraindication to lumbar puncture is raised.
   2. Performing a lumbar puncture in a patient with a CNS mass, elevated intracranial pressure, or a bleeding diathesis places the patient at risk for complications such as herniation, paraspinal hemorrhage, and death.
   3. CNS imaging should be performed before lumbar puncture in any patient in whom there is a suspicion of increased intracranial pressure.
   4. Findings associated with mass effect on CT scan are
      a. Age > 60 years
      b. Immunocompromise
      c. Preexisting CNS disease
      d. Seizure within the previous week
      e. Abnormal level of consciousness
      f. Inability to answer 2 consecutive questions or follow 2 consecutive commands correctly

Table 15–10. Common causes of meningitis in adults.

Organism	Characteristics
Viruses	Enteroviruses (echovirus and coxsackievirus) most common More common in children than adults Summer and Fall predominance
Streptococcus pneumoniae	Most common bacterial meningitis in adults of all ages. May occur de novo or by contiguous spread (sinuses, ears). Mortality rates $\cong$ 20%.
Neisseria meningitidis	Second most common cause overall. May occur in epidemics. Most commonly seen in young adults.
Listeria monocytogenes	Disease of older adults (older than 60 years) and immunosuppressed (including patients with diabetes and alcohol abuse)
Haemophilus influenzae	Previously very common cause of meningitis in children; now rare because of vaccination

   g. Gaze palsy, abnormal visual fields, facial palsy, arm or leg drift, aphasia

 Patients with an abnormal neurologic exam should undergo CNS imaging prior to lumbar puncture.

5. If CNS imaging is required, a patient with suspected meningitis should have blood cultures drawn and then receive empiric antibiotics immediately, undergo a CT scan, and then have the lumbar puncture.

Treatment

A. As with all infectious diseases, the specific treatment depends on the pathogen.

B. Because of the severity of meningeal infections, empiric therapy is recommended while waiting for Gram stain and culture results.

C. Antibiotic treatment should be ordered when the diagnosis of meningitis is suspected and given immediately after CSF begins to be collected.

D. In adult patients, the current recommendations are to treat empirically with a third-generation cephalosporin and vancomycin.

E. If *Listeria monocytogenes* is suspected, ampicillin is also added.

Headaches Associated with Head Trauma

Textbook Presentation

A common presentation of a posttraumatic headache would be a middle-aged person who recently suffered head trauma, usually without detectable cranial or neurologic injury, with a headache similar in quality to tension headaches. The headaches are often associated with symptoms such as irritability or anxiety.

Disease Highlights

A. Head trauma can cause serious cranial or neurologic injury including subdural, epidural or parenchymal hematoma, SAH, cerebral contusion, or depressed skull fracture.

B. More commonly, head trauma can cause new headaches or worsen preexisting headache syndromes.

C. Trauma-related headaches might occur after minor or major trauma. The IHS requires 2 of the following to qualify as major trauma:

   1. Loss of consciousness

   2. 10 minutes of posttraumatic amnesia

   3. 2 objective measures of cranial or neurologic trauma

D. There appears to be a significant amount of psychiatric distress and disability associated with posttraumatic headaches.

Evidence-Based Diagnosis

A. Acute evaluation of head trauma

1. In a patient with head trauma or a headache seemingly associated with head trauma, the first goal is to identify important and potentially treatable injury.

2. The initial test is usually a head CT scan. A difficult question is who can be clinically cleared without a CT scan.

3. One excellent study looked at over 900 patients after a minor head injury (defined as trauma resulting in loss of consciousness but not affecting the neurologic exam or Glasgow coma scale).

   a. 7 criteria were identified that yielded 100% sensitivity:

      (1) Headache

      (2) Vomiting

      (3) Age over 60 years

      (4) Drug or alcohol intoxication

      (5) Deficits in short-term memory

      (6) Physical evidence of trauma above the clavicles

      (7) Seizure

      (8) Many other authors have suggested that the presence of anticoagulation therapy be added to this list

   b. The specificity of these symptoms was poor (25%).

B. Diagnosis of posttraumatic headaches

1. The next step is to diagnose ongoing headaches as posttraumatic.

2. The IHS classifies these headaches into headaches following minor or major trauma (see above) and into acute (occurs within 14 days of the injury and resolves within 8 weeks) or chronic (occurs within 14 days of the injury and does not resolve within 8 weeks).

3. Headache develops in about 25% of patients following minor trauma.

   a. These headaches are most likely to be chronic.

   b. They are also most likely to meet criteria for tension-type headaches.

Treatment

A. The treatment of posttraumatic headaches is generally similar to the treatment of clinically similar headaches.

B. It does appear that associated psychological treatment, such as biofeedback and treatment of associated posttraumatic stress syndrome, might be beneficial.

Diagnostic Approach: Headache

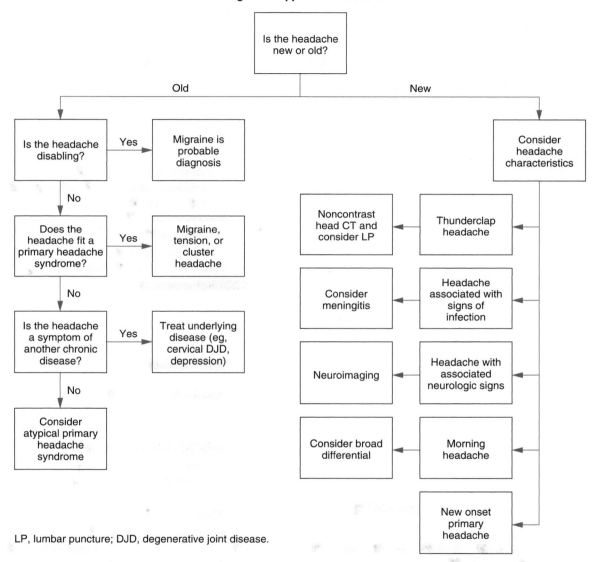

LP, lumbar puncture; DJD, degenerative joint disease.

I have a patient with hypercalcemia.
How do I determine the cause?

CHIEF COMPLAINT

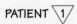 PATIENT 1

Mrs. D is a 60-year-old, African American woman who complains of longstanding constipation. Initial laboratory evaluation reveals a normal TSH, normal electrolytes, and a calcium level of 10.8 mg/dL (nl 8.4–10.2).

 What is the differential diagnosis of hypercalcemia? How would you frame the differential?

CONSTRUCTING A DIFFERENTIAL DIAGNOSIS

In general, hypercalcemia is detected in 1 of 3 clinical circumstances. First, hypercalcemia may be discovered during routine laboratory work-ups in patients with no symptoms or in at-risk patients, such as those with malignancy. In fact, most cases of hypercalcemia are diagnosed in asymptomatic persons. Second, hypercalcemia may be found during evaluation of patients with certain symptoms or findings that can be related to hypercalcemia, such as constipation, weakness, fatigue, depression, nephrolithiasis, or osteopenia. Third, severe, life-threatening hypercalcemia may present as altered mental status.

Because most cases of hypercalcemia are due to only a handful of conditions, it is easiest to divide the differential diagnosis into common and uncommon causes.

A. Common causes of hypercalcemia
  1. Primary hyperparathyroidism
  2. Hypercalcemia of malignancy
     a. Secretion of parathyroid hormone–related protein (PTHrP)

(1) Squamous cell carcinomas
(2) Adenocarcinoma of lung, pancreas, kidney, and others
  b. Osteolytic metastasis
     (1) Breast cancer
     (2) Multiple myeloma
  c. Production of calcitriol (Hodgkin disease)
  3. Milk-alkali syndrome (Mainly seen in patients with chronic renal failure who are taking calcium carbonate.)
B. Less common causes of hypercalcemia
  1. Drug related
     a. Lithium therapy (Causes hypercalcemia in about 10% of patients)
     b. Thiazide diuretic therapy
  2. Familial hypocalciuric hypercalcemia
  3. Related to renal failure
     a. Tertiary hyperparathyroidism
     b. Secondary hyperparathyroidism (in the setting of calcium supplementation)
  4. Secondary to other illnesses
     a. Hyperthyroidism
     b. Sarcoidosis and tuberculosis
C. Falsely elevated serum calcium (secondary to increased serum binding protein)
  1. Hyperalbuminemia
  2. Multiple myeloma

 1

Mrs. D comes to your office for an initial visit. Her constipation has been longstanding and severe enough to lead to physician visits over the past 5 years. Evaluation with colonoscopy had been normal. Results of laboratory tests drawn over the last few years by previous physicians show normal test results (including TSH), with the exception of calcium levels in the range of 11 mg/dL. Despite use of stool softeners and high-fiber supplements, she often needs laxatives to move her bowels more than once a week.

In addition to constipation, the patient's other medical problems are hypertension and tobacco use. She feels well. Her medications are atenolol and hydrochlorothiazide. Family history is notable only for hypertension in both parents. She is up-to-date on routine healthcare maintenance (mammography, colonoscopy, Pap smears) and her physical exam is unremarkable.

Following the laboratory results, she was told to stop taking the diuretic and return in 1 week to have her calcium level and BP rechecked.

 At this point, what is the leading hypothesis, and what are the active alternatives? What other tests should be ordered?

ORGANIZING THE DIFFERENTIAL DIAGNOSIS

There is no question that in a healthy, ambulatory patient with hypercalcemia, primary hyperparathyroidism must lead the list of possible diagnoses. This disease is common and often asymptomatic or minimally symptomatic. The apparent chronicity of this patient's hypercalcemia makes this diagnosis even more likely. Hypercalcemia related to thiazide use is also possible. However, thiazide diuretics should only cause chronic hypercalcemia in patients with other abnormalities in calcium metabolism. Most patients with hypercalcemia due to a malignancy have already been given a diagnosis of cancer when they seek care for hypercalcemia. Sarcoidosis is not a common cause of hypercalcemia but should probably be considered, given the patient's race, if another diagnosis is not made. Table 16–1 lists the differential diagnosis.

1

After withdrawing the thiazide, the calcium level is remeasured and remains unchanged. A PTH level is drawn.

(continued)

Table 16–1. Diagnostic hypotheses for Mrs. D.

Diagnostic Hypotheses	Clinical Clues	Important Tests
Leading Hypothesis		
Primary hyperparathyroidism	Elevated calcium level without evident underlying disease	PTH level
Active Alternative		
Thiazide diuretic use	Transient hypercalcemia or exacerbation of hypercalcemia in patient with underlying disease	Resolution with cessation of drug
Active Alternative—Must Not Miss		
Hypercalcemia of malignancy	Usually presents in patients with known malignancy	Diagnosis of malignancy Demonstration of PTHrP or skeletal metastasis
Other Alternative		
Sarcoidosis	Pulmonary disease with hilar lymphadenopathy or interstitial lung disease	Demonstration of noncaseating granulomas and exclusion of known causes of granulomatous disease

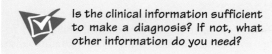

Is the clinical information sufficient to make a diagnosis? If not, what other information do you need?

Leading Hypothesis: Primary Hyperparathyroidism

Textbook Presentation

Primary hyperparathyroidism usually presents with hypercalcemia found during routine laboratory screening. Occasionally, it is detected during the evaluation of nonspecific symptoms, such as fatigue or constipation.

Disease Highlights

A. Primary hyperparathyroidism predominantly presents with modestly elevated calcium with few (if any) symptoms rather than the classic presentation of "stones, bones, groans, and psychiatric overtones."

Primary hyperparathyroidism accounts for more than 90% of cases of hypercalcemia in otherwise healthy ambulatory patients.

B. Etiology of primary hyperparathyroidism

   1. 85% of the cases of primary hyperparathyroidism are due to solitary parathyroid adenomas.

   2. Parathyroid hyperplasia, multiple adenomas, and the rare carcinoma cause the other 15% of cases.

      a. Parathyroid hyperplasia can be sporadic or inherited.

      b. Inherited syndromes of parathyroid hyperplasia include the multiple endocrine neoplasia type 1 (MEN 1) and MEN 2A syndromes and hypocalciuric hypercalcemia.

      c. Hypocalciuric hypercalcemia causes mild parathyroid hyperplasia but is associated with normal or only slightly elevated levels of PTH.

C. Clinical manifestations of primary hyperparathyroidism

   1. Nonspecific symptoms such as fatigue, irritability, and weakness are more common among patients with primary hyperparathyroidism.

   2. Decreased bone density is common in patients with primary hyperparathyroidism while classic osteitis fibrosis cystica is exceedingly rare today.

   3. Nephrolithiasis is present in 15–20% of patients with primary hyperparathyroidism.

   4. Other symptoms of primary hyperparathyroidism probably include increased frequency of hypertension, gout, and calcium pyrophosphate deposition disease.

D. Secondary and tertiary hyperparathyroidism

   1. Secondary hyperparathyroidism most commonly occurs in patients with renal failure.

      a. The chronic hypocalcemia of renal failure leads to parathyroid hyperplasia.

      b. Secondary hyperparathyroidism is usually associated with hypocalcemia.

      c. Hypercalcemia can develop in patients with secondary hyperparathyroidism if they are also receiving calcium or calcitriol or both.

   2. Tertiary hyperparathyroidism occurs when the parathyroid hyperplasia of secondary hyperparathyroidism begins to autonomously produce PTH. The high levels of secreted PTH cause hypercalcemia.

Evidence-Based Diagnosis

A. Hypercalcemia should be confirmed before evaluating a patient for primary hyperparathyroidism.

   1. The calcium level should be remeasured.

   2. Albumin or ionized calcium should be measured to account for plasma protein binding. If albumin is measured, then the corrected calcium = calcium (mg/dL) + 0.8(4-albumin (g/dL)).

B. Other effects of elevated PTH levels (hypercalciuria, hypophosphatemia, hyperphosphaturia) are seldom useful in differentiating primary hyperparathyroidism from hypercalcemia of malignancy—the second most common cause of hypercalcemia.

C. The diagnosis of primary hyperparathyroidism is usually not difficult.

   1. The diagnosis is extremely likely in an otherwise healthy patient with chronic hypercalcemia.

   2. An elevated PTH level is confirmatory; it distinguishes primary hyperparathyroidism from hypercalcemia of malignancy, which has low serum PTH levels.

   3. Other causes of hyperparathyroidism with an elevated PTH are usually easily excluded based on the history.

a. Patients with the MEN syndromes will have a family history.

b. Patients with hypocalciuric hypercalcemia usually have normal PTH levels and a family history.

c. Patients with tertiary hyperparathyroidism have renal failure.

MAKING A DIAGNOSIS

Final laboratory test results for Mrs. D follow:

Calcium: 10.9 mg/dL

Inorganic phosphate: 3.3 mg/dL (nl 2.5–4.4)

Ionized calcium: 6.20 mg/dL (nl 4.60–5.40)

PTH: 166 pg/mL (nl < 60)

A diagnosis of primary hyperparathyroidism was made.

 Have you crossed a diagnostic threshold for the leading hypothesis, primary hyperparathyroidism? Have you ruled out the active alternatives? Do other tests need to be done to exclude the alternative diagnoses?

The differential diagnosis of hypercalcemia in a patient with an elevated PTH is lithium use, MEN syndromes, secondary or tertiary hyperparathyroidism, or familial hypocalciuric hypercalcemia. Given the patient's medications, normal renal function and age at presentation, without a family history of hypercalcemia, primary hyperparathyroidism is clearly the most likely diagnosis. Although thiazide-induced hypercalcemia is not a cause of hyperparathyroidism per se, it is the only remaining possible diagnosis.

Alternative Diagnosis: Thiazide-Induced Hypercalcemia

Textbook Presentation

Thiazide-induced hypercalcemia is most commonly associated with only slightly elevated calcium levels and seen transiently soon after starting a thiazide diuretic.

Disease Highlights

A. Thiazide diuretics have hypocaliuric effects.

  1. Sodium depletion causes increased sodium and calcium retention in the proximal tubule.

  2. Thiazides probably also augment the effect of PTH.

B. Hypercalcemia is generally mild and should be short lived, as reduced PTH secretion will normalize calcium levels.

C. Some patients may have persistently, slightly elevated calcium levels.

D. Patients with hyperparathyroidism, or other causes of increased bone turnover, might have persistent and more pronounced degrees of hypercalcemia.

Evidence-Based Diagnosis

A. The diagnosis of thiazide-induced hypercalcemia depends on documenting hypercalcemia temporally related to beginning a diuretic.

B. Resolution of the abnormality with cessation of the drug makes the diagnosis.

C. Patients with more than slight ($\cong 0–.5$ mg/dL), persistent elevations of calcium while taking a thiazide should be evaluated for other causes of hypercalcemia, as should patients with thiazide-related hypercalcemia who also have an elevated PTH.

Treatment

Because the hypercalcemia is almost always mild and short lived, no treatment is necessary.

CASE RESOLUTION

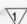

The patient's diuretic was stopped. Over the next 3 months, her calcium remained stable, confirming the diagnosis of primary hyperparathyroidism. Based on the patient's severe constipation, without another cause, the decision was made to treat her hyperparathyroidism. She underwent nuclear scanning of the parathyroid glands and results were normal. Surgical exploration of the neck was performed. A 3 × 3 cm, 4-gram, parathyroid adenoma was found and surgically removed without complication.

On follow-up, the patient had rapid normalization of her calcium levels. Her constipation, however, persisted. In the end, the constipation was considered to be functional and unrelated to the hypercalcemia.

As discussed below, the patient's symptoms are an indication for surgery. However, since the patient's symptoms were nonspecific, they failed to improve after surgery, which is not uncommon. The reported sensitivity of nuclear imaging of the neck for parathyroid adenomas is < 70%, so it is not surprising that the scan was normal.

Treatment of Hyperparathyroidism

A. Definitive treatment for primary hyperparathyroidism is surgical parathyroidectomy.

B. Who needs surgery?

  1. Because of the generally benign course of primary hyperparathyroidism, not everyone needs surgery.

  2. Recommendations from consensus panels are based on who is most likely to progress to symptomatic disease and who would benefit most from surgery.

  3. Indications for surgery

    a. Symptoms of hypercalcemia

    b. Elevated serum calcium > 1 mg/dL above normal

    c. Creatinine clearance reduction of 30%

    d. 24-hour urine calcium > 400 mg/d (nl < 150 mg/d)

    e. Bone mass > 2.5 standard deviations (SDs) below age-matched controls (Z score < −2.5)

    f. Age younger than 50

    g. Patient preference or patient inability to comply with long-term monitoring

C. Monitoring (for patients not undergoing surgery)

  1. Assessment of symptoms, calcium level, and renal function every 6–12 months.

  2. Bone density screening yearly of the hip, spine, and wrist.

  3. Monitoring, possibly radiographically, for development of nephrolithiasis

D. This approach to deciding which patients undergo surgery appears to be effective. A recent study observing 52 asymptomatic people for up to 10 years demonstrated the disease is usually not progressive.

  1. 38 (73%) had no progression of disease

  2. Patients who required surgery did so for the following reasons: 2 developed hypercalcemia, 8 developed hypercalciuria, and 6 developed low bone density.

E. Parathyroidectomy

  1. Parathyroidectomy is markedly effective at inducing normocalcemia (95–98%), improving bone density (100%) and improving symptoms (82%).

  2. Preoperative nuclear imaging of the parathyroid glands is very helpful in identifying abnormal glands, thus decreasing the need for detailed neck exploration.

    a. Sensitivity, 69%; specificity, 98%

    b. LR+, 34.5; LR−, 0.32

  3. Intraoperative PTH assays also serve to improve the surgical success rates.

CHIEF COMPLAINT

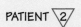
PATIENT 2

Mrs. W is an 80-year-old woman who is admitted to the hospital from her doctor's office because of lethargy, abdominal pain, and hypercalcemia. She complained to her doctor of 1 year of epigastric pain. The pain had been mild but had become severe and persistent over the last 6 weeks. Her daughter, who found her somewhat confused at their weekly lunch, brought her to the office.

On evaluation in the office she was found to be lethargic but oriented to person and place. Her vital signs were temperature, 36.9 °C; pulse, 94 bpm; BP, 110/90 mm Hg; RR, 14 breaths per minute. She was orthostatic. Her exam was remarkable for mild cachexia and tender hepatomegaly.

Initial laboratory test results in the physician's office were:

Sodium: 134 mEq/L

Potassium: 3.9 mEq/L

Chloride: 99 mEq /L

CO_2: 26 mEq /L

BUN: 24 mg/dL

Creatinine: 0.8 mg/dL

Glucose: 117 mg/dL

Calcium: 15.0 mg/dL

Albumin: 3.9 g/dL

Total bilirubin: 0.9 g/dL

Conjugated bilirubin: 0.6 g/dL

Alkaline phosphatase: 800 units/L

AST (SGOT): 124 units/L

ALT (SGPT): 86 units/L

Phosphate: 1.4 mg/dL

At this point, what is the leading hypothesis, and what are the active alternatives? What other tests should be ordered?

ORGANIZING THE DIFFERENTIAL DIAGNOSIS

This is an elderly woman with abdominal pain and significant hypercalcemia. Although primary hyperparathyroidism is a possibility, the high level of the calcium, the patient's symptoms, abnormal physical exam, and laboratory abnormalities strongly warrant consideration of other diseases. Hypercalcemia of malignancy needs to be considered given the patient's age and hepatomegaly. Most patients with hypercalcemia of malignancy have a previously diagnosed cancer, but it is possible for symptoms of cancer and hypercalcemia to present simultaneously or for symptoms of hypercalcemia to present alone. Malignancy primarily causes hypercalcemia through the elaboration of PTHrP or through osseous metastasis.

The milk-alkali syndrome should be considered. This syndrome is often caused by ingestion of large amounts of calcium carbonate in an effort to treat dyspepsia. This syndrome typically presents with hypercalcemia, metabolic alkalosis, and renal insufficiency. The presence of only 1 of the syndrome's 3 features makes this diagnosis less likely. The presence of other illnesses or medication use may suggest less common causes of hypercalcemia, such as granulomatous disease. Table 16–2 lists the differential diagnosis.

2

The patient reports no significant prior medical history but she has not seen a physician in over 5 years. She has been using calcium carbonate (Tums) for her abdominal pain but reports only intermittent use and none for the last few days. She is not taking any other medications. Review of systems is unremarkable other than the previously noted fatigue and abdominal pain.

An abdominal ultrasound done on the day of admission reveals multiple hepatic masses.

(continued)

Table 16–2. Diagnostic hypotheses for Mrs. W.

Diagnostic Hypotheses	Clinical Clues	Important Tests
Leading Hypothesis		
Hypercalcemia of Malignancy (elaboration of PTHrP)	Presence of malignancy, usually previously diagnosed Squamous cell carcinomas and adenocarcinoma of the lung most common	PTH-related peptide
Active Alternatives		
Hypercalcemia of Malignancy— Osseous metastases	Presence of malignancy, usually previously diagnosed Multiple myeloma and breast cancer most common	Demonstration of bony metastases
Primary hyperparathyroidism	Elevated calcium without evident underlying disease	PTH level
Other Alternative		
Milk-alkali syndrome	Hypercalcemia Metabolic alkalosis Renal insufficiency	Normal PTH level and history of calcium and absorbable alkali ingestion

Is the clinical information sufficient to make a diagnosis? If not, what other information do you need?

Leading Hypothesis: Hypercalcemia of Malignancy (Elaboration of PTHrP)

Textbook Presentation

Hypercalcemia of malignancy is most commonly detected in patients with previously diagnosed cancers. It is uncommon for symptomatic hypercalcemia to be the presenting symptom of a malignancy.

Disease Highlights

A. Hypercalcemia of malignancy is a heterogeneous process in which malignant cells elevate serum calcium in a number of ways.

   1. The most common cause of hypercalcemia is through elaboration of PTHrP.

   2. Tumors metastatic to bone may also cause hypercalcemia through direct osteolytic effects on the bones, sometimes via local elaboration of PTHrP. This syndrome is discussed below.

   3. It is likely there is a great deal of overlap between these first 2 causes.

   4. Rarely, tumors can cause hypercalcemia by elaborating vitamin D (seen most commonly with lymphoma).

B. The malignancies that commonly cause hypercalcemia are (in approximate order of frequency):

   1. Lung

   2. Breast

   3. Multiple myeloma

   4. Lymphoma

   5. Head and neck

   6. Renal

   7. Prostate

C. PTHrP is a normal, physiologic, protein that is produced by many non-neoplastic tissues.

   1. The protein shares considerable sequence homology to PTH and binds to the same receptor.

   2. PTH and PTHrP affect the bones and kidneys in the same way.

   3. Certain malignancies elaborate the protein in relatively large amounts.

   a. PTHrP is detectable in 80% of patients with hypercalcemia and malignancy.

   b. The most common tumors that produce this protein are squamous cell carcinomas and adenocarcinoma of the lung, pancreas, and kidney.

   4. In hypercalcemia of malignancy secondary to PTHrP, hypercalcemia commonly precedes bony metastasis.

Evidence-Based Diagnosis

A. Similar to primary hyperparathyroidism, hypercalcemia of malignancy seldom presents significant diagnostic confusion.

B. In patients without bony metastasis, the diagnosis (and differentiation from primary hyperparathyroidism) is made by detecting high PTHrP and low PTH levels.

C. In patients with bony metastases, a low serum PTH confirms the diagnosis.

MAKING A DIAGNOSIS

Given the results of the patient's ultrasound, it is highly likely that she has a malignancy that is causing the hypercalcemia. The next step is to make a definitive diagnosis of the malignancy so that specific treatment can be instituted. Determining how the malignancy is causing hypercalcemia will be part of this evaluation; is the hypercalcemia a result of osseous metastasis or of PTHrP?

The patient was given normal saline for hydration and furosemide for diuresis when mild peripheral edema developed. Her calcium dropped over the first 3 days in the hospital to 11.2 mg/dL, where it remained stable.

As a follow-up to the ultrasound, a torso CT was ordered. This revealed a large lung mass and multiple liver masses. CT guided biopsy of the liver was consistent with metastatic squamous cell carcinoma, likely of pulmonary origin.

 Have you crossed a diagnostic threshold for the leading hypothesis, hypercalcemia of malignancy (elaboration of PTHrP)? Have you ruled out the active alternatives? Do other tests need to be done to exclude the alternative diagnoses?

Alternative Diagnosis: Hypercalcemia of Malignancy (Osseous Metastasis)

Textbook Presentation

Similar to hypercalcemia of malignancy caused by PTHrP, hypercalcemia due to malignancies metastatic to bone generally presents in patients with previously diagnosed cancer. Breast cancer and multiple myeloma (discussed in detail here) are the most common causes.

Multiple myeloma commonly presents with bone pain (often back pain), anemia, hypercalcemia, or renal insufficiency in patients in their 60s. Plain radiographs commonly demonstrate osteolytic lesions and the diagnosis is made by the demonstration of paraproteinemia and increased plasma cells on bone marrow examination.

Disease Highlights

A. Breast cancer and multiple myeloma only cause hypercalcemia after metastasizing to bone.

B. The hypercalcemia is due to local osteolytic effects on bone, sometimes related to PTHrP secretion, sometimes related to other mediators.

C. Multiple myeloma is caused by a malignant proliferation of plasma cells. The plasma cells usually secrete a single immunoglobulin, called the M component (monoclonal component) that is detected on serum or urine protein electrophoresis.

D. Multiple myeloma most commonly affects patients in the seventh decade of life. Blacks are affected at twice the rate as whites.

E. Symptoms are varied and result from the effect of plasma cell proliferation on multiple systems.

   1. Anemia: Secondary to plasma cell bone marrow infiltration

   2. Infections: When the M component is excluded, patients with myeloma usually have hypogammaglobulinemia.

   3. Bone pain and hypercalcemia: Proliferation of plasma cells in the bone cause osteolytic lesions.

   4. Renal insufficiency: Multiple myeloma can cause renal insufficiency in multiple ways:

      a. Light chain associated injury to the kidney. Injury may occur in a variety of ways, including toxic effect of light chains on the renal tubules and obstruction secondary to the heavy burden of filtered light chains.

      b. Hypercalcemia

      c. Amyloid deposition in the kidney

      d. Urate nephropathy

   5. Serum hyperviscosity may occur from hypergammaglobulinemia. This commonly causes headache and visual disturbances.

F. Symptoms at presentation as reported in a recent study

   1. Anemia was present in 73% of patients. The anemia was usually mild, normochromic, normocytic.

   2. 58% of patients had bone pain at presentation and 67% had lytic bone lesions on x-ray films.

   3. 19% had renal insufficiency

   4. 13% had hypercalcemia > 11 mg/dL

   5. M component

      a. 82% of patients had an abnormal serum protein electrophoresis. Of the 18% with a normal serum electrophoresis, 97% had an abnormal urine protein electrophoresis.

      b. The M component most commonly appears in the gamma range and is most commonly IgG.

      c. 16% have only free light chains.

   6. A sizable minority (36%) had another plasma cell abnormality present at the time of diagnosis (monoclonal gammopathy of unknown significance, plasmacytoma, amyloidosis).

Evidence-Based Diagnosis

A. The diagnosis of multiple myeloma is based on the identification of:

   1. Marrow plasmacytosis (> 10%)

   2. Lytic bone lesions

   3. A serum or urine M component or both.

B. Clues to the diagnosis are the presence of normocytic anemia, bone pain, and elevated immunoglobulins.

C. There are a few important issues that may confuse the diagnosis.

   1. Filtered light chains are not detected on traditional urine dipsticks. A patient with light chain only myeloma may have normal amounts of serum protein and, apparently, no proteinuria. The presence of a monoclonal gammopathy will be easily detected with serum and urine protein electrophoresis.

   2. The bone lesions of multiple myeloma are almost exclusively osteolytic. They will usually be missed on bone scans but are easily seen on plain x-ray films.

Alternative Diagnosis: Milk-Alkali Syndrome

Textbook Presentation

Most commonly seen in patients with end-stage renal disease who are treated with calcium carbonate to combat hyperphosphatemia.

Disease Highlights

A. The milk-alkali syndrome is a syndrome of hypercalcemia, metabolic alkalosis, and renal insufficiency caused by the ingestion of calcium and an absorbable alkali.

B. In addition to patients with end-stage renal disease, milk-alkali syndrome is seen in patients who take large amounts of calcium carbonate for dyspepsia.

C. Milk-alkali syndrome in renal failure

   1. Patients with end-stage renal disease (especially those receiving hemodialysis) often have hyperphosphatemia.

      a. Hyperphosphatemia develops in patients with renal failure as renal clearance of phosphate falls.

      b. Early in the course of renal failure, hypocalcemia and hyperphosphatemia induce secondary hyperparathyroidism. This elevated PTH serves to increase calcium release from the bones and enhance renal phosphate excretion.

      c. As renal failure worsens, hyperparathyroidism becomes counterproductive as the kidneys no longer respond to PTH by excreting phosphate while phosphate continues to be released, with calcium, from the bones.

   2. Treatment of hyperphosphatemia in renal failure

      a. In patients receiving hemodialysis, phosphate binders are given orally to reduce the amount of phosphate absorbed.

      b. Calcium carbonate is the most widely used phosphate binder. Calcium acetate is also effective.

      c. Aluminum hydroxide and sevelamer (RenaGel) are also effective, but their use is limited by side effects and cost, respectively.

      d. In the future, calcium mimetics may be effective in combating the secondary hyperparathyroidism that caused the hyperphosphatemia.

   3. The milk-alkali syndrome has become quite common as calcium carbonate has become the preferred binder.

   4. One study reported a 36% incidence of hypercalcemia in hemodialysis patients beginning calcium carbonate therapy.

D. Milk-alkali syndrome unrelated to renal failure

   1. Predominantly a disease of women who use high doses of calcium carbonate

   2. Probably the most common cause of hypercalcemia in hospitalized patients after malignancy and primary hyperparathyroidism

Evidence-Based Diagnosis

A. The diagnosis of milk-alkali syndrome is based on history with supporting laboratory test results.

B. In patients with renal failure, an elevated calcium level, in the setting of calcium carbonate use and an elevated PTH, is diagnostic.

C. In patients without renal failure, the common presentation is a patient consuming large amounts of calcium carbonate with a normal PTH and normal phosphate.

Treatment

A. In the setting of renal failure, treatment of the milk-alkali syndrome calls for reduction of calcium carbonate intake.

   1. Other means of controlling hyperphosphatemia must then be used.

   2. This may include use of sevelamer, prolonged dialysis, or parathyroidectomy.

B. Patients without renal failure need only to discontinue taking calcium carbonate.

   1. In patients with symptomatic hypercalcemia, cessation of calcium carbonate intake and hydration is usually sufficient treatment.

   2. Caution should be taken when treating patients with severe milk-alkali syndrome with fluid and loop diuretics. These patients appear to be at particular risk for subsequent, transient, hypocalcemia.

CASE RESOLUTION

2

The patient's laboratory test results follow:

PTHrP: 3.3 (nl 0–1.9)

PTH: 13 pg/mL (nl < 60)

Mrs. W's hypercalcemia was presumed to be secondary to malignancy with an elevated PTHrP. She was treated with zoledronic acid, while she received hydration. After a long discussion, the patient opted to be treated with palliative chemotherapy. Although she did quite well initially, her condition declined markedly over the next 12 weeks. Chemotherapy was discontinued, and she was transferred to a hospice center where she died 4 weeks later.

Because the patient had metastatic squamous cell lung cancer, her rapid decline was not unexpected. The average life expectancy of patients with squamous cell carcinoma and extensive disease is a little less than 1 year. In general, patient prognosis depends much more on the type and stage of cancer rather than the presence or absence of hypercalcemia.

Treatment of Hypercalcemia of Malignancy

A. All patients with hypercalcemia of malignancy benefit from treatment of the underlying disease.

B. Beyond treatment of the malignancy, treatment aimed directly at hypercalcemia depends on its severity.

C. The mainstays of treatment for moderate and severe elevations of calcium are the bisphosphonates.

   1. Bisphosphonates work by inhibiting osteoclast activity.

   2. Pamidronate is indicated for the treatment of hypercalcemia of malignancy of any type. It is likely more effective in patients with bony metastasis than in those with PTHrP-related hypercalcemia.

   3. Zoledronic acid is indicated for the treatment of hypercalcemia of malignancy related to osseous metastasis. It is probably more effective than pamidronate in this population.

D. For patients with severe, symptomatic hypercalcemia, therapy must be more rapidly effective than treatment of the underlying disease or bisphosphonates therapy (which takes about 48 hours to reach full effectiveness).

   1. Saline hydration treats the dehydration that frequently accompanies hypercalcemia and decreases reabsorption of calcium in the proximal tubule of dehydrated, hypercalcemic patients.

   2. Once hydration is attained, a loop diuretic can further assist in achieving calciuresis.

   3. Calcitonin also affects rapid decreases in serum calcium.

   4. While immediate therapy for hypercalcemia is instituted, a bisphosphonate should be given and long-term treatment of the malignancy should be planned.

Diagnostic Approach: Hypercalemia

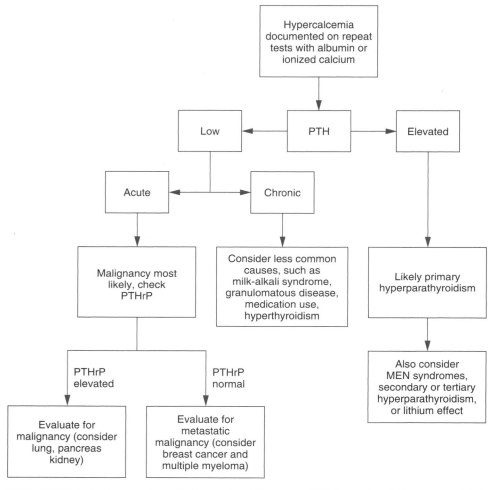

MEN, multiple endocrine neoplasia; PTH, parathyroid hormone; PTHrP, parathyroid hormone–related protein.

I have a patient with hyponatremia. I have a patient with hypernatremia. How do I determine the cause?

HYPONATREMIA

CHIEF COMPLAINT

PATIENT 1

Mr. D is a 42-year-old man who is brought to the emergency department by the police department. He is disoriented and confused. Initial labs reveal a serum sodium concentration of 118 mEq/L.

What is the differential diagnosis of hyponatremia? How would you frame the differential?

CONSTRUCTING A DIFFERENTIAL DIAGNOSIS

Hyponatremia develops when the body is unable to excrete free water. Hyponatremia is defined as serum sodium concentration < 134 mEq/L and is significant when the concentration is < 130 mEq/L. The first step in evaluating the hyponatremic patient is to determine the patient's volume status and identify who is clinically hypervolemic, euvolemic, or hypovolemic (Figure 17–1). This step narrows the differential diagnosis and is necessary to properly interpret test results. Correct classification of the patient's volume status requires a review of the history, physical exam findings, and laboratory results. After the patient's volume status has been determined, the different etiologies can be considered (Figure 17–2). This chapter will focus on true (hypoosmolar) hyponatremia. Pseudohyponatremia is discussed briefly at the end.

Differential Diagnosis of Hyponatremia

A. Hypervolemia
  1. Congestive heart failure (CHF)
  2. Cirrhosis
  3. Nephrotic syndrome
  4. Renal failure (Glomerular filtration rate [GFR] < 5 mL/min)
B. Euvolemia
  1. Syndrome of inappropriate antidiuretic hormone (SIADH)
    a. Cancers (eg, pancreas, lung)
    b. CNS disease (eg, cerebrovascular accident, trauma, infection, hemorrhage, mass)
    c. Pulmonary diseases (eg, infections, respiratory failure)
    d. Drugs
      (1) Thiazides
      (2) Antidiuretic hormone (ADH) analogues (vasopressin, desmopressin acetate [DDAVP], oxytocin)
      (3) Chlorpropamide (6–7% of treated patients)
      (4) Carbamazepine
      (5) Antidepressants (tricyclics and selective serotonin reuptake inhibitors) and antipsychotics
      (6) Nonsteroidal anti-inflammatory drugs (NSAIDs)
      (7) Ecstasy
      (8) Others (cyclophosphamide, vincristine, nicotine, opiates, clofibrate)
  2. Hypothyroidism

Determining Volume Status in Hyponatremia

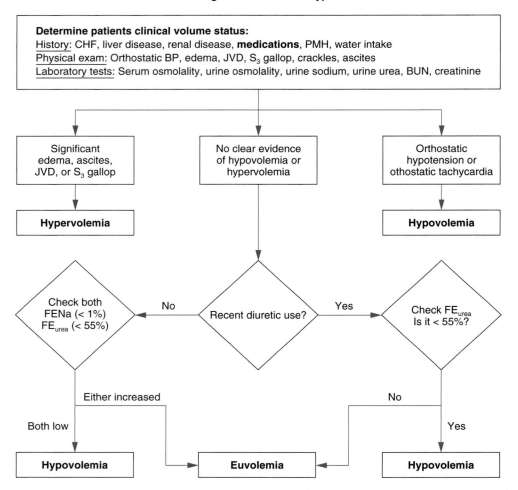

CHF, congestive heart failure; PMH, past medical history; JVD, jugular venous distention; BUN, blood urea nitrogen; FENa, fractional excretion of sodium.

Figure 17–1.

3. Psychogenic polydipsia

4. Glucocorticoid deficiency

C. Hypovolemia

    1. Salt and water loss with free water replacement

      a. Severe diarrhea with free water ingestion

      b. Prolonged exertion with free water ingestion

      c. Large burns with free water replacement

      d. Third-spacing with free water replacement

2. Mineralcorticoid deficiency

3. Renal disease

    a. Diuretics

    b. Salt-wasting nephropathy

Before proceeding, it is useful to briefly review the pathophysiology of hyponatremia. Hyponatremia develops when patients do not excrete their daily ingested excess (or free) water. Free water excretion requires 3 distinct mechanisms (Figure 17–3):

Differential Diagnosis of True Hyponatremia by Volume Status

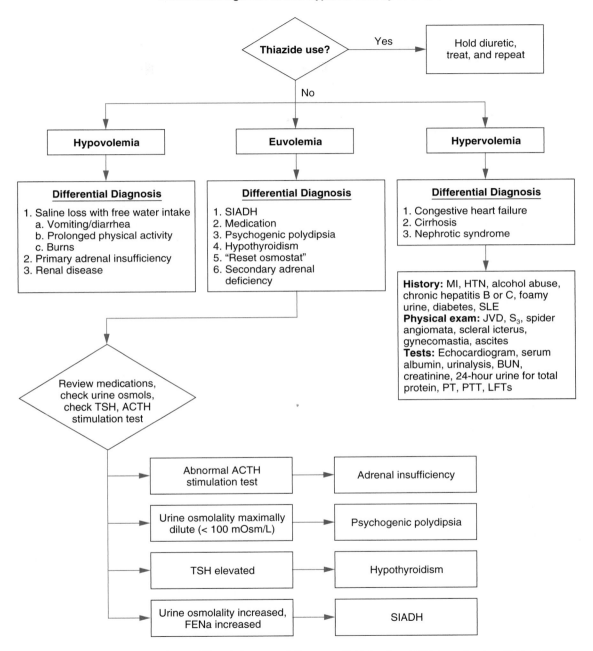

SIADH, syndrome of inappropriate antidiuretic hormone; MI, myocardial infarction; HTN, hypertension; SLE, systemic lupus erythematosus; JVD, jugular venous distention; BUN, blood urea nitrogen; PT, prothrombin time; PTT, partial thromboplastin time; LFTs, liver function tests; ACTH, corticotropin; FENa, fractional excretion of sodium.

Figure 17–2.

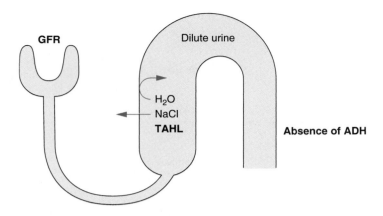

Figure 17–3. Pathophysiology of free water excretion. Free water diuresis requires (1) GFR, (2) functioning TAHL, and (3) absence of ADH. (GFR, glomerular filtration rate; TAHL, thick ascending loop of Henle; ADH, antidiuretic hormone.)

1. Glomerular filtration

2. Separation of water from solute so that free water can be excreted. This occurs in the thick ascending loop of Henle. This section of the tubule is impermeable to water. Therefore, sodium pumped out of the lumen leaves free water within the tubule.

3. Excretion of free water. Finally, water must travel through the tubules without being reabsorbed into the kidney. This requires absent or low levels of ADH. (ADH *increases* the permeability of the distal tubule to water, allowing water to move from the lumen of the tubule back into the renal interstitium.)

In short, free water excretion requires glomerular filtration, a functioning thick ascending loop of Henle, and low levels of ADH. Interference with these 3 mechanisms contributes to hyponatremia.

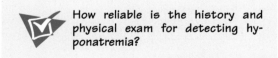

How reliable is the history and physical exam for detecting hyponatremia?

The adverse effects and manifestations of hyponatremia depend on its severity and rapidity of development. Acute hyponatremia leaves the brain hypertonic relative to the serum. This osmotic gradient drives water into the brain, resulting in cerebral edema and CNS symptoms.

Typically, patients with serum sodium levels > 130 mEq/L are asymptomatic; those with levels from 125 mEq/L to 130 mEq/L may have nausea, vomiting, or abdominal symptoms. Agitation and confusion may develop in patients with levels < 125 mEq/L. Levels below 115 mEq/L have been associated with seizures and coma. More severe degrees of hyponatremia may cause brain damage, brainstem herniation, and death.

Because the classification scheme of hyponatremia relies on the correct determination of the patient's volume status, it is important to ask, "How reliable is the physical exam for classifying the patient's volume status?"

A. In patients with hyponatremia, *hypervolemic* states are easily distinguished from euvolemic or hypovolemic states. In such patients, the hyponatremia develops only in advanced disease (ie, CHF, cirrhosis, or nephrotic syndrome). By this time, there is often a known history of CHF, cirrhosis, or nephrosis. Furthermore, physical findings of volume overload (eg, edema, jugular venous distention [JVD], S_3, and ascites) are usually present.

B. Separating euvolemic patients from hypovolemic patients is more difficult. Hypovolemic patients may have a history of volume loss (ie, diarrhea, intense prolonged sweating) or physical findings of hypotension, tachycardia, or orthostatic hypotension. However, the history and physical findings are less accurate:

1. Sensitivity, 25–47%; specificity 48–77%

2. Positive and negative LRs, approximately 1

C. Given the limitations of the history and physical exam, certain laboratory tests are critical to distinguish euvolemic patients from hypovolemic patients. The 3 most accurate biochemical parameters are spot urine sodium, fractional excretion of sodium (FENa), and fractional excretion of urea (FE$_{urea}$). All parameters were studied in patients who were either euvolemic or hypovolemia. Hypervolemic patients (with ascites or edema) were excluded because hyponatremia in these patients is usually due to *ineffective circulating volume.* Such patients usually avidly reabsorb sodium. Obtaining urine sodium measurements in clinically hypervolemic patients may mislead clinicians into thinking these patients are hypovolemic.

1. Spot urine sodium
   a. Hypovolemic patients should avidly reabsorb sodium resulting in decreased urine sodium.
   b. Sensitivity of low urine sodium for hypovolemia is 62–80% and specificity is 72–100%. LR+, 2.2–∞; LR–, 0.2–0.5
   c. Urine sodium may be spuriously low in some euvolemic patients.
      (1) Patients with psychogenic polydipsia (see below) are euvolemic but may have low urine sodium *concentration* due to dilution of the excreted sodium in vast quantities of water.
      (2) Some patients with SIADH *ingest* little sodium causing decreased urinary sodium output.
   d. Urine sodium is spuriously high in some volume-depleted patients. Patients with vomiting and metabolic alkalosis may have some obligatory sodium loss with bicarbonate. Urine chloride is low in such cases.

2. FENa = $(U_{Na^+} \times P_{Cr})/(P_{Na^+} \times U_{Cr})$
   a. Compares fraction of sodium excreted to fraction of sodium filtered. In hypovolemic states, fraction excreted should be low (< 0.5–1%)
   b. Sensitivity is improved (compared with spot urine sodium determination) but specificity still imperfect due to low FENa in some patients with psychogenic polydipsia and SIADH.
   c. 100% sensitive, 77% specific; LR+ 4.3, LR– 0
3. (FE_{urea}) = $(U_{urea} \times P_{Cr})/(P_{urea} \times U_{Cr})$
   a. Compares fraction of urea excreted to urea filtered. In euvolemic states, urea is rapidly excreted (FE_{urea} > 55%)
   b. One study suggests a combination of low fractional excretion of both sodium (< 1%) and urea (< 55%) was 100% sensitive and specific for hypovolemia.

 Urine sodium and FENa help properly classify patients as euvolemic or hypovolemic.

 Due to his confusion, Mr. D is unable to relate his past medical history. His chart is requested. Physical exam reveals a disheveled man appearing older that his stated age. He is unshaven and smells of alcohol. His vital signs are BP, 90/50 mm Hg; pulse, 90 bpm; temperature, 36.0 °C; RR, 18 breaths per minute. He has no orthostatic change in BP. Neck veins are flat. His lungs are clear to auscultation. Cardiac exam reveals a regular rate and rhythm. There is no JVD, S_3 gallop, or murmur. His abdomen is distended, and his flanks are bulging. Extremity exam reveals 3+ pitting edema extending all the way up his thighs.

Lab studies reveal a glucose of 100 mg/dL, a BUN of 28 mg/dL, and a serum osmolality of 252 mOsm/L.

 At this point, what is the leading hypothesis, and what are the active alternatives? What other tests should be ordered?

ORGANIZING THE DIFFERENTIAL DIAGNOSIS

The first step is to determine whether Mr. D is hypervolemic, euvolemic, or hypovolemic. Mr. D's marked peripheral edema clearly indicates that he is *hypervolemic.* The 3 causes of hypervolemic hyponatremia include CHF, nephrotic syndrome, and cirrhosis. Of these, cirrhosis seems most likely. The smell of alcohol raises the suspicion of alcohol abuse and liver disease and the bulging flanks suggest ascites, which in turn suggests cirrhosis. CHF is possible although Mr. D has neither an S_3 gallop nor JVD. Despite their absence, CHF should still be considered since neither finding is terribly sensitive for CHF. Finally, we do not have any information yet about renal function or proteinuria. Table 17–1 lists the differential diagnosis.

 Review of Mr. D's past medical record reveals that he has a long history of alcohol-related complications. Six months ago he was hospitalized for bleeding esophageal varices.

Table 17–1. Diagnostic hypotheses for Mr. D.

Diagnostic Hypothesis	Clinical Clues	Important Tests
Leading Hypothesis		
Cirrhosis	*History:* Heavy alcohol use, hepatitis C or chronic hepatitis B, esophageal varices *Physical exam:* Scleral icterus, spider angiomata, gynecomastia, ascites (bulging flanks, shifting dullness)	Serum albumin ALT, AST Bilirubin, PT, PTT Hepatitis B surface antigen Hepatitis C antibody Liver ultrasound and Doppler
Active Alternatives—Most Common		
Nephrotic syndrome	*History:* Foamy urine, diabetes, SLE	Serum albumin Urinalysis 24-hour urine total protein BUN, creatinine
Active Alternatives—Must Not Miss		
Congestive heart failure	History of MI, poorly controlled hypertension S_3 gallop, JVD, crackles on lung exam Peripheral edema	Echocardiogram ECG

Is the clinical information sufficient to make a diagnosis of cirrhosis? If not, what other information do you need?

Leading Hypothesis: Cirrhosis

Textbook Presentation

See Chapter 12, Edema for a full discussion. Patients with cirrhosis may have ascites, variceal hemorrhage, encephalopathy, jaundice, hypoalbuminemia, coagulopathy, and elevated transaminases).

Disease Highlights

A. No clinical finding is terribly sensitive for cirrhosis.

   1. Jaundice, 14%

   2. Variceal bleeding, 50%

   3. Ascites, 30%

   4. Encephalopathy, 50–70%

   5. Splenomegaly, 36–92%

B. Pathogenesis of hyponatremia in cirrhosis

   1. Hypoalbuminemia and splanchnic dilatation (possibly secondary to elevated nitric oxide)

causes decreased effective circulating volume and decreased systemic vascular resistance respectively, which leads to decreased mean arterial pressure, resulting in

   a. Elevated ADH (particularly important)

   b. Decreased GFR

   c. Increased proximal reabsorption of solute causing decreased solute delivery to loop of Henle

   2. NSAIDs may worsen edema by reducing GFR and worsen hyponatremia. NSAIDs also lower renal PGE_2, which normally antagonizes ADH.

   3. Renal arteriolar vasoconstriction further decreases GFR and increases proximal sodium reabsorption.

C. Prevalence of hyponatremia in patients with cirrhosis and ascites is $\cong$ 30%.

D. Hyponatremia is associated with more severe cirrhosis and worse outcome, especially if there is no clear precipitant (Table 17–2).

E. Hyponatremia may worsen hepatic encephalopathy.

Evidence-Based Diagnosis

A. Physical exam findings in cirrhotic patients *with* hyponatremia

   1. Ascites present in 89%

   2. Peripheral edema seen in 59%

Table 17–2. Comparison of findings in patients who have cirrhosis with and without hyponatremia.

Finding	Patients without Hyponatremia	Patients with Hyponatremia
Small liver size	5%	85%
BP	112/59 mm Hg	99/54 mm Hg
Hepatorenal syndrome	5%	85%
Death	25%	93%

B. Lab studies: Mean urine sodium 4.8 mEq/L (measurements made off diuretics for 5 days). (Decreased effective circulating volume causes increased renal reabsorption of sodium.)

MAKING A DIAGNOSIS

Lab studies reveal an albumin of 2.1 g/dL, bilirubin 6.2 mg/dL, AST (SGOT) 85 units/L, ALT (SGPT) 45 units/L, INR of 1.8. An abdominal ultrasound reveals moderate ascites and a small liver with coarse architecture suggestive of cirrhosis.

 Have you crossed a diagnostic threshold for the leading hypothesis, cirrhosis? Have you ruled out the active alternatives? Do other tests need to be done to exclude the alternative diagnoses?

Mr. D's findings point fairly conclusively to hypervolemic hyponatremia secondary to cirrhosis. The prior history of varices and ascites point to portal hypertension while the jaundice, hypoalbuminemia, and increased INR suggest synthetic failure by the liver. CHF secondary to an alcoholic cardiomyopathy is still possible. Other causes of hypervolemia hyponatremia, such as nephrotic syndrome, are less likely but possible.

Alternative Diagnosis: CHF & Hyponatremia

Textbook Presentation

Typically, patients with CHF complain of shortness of breath, dyspnea on exertion, fatigue, and orthopnea. (See Chapter 11, Dyspnea for a complete discussion of CHF.)

Disease Highlights

A. Patients with CHF and hyponatremia have marked *increases* in total body sodium content.

B. Fall in cardiac output is sensed at carotid baroreceptors and leads to increased ADH. GFR is decreased. Elevated ADH and reduced GFR both interfere with free water clearance. In patients with hyponatremia, water retention *exceeds* sodium retention.

C. Hyponatremia is observed in patients with severe CHF and portends a worse prognosis.

D. Diuretic therapy (particularly thiazides) can worsen the hyponatremia.

Evidence-Based Diagnosis

See CHF discussion in Chapter 11, Dyspnea.

Treatment

A. Treatment of underlying CHF

1. Similar to other patients with CHF (See Chapter 11, Dyspnea).

2. ACE inhibitors: Hyponatremia suggests activation of renin angiotensin system; such patients who are taking ACE inhibitors are susceptible to hypotension. Therefore, therapy with ACE inhibitors should be initiated at *low* doses. ACE inhibitors can help restore sodium levels to normal.

3. Avoid NSAID use, which can decrease prostaglandin-dependent renal blood flow and worsen renal function.

B. Treatment of hyponatremia

1. Exclude overdiuresis with free water replacement

2. Restrict water intake < 1000 mL/d

3. Discontinue thiazide diuretics

4. Furosemide in symptomatic, volume-overloaded patients

5. Short-term, preliminary studies suggest tolvaptan, an ADH V2 receptor antagonist, can help correct hyponatremia in patients with CHF (40% of patients treated with tolvaptan became normonatremic, compared with 1% of patients who received placebo).

Alternative Diagnosis: Nephrotic Syndrome

Textbook Presentation
See Chapter 12, Edema for full discussion. Patient's typically complain of edema.

Disease Highlights

A. Lesions may be primary and idiopathic (ie, minimal change lesion) or secondary to systemic disease (eg, diabetes mellitus, malignancy).

B. Glomerular lesion leads to albuminuria and hypoalbuminemia. Patients with nephrotic syndrome are total body sodium *overloaded*. The effective *intravascular* volume may be decreased or increased.

   1. In some patients, hypoalbuminemia and decreased oncotic pressures lead to edema and ineffective circulating volume.

   2. In other patients, primary sodium retention and hypervolemia precipitate edema.

C. In patients with decreased effective circulating volume, decreased renal perfusion and elevated ADH can produce hyponatremia.

D. Pseudohyponatremia may be seen secondary to marked hypertriglyceridemia.

Evidence-Based Diagnosis

A. Nephrotic syndrome is characterized by urine protein excretion ≥ 3.5 g protein/d, edema, hypoalbuminemia, and hyperlipidemia.

B. Renal biopsy can help identify certain underlying disease states.

Treatment
Free water restriction.

CASE RESOLUTION

An echocardiogram reveals normal left ventricular function and a urinalysis reveals only 1+ proteinuria not suggestive of nephrotic range proteinuria. A paracentesis is performed to rule out spontaneous bacterial peritonitis and is normal.

Mr. D's history, physical exam, and laboratory findings clearly point to severe cirrhosis. CHF and nephrotic syndrome are effectively ruled out by the echocardiogram and urinalysis. An important aspect of his care is to ensure a safe and gradual return of his serum sodium to normal.

Treatment of Hyponatremia Associated with Hypervolemia

 Correction of hyponatremia must be done carefully. Rapid correction may result in permanent brain damage.

A. In longstanding hyponatremia, physiologic adaptations protect the brain from cerebral edema by lowering intraneuronal osmolality.

B. Rapid *correction* of hyponatremia leaves the brain hypotonic relative to plasma.

C. Subsequent efflux of water from the cells can lead to intramyelinic edema and injury, resulting in demyelinization and central pontine myelinolysis.

   1. Typically, patients have severe chronic hyponatremia that is rapidly corrected; 2–6 days later spastic quadriparesis and pseudobulbar palsy develop. Death may occur.

   2. May occur when hyponatremia is corrected too rapidly (> 0.5 mEq/L/h).

   3. Pons is most commonly affected but other areas of white matter may be affected.

   4. Several therapeutic approaches to central pontine myelinolysis have been used.

      a. Discontinuation of hypertonic saline (if used to treat hyponatremia)

      b. DDAVP

      c. Hypotonic fluid administration (ie, D5W)

D. Therefore, patients with *asymptomatic* hyponatremia should be corrected more gradually than patients with symptomatic hyponatremia and severe neurologic symptoms (eg, coma, seizures).

E. Asymptomatic or mildly symptomatic patients

   1. Free water restriction is the therapy of choice.

2. The goal of therapy is to correct the serum sodium by ≤ 0.5 mEq/L/h. Some authorities suggest a maximum correction of 10 mEq/L/d.

F. Patients with **severe** neurologic symptoms from hyponatremia (seizures, coma)

1. Renal consultation is advised.

2. ICU monitoring is usually appropriate.

3. Hypertonic saline (3%) can be given to such patients.

4. For patients with severe symptoms, the goal is an initial correction rate of 1–2 mEq/L/h for 3–4 hours or until symptoms (ie, seizures or coma) abate.

5. A maximum of 8–12 mEq/L/d (0.33 mEq/L/h) correction is still recommended.

6. Formulas can help estimate the initial rate of infusion. However, actual responses may vary, and patients must have frequent sodium measurements to ensure an appropriate rate of correction.

7. The impact of 1 L of fluid can be calculated as follows:

    a. {(Infusate Na − Plasma [Na⁺])/(TBW + 1)}

      (1) Total body water (TBW) = 0.6 × weight (kg) men

      (2) TBW = 0.5 × weight (kg) women

      (3) Infusate Na = 154 mEq/L for normal saline

      (4) Infusate Na = 513 mEq/L for 3% normal saline

    b. Assume an asymptomatic 70 kg male. Initial [Na] = 110 mEq/L

      (1) TBW = 0.6 × 70 (kg) = 42 L

      (2) Using *normal saline* [Na⁺] = 154 mEq/L

        (a) Increase in [Na⁺] = {(154 − 110)/(42 + 1)} = 1 mEq per liter infused

        (b) If the desired correction rate is 0.33 mEq/L/h, then the 1 L would be administered over 3 hours.

      (3) If the patient was seizing, more rapid correction would be advised using *3% normal saline* [Na⁺] = 513 mEq/L

        (a) Increase in [Na⁺] = {(513 − 110)/(42 + 1)} = 9.3 mEq/L infused

        (b) If the desired rate of correction for the first 3 hours was 2 mEq/L/h, then 2/9.3 × 1000 (= 215 mL/h) would be administered per hour for the first 3 hours

    c. Electrolytes should be monitored every 2 hours.

    d. Furosemide is often administered to prevent intravascular volume overload. Furosemide may also increase free water loss.

    e. Hypertonic saline should be stopped if *any* of the following criteria are met:

      (1) Life-threatening symptoms abate (regardless of the persistence of hyponatremia)

      (2) Serum sodium > 120 mEq/L

      (3) Total magnitude of correction > 25 mEq/L

      (4) Additionally, the rate of change should be < 12 mEq/L/d

Treatment of Hyponatremia in Cirrhosis

A. Fluid restriction (free water restriction)

B. Opioid kappa-agonists (ie, naloxone, niravoline) block the release of ADH from the hypothalamus.

C. Demeclocycline can antagonize the effects of ADH. Nephrotoxicity, exacerbated by hepatic dysfunction, limits its use.

D. ADH receptor antagonists VPA-985 combined with free water restriction is promising, but only short-term studies have been published to date.

The patient has mild, not severe, symptoms from hyponatremia. Rapid correction of hyponatremia must be avoided. Hypertonic saline is not indicated.

Mr. D is begun on free water restriction and his sodium gradually improves to 128 mEq/L. His mental status returns to normal.

CHIEF COMPLAINT

PATIENT 2

Mrs. L is a 60-year-old woman who comes to see you for a follow-up of her hypertension. She reports no specific complaints except perhaps some mild fatigue. On physical exam, her BP is well controlled at 126/84 mm Hg. Routine chemistries reveal a serum sodium of 128 mEq/L. Her other electrolytes and creatinine are normal. Her glucose is 108 mg/dL and BUN 28 mg/dL.

At this point, what is the leading hypothesis, and what are the active alternatives? What other tests should be ordered?

ORGANIZING THE DIFFERENTIAL DIAGNOSIS

The first step is to classify Mrs. L's clinical status as hypervolemic, euvolemic, or hypovolemic. A careful exam should search for signs of hypervolemia (edema, JVD, ascites, S_3 gallop, or crackles) and for signs of hypovolemia (hypotension, tachycardia, and orthostatic hypotension). If Mrs. L is not hypervolemic, urine sodium and FENa can further help distinguish euvolemia from hypovolemia.

Mrs. L denies any history that suggests volume loss (vomiting, diarrhea, or excessive perspiration). Furthermore, she has no history of any diseases associated with hypervolemic states (CHF, cirrhosis, renal failure, or nephrotic syndrome). She denies any dyspnea on exertion or orthopnea. On physical exam, BP is normal with no significant change going from lying to standing. There is no pretibial or pedal edema. Cardiovascular exam reveals no JVD, S_3 gallop, or crackles. There are no signs of ascites (bulging flanks, shifting dullness).
   Mrs. L's urine studies reveal a urine sodium concentration of 60 mEq/L and a FENa of 5%.

Mrs. L's history and exam do not suggest hypervolemia. Her exam does not suggest hypovolemia. Furthermore, neither her urine sodium nor her FENa are low (as would be expected if she were hypovolemic). Therefore,

Mrs. L has euvolemic hyponatremia. The differential diagnosis of euvolemic hyponatremia includes SIADH, adverse effect of medication, glucocorticoid insufficiency, hypothyroidism, and psychogenic polydipsia. At this point the leading hypothesis is uncertain. Table 17–3 lists the differential diagnosis. Further history may help prioritize the differential diagnosis.

Mrs. L has no history of psychiatric illness and denies excessive water ingestion. Past medical history: Hypertension treated with amlodipine. Social history: 40-pack-year history of smoking. Alcohol use is minimal. Review of systems: Cough has been present over the last 1–2 months. Otherwise normal.

Mrs. L's history is not particularly diagnostic. She is not on a thiazide diuretic, one of the most common medications causing hyponatremia. She denies a history of unusual water ingestion. Her recent cough and tobacco history raises the possibility of SIADH from a lung cancer. Adrenal insufficiency may become life-threatening and should be considered a "must not miss" diagnosis.

Is the clinical information sufficient to make a diagnosis? If not, what other information do you need?

Leading Hypothesis: SIADH

Textbook Presentation

Patients are often (although not always) elderly, with a chief complaint of confusion or weakness. Alternatively, mild hyponatremia may be discovered incidentally on serum chemistries.

Disease Highlights

A. Secondary to inappropriate ADH release despite euvolemia and hypotonicity.

B. Patients are clinically euvolemic. Clinically inapparent volume expansion due to water retention leads to urinary sodium loss.

C. Etiologies

   1. Cancer, 15%

      a. Ectopic production by small cell carcinoma of the lung is the most common malignancy.

Table 17–3. Diagnostic hypotheses for Mrs. L.

Diagnostic Hypotheses	Clinical Clues	Important Tests
Leading Hypothesis		
SIADH	History of cancer (or cancer risks) Unusual cough Hemoptysis or lymphadenopathy Neurologic or pulmonary disease HIV	Urine sodium > 40 mEq/L FENa > 1% Urine osmolality > 300 mOsm/L Exclusion of hypothyroidism and adrenal insufficiency
Active Alternative—Most Common		
Medication	Medication history	Response to discontinuation of drug
Hypothyroidism	Fatigue Cold intolerance	TSH
Psychogenic polydipsia	Psychiatric history Water ingestion	Urine osmolality < 100 mOsm/L Response to water restriction
Active Alternative—Must Not Miss		
Adrenal insufficiency	Withdrawal of long-term corticosteroid therapy Pituitary disease HIV Sarcoidosis	Corticotropin stimulation test

b. Pancreatic cancer, lymphoma, endometrial cancer, leukemia, and other tumors may cause SIADH.

2. Neurologic disease (eg, meningitis, tumors, trauma, cerebrovascular accidents)

3. Intrathoracic disease (eg, pneumonia, tuberculosis, HIV)

4. Drugs

a. Thiazides

b. ADH analogues (vasopressin, DDAVP, oxytocin): hyponatremia develops in 5% of women who are given oxytocin to induce labor

c. Chlorpropamide: 6–7% of treated patients

d. Carbamazepine

(1) Rates of 20–30% have been recorded

(2) Advanced age increases risk

(3) Elevated serum levels increase risk

e. Antidepressants (tricyclics and selective serotonin reuptake inhibitors) and antipsychotics

(1) Hyponatremia may be multifactorial including:

(a) SIADH

(b) Psychogenic polydipsia

(c) Psychosis-induced elevated ADH

(d) Increased water ingestion due to dry mouth from anticholinergic effects

(2) Incidence 0.8% with fluoxetine

f. NSAIDs

g. Ecstasy

h. Others (cyclophosphamide, vincristine, nicotine, opiates, clofibrate)

5. AIDS

a. SIADH may be secondary to *Pneumocystis* pneumonia, CNS infections, or cancer.

b. Hyponatremia may also be due to adrenal insufficiency or diarrhea (with free water ingestion).

6. Hypothyroidism

a. Hyponatremia may occur in 10% of patients with hypothyroidism but is rarely symptomatic.

b. In part secondary to ADH release.

c. Elevated ADH levels may be secondary to decreased cardiac output.

7. Idiopathic

D. Reset osmostat

1. A variant of SIADH in which ADH control is modulated to maintain serum sodium levels at a lower range than normal. Patients retain ability to excrete water load at new equilibrium point.

2. Therefore, hyponatremia is not progressive.

3. Patients typically have serum sodium levels between 125 mEq/L and 135 mEq/L.

4. Very dilute urine osmolality may be seen following water load (< 100 mOsm/L).

5. Etiology is similar to SIADH.

6. Treatment is directed at the underlying disorder.

Evidence-Based Diagnosis

A. Standard criteria:

1. Plasma osmolality < 270 mOsm/L

2. Urine sodium is typically > 40 mEq/L.

3. FENa is usually > 1%.

4. Urine osmolality not maximally dilute due to active ADH (urine osmolality > 100 mOsm/L, usually > 300 mOsm/L)

5. Other causes of euvolemic hyponatremia excluded (hypothyroidism, psychogenic polydipsia, adrenal insufficiency)

B. 13–20% of patients have low urine sodium and low FENa due to low sodium intake.

C. All patients had elevated FE_{urea} (> 55%).

MAKING A DIAGNOSIS

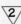

The urine osmolality is 500 mOsm/L. The serum osmolality is 266 mOsm/L. Her TSH is normal at 2.3 mU/L.

Have you crossed a diagnostic threshold for the leading hypothesis, SIADH? Have you ruled out the other active alternatives that cause euvolemic hyponatremia? Do other tests need to be done to exclude the alternative diagnoses?

Mrs. L's elevated FENa (5%) and urine osmolality are consistent with SIADH. It is important to consider the alternative diagnosis before concluding that she in fact has SIADH. If SIADH is confirmed, a search for the underlying cause is appropriate.

Alternative Diagnosis: Diuretic Hyponatremia

Textbook Presentation

The most common clinical situation is a small elderly woman who started taking a thiazide diuretic for hypertension. Several days later, she returns to your office with confusion or seizures, or both due to hyponatremia.

Disease Highlights

A. Most commonly seen with thiazide diuretics; rarely seen with loop diuretics

B. Hyponatremia can be multifactorial; pathogenesis may vary in different patients

1. Most patients are hypovolemic

a. Thiazide diuretics interfere with NaCl transport in cortical diluting segments. This limits NaCl transport out of the tubule, reducing formation of free water within the tubule, which leads to decreased free water excretion.

b. Decreased GFR causes increased proximal sodium reabsorbtion leading to reduced distal sodium delivery and free water clearance.

c. Volume depletion may elevate ADH levels.

d. Sodium losses are occasionally marked.

2. Some patients are hypervolemic or euvolemic.

a. Thiazides can increase ADH without volume depletion (ie, SIADH).

b. Increased water intake with impaired free water excretion

C. Usually occurs within 14 days of initiating thiazide therapy but can occur at any time.

D. Hyponatremia often develops rapidly (< 2 days).

E. NSAID use may increase the risk of thiazide-induced hyponatremia.

F. Hyponatremia may persist for 1 month after discontinuation of thiazide.

Evidence-Based Diagnosis

A. Despite volume depletion, urine sodium concentration and FENa may be elevated if diuretic action is still present.

B. FE_{urea} is usually low due to true volume depletion.

C. Patients treated with a diuretic who have high FENa and high FE_{urea} are not likely to be volume depleted. In these patients, an SIADH like syndrome is most likely. Treat accordingly.

Treatment

A. Stopping the diuretic is usually adequate.

B. Hypovolemic patients

1. Consider careful volume resuscitation with normal saline.

2. Correct sodium concentration at rate < 0.5 mEq/L/h (see formulas above to calculate correct rate).

3. Unlike hypervolemic patients, the correction of the fluid deficit in a hypovolemic patient may lead to a drop in ADH levels. This may result in rapid water losses and rapid and dangerous correction of serum sodium concentration. Serum sodium levels should be followed closely and electrolyte replacement may need to be terminated if serum sodium levels or urinary output rise abruptly.

4. Hypertonic saline can be used if severe neurologic symptoms are present (see calculations above; common estimate is 2 mL/kg/h of 3% normal saline for 3–4 hours.)

C. Patients euvolemic and SIADH likely: restrict free water.

D. Some authorities recommend checking serum sodium in elderly women 1–3 days after initiating thiazide diuretic, particularly if they take NSAIDs.

Alternative Diagnosis: Psychogenic Polydipsia

Textbook Presentation

Psychogenic polydipsia typically occurs in patients with psychiatric history and unexplained hyponatremia. Patients do not usually admit to excessive water intake. SIADH may also be seen in psychiatric patients.

Disease Highlights

A. Requires massive water ingestion > 8–10 L/d

B. Urine osmolality maximally dilute ($\cong$ 100 mOsm/L)

C. Reported in 5% of chronically ill hospitalized psychiatric patients

D. Since volume status is normal, renal excretion of sodium is usually normal and FENa is usually > 1%. However, spot urine sodium *concentration* is low due to dilution by massive water intake.

E. Complications include those of hyponatremia and incontinence, hydronephrosis (from massive urinary output), hypocalcemia, and CHF.

Evidence-Based Diagnosis

A. Water restriction test can prove the diagnosis by demonstrating rapid resolution of hyponatremia.

B. Mean urine sodium concentration is 18 mEq/L.

C. FENa > 0.5% in 66%

D. FE_{urea} > 55% in 100%

E. Mean urine osmolality 144 ± 23 mOsm/L

Treatment

A. Careful free water restriction allows gradual restoration of serum sodium concentration.

B. For severe neurologic symptoms (eg, seizures, coma), hypertonic saline can be used.

Alternative Diagnosis: Adrenal Insufficiency

Textbook Presentation

Classically, fatigue, weight loss, nausea, vomiting, and abdominal pain are the presenting symptoms. Primary or secondary adrenal insufficiency may cause hyponatremia. Hypotension, orthostasis, and fever may be seen.

Disease Highlights

A. Etiology

1. Adrenal insufficiency may occur secondary to damage to the adrenal gland (primary adrenal insufficiency) or secondary to hypothalamic-pituitary insufficiency, which decreases corticotropin (ACTH).

2. Both primary and secondary adrenal insufficiency cause hypocortisolism. Cortisol normally suppresses ADH release. Decreased cortisol causes increased ADH levels and hyponatremia.

3. Primary adrenal insufficiency is also associated with hypoaldosteronism.

a. Results in cortisol, aldosterone, and DHEA deficiency

b. Aldosterone deficiency results in salt losses and clinical hypovolemia.

c. Catecholamine synthesis is also usually impaired (except in autoimmune adrenal disease).

d. DHEA deficiency may decrease libido in women and impact quality of life.

e. Etiologies of primary adrenal insufficiency

(1) Autoimmune adrenalitis (80–90% of cases in developed nations)

(2) HIV infection: 33% of HIV patients admitted to ICUs have adrenal insufficiency.

(3) Tuberculosis

(4) Less common etiologies: Fungal infection, cytomegalovirus, bilateral adrenal hemorrhage (seen in septic shock), infiltration or inherited disorders, ketoconazole

4. Secondary adrenal insufficiency (hypothalamic-pituitary insufficiency)

  a. Results in isolated cortisol deficiency (aldosterone is primarily under control by the renin-angiotensin system and is still secreted) and causes elevated ADH levels and hyponatremia.

  b. Patients are often euvolemic.

  c. Etiologies

   (1) Iatrogenic due to corticosteroid therapy

     (a) Up to 50% of patients taking long-term corticosteroid therapy have adrenal insufficiency.

     (b) Recovery of hypothalamic-pituitary-adrenal axis may take 9–12 months.

   (2) Sepsis

   (3) Pituitary tumors (30% of patients with pituitary macroadenoma)

   (4) Less common etiologies: Pituitary infarction, irradiation and autoimmune hypophysitis, HIV, sarcoidosis, hemochromatosis

  d. Hyponatremia may be precipitated by intercurrent illness, leading to inadequate cortisol response; 43% of patients with secondary adrenal insufficiency had superimposed infection when presenting with hyponatremia.

 Suspect hypopituitarism as the cause of hyponatremia in any patient with a history of pituitary disease (eg, macroadenoma, infarction, empty sella syndrome).

B. Adrenal crisis

  1. 3% of patients per year

  2. Often secondary to insufficient increases in glucocorticoid during times of stress

Evidence-Based Diagnosis

A. History and physical

  1. Acute adrenal insufficiency presents similar to septic shock with hypotension, abdominal pain, vomiting, and fever.

  2. Chronic adrenal insufficiency

    a. May present with a variety of nonspecific symptoms (eg, fatigue, weakness, weight loss).

    b. Orthostatic hypotension may be seen.

    c. Skin darkening (palmer creases, scars, knuckles) can be seen in primary adrenal insufficiency due to increased ACTH levels.

  3. Findings in secondary adrenal insufficiency

    a. Decreased libido, 100% of men

    b. Reduced pubic/axillary hair, 86%

    c. Nausea and vomiting, 75%

    d. Weight loss, 32%

    e. Abdominal pain, 29%

    f. Diarrhea, 18%

B. Laboratory tests

  1. ACTH measurements (8 AM) differentiate primary from secondary adrenal insufficiency

    a. ACTH is elevated in primary adrenal insufficiency.

    b. ACTH is low in adrenal insufficiency secondary to hypothalamic-pituitary dysfunction.

  2. Primary adrenal insufficiency

    a. Cosyntropin stimulation test is the test of choice.

     (1) 250 mcg given IM or IV

     (2) Serum cortisol measured 30–60 minutes later

     (3) Level > 415 nmol/L rules out adrenal insufficiency

     (4) Sensitivity, 97.5%; specificity, 95%; LR+, 19.5; LR−, 0.026

     (5) Specificity in acute settings (ICU) such as septic shock is markedly reduced.

       (a) Severe stressors should elevate cortisol levels.

       (b) Corticotropin stimulation tests are unnecessary in these situations.

       (c) Baseline cortisol levels < 25 mcg/dL suggest adrenal insufficiency.

    b. Adrenal imaging with CT scanning is appropriate in patients with an abnormal cosyntropin stimulation test.

    c. HIV testing should be considered.

    d. Adrenal cortex autoantibodies or antibodies against 21-hydroxylase are present in > 80% of patients with autoimmune adrenalitis.

3. Secondary adrenal insufficiency

    a. Decreased cortisol causes lack of suppression of ADH leading to increased ADH resulting in urine sodium and osmol values similar to SIADH: Average urinary sodium, 110 mmol/L; average urine osmolality, 399 mOsm/L

    b. *Longstanding* (but not recent) pituitary insufficiency causes adrenal atrophy. When present, adrenal atrophy may reduce response to cosyntropin stimulation test.

        (1) 250 mcg given IM or IV

        (2) Serum cortisol measured 30–60 minutes later

        (3) Levels > 500–600 nmol/L argue against longstanding adrenal insufficiency.

        (4) Sensitivity, 57%; specificity, 95%; LR+, 11.5; LR−, 0.45

        (5) Normal cosyntropin stimulation test does not rule out secondary adrenal insufficiency if the pretest probability is moderate to high.

        (6) Sensitivity is likely to fall with recent onset of secondary adrenal insufficiency because of the lesser degrees of adrenal atrophy.

    c. Suspected recent onset pituitary insufficiency

        (1) Adrenal atrophy may not occur.

        (2) Cosyntropin stimulation tests may be normal.

        (3) Provocative tests that require an intact axis, such as the insulin tolerance test, can be used. Induced hypoglycemia provokes the hypothalamic pituitary axis to release cortisol. Cortisol levels > 500 nmol/L suggest an intact axis. Experience is required to avoid complications of hypoglycemia. Endocrine consultation is advised.

    d. Pituitary MRI is indicated in patients with adrenal insufficiency and low ACTH levels.

Treatment

A. Corticosteroid replacement

    1. In both primary and secondary insufficiency, therapy must replace normal corticosteroid output *and dosage must be automatically increased at times of stress to prevent life-threatening adrenal crisis.*

    2. Primary adrenal insufficiency

        a. Hydrocortisone

            (1) Daily dose: 15–25 mg/d; half to two-thirds in the morning; the rest taken 6–8 hours later

            (2) Prevention of adrenal crisis

                (a) Strenuous physical activity: Add 5–10 mg hydrocortisone

                (b) Pregnancy: Increase dose by 50% during third trimester with peripartum stress coverage. Endocrine consultation is advised.

                (c) Hyperthyroidism: Double or triple daily dose

                (d) Febrile illness: Double daily dose

                (e) Major surgery or trauma: 100–150 mg/d of IV hydrocortisone

            (3) Treatment of adrenal crisis

                (a) Hydrocortisone 100 mg IV and then 100–200 mg/d IV up to 100 mg every 8 hours

                (b) Normal saline (often up to 1 L/h)

 When adrenal crisis is suspected, blood tests should be drawn for cortisol and ACTH. Treatment should commence immediately and not await laboratory results.

        b. Mineralcorticoid

            (1) 0.05–0.2 mg/d of fludrocortisone

            (2) Monitor sodium and potassium levels as well as BP

        c. DHEA can be considered for women with impaired sense of well being despite glucocorticoid and mineralcorticoid replacement.

    3. Secondary adrenal insufficiency

        a. Hydrocortisone as for primary adrenal insufficiency

        b. For hyponatremia: Fluid restriction is appropriate. For severe symptoms (coma, seizures), hypertonic saline may be necessary.

CASE RESOLUTION

The serum cortisol level following 250 mcg of corticotropin is 800 nmol/L. Her glucose is 100 mg/dL.

Mrs. L's urine osmolality is not dilute, effectively ruling out psychogenic polydipsia. Her TSH and corticotropin stimulation tests are also normal, ruling out hypothyroidism and adrenal insufficiency. (Secondary adrenal insufficiency of recent onset is still theoretically possible, but nothing in the history suggests the patient is at risk for pituitary disease.) Therefore, Mrs. L has SIADH. The final step will be to determine the etiology of the SIADH. As noted above, SIADH can result from a variety of pulmonary, neurologic, or malignant causes. Following clinical clues is important. Her recent cough and long history of tobacco use suggests an underlying pulmonary etiology.

A chest film reveals a 5-cm pulmonary mass adjacent to the right hilum. Bronchoscopy and biopsy confirms small cell carcinoma of the lung. Mrs. L is referred to medical oncology. Her hyponatremia is controlled with free water restriction.

Treatment of SIADH

A. Determine etiology
   1. Review medications, consider CT scan of the chest and head
   2. Water restriction is the cornerstone of therapy.

B. Asymptomatic
   1. Fluid restriction < 1 L/d
   2. Discontinue any medication that may cause SIADH.
   3. Give demeclocycline if fluid restriction is inadequate to restore normal sodium levels.
      a. Blocks the intracellular effect of ADH by interfering with the generation and action of cyclic adenosine monophosphate (cAMP)
      b. Can cause photosensitivity and nephrotoxicity
   4. Urea 30 mg/d has also been used to enhance water excretion unresponsive to the above modalities.
   5. Antagonists of ADH have been used.

C. Symptomatic
   1. In patients with moderate symptoms, normal saline with furosemide (20 mg once or twice daily) to correct sodium at a rate < 0.5 mEq/L/h
   2. Normal saline without furosemide may worsen hyponatremia. Since sodium handling is intact (but water is not), the administered sodium may be excreted but the accompanied water is retained, causing decreased serum sodium.
   3. In patients with severe symptoms (eg, seizures or coma) 3% normal saline to correct sodium at a rate of 1–2 mEq/L/h can be used until serum sodium reaches 125 mEq/L or symptoms improve (see calculations above). Authorities recommend limiting sodium correction to 8–12 mEq/L/d.

Hypovolemic Hyponatremic Syndromes

Textbook Presentation

Hyponatremia typically develops in volume depletion when sodium losses from the GI tract or skin (vomiting, diarrhea, excessive perspiration) are replaced with free water. Patients may have orthostatic hypotension or dry mucous membranes.

Disease Highlights

A. Primary control of ADH release is serum osmolality. Hypo-osmolality normally inhibits ADH release leading to free water diuresis.

B. *Significant* hypovolemia can stimulate ADH release independent of serum osmolality.

C. Free water ingestion in face of elevated ADH levels causes hyponatremia.

D. Exercise-induced hyponatremia
   1. Typically follows prolonged workout (≥ 6 hours)
   2. Hyponatremia has been reported in 29% of Hawaiian Ironman triathletes.
   3. Symptomatic hyponatremia develops in 0.1–4% of participants in ultramarathon events (9–12 hours).
   4. Excessive perspiration in the absence of adequate salt repletion leads to hypovolemia.
   5. In hypovolemia, ADH is elevated, GFR is decreased, and proximal sodium reabsorption is increased, resulting in decreased free water excretion.
   6. Thirst and free water ingestion are increased in patients who are hypovolemic.
   7. Free water ingestions combined with decreased free water elimination causes hyponatremia.
   8. Some clinicians favor excessive free water intake as fundamental problem.
   9. Elevated sweat sodium content increases the risk of hypovolemia and hyponatremia.
   10. Cystic fibrosis has been discovered in several persons who were being evaluated for exercise-induced hyponatremia.

11. Rapid onset of hyponatremia renders plasma hypotonic relative to the brain leading to cerebral edema.

12. Hyponatremia and cerebral edema cause neurologic symptoms.

13. Compared with water, sodium-containing sports drinks have been shown to protect persons from hyponatremia.

E. Typical urine findings include

1. Decreased urine sodium concentration (< 30 mEq/L)

2. Decreased FENa (< 1%)

3. Increased urine osmolality (> 450 mOsm/L)

4. Prerenal azotemia (BUN/Cr > 20)

5. Elevated uric acid

Treatment

A. For mildly symptomatic patients, normal saline can be used (see calculations above).

B. For severely symptomatic patients, 3% normal saline can be used.

C. Correction of hyponatremia in hypovolemic patients may be more rapid than predicted by calculations due to the suppression of ADH by volume resuscitation.

D. Frequent monitoring of serum sodium is mandatory.

REVIEW OF OTHER IMPORTANT DISEASES

Pseudohyponatremia

Textbook Presentation

Since sodium is the major extracellular osmol, true hyponatremia is associated with hypo-osmolality. Cer-

tain rare conditions interfere with the accurate measurement of sodium and cause the sodium concentration to appear *spuriously* low. These conditions are referred to as **pseudohyponatremia.** Causes include *marked* hyperlipidemia and *marked* hyperproteinemia. In these cases, the true serum sodium concentrations and serum osmolality are normal. Marked hyperglycemia works somewhat differently. Marked hyperglycemia draws water into the intravascular space and also produces hyponatremia. In this situation, the hyperglycemia makes the serum hyperosmolar. This discussion will be limited to patients with hyponatremia secondary to marked hyperglycemia.

Disease Highlights

A. In poorly controlled diabetes, intravascular glucose acts as an osmotic agent drawing water from the cells into the plasma resulting in hyponatremia.

B. Serum osmolality is elevated.

C. Correction factors can help predict the serum sodium concentration after the hyperglycemia is treated (and the intravascular water relocates to the intracellular space). The optimal correction factor is controversial.

D. Experiments suggest that the sodium concentration will increase by 2.4 mEq/L for every 100 mg/dL that glucose falls with treatment. A sodium of 129 mEq/L in a patient with a serum glucose of 1000 mg/dL would correct as follows:

1. Serum glucose will fall 900 mg/dL with treatment (to about 100 mg/dL).

2. Correct sodium concentration by 2.4 per 100 mg/dL fall in glucose.

3. $9 \times 2.4 = 21.6$

4. Corrected sodium = 129 + 21.6 = 150.6

HYPERNATREMIA

CHIEF COMPLAINT

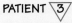

Mr. R is an 80-year-old nursing home resident with a history of severe dementia brought to the emergency department with lethargy and confusion. Serum chemistries reveal a sodium level of 168 mEq/L.

  What is the differential diagnosis of hypernatremia? How would you frame the differential?

CONSTRUCTING A DIFFERENTIAL DIAGNOSIS

Hypernatremia is almost always secondary to a free water deficit. Hypernatremia causes an osmotic water shift from the intracellular to extracellular space producing intracellular dehydration. The differential diagnosis of hypernatremia is markedly simpler than that of hyponatremia.

Hypernatremia and hyperosmolality are potent stimulators of thirst. Therefore, hypernatremia occurs almost exclusively in patients with a depressed sensorium who have *impaired water intake* because they are either unaware of their thirst or physically unable to get to water. The most common clinical scenarios involve infants or the elderly with severe dementia. In such patients, normal insensible water losses or increased water loss (ie, from diarrhea) are not matched by oral intake and hypernatremia develops. The urine osmolality in such patients is typically high (> 700 mOsm/L).

Hypernatremia may also develop in patients with marked hyperglycemia. The osmotic diuresis results in a free water loss and may result in hypernatremia if free water intake is impaired due to an altered sensorium. This may not be obvious when the patient presents because the hyperglycemia draws water from the intracellular compartment into the extracellular compartment diluting the sodium concentration. With treatment of the hyperglycemia, the hypernatremia can worsen as water moves back to the intracellular space.

Other causes of hypernatremia are rare and will be touched upon here only briefly. Hypernatremia may develop in patients who have an impairment in renal *water conservation* (ie, diabetes insipidus [DI]). Even in these patients, increased thirst normally prompts increased water intake and allows such patients to compensate and maintain normonatremia. (These patients complain of polydipsia and polyuria.) Hypernatremia may develop when a superimposed process limits water intake. The urine osmolality in such patients is inappropriately low (< 700 mOsm/L). DI can result from either pituitary processes, which cause decreased ADH, or renal processes, which cause resistance to ADH. Finally, very rare causes of hypernatremia include hypothalamic lesions, which render patients unaware of thirst despite a normal sensorium, or increased salt intake (ie, infusion of hypertonic saline or salt water ingestion).

Symptoms develop due to dehydration (tachycardia, orthostatic hypotension, dry mucous membranes and axilla) and due to the hypernatremia (depressed sensorium, coma, focal deficits and seizures). Symptoms are more severe with rapidly developing hypernatremia.

Differential Diagnosis of Hypernatremia

A. Impaired water intake: urine osmolality > 700 mOsm/L
  1. Neurologic disease (eg, dementia, delirium, coma, stroke)
  2. Water unavailable (ie, desert conditions)
B. Osmotic diuresis with impaired water intake
  1. Hyperosmolar hyperglycemia
  2. Postobstructive diuresis
C. Rare etiologies
  1. DI (if associated with decreased water intake)
    a. Neurogenic DI associated with decreased ADH production
    b. Nephrogenic DI (ADH resistance)
      (1) Chronic lithium ingestion
      (2) Hypercalcemia
  2. Hypothalamic lesions cause decreased thirst
  3. Increased salt intake
    a. Salt water ingestion
    b. Hypertonic saline

ORGANIZING THE DIFFERENTIAL DIAGNOSIS

In the face of severe neurologic dysfunction (ie, dementia), the most common cause of hypernatremia is inadequate water intake. Often, some other illness has supervened to further compromise the patient's state of alertness and oral intake. Marked hyperglycemia should always be considered a "must not miss" alternative. Inadequate water conservation due to DI is possible but far less common. Table 17–4 lists the differential diagnosis.

The nursing home reports that Mr. R has had a cough for the last 3 days with low-grade fever. Over the last 48 hours, he has become progressively less responsive and his oral intake and urinary output have dropped dramatically.

Mr. R is minimally responsive to stimuli. Vital signs are BP, 110/70 mm Hg; pulse, 110 bpm; temperature, 38.1 °C; RR, 20 breaths per minute. His oral mucosa is parched and his axilla dry. Lung exam is difficult to evaluate due to poor effort. Cardiac exam reveals tachycardia;

Table 17–4. Diagnostic hypotheses for Mr. R.

Diagnostic Hypotheses	Clinical Clues	Important Tests
Leading Hypothesis		
Inadequate water consumption	Altered sensorium History of neurologic or physical disability limiting access to or ingestion of water Concomitant illness	Urine osmolality > 700–800 mOsm/L
Active Alternative—Most Common		
Diabetes insipidus (DI)	Complaints of polydipsia, polyuria	Urine osmolality < 700 mOsm/L
Neurogenic DI	History of CNS trauma, surgery, CVA, sarcoidosis	ADH levels low Exogenous ADH leads to marked increase in urine osmolality
Nephrogenic DI	Lithium ingestion	ADH levels elevated Exogenous ADH leads to minimal increase in urine osmolality
Active Alternative—Must Not Miss		
Hyperglycemia	Diabetes mellitus Concurrent illness	Markedly elevated serum glucose

neck veins are flat. There is no S_3 or S_4. Chest x-ray reveals a right lower lobe infiltrate. Labs: Na, 168 mEq/L; K, 4.2 mEq/L; HCO_3^-, 24 mEq/L; chloride, 134 mEq/L; BUN, 45 mg/dL; creatinine, 1 mg/dL. Serum glucose is 150 mg/dL.

 Is the clinical information sufficient to make a diagnosis? If not, what other information do you need?

Leading Hypothesis: Hypernatremia Secondary to Inadequate Water Intake

Textbook Presentation

Patients with hypernatremia due to inadequate water ingestion usually have an altered neurologic status or physical disability. A superimposed illness may worsen cognitive function, worsening oral intake and promote hypernatremia. Mental status on evaluation is almost always impaired and may vary from confusion to frank coma.

Evidence-Based Diagnosis

The diagnosis is easily confirmed by the presence of hypernatremia, increased urine osmolality, and absence of hyperglycemia.

MAKING A DIAGNOSIS

An elevated urine osmolality can confirm urinary concentrating ability and establish inadequate fluid intake (versus inadequate conservation) as the etiology. An evaluation of the underlying precipitant is also important.

 Mr. R's urine osmolality is 850 mOsm/L. Blood cultures grow *Streptoccocus pneumoniae*.

As in the overwhelming majority of cases of hypernatremia, the diagnosis is straightforward. The history, exam, and elevated urine osmolality all confirm hypernatremia due to decreased intake. Urine concentrating ability is intact. Serum glucose is normal. Further diagnostic testing is not required.

CASE RESOLUTION

 Mr. R is given D5W. His body weight is measured at 140 lbs (63 kg). The rate of free water ad-

(continued)

ministration must be determined. He is started on ceftriaxone to treat his pneumonia.

Treatment of Hypernatremia

A. The brain adapts to hypernatremia by increasing intracellular osmolality to minimize cellular dehydration.

B. Rapid correction of hypernatremia leaves the brain hypertonic relative to the plasma. This promotes osmotic movement of water into the brain and cerebral edema. Seizures and death can occur.

C. Hypernatremia should be corrected slowly $\cong 0.5$ mEq/L/h; maximum of < 0.7 mEq/L/h.

D. The total water deficit can be calculated and then delivered at a rate to ensure the correction of hypernatremia is gradual.

1. Water deficit = TBW $\times$ ((Na$_{Patient}$ − 140)/140)

2. In hypernatremic patients, TBW = 0.5 $\times$ weight (men); TBW = 0.4 $\times$ weight (women)

3. Example: Suppose a 70-kg man has a serum sodium of 165 mEq/L

   a. TBW = 0.5 $\times$ 70 = 35 L

   b. Water deficit = 35 ((165 − 140)/140) = 6.3 L of D5W

   c. To correct from 165 to 140 at 0.5 mEq/L/h would require (165 − 140)/0.5 hours = 25/0.5 = 50 hours

   d. Therefore, 6.3 L administered over 50 hours = 125 mL of D5W per hour.

   e. Substituting D5 0.45 normal saline would cut the free water by half. Therefore, the infusion rate would need to double.

   f. Ongoing losses must be added.

4. Many such patients are markedly hypovolemic on presentation. Patients who are hypotensive should initially receive normal saline to restore adequate perfusion and then be switched to D5W at the appropriate rate.

Three days after D5W is started, his electrolytes are normal. He gradually returns to his baseline neurologic function and is discharged after 6 days of therapy to continue his oral antibiotics at the nursing home.

I have a patient with jaundice or abnormal liver enzymes. How do I determine the cause?

CHIEF COMPLAINT

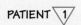

PATIENT 1

Ms. B is a 56-year-old woman who comes to your office because her skin and eyes have been yellow for the past 2 weeks.

What is the differential diagnosis of jaundice? How would you frame the differential?

CONSTRUCTING A DIFFERENTIAL DIAGNOSIS

The differential diagnosis of jaundice, or hyperbilirubinemia, is often organized pathophysiologically. It is helpful to review some basic physiology first:

A. Oxidation of the heme moiety of Hgb generates biliverdin, which is metabolized into **unconjugated bilirubin,** which is bound to albumin.

B. **Uptake:** The unconjugated bilirubin-albumin complex reaches the liver cell, and bilirubin dissociates, entering the hepatocyte.

C. **Conjugation:** Unconjugated bilirubin + glucuronic acid = **conjugated bilirubin.**

D. **Excretion** of conjugated bilirubin into the bile

    1. The rate limiting step of bilirubin metabolism in the liver

    2. If excretion is impaired, conjugated bilirubin travels back through the sinusoidal membrane of the hepatocyte into the bloodstream.

E. Conjugated bilirubin in the bile is transported through the biliary ducts into the duodenum; it is not reabsorbed by the intestine.

    1. Can be excreted unchanged in the stool

    2. Can be converted to **urobilinogen** by colonic bacteria

        a. Urobilinogen can be reabsorbed, entering the portal circulation.

        b. Some is taken up by the liver and reexcreted into the bile.

        c. Some bypasses the liver and is excreted by the kidney, thus appearing in the urine in small amounts.

F. **Unconjugated bilirubin is not found in the urine** because it is bound to albumin and cannot be filtered by the glomeruli.

G. **Conjugated bilirubin is filtered and excreted in the urine** when there is hyperbilirubinemia.

The first key point in the differential diagnosis of hyperbilirubinemia is determining which kind of bilirubin is elevated.

Dark, tea-colored urine means the patient has conjugated hyperbilirubinemia.

Light stools, often described as "clay colored," occur when extrahepatic obstruction prevents bilirubin from entering the intestine.

If there is unconjugated hyperbilirubinemia (when > 80% of the bilirubin is unconjugated), use a pathophysiologic framework:

A. Increased bilirubin production

    1. Hemolysis

    2. Dyserythropoiesis

    3. Extravasation of blood into tissues

B. Impaired hepatic bilirubin uptake
   1. Congestive heart failure
   2. Sepsis
   3. Drugs (rifampin, probenecid, chloramphenicol)
   4. Fasting
   5. Portosystemic shunts
C. Impaired bilirubin conjugation (decreased hepatic glucuronosyltransferase activity)
   1. Hereditary
      a. Gilbert syndrome
      b. Crigler-Najjar syndrome
   2. Acquired
      a. Neonates
      b. Hyperthyroidism
      c. Ethinyl estradiol
      d. Liver disease (causes mixed hyperbilirubinemia; usually predominantly conjugated)
      e. Sepsis

 Most patients with unconjugated hyperbilirubinemia have hemolysis, Gilbert syndrome, congestive heart failure, or sepsis.

Although many sources organize the differential diagnosis for conjugated hyperbilirubinemia (when > 50% is conjugated) using a pathophysiologic framework, a more practical, clinical approach uses the results of other liver function tests:

A. Normal liver enzymes (ALT [SGPT], AST [SGOT])
   1. Sepsis or systemic infection
   2. Rotor syndrome
   3. Dubin-Johnson syndrome
B. Elevated liver enzymes
   1. Transaminases more elevated than alkaline phosphatase: hepatocellular jaundice
      a. Acute viral or alcoholic hepatitis
      b. Alcoholic or nonalcoholic steatohepatitis
      c. Chronic hepatitis (viral, alcoholic, autoimmune)
      d. Cirrhosis of any cause
      e. Primary sclerosing cholangitis
      f. Primary biliary cirrhosis
      g. Drugs
   2. History suggestive of obstruction or alkaline phosphatase more elevated than transaminases, or both: cholestatic jaundice

   a. Extrahepatic cholestasis (biliary obstruction)
   b. Intrahepatic cholestasis (primarily due to impaired excretion)
      (1) Viral hepatitis
      (2) Alcoholic hepatitis
      (3) Cirrhosis
      (4) Drugs and toxins
      (5) Sepsis
      (6) Total parenteral nutrition
      (7) Postoperative jaundice
      (8) Infiltrative diseases (amyloidosis, lymphoma, sarcoidosis, tuberculosis)

So regardless of how you organize this differential, the first step is to determine whether the hyperbilirubinemia is primarily unconjugated or conjugated. The differential of unconjugated hyperbilirubinemia is limited. If the hyperbilirubinemia is conjugated, the second step is to determine whether there is extrahepatic obstruction or intrinsic liver dysfunction due to 1 of many possible etiologies. Although other liver function tests can serve as a guide, it is clear from the way the above differentials overlap that these tests are not very specific.

 Ms. B also tells you she has dark urine, light-colored stools, anorexia, and fatigue. She has no nausea, vomiting, abdominal pain, or fever. Ms. B's physical exam shows scleral icterus and jaundice as well as marked hepatomegaly, with her liver edge palpable 6–7 cm below the costal margin. The liver extends across the midline. There is a palpable organ in the left upper quadrant that is either the liver or the spleen. There is no abdominal tenderness or distention. There is no peripheral edema, and the rest of her exam is normal.

 How reliable is the physical exam for detecting hyperbilirubinemia?

A. Jaundice
   1. Detectable on physical exam when total bilirubin is > 2.5–3.0 mg/dL

 Scleral icterus is detectable before jaundice of the skin.

2. For bilirubin > 3.0 mg/dL, sensitivity of physical exam is 78.4% and specificity is 68.8% (LR+ = 2.5, LR− = 0.31).

3. For bilirubin > 15.0 mg/dL, sensitivity of physical exam is 96.4%.

B. Hepatomegaly: The test characteristics of the physical exam for finding hepatomegaly are not well established.

C. Splenomegaly

1. Percussion looks for loss of tympany as the enlarged spleen impinges on the air filled lung, stomach, and colon.

    a. Dullness instead of tympany in Traube space (six rib superiorly, midaxillary line laterally, and left costal margin inferiorly); **in nonobese patients who have not eaten recently,** has an LR+ of 4.3 and an LR− of 0.26.

    b. Dullness by the Castell method (percussing at the lowest intercostal space in the left anterior axillary line in both expiration and inspiration) has an LR+ of 4.8 and an LR− of 0.21.

2. Palpation (combining studies with a variety of palpation methods) has LR+ of 7.25–13.5 and an LR− of 0.45–0.74.

D. Ascites

1. The best 2 historical findings are

    a. Increased abdominal girth (LR+ = 4.16, LR− = 0.17)

    b. Ankle swelling (LR+ = 2.80, LR− = 0.10)

2. The best physical exam findings are

    a. Fluid wave (LR+ = 6.0, LR− = 0.4)

    b. Shifting dullness (LR+ = 2.7, LR− = 0.3)

    c. Proper physical exam technique must be used to obtain these LRs.

3. Ultrasound can detect 100 mL of ascites

Given the history and the physical exam findings of jaundice, massive hepatomegaly, and possible splenomegaly, you are confident that Ms. B has hyperbilirubinemia and suspect that it will be primarily conjugated. You obtain the following initial tests: total bilirubin, 13 mg/dL; direct bilirubin, 9.6 mg/dL; AST, 301 units/L; ALT, 113 units/L; alkaline phosphatase, 503 units/L; albumin, 2.8 g/dL; prothrombin time (PT), 15.4 s (control 11.1 s). WBC = 22,000 cells/mcL with 80% PMNs, 16% lymphocytes, and 4% monocytes.

At this point, what is the leading hypothesis, and what are the active alternatives? What other tests should be ordered?

ORGANIZING THE DIFFERENTIAL DIAGNOSIS

The alkaline phosphatase is more elevated than the transaminases, pointing toward either extrahepatic obstruction or intrahepatic cholestasis. The markedly enlarged liver suggests chronic liver disease, most likely due to the common etiologies of alcohol abuse or chronic hepatitis C, or both. It is necessary to test for hepatitis and to image to rule out extrahepatic obstruction, since cancer or stricture are a more likely cause of painless jaundice than stones. Pancreatic cancer is the most common malignancy that causes extrahepatic obstruction; cholangiocarcinoma and ampullary carcinoma are 2 other possibilities. Occasionally, obstruction is due to benign polyps in the biliary tree. Table 18–1 lists the differential diagnosis.

Ms. B had a blood transfusion in Latvia in 1996. She has no history of injection drug use or smoking; she has consumed between 2 glasses and 1 bottle of wine daily for years. Her past medical history is notable only for *Helicobacter pylori*–positive gastric and duodenal ulcers 6 years ago, treated with eradication therapy. She is on no medications.

Is the clinical information sufficient to make a diagnosis? If not, what other information do you need?

Leading Hypothesis: Alcoholic Liver Disease

Textbook Presentation

Alcoholic liver disease encompasses a broad spectrum of abnormalities, beginning with steatosis, progressing to

Table 18–1. Diagnostic hypotheses for Ms. B.

Diagnostic Hypotheses	Clinical Clues	Important Tests
Leading Hypothesis		
Alcoholic hepatitis	Alcohol history Hepatomegaly Signs of cirrhosis (palmar erythema, angiomata) AST > ALT	CT scan Liver biopsy
Active Alternative—Most Common		
Viral hepatitis	Exposure to body fluids, needles, or contaminated food Signs of cirrhosis if chronic hepatitis B or C	Hepatitis A antibody Hepatitis B antigen and antibodies Hepatitis C antibody
Active Alternative—Must Not Miss		
Pancreatic cancer	Jaundice (with or without pain) Weight loss Alkaline phosphatase elevation > transaminase elevation	CT scan MRI ERCP Endoscopic ultrasound
Other Hypotheses		
Common bile duct stones	Lack of pain makes gallstones unlikely, although multiple CBD stones can present painlessly	CT scan MRI Endoscopic ultrasound ERCP
Strictures or polyps	Painless jaundice	CT scan MRI Endoscopic ultrasound ERCP
Ampullary carcinoma or cholangiocarcinoma	Painless jaundice	CT scan MRI Endoscopic ultrasound ERCP

steatohepatitis and sometimes cirrhosis. The amount of alcohol necessary to develop advanced alcoholic liver disease varies among individuals, but in general, is about 80 g (6–8 drinks) daily for several years. The risk is higher for women at any given level of alcohol consumption.

1. Steatosis

Textbook Presentation

Steatosis is usually asymptomatic, with normal or mildly elevated transaminases. Hepatomegaly is present in 70% of patients with biopsy proven steatosis.

Disease Highlights

A. Potentiates liver damage from other insults, such as viral hepatitis or acetaminophen toxicity, and promotes obesity-related liver disease.

B. Completely reversible with abstinence from alcohol

2. Alcoholic Steatohepatitis

Textbook Presentation

The classic manifestations of alcoholic steatohepatitis (also called alcoholic hepatitis) are fever, malaise, jaundice, and tender hepatomegaly.

Disease Highlights

A. In reality, there is a broad range of presentations, including asymptomatic or isolated hepatomegaly.

B. Since cirrhosis can coexist, alcoholic hepatitis can also present with complications of portal hypertension, such as ascites, varices, and encephalopathy.

C. 1-month mortality between 0% and 50% in hospitalized patients

1. Can use the *discriminant function (DF)* to refine the prognosis: DF = 4.6 × (patient PT − control PT) + serum bilirubin level

2. If the DF is > 32, the patient's chance of dying in the hospital exceeds 50%.

D. Cirrhosis develops in 50% of patients by 5 years.

Evidence-Based Diagnosis

A. Transaminases are generally < 5–10 times normal.

B. GGT (gamma-glutamyl transpeptidase) is often elevated.

C. AST:ALT ratio often, but not always, > 2

    1. 70% of patients in 1 study

    2. Another study showed mean ratio of 2.6 for patients with alcoholic liver disease, compared with mean of 0.9 for patients with nonalcoholic steatohepatitis; however, there was some overlap.

You cannot use the AST:ALT ratio to definitively rule in or rule out alcoholic liver disease.

D. Imaging (with ultrasound or CT) is most helpful for ruling out other diagnoses; can variably see fatty infiltration, hepatomegaly, ascites, or cirrhosis.

E. Liver biopsy is the gold standard for diagnosis but is not always necessary.

3. Cirrhosis

A. See Chapter 12, Edema for a discussion of cirrhosis.

B. The prognosis of alcoholic cirrhosis varies, depending on whether the patient stops consuming alcohol.

    1. 5-year survival of 90% if patient becomes abstinent

    2. 5-year survival of 70% if patient continues to consume alcohol

    3. 5-year survival of 30–50% once complications of cirrhosis appear

MAKING A DIAGNOSIS

Ms. B's transaminases are consistent with, but not diagnostic of, alcoholic liver disease. An imaging study is necessary not to rule in alcoholic liver disease, but rather to exclude alternative diagnoses. As discussed in Chapter 2, Abdominal Pain, ultrasound is the best first test to look for stones. However, in this patient, pancreatic or other malignancies are more likely causes of extrabiliary obstruction than stones; therefore, an abdominal CT scan is the best first test. Tests for hepatitis are necessary in all patients with liver disease and are especially important in Ms. B because of her history of a blood transfusion.

Ms. B has an abdominal CT scan, which shows an enlarged, nodular liver, moderate ascites, and a normal pancreas. Her hepatitis A IgM antibody, HBsAg and hepatitis B IgM core antibody, and hepatitis C antibody are all negative.

Have you crossed the diagnostic threshold for the leading hypothesis, alcoholic hepatitis? Have you ruled out the active alternatives? Do other tests need to be done to exclude the alternative diagnoses?

Alternative Diagnosis: Pancreatic Cancer

Textbook Presentation

Patients with pancreatic cancer often have vague abdominal pain for weeks or months, followed by weight loss and perhaps the abrupt onset of painless jaundice.

Disease Highlights

A. > 90% of cases are ductal carcinomas; 70–80% are in pancreas head and 20–25% in pancreas body or tail

B. Clinical presentation

    1. Symptoms are insidious and often present for more than 2 months.

    2. Abdominal pain is the most common presenting complaint, occurring in up to 80% of patients.

        a. Often described as gnawing, visceral pain, sometimes radiating from the epigastrium to the sides or back

        b. Sometimes improves with bending forward; worse at night or after eating

        c. Back pain is prominent if splanchnic nerve or celiac plexus infiltration occurs

    3. Weight loss is common.

    4. Jaundice

        a. In 80% of patients with cancers in the head; more if mass is > 2 cm

        b. Can occur when the cancer is in the body or tail but is then due to liver metastases

        c. Can be painless or associated with abdominal pain

    5. Rare presentations include acute pancreatitis, malabsorption, migratory thrombophlebitis, and GI bleeding.

Evidence-Based Diagnosis

A. CT scan

    1. Sensitivity, 53–92%; specificity 64–100%, with averages about 85% for sensitivity and 90% for specificity

    2. LR+ = 8.5; LR– = 0.17

B. MRI scan

    1. Sensitivity, 83%; specificity, 100%

    2. LR+ = ∞; LR– = 0.17

C. Endoscopic ultrasound

    1. Sensitivity, 93–100%; specificity, 75–100%

    2. LR+ = 3.72–∞; LR– = 0–0.09

D. Endoscopic retrograde cholangiopancreatography (ERCP)

    1. Sensitivity, 95%; specificity, 97%

    2. LR+ = 32, LR– = 0.05

Treatment

A. Complete resection is possible in ~15% of patients; 5-year survival is still only 10%.

B. Palliative approach for patients with nonresectable cancer

    1. Biliary diversion, either percutaneous or surgical

    2. Radiation therapy for pain relief

    3. Gemcitabine for improved quality of life, but not increased survival

    4. Median survival is 6 months.

CASE RESOLUTION

With an LR– of 0.17 at best, a normal CT scan does not always rule out pancreatic cancer. However, in this patient, given that her CT scan shows evidence of advanced liver disease (a more likely diagnosis for her), it is not necessary to do further imaging studies. The other active alternative, chronic hepatitis, is ruled out by her negative serologies. These test results, combined with her alcohol intake history, makes alcoholic liver disease the most likely diagnosis. At this point, some clinicians would proceed with treatment for alcoholic hepatitis, while others would confirm the diagnosis and, for prognostic purposes, establish the presence or absence of cirrhosis with a liver biopsy.

Her liver biopsy showed acute alcoholic hepatitis with cirrhosis. Because her DF was > 32, she was treated with prednisone. She was also advised to abstain from alcohol. She completed the course of prednisone and has remained abstinent. Several weeks later, her bilirubin was normal and she felt well.

Treatment of Alcoholic Steatosis & Steatohepatitis

A. Alcoholic steatosis: abstain from alcohol

B. Alcoholic steatohepatitis

    1. Abstain from alcohol.

    2. Consider selected medications in severe, acute steatohepatitis.

        a. In 1 study, pentoxifylline was shown to reduce mortality and development of hepatorenal syndrome in hospitalized patients with DF > 32.

        b. There are conflicting data on corticosteroids, but there is some evidence of mortality benefit in selected patients: specifically, those with DF > 32 or spontaneous encephalopathy (or both), in the absence of infection, GI bleeding, and renal failure.

CHIEF COMPLAINT

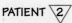

PATIENT 2

Mr. R is a 24-year-old graduate student who comes to see you because his girlfriend thought his eyes looked yellow yesterday. He has felt tired and a bit queasy for the last couple of weeks but thought he was just overworked and anxious. He has had some aching pain in the right upper quadrant and epigastrium, not related to eating or bowel movements. He has had no fevers, chills, or sweats. He has noticed dark urine for 1 or 2 days but attributed it to not drinking enough.

On physical exam, he appears tired. He has scleral icterus, and his liver is palpable 2 cm below the costal margin and is mildly tender. The spleen is not palpable, and the rest of his abdomen is nontender and nondistended. He has no edema, and the rest of his exam is normal.

 At this point, what is your leading hypothesis, and what are the active alternatives? What other tests should be ordered?

ORGANIZING THE DIFFERENTIAL DIAGNOSIS

The differential diagnosis for fatigue, nausea, and vague abdominal pain is broad, but the findings of scleral icterus and tender hepatomegaly point toward a hepatic source. More than 90% of patients with viral hepatitis have a history of anorexia, malaise, and nausea, with the physical exam showing hepatomegaly, hepatic tenderness, or both.

 Hepatitis is unlikely in the absence of nausea, anorexia, malaise, hepatomegaly, or hepatic tenderness.

Mr. R's clinical picture is consistent with viral hepatitis. Hepatitis A is the most frequent cause of acute viral hepatitis; hepatitis C is the second most frequent but is usually asymptomatic acutely. By virtue of being common, alcoholic hepatitis is another active alternative diagnosis; the presentation can mimic that of viral hepatitis. Biliary obstruction is always a consideration in patients with jaundice, but the prodrome and type of abdominal pain are not typical. Table 18–2 lists the differential diagnosis.

 He has no past medical history and takes no medicines; he does not smoke or use illicit drugs. He drinks 1–2 beers most weeks, and oc-

(continued)

Table 18–2. Diagnostic hypotheses for Mr. R.

Diagnostic Hypotheses	Clinical Clues	Important Tests
Leading Hypothesis		
Acute hepatitis A	Exposure to potentially contaminated food, travel Right upper quadrant pain Nausea with or without vomiting Malaise	IgM anti-HAV
Active Alternative—Most Common		
Acute alcoholic steatohepatitis	History of binge drinking Alcohol history Hepatomegaly Signs of cirrhosis (palmar erythema, angiomatia) AST > ALT	CT scan Liver biopsy
Active Alternative—Must Not Miss		
Hepatitis B or C	Exposure to needles or body fluids Right upper quadrant pain Nausea with or without vomiting Malaise	*Hepatitis B:* HBsAg, IgM anti-HBc *Hepatitis C:* anti-HCV, viral load
Other Hypotheses		
Epstein-Barr or cytomegalovirus hepatitis	Adenopathy Pharyngitis	EBV, CMV antibodies
Biliary obstruction	Biliary colic	Ultrasound

casionally shares a bottle of wine with friends. He has never had a blood transfusion or a tattoo. He enjoys trying different restaurants, and frequently eats sushi and ceviche. Initial lab tests include the following: total bilirubin, 6.5 mg/dL; conjugated bilirubin, 4 mg/dL; ALT, 1835 units/L; AST, 1522 units/L; alkaline phosphatase, 175 units/L; WBC, 9,800 cells/mcL (normal differential); Hgb, 14.5 g/dL; Hct, 44%.

 Is the clinical information sufficient to make a diagnosis? If not, what other information do you need?

Leading Hypothesis: Hepatitis A

Textbook Presentation

The classic presentation is the gradual onset of malaise, nausea, anorexia, and right upper quadrant pain, followed by jaundice.

Disease Highlights

A. Prevalence: Accounts for 20–40% of cases of viral hepatitis in the United States.

B. Clinical manifestations
   1. Often subclinical in children and generally symptomatic in adults
   2. Average incubation period is 30 days (range 15–49 days), followed by prodromal symptoms of fatigue, malaise, nausea, vomiting, anorexia, fever, and right upper pain; about 1 week later, jaundice appears.
   3. 70% of patients have jaundice; 80% have hepatomegaly
   4. Other physical findings include splenomegaly, cervical lymphadenopathy, rash, arthritis, and leukocytoclasic vasculitis.
   5. Uncommon extrahepatic manifestations include vasculitis, arthritis, optic neuritis, transverse myelitis, thrombocytopenia, and aplastic anemia.

C. Transmission
   1. Fecal-oral transmission, either sporadically or in an epidemic form
      a. Contaminated water, shellfish, frozen strawberries, etc.
      b. Contamination from infected restaurant worker
      c. Exposure history not always clear

   2. No maternal-fetal transmission

D. Clinical course
   1. Generally self-limited, with rare cases of fulminant hepatic failure
      a. Fulminant course is more common in patients with underlying hepatitis C.
      b. 1.1% fatality rate in adults > age 40
   2. 85% fully recover in 3 months, and nearly all by 6 months
   3. Transaminases normalize more rapidly than serum bilirubin

E. Prevention
   1. Vaccination is available for preexposure prophylaxis.
   2. Can use immune serum globulin with or without vaccination for postexposure prophylaxis

Evidence-Based Diagnosis

A. Liver function tests
   1. ALT and AST are generally over 1000 units/L; ALT is generally > AST.
   2. Bilirubin commonly > 10 mg/dL
   3. Alkaline phosphatase is usually elevated.

B. Antibody tests (see Figure 18–1)
   1. Serum IgM anti-HAV detects acute illness, being positive at the onset of symptoms and remaining positive for 4–6 months
   2. LR+ = 99, LR− = 0.01
   3. Serum IgG anti-HAV appears in the convalescent phase of the disease and remains positive for decades.

MAKING A DIAGNOSIS

The pretest probability for some form of viral hepatitis is so high that it is not necessary to consider other diagnoses at this point. Although Mr. R's history of food exposure suggests hepatitis A, it is generally necessary to test for all 3 of the primary hepatitis viruses. Hepatitis C can sometimes be spread through fecal-oral contamination, and the exposure history for both hepatitis B and C is often unclear.

 His hepatitis A IgM antibody is positive, with negative HBsAg, IgM anti-HBc, and anti-HCV.

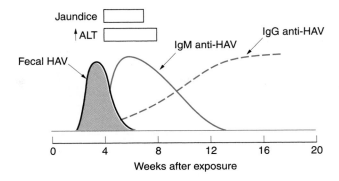

Figure 18–1. Natural history of hepatitis A symptoms and antibodies. HAV, hepatitis A virus; ALT, alanine amino-transferase.

Have you crossed a diagnostic threshold for the leading hypothesis, acute hepatitis A? Have you ruled out the active alternatives? Do other tests need to be done to exclude the alternative diagnoses?

Alternative Diagnosis: Acute Hepatitis B

Textbook Presentation

The classic presentation is the gradual onset of malaise, nausea, anorexia, right upper quadrant pain, followed by jaundice. Hepatitis B is often subclinical.

Disease Highlights

A. Prevalence of hepatitis B virus (HBV) carriers
   1. 0.1–2% (low prevalence) in the United States, Canada, and Western Europe
   2. 3–5% (medium prevalence) in Mediterranean countries, Japan, central Asia, the Middle East, and Latin and South America
   3. 10–20% (high prevalence) in southeast Asia, China, and subSaharan Africa

B. Clinical manifestations
   1. 70% of patients have subclinical infection or are anicteric; 30% of patients have icteric hepatitis
   2. Incubation period is 1–4 months.
   3. Symptoms are similar to those of hepatitis A, but serum sickness-like syndrome can be part of the prodrome (fever, rash, arthralgias).

C. Transmission
   1. In high prevalence areas, transmission is primarily perinatal, occurring in 90% of babies born to HBeAg-positive mothers; it can be prevented by neonatal vaccination.
   2. In medium prevalence areas, childhood infection occurs from contaminated household objects, via minor breaks in the skin or mucous membranes.
   3. In low prevalence areas, transmission is most often sexual, via percutaneous inoculation (eg, injection drug use, accidental needlestick, tattooing, body piercing, acupuncture), or from contaminated blood transfusion.

D. Clinical course
   1. Fulminant hepatic failure occurs in 0.1–0.5% of patients.
   2. Transaminases normalize in 1–4 months if acute infection resolves.
   3. Elevation of ALT for > 6 months indicates progression to chronic hepatitis.
      a. < 5% of adult acute infections progress to chronic hepatitis
      b. 90% for perinatally acquired infection
      c. 20–50% for infection acquired between ages 1 and 5

E. Prevention of hepatitis B
   1. Vaccination for preexposure prophylaxis
   2. Vaccination and HB immune globulin within 12 hours for postexposure prophylaxis

Evidence-Based Diagnosis

A. Liver function tests: similar to hepatitis A
B. **Hepatitis B surface antigen (HBsAg)** appears 1–10 weeks after acute exposure, prior to symptoms or elevations of transaminases (Figure 18–2).

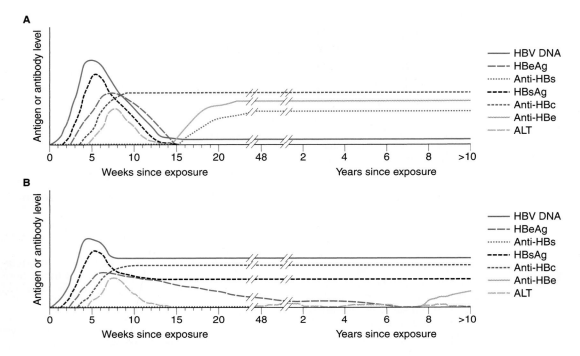

A

B

Figure 18–2. Natural history of acute (**A**) and chronic (**B**) hepatitis B infections. (Reproduced with permission from Ganem D, Prince AM. Hepatitis B virus infection—natural history and clinical consequences. *NEJM.* 2004;350:1118–1129.)

1. Should be present in patients with acute symptoms
2. Should clear in 4–6 months
3. LR+ = 27, LR− = 0.2

C. **Hepatitis B surface antibody (HBsAb)** appears after disappearance of HBsAg; there can be a "window period" of several weeks to months between the disappearance of HBsAg and the appearance of HBsAb.

D. **IgM hepatitis B core antibody (IgM anti-HBc)** appears shortly after HBsAg and is the only marker of acute infection detectable during the "window period."

1. LR+ = 45, LR− = 0.1
2. However, IgM anti-HBc can remain detectable for 2 years, and titer can increase during exacerbations of chronic hepatitis B.

Treatment

A. Supportive therapy: rest, oral hydration, and antiemetic medications as needed

B. Admit if INR is elevated or patient is unable to hydrate orally.

C. Liver transplant if fulminant hepatitis occurs

Alternative Diagnosis: Chronic Hepatitis B

Textbook Presentation

Manifestations can range from asymptomatic, to isolated fatigue, to cirrhosis with portal hypertension. There is often no history of acute hepatitis B.

Disease Highlights

A. Defined as presence of HBsAg for more than 6 months (see Figure 18–2)

B. 10–20% have extrahepatic findings (eg, polyarteritis nodosa, glomerular disease)

C. Can have periodic exacerbations that can be asymptomatic or appear to be acute hepatitis or hepatic failure, with elevations of transaminases and sometimes IgM anti-HBc titers

D. HBsAb is generally detectable for life (0.5–2%/year become HBsAg negative)

E. 5–10% of patients per year become HBeAg negative and anti-HBe antibody positive

1. Disappearance of HBeAg is accompanied by a "flare," a transient rise in transaminases

2. 75–80% of patients with anti-HBe antibodies have detectable HBV DNA

3. HBeAg negative patients with relatively normal transaminases have a good prognosis; those with elevated transaminases and viral loads have a worse prognosis.

F. Prognosis

1. Asymptomatic chronic carriers do well (cirrhosis develops in ~1%)

2. Patients from endemic areas and those with chronic active hepatitis have significant complication rates.

  a. Rate of developing cirrhosis is 12–20%

  b. Rate of developing hepatocellular carcinoma is 6–15%

    (1) Relative risk is 100 times that of noncarriers.

    (2) HBeAg-positive carriers have the highest risk.

    (3) Screening with ultrasound and alpha-fetoprotein levels is controversial.

Evidence-Based Diagnosis

A. HBsAg is always positive.

B. Early: HBeAg positive, anti-HBe negative, HBV DNA positive

C. Late (but not in all patients): HBeAg negative, anti-HBe positive, HBV DNA positive

Treatment

A. HBeAg positive patients have high rates of early progression to chronic active hepatitis and cirrhosis and should be treated.

B. Asymptomatic HBeAg negative patients with viral loads below 10^5 genomes/mL and normal transaminases are usually not treated; those with higher viral loads and abnormal transaminases are sometimes treated.

C. Markers of successful therapy include loss of HBeAg, seroconversion to anti-HBe antibodies, and reduction of the viral load.

D. True cure is rare (1–5% of patients).

E. Current treatment options include interferon alfa, lamivudine, and adefovir.

Alternative Diagnosis: Hepatitis C

Textbook Presentation

Most patients are asymptomatic, with jaundice developing in less than 25%. When present, symptoms are similar to those of other viral hepatitis and last 2–12 weeks.

Disease Highlights

A. Prevalence

1. 20% of cases of acute hepatitis; most are asymptomatic

2. Prevalence of anti-HCV antibody is 1.4–1.8% in the United States

B. Transmission

1. Currently, 1/1,900,000 blood transfusions transmit hepatitis C; up to 10% of transfusion recipients prior to 1990 were infected

2. Now, hepatitis C is primarily transmitted through injection drug use, with occasional cases due to ear or body piercing, sex with an injection drug user, or accidental needlesticks.

3. Rarely, transmission can occur to household contacts

4. Transmission between monogamous partners is about 1%/year; risk of sexual transmission is higher if index carrier also has HIV or multiple partners.

C. Clinical course

1. Average incubation period is 7–8 weeks

2. Fulminant hepatitis is rare.

3. ALT normalizes in up to 40% of patients, but < 15% actually clear the infection.

4. Depending on the series, chronic infection develops in 80–100% of patients.

5. Extrahepatic manifestations are common, being found in about 75% of patients.

  a. Fatigue, arthralgias, paresthesias, myalgias, pruritus, and sicca syndrome are found in > 10% of patients.

  b. Vasculitis secondary to cryoglobulinemia is found in 1% of patients, although cryoglobulinemia is present in about 40%.

  c. Depression and anxiety are more common than in uninfected persons.

D. Chronic hepatitis C

1. 30% of patients have stable chronic hepatitis, 40% have variable progression, and 30% have severe progression

2. 6 genotypes have been identified: type 1 is most common in United States but is less responsive to current therapy than types 2 and 3.

3. There is no correlation between ALT levels and liver histology.

 It is necessary to do a liver biopsy to determine the activity and severity of the disease.

4. Over 20 years, cirrhosis develops in 20–50%, depending on the population.

   a. Liver histology is the best predictor of progression to cirrhosis.

   b. Other predictors of progression to cirrhosis include age at infection, duration of infection, consumption of alcohol > 50 g/d, HIV coinfection, CD4 count < 200/mcL, male sex, higher body mass index (BMI), diabetes, steatosis, and possibly genotype 3, smoking, and hemochromatosis heterozygosity.

   c. 5-year survival for compensated cirrhosis is 80% but drops to 50% once decompensation occurs.

   d. Hepatocellular carcinoma develops in up to 3% of patients per year.

E. Prevention: no vaccine available; no role for immunoglobulin

Evidence-Based Diagnosis

A. Anti-HCV antibody tests

   1. Main screening assay is an **enzyme immunoassay (EIA)**

   a. Sensitivity of 92–95% for second-generation test (EIA-2) and 97% for third-generation test (EIA-3)

   b. Positive predictive value (true positive EIAs/all positive EIAs) is 50–61% in low prevalence populations, such as blood donors, and 88–95% in high prevalence populations.

   c. Can be negative in immunocompromised patients, such as organ transplant recipients, HIV-infected patients, or hemodialysis patients, even in presence of active viral infection

   d. Positive in 50% of patients with acute hepatitis C at time of presentation; mean time to seroconversion is 10 weeks but can occur within 4 weeks

   2. A more specific, confirmatory antibody test is a **RIBA immunoblot** test, which is read as positive, indeterminate, or negative; it will stay positive in patients who have recovered from HCV infection.

B. HCV RNA tests

   1. Qualitative HCV PCR assay

   a. Can detect HCV RNA at a level of < 100 copies/mL

   b. Specificity as high as 97–99% in some laboratories

   c. Can have a lot of variability in results, even with standardized kits

2. Quantitative HCV RNA tests ("viral load")

   a. Quantitative polymerase chain reaction (PCR) can have a lot of variability. It is not as sensitive as qualitative PCR, with detection limit of about 1000 copies/mL.

   b. Quantitative branched DNA test is more reproducible than PCR, but much less sensitive, with detection limit of 200,000 copies/mL.

C. Genotype testing

   1. Used for prediction of response to treatment and choice of treatment duration

   2. Genotypes do not change, so this test needs to be done only once.

D. When should you order the different antibody and RNA tests?

   1. In a patient with **acute hepatitis,** order the anti-HCV EIA first; if it is negative, order a qualitative HCV RNA, which is detectable within days of exposure.

   2. In a patient with **chronic liver disease or an elevated ALT,** order the anti-HCV EIA.

   a. Nearly all results are true positives, so confirmatory testing is not required.

   b. If you choose to do a confirmatory test, the best is a quantitative HCV RNA, since viral load predicts response to treatment; if the quantitative HCV RNA is negative, order the more sensitive qualitative HCV RNA.

   3. When a positive anti-HCV EIA is found in blood donors, or in patients with normal ALT levels, confirmatory testing is necessary.

   a. In 1 strategy, all such patients get retested for anti-HCV using the RIBA test; patients with positive and indeterminate results then get tested using qualitative HCV PCR.

   b. In another strategy, all patients just get tested using qualitative HCV PCR.

   c. Both strategies have the potential to produce false-negative results; in such cases, patients should be retested at 6–12 months.

   4. Immunocompromised patients with suspected hepatitis C who are EIA antibody negative should have a qualitative PCR.

Treatment

A. Goals of treatment: Prevention of cirrhosis and its complications, reduction of extrahepatic manifestations, and reduction of transmission

B. Response rates (defined as at least a 2 log decrease from baseline viral load after 12 weeks of treatment)

are about 88% for genotypes 2 and 3, compared with about 48% for genotypes 1, 4, 5, and 6.

C. Patients with higher viral loads have higher relapse rates and are often treated longer than those with lower viral loads.

D. Currently, the best results are seen with a combination of pegylated interferon and ribavirin.

CASE RESOLUTION

Mr. R clearly has acute hepatitis A, presumably from contaminated food. Although he is nauseated, he is able to drink adequate fluid. His INR is normal at 1.1. You recommend rest and oral

hydration for Mr. R, and serum immune globulin for his girlfriend. He feels much better when he returns 1 month later.

 The best test of the liver's synthetic function is the PT. It is important to check the INR in all patients with hepatitis to look for signs of liver failure.

Treatment of Hepatitis A

A. Supportive therapy: rest, oral hydration, and antiemetic medications as needed

B. Admit if INR is elevated or patient is unable to hydrate orally.

C. Liver transplant if fulminant hepatitis occurs

CHIEF COMPLAINT

Mr. H is a 55-year-old man with unexpected transaminase abnormalities.

 What is the differential diagnosis of asymptomatic elevation transaminases? How would you frame the differential?

CONSTRUCTING A DIFFERENTIAL DIAGNOSIS

The basic framework is to separate hepatic from nonhepatic causes.

A. Hepatic causes
1. Alcohol abuse
2. Medication
3. Chronic hepatitis B or C
4. Steatosis and nonalcoholic steatohepatitis (nonalcoholic fatty liver disease [NAFLD])
5. Autoimmune hepatitis
6. Hemochromatosis

7. Wilson disease (in patients < 40 years old)
8. α_1-Antitrypsin deficiency

B. Nonhepatic causes
1. Celiac sprue
2. Inherited disorders of muscle metabolism (AST elevation only)
3. Acquired muscle disease (AST elevation only)
4. Strenuous exercise (AST elevation only)

Mr. H comes in for a routine appointment. He feels fine. His past medical history is notable for type 2 diabetes and hypertension. His medications include metformin, atorvastatin, hydrochlorothiazide, and lisinopril. He does not smoke, and he has a beer with dinner occasionally. His physical exam shows a BP of 125/80 mm Hg, pulse of 80 bpm, RR of 16 breaths per minute, weight 230 lbs, height 5 ft 9 in (BMI = 34.0). Pulmonary, cardiac, and abdominal exams are all normal.

Laboratory test results from his last visit include a creatinine of 0.9 mg/dL, a Hgb A1C of 6.8%, an LDL of 95 mg/dL, a bilirubin of 0.8

(continued)

mg/dL, an AST of 85 units/L, an ALT of 92 units/L, and a normal alkaline phosphatase. You then note that his transaminases were 45 units/L and 53 units/L, respectively, when last checked a year earlier.

 At this point, what is your leading hypothesis, and what are your active alternatives? What other tests should be ordered?

ORGANIZING THE DIFFERENTIAL DIAGNOSIS

In the absence of an obvious nonhepatic cause of liver enzyme elevations, the initial approach is to focus on the hepatic causes. The prevalence of the liver diseases in the differential diagnosis varies widely, depending on the population studied. For example, in a study of over 19,000 young, healthy military recruits, of whom 99 had enzyme elevations, only 11 were found to have any liver disease (4 had hepatitis B, 4 had hepatitis C, 2 had autoimmune hepatitis, 1 had cholelithiasis). A study of 100 blood donors with elevated enzymes found that 48% had alcoholic liver disease, 22% had NAFLD, and 17% had hepatitis C. In another study, patients with elevated enzymes in whom a diagnosis could not be made by history or blood tests underwent liver biopsy; NAFLD was found in over 50% of them.

NAFLD is extremely common in obese, diabetic patients, so Mr. H is at high risk for this disease. He has no specific risk factors for chronic hepatitis, but often the exposure history is unclear. His alcohol intake is minimal, but sometimes even small amounts of alcohol can cause liver enzyme elevations. He is also on 2 medications, metformin and atorvastatin, that can cause elevation of liver enzymes. (Although statins cause transaminase elevation in 0.5–2.0% of patients, the clinical significance is unclear, and progression to liver failure is rare. The American College of Cardiology recommends measuring transaminases at baseline, at 12 weeks, and then annually.) The final possibility to consider at this point is hemochromatosis, a fairly common gene mutation that can present with liver enzyme abnormalities and diabetes. Table 18–3 lists the differential diagnosis.

 Mr. H first abstains from alcohol for 2 weeks; his repeat liver enzymes show AST = 90 units/L

and ALT = 95 units/L. He then stops his atorvastatin and metformin for 1 week, with no change in his transaminases. PT, albumin, and CBC are all normal.

 Is the clinical information sufficient to make a diagnosis? If not, what other information do you need?

Leading Hypothesis: NAFLD

Textbook Presentation

Patients are often asymptomatic but sometimes complain of vague right upper quadrant discomfort. It is common to identify patients by finding hepatomegaly on exam or asymptomatic transaminase elevations.

Disease Highlights

A. Epidemiology and etiology
1. Risk factors include obesity, type 2 diabetes, hypertriglyceridemia, and family history.
2. NAFLD is found in up to 75% of obese patients, 50% of diabetics, and close to 100% of patients with diabetes and obesity.
3. Most common cause of abnormal liver test results in the United States.
4. Multiple secondary causes
   a. Nutritional (eg, total parenteral nutrition, starvation, rapid weight loss, malnutrition, bariatric surgery)
   b. Drugs (eg, methotrexate, amiodarone, estrogens, glucocorticoids, aspirin, cocaine, antiretroviral agents)
   c. Metabolic or genetic
   d. Other (eg, inflammatory bowel disease, HIV, environmental hepatotoxins)

B. Clinical course
1. Natural history is not well defined.
2. A small series of patients who underwent biopsy found 28% had progression of liver damage, 59% were unchanged, and 13% had improvement.
3. Patients who are found to have pure steatosis on biopsy have best prognosis.
4. Patients with steatohepatitis or advanced fibrosis have worse prognosis and can progress to cirrhosis; the rate of progression is unclear.

Table 18–3. Diagnostic hypotheses for Mr. H.

Diagnostic Hypotheses	Clinical Clues	Important Tests
Leading Hypothesis		
Nonalcoholic fatty liver disease	Obesity (BMI > 30) Diabetes	Ultrasound Liver biopsy
Active Alternatives—Most Common		
Hemochromatosis	Family history Diabetes	Serum iron/TIBC, ferritin
Alcohol	Intake history AST > ALT	Abstinence
Medication	Medication history (prescriptions and nonprescription)	Stopping the medication
Active Alternatives—Must Not Miss		
Hepatitis B or C	Exposure to body fluids, needles	HBsAg Anti-HBc Anti-HBs Anti-HCV
Other Hypotheses		
Autoimmune hepatitis	Other autoimmune disease	Serum protein electrophoresis Antinuclear antibodies Liver biopsy
Wilson disease	Age < 40 Neuropsychiatric symptoms	Ceruloplasmin
α_1-Antitrypsin deficiency	Emphysema	AAT level

5. Predictors of severe fibrosis or cirrhosis include age > 45 (OR = 5.6), BMI > 30 (OR = 4.3), AST:ALT ratio > 1 (OR = 4.3), type 2 diabetes mellitus (OR = 3.5).

Evidence-Based Diagnosis

A. Blood tests

   1. Transaminase elevation is usually < 4 times normal; AST:ALT ratio is usually less than 1, but not if there is advanced disease

   2. Serum ferritin is elevated in 50% of patients.

   3. Alkaline phosphatase and GGT are often mildly elevated.

B. Imaging

   1. Ultrasound

      a. For steatosis

         (1) Sensitivity, 89%; specificity, 93%

         (2) LR+, 12.7; LR–, 0.12

      b. For fibrosis

         (1) Sensitivity, 77%; specificity, 89%

         (2) LR+, 7; LR–, 0.37

   2. CT scan is similar to ultrasound.

   3. No imaging study can reliably distinguish steatosis from more advanced NAFLD.

   4. On ultrasound and CT scan, fatty infiltration occasionally has a nodular appearance suggestive of metastatic disease; MRI can then distinguish between these 2 possibilities.

C. Liver biopsy is the gold standard for diagnosis, staging, and measuring response to treatment.

It is necessary to rule out other causes of liver disease listed in the above differential before diagnosing NAFLD.

MAKING A DIAGNOSIS

You should take somewhat of a stepwise approach to evaluating asymptomatic liver enzyme abnormalities. As was done with Mr. H, the first step is to stop alcohol and, if possible, potentially hepatotoxic medications, and then remeasure the liver enzymes. Although aspects of the history can increase the likelihood of a specific diagnosis, the history is not sensitive or specific enough to make a diagnosis, and it is necessary to test somewhat broadly. If liver enzyme abnormalities persist after stopping alcohol and potentially hepatotoxic medications, the American Gastroenterological Association recommends beginning with a PT; serum albumin; CBC; hepatitis A, B, and C serologies; and iron studies (serum iron, total iron-binding capacity [TIBC], ferritin).

IgM and IgG anti-HAV are both negative. HBsAg and IgM anti-HBc are negative; IgG anti-HBc and anti-HBs are positive. Anti-HCV is negative. The transferrin saturation is 35%, and the serum ferritin is 190 ng/mL.

Have you crossed a diagnostic threshold for the leading hypothesis, NAFLD? Have you ruled out the active alternatives? Do other tests need to be done to exclude the alternative diagnoses?

Alternative Diagnosis: Hereditary Hemochromatosis

Textbook Presentation

Most patients are asymptomatic, but a few have extrahepatic manifestations of iron overload (see below). Some patients are identified by screening the family members of affected individuals.

Disease Highlights

A. Autosomal recessive with homozygote frequency of 1:200 to 1:400 in whites; much less frequent in Hispanics and African Americans

B. Iron deposition occurs throughout the reticuloendothelial system, leading to a broad range of potential manifestations

    a. In the liver leads to cirrhosis and then to hepatocellular carcinoma

    b. In the heart leads to dilated cardiomyopathy

    c. In the pituitary leads to secondary hypogonadism

    d. In the pancreas leads to diabetes

    e. In the joints leads to arthropathy

    f. In the thyroid leads to hypothyroidism

C. Clinical presentation

    1. Up to 75% of patients are asymptomatic.

    2. Liver function abnormalities are present in 75%.

    3. Weakness and lethargy are present in 74%.

    4. Skin hyperpigmentation is seen in 70%.

    5. Diabetes mellitus occurs in 48%.

    6. Arthralgias are present in 44%.

    7. Impotence is seen in 45%.

    8. Electrocardiographic abnormalities are present in 31%.

Evidence-Based Diagnosis

A. Liver biopsy with measurement of hepatic iron index is the gold standard.

B. Initial screening should be done with a fasting transferring saturation (serum iron/TIBC) and ferritin.

    1. Transferrin saturation ≥ 45%

        a. Men

            (1) Sensitivity, 81%; specificity, 94%

            (2) LR+ = 13.5, LR− = 0.2

        b. Women

            (1) Sensitivity, 48%; specificity, 97%

            (2) LR+ = 16, LR− = 0.53

    2. Ferritin ≥ 200 ng/mL

        a. Men

            (1) Sensitivity, 78%; specificity, 76%

            (2) LR+ = 3.25, LR− = 0.23

        b. Women

            (1) Sensitivity, 54%; specificity, 95%

            (2) LR+ = 20, LR− = 0.48

C. Patients who have a transferrin saturation ≥ 45% and an elevated ferritin should undergo HFE gene testing, looking for the hereditary hemochromatosis mutations.

All first-degree relatives of patients with hereditary hemochromatosis should undergo gene testing, regardless of the results of the iron studies.

1. If C282Y/C282Y homozygous mutation is found

   a. If age is < 40 years, ferritin < 1000 ng/mL, and transaminases are normal, proceed to treatment

   b. Otherwise, perform liver biopsy to determine severity

2. If other mutations or no mutations are found, look for other causes of iron overload or perform liver biopsy for diagnosis.

Treatment

Periodic phlebotomy—to reduce the iron overload—has been shown to reduce the risk of progression to cirrhosis.

CASE RESOLUTION

Mr. H's transaminase levels remained elevated after abstaining from alcohol and discontinuing medications, making those diagnoses unlikely. His hepatitis A and C serologies are negative; his hepatitis B serologies are consistent with a previous infection and not chronic hepatitis B. His transferrin saturation is normal, and the slightly elevated ferritin is not specific for any particular disease.

At this point, you could order an antinuclear antibody (ANA), smooth muscle antibody (SMA), ceruloplasmin, and α_1-1 antitrypsin (AAT) levels. However, considering his age, gender, and lack of other symptoms or illnesses, autoimmune hepatitis, Wilson disease, and α_1-antitrypsin deficiency are all very unlikely. At this point, NAFLD is by far the most likely diagnosis. An ultrasound is not absolutely necessary, but it could confirm the diagnosis of NAFLD.

Mr. H has an ultrasound, which shows an enlarged liver with diffuse fatty infiltration. He begins to walk 20 minutes 4 times/week, and reduces his portion sizes. His transaminases remain stable for the next several months. One year later, he has lost 20 pounds, and his transaminases have decreased to around 40.

Treatment of NAFLD

A. Weight loss

B. Exercise

C. Control of diabetes

Summary table of serologic markers in hepatitis B.

HBsAg	HBeAg	IgM anti-HBc	IgG anti-HBc	Anti-HBs	Anti-HBe	HBV DNA	
+	+	+				+	Acute -early
		+			+/−		-window period
			+	+	+	−	-recovery phase
+	+		+			+	Chronic -early
+			+		+	+	-late[a]
+	+/−	+				+	-flare

[a]In some, but not all, patients.

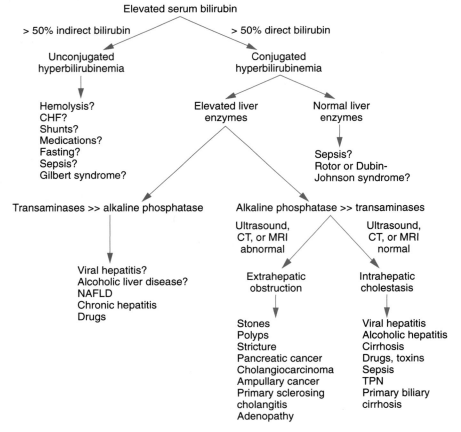

Approach to Hyperbilirubinemia

Elevated serum bilirubin

> 50% indirect bilirubin

> 50% direct bilirubin

Unconjugated hyperbilirubinemia

Conjugated hyperbilirubinemia

Hemolysis?
CHF?
Shunts?
Medications?
Fasting?
Sepsis?
Gilbert syndrome?

Elevated liver enzymes

Normal liver enzymes

Sepsis?
Rotor or Dubin-Johnson syndrome?

Transaminases >> alkaline phosphatase

Alkaline phosphatase >> transaminases

Viral hepatitis?
Alcoholic liver disease?
NAFLD
Chronic hepatitis
Drugs

Ultrasound, CT, or MRI abnormal

Ultrasound, CT, or MRI normal

Extrahepatic obstruction

Intrahepatic cholestasis

Stones
Polyps
Stricture
Pancreatic cancer
Cholangiocarcinoma
Ampullary cancer
Primary sclerosing cholangitis
Adenopathy

Viral hepatitis
Alcoholic hepatitis
Cirrhosis
Drugs, toxins
Sepsis
TPN
Primary biliary cirrhosis

CHF, congestive heart failure; NAFLD, nonalcoholic fatty liver disease; TPN, total parenteral nutrition.

Figure 18–A.

Serologic Testing in Hepatitis C

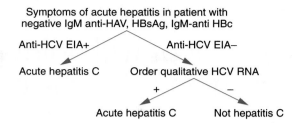

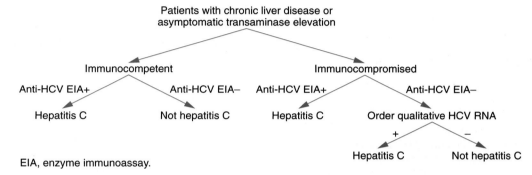

EIA, enzyme immunoassay.

Figure 18–B.

Approach to Asymptomatic AP Elevation

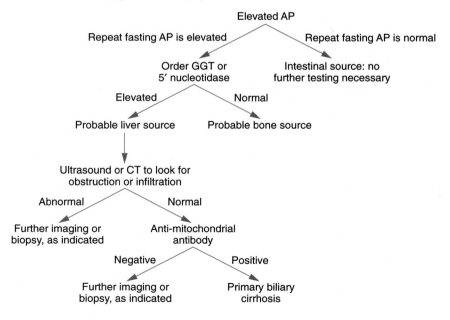

AP, alkaline phosphatase; GGT, gamma-glutamyl transpeptidase.

Figure 18–C.

I have a patient with joint pain.
How do I determine the cause?

CHIEF COMPLAINT

PATIENT 1

Mrs. K is a 75-year-old woman who complains of a painful left knee.

What is the differential diagnosis of joint pain? How would you frame the differential?

CONSTRUCTING A DIFFERENTIAL DIAGNOSIS

The causes of joint pain range from common to rare and from not particularly dangerous to joint- and life-threatening. Even the most benign causes of joint pain can lead to serious disability. The evaluation of a patient with joint pain calls for a detailed history and physical exam (often focusing on extra-articular findings) and frequently the sampling of joint fluid. The diagnosis of a particular illness may be made based on history, joint fluid abnormalities or, in the case of many rheumatologic diseases, on the presence of abnormalities in multiple organ systems and serologies.

The differential diagnosis below is organized by the number of joints involved (monoarticular vs polyarticular) and the appearance of the joint (inflammatory vs noninflammatory). Recognize that all of the monoarticular arthritides can present in a polyarticular distribution, and classically polyarticular diseases may occasionally only affect a single joint. Recognize also that abnormalities of periarticular structures may sometimes mimic articular disease.

The joint distribution of diseases that cause joint pain is variable; monoarticular arthritides may present with polyarticular findings and vice versa.

A. Monoarticular arthritis
  1. Inflammatory
    a. Infectious
      (1) Gonococcal arthritis
      (2) Nongonococcal septic arthritis
      (3) Lyme disease
    b. Crystalline
      (1) Monosodium urate (gout)
      (2) Calcium pyrophosphate dihydrate deposition disease (CPPDD or pseudogout)
    c. Traumatic
  2. Noninflammatory
    a. Osteoarthritis (OA)
    b. Traumatic
B. Polyarticular arthritis
  1. Inflammatory
    a. Rheumatologic
      (1) Rheumatoid arthritis (RA)
      (2) Systemic lupus erythematosis (SLE)
      (3) Psoriatic arthritis
      (4) Other rheumatic diseases
    b. Infectious
      (1) Bacterial
        (a) Bacterial endocarditis
        (b) Lyme disease

(2) Viral

    (a) Rubella

    (b) Hepatitis B

    (c) HIV

    (d) Parvovirus

(3) Postinfectious

    (a) Enteric

    (b) Urogenital

    (c) Rheumatic fever

2. Noninflammatory: OA

Mrs. K's symptoms started after she stepped down from a bus with unusual force. The pain became intolerable within about 6 hours of onset and has been present for 3 days now. She otherwise feels well. She reports no fevers, chills, dietary changes, or sick contacts.

On physical exam she is in obvious pain, limping into the exam room on a cane. Her vital signs are temperature, 37.0 °C; RR, 12 breaths per minute; BP, 110/70 mm Hg; pulse, 80 bpm. The only abnormality on exam is the right knee. It is red, warm to the touch, and tender to palpation. The range of motion is limited to only about 20 degrees.

 At this point, what is the leading hypothesis, and what are the active alternatives? What other tests should be ordered?

ORGANIZING THE DIFFERENTIAL DIAGNOSIS

The patient's symptoms clearly localize to articular, rather than periarticular, structures since the exam reveals an inflamed joint with limited range of motion. Therefore, the differential diagnosis focuses primarily on the causes of inflammatory monoarticular arthritis, such as septic arthritis, gout, pseudogout, and trauma.

Salient points of the patient's presentation are the rapid onset of the pain; the mild, antecedent trauma; and the lack of systemic symptoms, such as fever, fatigue, or weight loss.

Given the patient's age, the single inflamed joint, and high incidence of gout, this diagnosis must lead the list. CPPDD (also called pseudogout) is common in the

knee of elderly patients, so this must also be high in the differential diagnosis. Traumatic injury to the knee such as a meniscal injury or intra-articular fracture are probably less likely given the mild nature of the injury and intensity of the inflammation of the joint.

An infectious arthritis is probably less likely, given the sudden onset and lack of systemic symptoms, but needs to be considered, as it is potentially disastrous if left untreated. Gonococcal and nongonococcal septic arthritis are possibilities. Lyme disease can affect multiple joints but most commonly causes a monoarticular arthritis of the knee. Table 19–1 lists the differential diagnosis.

Mrs. K's other medical problems include diabetes with diabetic nephropathy, hypertension, and hypercholesterolemia. Her medications are insulin, enalapril, atorvastatin, and hydrochlorothiazide. There is no history of alcohol or drug abuse.

 Is the clinical information sufficient to make a diagnosis? If not, what other information do you need?

Leading Hypothesis: Gout

Textbook Presentation

Gout classically presents in older patients with acute and severe pain of the great toe. The pain generally begins acutely and becomes unbearable within hours of onset. Patients often say that they are not even able to place a bed sheet over the toe. On physical exam, the first metatarsophalangeal (MTP) joint is warm, swollen, and red.

Disease Highlights

A. Gout is the most common crystal-induced arthropathy.

B. Gouty attacks occur when sodium urate crystallizes in synovial fluid inducing an inflammatory response and causing an abrupt, remarkably painful arthritis.

C. The primary risk factor for gout is hyperuricemia.

D. Location

    1. The classic location for gout is the first MTP joint (podagra).

Table 19–1. Diagnostic hypotheses for Mrs. K.

Diagnostic Hypotheses	Clinical Clues	Important Tests
Leading Hypothesis		
Gout	Previous episodes Rapid onset Involvement of first MTP joint	Classic presentation or demonstration of sodium urate crystals in synovial fluid
Active Alternative		
CPPDD (pseudogout)	May present as chronic or acute arthritis	Demonstration of crystals in synovial fluid or classic x-ray findings
Active Alternative—Must Not Miss		
Bacterial arthritis (gonococcal or nongonococcal)	Fever with monoarticular or polyarticular arthritis	Positive synovial (or other body) fluid cultures
Lyme disease	Exposure to endemic area History of tick bite Rash	Clinical history Serologies Response to treatment
Other Alternative		
Traumatic injury	Usually history of severe trauma	Appropriate imaging (x-ray film for fracture, MRI for cartilaginous injury)

2. The joints of the lower extremities and the elbows are also common sites.

E. Gouty attacks often occur after abrupt changes in uric acid levels. Common causes are:

   1. Large protein meals
   2. Alcohol binges
   3. Initiation of thiazide or loop diuretics
   4. New renal failure

F. Gouty attacks can also be induced by trauma.

G. The initial attack nearly always involves a single joint, while later attacks may be polyarticular.

H. Forms of gout

   1. Acute gouty arthritis is by far the most common type of gout.
   2. Chronic arthritis can develop in patients who have untreated hyperuricemia.
   3. Tophaceous gout occurs when there is deposition of sodium urate crystals in and around joints.
   4. The kidney can also be affected by gout. Patients can develop sodium urate stones or a urate nephropathy.

I. Evaluation of a patient with gout

   1. Patients with a new diagnosis of gout should be evaluated for alcoholism, renal insufficiency, myeloproliferative disorders, and hypertension.
   2. Patients in whom gout first occurs in their teens and twenties should be evaluated for disorders of purine metabolism.

Evidence-Based Diagnosis

A. Acute monoarticular arthritis is an absolute indication for arthrocentesis.

B. Sampling synovial fluid will not only rule out potentially joint destroying septic arthritis but will also usually make a diagnosis.

 Every acute, inflammatory joint effusion should be tapped.

C. Arthrocentesis

   1. Joint fluid is routinely sent for cell count, Gram stain, and culture.

2. Normal joint fluid is small in volume and clear with a very low cell count and glucose similar to plasma.

3. Characteristics of abnormal synovial fluid are shown in Table 19–2. These numbers should be used as estimates.

4. Joint fluid obtained during an acute flare of gout will have a WBC consistent with an inflammatory effusion or sometimes a septic joint.

5. The only setting in which it is reasonable not to tap a monoarticular effusion is when a septic joint is extremely unlikely and there is truly no diagnostic question. This may be the case.

   a. When a patient has recurrent effusions secondary to documented process (gout).

   b. When the diagnosis is clear (podagra for gout or joint trauma in a patient with a bleeding diathesis for hemarthrosis).

D. Clinical diagnosis

1. Despite the crucial role of arthrocentesis in the diagnosis of acute monoarticular arthritis, the diagnosis of gout can occasionally be made with some certainty without joint aspiration.

2. The following clinical points make a diagnosis of gout probable:

   a. More than 1 attack of acute arthritis

   b. Maximal inflammation in < 1 day

   c. Monoarthritis

   d. Joint erythema

   e. First MTP involvement

   f. Unilateral MTP arthritis

   g. Unilateral tarsal acute arthritis

   h. Tophus

   i. Asymmetric joint swelling

   j. Hyperuricemia

   k. Bone cysts without erosion on x-ray film

   l. Negative joint fluid culture

3. The test characteristics of a combination of these findings are provided in Table 19–3.

4. Fever may accompany acute attacks.

   a. Present in 44% of patients

   b. 10% of patients have fevers > 39.0 °C

5. Other findings that make gout more probable are:

   a. Hypertension

   b. Use of thiazide or loop diuretics

   c. Obesity

   d. Alcohol use

MAKING A DIAGNOSIS

The evaluation of this patient clearly requires joint aspiration. Septic arthritis is in the differential of any acutely inflamed joint. Although Mrs. K has only 4 criteria for gout (maximal inflammation in < 1 day, monoarthritis, joint erythema, and asymmetric joint swelling), gout remains likely given the presence of hypertension and her use of a thiazide.

X-ray films of the knee demonstrate evidence of mild OA but no evidence of fracture. Joint fluid is aspirated from the patient's knee.

Have you crossed a diagnostic threshold for the leading hypothesis, gout? Have you ruled out the active alternatives? Do other tests need to be done to exclude the alternative diagnoses?

Table 19–2. Characteristics of abnormal synovial fluid.

Characteristic	Noninflammatory	Inflammatory	Septic
Color and clarity	Yellow and clear	Yellow and cloudy	Yellow to green and opaque
WBC count	< 2000/mcL	200–10,000/mcL	> 90,000/mcL
%PMN	< 25	< 50	> 75
Glucose	Equal to plasma	Less than plasma	< 20

Table 19–3. Test characteristics of combined findings for the diagnosis of gout.

Criteria	Sensitivity	Specificity	LR+	LR−
6 or more of the clinical points[a]	87%	96%	22	0.13
5 or more of the clinical points[a]	95%	89%	8.6	0.05
Serum uric acid > 7 mg/dL	90%	54%	1.9	0.19

[a]See text for list of clinical points.

Modified from Black ER. *Diagnostic Strategies for Common Medical Problems.* Philadelphia: American College of Physicians, 1999: p. 396.

Alternative Diagnosis: CPPDD

Textbook Presentation

CPPDD generally presents in older patients. It may present with an acute flare (pseudogout) or, more commonly, as a degenerative arthritis with suspicious x-ray findings that distinguish it from OA. Patients often have other diseases associated with CPPDD, such has hyperparathyroidism.

Disease Highlights

A. CPPDD is a crystal-induced arthropathy that can be clinically indistinguishable from gout, except for the presence of calcium pyrophosphate dihydrate crystal in the joint fluid.

B. Like gout, it is caused by the inflammatory response to crystal in the synovial space.

C. There are many other similarities between pseudogout and gout.

1. Both cause acute painful monoarticular attacks.

2. Both can cause polyarticular flares.

3. Flares can be induced by trauma or illness.

4. Both can potentially cause destructive arthropathy.

5. Incidence increases with age.

D. There are some aspects of the disease quite distinct from gout.

1. Episodic "gout-like" flares only occur in a minority of patients.

2. CPPDD commonly manifests as a degenerative arthritis (in about 50% of patients).

3. It has highly specific radiologic features.

4. It most commonly affects the knee.

 Although CPPDD is commonly thought of as pseudogout, it more commonly presents as a chronic degenerative arthritis.

E. Pseudogout has been associated with a number of diseases, the most common of which are:

1. Hyperparathyroidism

2. Hypocalciuric hypercalcemia

3. Hemochromatosis

4. Hypothyroidism

5. Gout

6. Hypomagnesemia

7. Hypophosphatasia

8. Amyloidosis

Evidence-Based Diagnosis

A. Definite diagnosis of CPPDD arthritis requires demonstrations of the calcium pyrophosphate crystals in synovial fluid.

B. Certain x-ray findings are quite suggestive. The classic findings are punctate and linear calcific densities, most commonly seen in the cartilage of the knees, hip, pelvis, and wrist.

C. Proposed criteria offer findings that should alert the physician to the possibility of CPPDD:

1. Acute arthritis of a large joint, especially the knees, in the absence of hyperuricemia.

2. Chronic arthritis with acute flares.

3. Chronic arthritis that would be atypical for OA because of certain associated findings.

   a. Presence in atypical joints (wrist, shoulder)

   b. Subchondral cyst formation

   c. Tendinous calcifications

D. Evaluation of a patient with pseudogout should include testing for related diseases. The evaluation generally includes measuring the levels of the following:

1. Calcium

2. Magnesium

3. Phosphorus
4. Alkaline phosphatase
5. Iron, ferritin, and TIBC
6. Glucose
7. TSH
8. Uric acid

Treatment

A. Treat an associated underlying disease, when present.
B. Acute attacks can be managed with
1. Nonsteroidal anti-inflammatory drugs (NSAIDs)
2. Joint aspiration with corticosteroid injection
3. Colchicine
C. Chronic degenerative arthritis is difficult to treat. NSAIDs are usually used.

Alternative Diagnosis: Septic Arthritis

Textbook Presentation

Septic arthritis usually presents as subacute joint pain, the knee being most common, associated with low-grade fever and progressive pain and disability. Because the infection usually begins with hematogenous spread, a risk factor for bacteremia (such as injection drug use) is sometimes present.

Disease Highlights

A. Septic arthritis usually occurs via hematogenous spread of bacteria.
B. Joint distribution
1. The knee is the most commonly affected joint.
2. Monoarticular arthritis is the rule, with multiple joints involved in < 15% of patients.
3. Infection is most common in previously abnormal joints, such as those affected by OA or RA.
C. *Staphylococcus aureus* is the most common organism followed by species of streptococcus.

Evidence-Based Diagnosis

A. Clinical findings
1. Fever is common, occurring in about 80% of patients.
2. Fever > 39.0 °C is rare.
3. WBC > 10,000/mcL is seen in only 50% of patients.

Fever cannot distinguish septic arthritis from other forms of monoarticular arthritis. Patients with gout may be febrile while those with septic joints may not.

B. Laboratory findings
1. Definitive diagnosis is made by Gram stain and culture.
2. Gram stain of synovial fluid is positive in about 75% of patients with septic arthritis. The yield is highest with *S aureus*.
3. Joint fluid culture is positive in about 90% of cases.
4. Other fluid should also be cultured because blood and sputum may help identify an organism if one is not isolated from the synovium. About 50% of patients will have positive blood cultures.

Because of the potential for septic arthritis to cause joint destruction, a single, acutely inflamed joint should be assumed infected until proved otherwise.

Treatment

A. Antibiotic therapy is directed by Gram stain findings.
B. Empiric therapy should cover *S aureus*.
C. The affected joint should also be drained, either with a needle, arthroscope, or arthrotomy (opening the joint in the operating room).
D. In general, larger joints (eg, knees, hips, shoulder) require more than needle drainage.
E. Patients who receive treatment within 5 days of symptom onset have the best prognosis.

Alternative Diagnosis: Disseminated Gonorrhea

Textbook Presentation

Disseminated gonorrhea is classically seen in young, sexually active women who have fever and joint pain. The most common presentation is severe pain of the wrists, hands, and knees with warmth and erythema diffusely over the backs of the hands. A rash may sometimes be present.

Disease Highlights

A. Disseminated gonorrhea is a disease with rheumatologic manifestations that is seen in young, sexually active persons.

B. Women are 3 times more likely to have the disease than men.

 Disseminated gonorrhea usually occurs in patients without a history of a recent sexually transmitted disease.

C. Disseminated gonorrhea seems to present in 1 of 2 ways (with a good deal of overlap): a classic septic arthritis or a triad of tenosynovitis, dermatitis, and arthralgia.

1. The triad presentation seems to reflect a high-grade bacteremia with reactive features.

2. The tenosynovitis presents predominantly as a polyarthralgia of the hands and wrists.

3. The rash is a scattered, papular, or vesicular rash.

4. The more classic, monoarticular septic joint presentation occurs in about 40% of patients.

5. Table 19–4 gives the frequency of various findings in these 2 types of presentation.

Evidence-Based Diagnosis

A. Diagnosis is based on isolating the organism.

B. In patients with negative synovial cultures or no ef-

fusions, the blood, pharynx, and genitals should be cultured.

C. If all cultures are negative, the disease can still be diagnosed if there is a high clinical suspicion and a rapid response to appropriate antibiotics.

 Negative cultures do not necessarily exclude the diagnosis of disseminated gonorrhea.

Treatment

A. Ceftriaxone 1 g IV or IM every 24 hours or cefotaxime 1 g IV every 8 hours

B. IV therapy is generally recommended for 24–48 hours after improvement.

Alternative Diagnosis: Lyme Disease

Textbook Presentation

Lyme disease may present in different ways at different stages of the disease. A classic presentation of the joint symptoms present in the later stages would be a patient with knee pain who is from an area where the disease is endemic. There may be a history of a previous tick bite, rash, or nonspecific febrile illness.

Disease Highlights

A. Lyme disease is caused by the spirochete *Borrelia burgdorferi,* transmitted by a number of species of *Ixodes* ticks.

B. The tick most commonly transmits the disease during its nymphal stage.

C. The disease is endemic only in certain places. In the United States, it is most common along the northern Atlantic Coast, Wisconsin, and Minnesota.

D. Peak incidence is in June and July, with disease occurring from March through October.

E. The disease is generally divided into 3 stages.

1. Early localized diseased

a. Skin findings are most common, usually an area of localized erythema.

(1) 80% of patients have an acute rash.

(2) 50% of the rashes occur below the waist.

(3) The mean diameter of the rash is 10 cm.

Table 19–4. Physical signs and culture results in patients with disseminated gonorrhea.

Characteristic	Septic Arthritis	Triad
% Female	63%	77%
Tenosynovitis	21%	87%
Fever	32%	50%
Skin lesions	42%	90%
Positive blood cultures	0%	43%
"Tapable" joint effusion[a]	100%	0%

[a]Note that this is how the groups were distinguished.
Modified from O'Brien JP, Goldenberg DL, Rice PA. Disseminated gonococcal infection: a prospective analysis of 49 patients and a review of pathophysiology and immune mechanisms. *Medicine (Baltimore).* 1983;62:395–406.

(4) About 60% of the rashes are an area of homogeneous erythema.

(5) About 30% of rashes are the more classic target lesion.

(6) About 10% of the patients have multiple lesions.

 Only about 33% of patients with Lyme disease have the classic target rash on presentation.

b. Other symptoms include

(1) Myalgias and arthralgias (59%)

(2) Fever (31%)

(3) Headache (28%)

2. Early disseminated disease can involve the heart and the CNS.

a. AV node block is the most common cardiac manifestation.

b. Headache is the most common CNS finding, while meningitis and cranial nerve palsies (especially CN7) also occur.

3. Joint symptoms predominate late in the disease.

a. Occurs in about 10% of patients months after infection.

b. Monoarticular knee arthritis is the most common.

Evidence-Based Diagnosis

A. Definitive diagnosis of Lyme disease is based on clinical characteristics, exposure history, and antibody titers.

B. Antibodies may be negative early in the disease and are thus not helpful in the setting of acute infection.

C. Antibodies are nearly 100% sensitive in the setting of arthritis.

Treatment

A. There are multiple antibiotic regimens effective in the treatment of localized and disseminated Lyme disease.

B. Prophylactic treatment with a single dose of doxycycline given after a tick bite is effective at preventing Lyme disease but is generally not recommended.

C. Chronic and debilitating symptoms from Lyme disease rarely develop after appropriate treatment and, when they do occur, the etiology of these symptoms is not clear.

CASE RESOLUTION

Mrs. K's synovial fluid aspiration yielded 25 mL of translucent, yellow fluid. The WBC was about 15,000/mcL with 56% PMNs. The Gram stain was negative, and crystal exam with polarized light microscopy demonstrates negatively bire-fringent crystals consistent with sodium urate crystals, thus making the diagnosis of gout.

The inflammatory joint fluid could have been predicted by the exam. Acute gout is commonly associated with very inflamed joints, often with WBC counts higher than usually seen with other inflammatory joint conditions. The positive crystal exam makes the diagnosis of gout. This is the patient's first flare so the primary decision is how the patient's symptoms should be treated.

Treatment of Gout

A. Therapy for gout is classified as either abortive (to treat an acute flare) or prophylactic (to prevent flares and the destructive effects on the joints and kidneys).

B. Abortive therapy is outlined in Table 19–5.

1. All of the therapies are effective, and the choice is usually made by the potential adverse effect.

2. Most frequently, patients will be treated with a combination of a potent NSAID and colchicine.

Table 19–5. Immediate therapies for gout with potential adverse effects.

Therapy	Potential Adverse Effects
NSAIDs	Nephrotoxicity GI toxicity
Colchicine	GI toxicity (diarrhea)
Oral corticosteroids	GI toxicity Hyperglycemia
Intra-articular corticosteroids	Complications of joint injection Hyperglycemia

C. Prophylactic therapy

1. There are 5 basic indications for prophylactic therapy:

   a. Frequent attacks

   b. Disabling attacks

   c. Urate nephrolithiasis

   d. Urate nephropathy

   e. Tophaceous gout

2. Prophylactic therapy should begin with non-pharmacologic interventions to decrease uric acid levels and decrease the risk of gouty flares.

   a. Abstinence from alcohol use.

   b. Weight loss

   c. Discontinuation of medications that impair urate excretion (eg, aspirin, thiazide diuretics).

3. Potential prophylactic treatments are listed below:

   a. NSAIDs

   b. Colchicine

   c. Allopurinol

   d. Probenecid

   e. Sulfinpyrazone

4. Colchicine should be used during the initiation of urate-lowering therapy to prevent recurrent gouty flares.

   a. NSAIDs may be added if necessary.

   b. Colchicine is usually continued for the first 6 months of urate-lowering therapy.

5. Allopurinol is usually the first antihyperuricemic drug used.

6. If allopurinol is ineffective, uric acid excretion should be measured. Patients with low uric acid excretion should be placed on a uricosuric agent, such as probenecid.

CHIEF COMPLAINT

PATIENT 2

Mrs. C is a 50-year-old woman who comes to your office complaining of joint pain. She reports the pain has been present for about 2 years. The pain affects her hands and her wrists. She describes the pain as "a dull aching" and "a stiffness." It is worst in the morning and improves over 2 to 3 hours. She says that on particularly bad days she uses NSAIDs with moderate relief.

At this point, what is the leading hypothesis, and what are the active alternatives? What other tests should be ordered?

ORGANIZING THE DIFFERENTIAL DIAGNOSIS

Although morning stiffness is common with most types of arthritis, Mrs. C's prolonged symptoms are suggestive of an inflammatory arthritis. She does not seem to have other systemic symptoms, and she has no history of a recent infection. Even considering these facts, the differential diagnosis is broad.

RA has to lead the differential diagnosis for a middle-aged woman with a symmetric, inflammatory arthritis. The chronicity, age at onset, and joint distribution all support this diagnosis. Psoriatic arthritis can be indistinguishable from RA, especially early in its course, and needs to be considered. SLE can also present as a chronic, inflammatory arthritis. The patient is older than the average age of onset for SLE, and we have not heard about other organ system involvement.

Degenerative arthropathies such as OA and CPPDD should be considered, but the joint distribution and inflammatory nature of the arthritis makes these less likely. Table 19–6 lists the differential diagnosis.

2

Mrs. C is otherwise well, except for a history of mild hypertension managed with an angiotensin-receptor blocker. She reports no other joint pains. She does not have a history of psoriasis.

Her vitals signs are temperature, 37.1 °C; BP, 128/84 mm Hg; pulse, 84 bpm; RR, 14 breaths per minute. Her general physical exam is essentially normal. There is a 2/6 systolic ejection

Table 19–6. Diagnostic hypotheses for Mrs. C.

Diagnostic Hypotheses	Clinical Clues	Important Tests
Leading Hypothesis		
Rheumatoid arthritis	Morning stiffness Symmetric polyarthritis Commonly involves the MCP joints	Clinical diagnosis and diagnostic criteria
Active Alternative		
Psoriatic arthritis	Psoriasis Dactylitis Spinal arthritis Often asymmetric Often involves the DIP joints	Clinical diagnosis
Systemic lupus erythematosis	Multisystem disease Most common in young, African American women	Clinical diagnosis aided by serologies and diagnostic criteria
Other Alternative		
Osteoarthritis	Chronic arthritis in weight-bearing joints In the hands, DIP and PIP involvement more common than MCP involvement	X-ray film of affected joints

murmur. Joint exam reveals limited range of motion of the MCPs and wrists bilaterally. There is swelling of the third and fourth MCP on the right and the third on the left. There is pain at the extremes of motion and a boggy quality to the joints. A detailed skin exam is normal. The patient is wearing nail polish on the day of the visit.

 Is the clinical information sufficient to make a diagnosis? If not, what other information do you need?

Leading Hypothesis: RA

Textbook Presentation

RA is most commonly seen in middle-aged patients with painful, stiff, and swollen hands. Morning stiffness is often a predominant symptom. Swollen and tender metacarpophalangeal (MCP) and proximal interphalangeal (PIP) joints are usually seen on exam. Laboratory evaluation may reveal an anemia of chronic inflammation and a positive rheumatoid factor (RF).

Disease Highlights

A. RA is the paradigm for idiopathic inflammatory arthritides.

B. The sine qua non of RA is the presence of an inflammatory synovitis, most commonly involving the hands. This synovitis eventually forms a destructive pannus that injures articular and periarticular tissue.

C. RA is fairly common, present in about 1% of the population, so the diagnosis should be considered in any adult patient presenting with joint symptoms and true findings of arthritis on exam.

 RA should be considered in any adult with a chronic, symmetric polyarthritis.

D. Common findings in RA, all included in The American College of Rheumatology (ACR) diagnostic criteria for RA are:

1. Symmetric arthritis of the hands

2. Presence of serum RF

3. Presence of radiographic changes typical of RA on hand and wrist x-rays.

E. Morning stiffness is a classic finding.

1. Although many people are stiff upon awakening, those with inflammatory arthritis can experience stiffness for an hour or more.

2. Morning stiffness improves with therapy.

Morning stiffness is a good clue to an inflammatory arthritis.

F. The joints most commonly involved are

1. Hand

a. MCP and PIP joints are most commonly affected.

b. Distal interphalangeal (DIP) joints are often spared.

c. Ulnar deviation of the MCPs as well as swan neck and boutonnière deformities are classic findings.

2. Elbow

3. Knee

4. Ankle

5. Cervical spine

a. Usually presents as neck pain and stiffness

b. C1–C2 instability can occur secondary to associated tenosynovitis.

(1) This can produce cervical myelopathy.

(2) Advisable to x-ray the cervical spines of patients with RA prior to elective endotracheal intubation.

G. Once RA is established, joint destruction begins to occur and can be seen on x-rays. The chronic synovitis causes erosions of bone and cartilage.

H. Longstanding RA can cause severe joint deformity through destruction of the joint and injury to the periarticular structures.

I. Nonarticular findings are common with RA.

1. Rheumatoid nodules are usually seen over extensor surfaces.

2. Dry eyes are common.

3. Pulmonary disease (eg, pulmonary nodules or interstitial lung disease) is more common in RA than in most other rheumatologic diseases.

4. Pericardial disease

a. Asymptomatic pericardial effusion is most common.

b. Restrictive pericarditis can occur.

5. Anemia

a. RA is the textbook cause of anemia of chronic disease.

b. See Chapter 4, Anemia for a more complete discussion.

J. Still disease

1. Rarely, young adults can have acute symptoms that resemble systemic juvenile RA.

2. The classic presentation involves fevers, rash, myalgia, arthralgia and arthritis, predominantly of the knees and wrist.

3. The acuity of the presentation and associated symptoms may make differentiation from a viral arthritis difficult.

4. The diagnostic criteria require the presence of a through d and the presence of 2 from e through h.

a. Fever > 39.0 °C

b. Arthralgia or arthritis

c. RF < 1:80

d. Antinuclear antibody (ANA) < 1:100

e. WBC > 15,000/mcL

f. Classic rash

g. Pleuritis or pericarditis

h. Hepatomegaly, splenomegaly, pericarditis

Evidence-Based Diagnosis

A. The diagnosis of RA can be difficult because it may resemble other causes of inflammatory arthritis around the time of onset.

B. RF is a nonspecific test.

1. It is occasionally present in healthy people and in a number of inflammatory states such as:

a. Chronic bacterial infections

b. Viral infections

c. Parasitic diseases

d. Sarcoidosis

e. Periodontal disease

2. The test characteristics of RF are not well established with sensitivities ranging from 25% to 90% and specificities of about 95%.

C. The ACR has developed diagnostic criteria for RA.

1. A patient must have 4 of the following to make a diagnosis. If present, any 1 of the first 4 must have been present for at least 6 weeks.

a. Morning stiffness (lasting at least 1 hour before maximal improvement)

b. Simultaneous arthritis of more than 2 joint areas

    c. Arthritis of hand joints

    d. Symmetric arthritis

    e. Rheumatoid nodules

    f. Serum RF

    g. Radiographic changes (typical of RA on hand and wrist x-rays)

  2. Although meant to standardize research and not to be used as diagnostic criteria, they are helpful in highlighting the clinical characteristics of RA.

D. The ACR criteria can be used to help guide diagnosis.

  1. One recent study compared these criteria with the diagnosis of a panel of rheumatologists in patients referred for a new diagnosis of arthritis.

  2. The test characteristics for the criteria are shown in the first 2 lines of Table 19–7. They demonstrate that the criteria are only moderately helpful in making a diagnosis.

  3. The criteria can be made more helpful by changing the requirements for the diagnosis.

  4. As seen in the lower rows of Table 19–7, a patient with 6 or more criteria at any point in time essentially has RA while a patient with fewer than 2 criteria at 2 years is very unlikely to have disease.

MAKING A DIAGNOSIS

The presentation of Mrs. C's symptoms is typical for RA. She already fulfills 4 of the ACR criteria for RA. Further evaluation should be directed toward gathering other information that might suggest RA and make other diagnoses less likely.

A CBC with iron studies, RF, and ANA are done. X-ray films are ordered with fine details of the hands.

Have you crossed a diagnostic threshold for the leading hypothesis, RA? Have you ruled out the active alternatives? Do other tests need to be done to exclude the alternative diagnoses?

Alternative Diagnosis: Psoriatic Arthritis

Textbook Presentation

Psoriatic arthritis most commonly presents as joint pain in middle-aged patients with a history of psoriasis. There are signs and symptoms of an inflammatory arthritis often involving the wrists, MCP, PIP, and DIP joints symmetrically. Exam of the skin reveals psoriasis and psoriatic nail changes.

Disease Highlights

A. Psoriasis is a very common skin disease that can be complicated by arthritis.

B. Psoriatic arthritis is one of the seronegative spondyloarthropathies.

  1. The American College of Rheumatology defines the seronegative spondyloarthropathies as diseases characterized by inflammatory axial spine

Table 19–7. Test characteristics for the ACR criteria for the diagnosis of RA.

No. of Criteria	Time Frame	Sensitivity	Specificity	LR+	LR−
≥ 4 (ACR criteria)	Within 1 year of symptoms	66%	82%	3.67	0.41
≥ 4 (ACR criteria)	After 2 years of follow-up	91%	75%	3.64	0.12
≤ 1	Within 1 year	91%	50%	1.82	0.18
≤ 1	After 2 years	98%	42%	1.69	0.05
≥ 6	Within 1 year	9%	100%	∞	0.91
≥ 6	After 2 years	37%	100%	∞	0.63

ACR, American College of Rheumatology; RA, rheumatoid arthritis.

involvement, asymmetric peripheral arthritis, enthesopathy, and inflammatory eye diseases.

2. Patients with these diseases classically have a negative ANA and RF, giving the group the "seronegative" moniker.

3. Other seronegative spondyloarthropathies are ankylosing spondylitis, reactive arthritis, and the arthritis of inflammatory bowel disease.

C. The distribution of the arthritis in psoriatic arthritis is quite variable but follows 3 general presentations:

1. Oligoarthritis often involving large joints and the hands. Dactylitis, a swelling of the entire finger causing a "sausage digit" secondary to both arthritis and tenosynovitis, is a classic finding.

2. A polyarthritis similar to RA

3. A spinal arthritis

D. The arthritis can be indistinguishable from RA, especially early in the course of both diseases.

1. X-ray films of the hands can show erosions early in the disease.

2. About 10% of patients with psoriatic arthritis have a positive RF.

E. Distinguishing features include

1. Common involvement of DIP joints

2. Spine involvement that is uncommon in RA

3. Arthritis mutilans, a syndrome in which there is destruction of a finger and associated MCP causing near loss of a finger.

Evidence-Based Diagnosis

A. The most diagnostic feature of psoriatic arthritis is the presence of psoriasis.

B. Although there are reports of the arthritis preceding the skin disease, psoriasis must be present to make the diagnosis.

C. A very careful skin exam should be done in all patients in whom the diagnosis is suspected.

D. Nail findings

1. Psoriasis can cause recognizable changes in the nails (eg, pitting, oil staining).

2. Nail changes occur in only about 20% of people with psoriasis but in about 80% of people with psoriasis and arthritis.

3. Nail changes are especially common in people with DIP arthritis.

A nail exam is important when considering the diagnosis of PA. Nail polish should be removed for the visit.

Treatment

The treatment of psoriatic arthritis is similar to the treatment of RA outlined below.

Alternative Diagnosis: SLE

Textbook Presentation

SLE would classically present in a young woman with fatigue and arthritis, commonly of the hands. There are often suspicious findings in the history such as an episode of pleuritis or undiagnosed anemia.

Disease Highlights

A. SLE is a truly systemic autoimmune disease primarily affecting women of childbearing age.

B. Various groups are more prone to disease.

1. Female:male ratio is about 9:1.

2. There is a strong genetic component with resulting familial clustering.

3. African Americans are the most commonly affected ethnic group.

C. Almost every organ can be involved, although the joints, skin, and kidneys are most commonly affected.

D. The pathogenesis of the disease is related to the formation of autoantibodies to a number of nuclear antigens. The ANA is the most common.

E. The most common features of SLE, both at presentation and later in follow-up, are listed in Table 19–8.

Evidence-Based Diagnosis

A. The diagnosis of SLE, especially in people with mild disease, can be difficult.

B. The ACR has developed criteria to help in the diagnosis.

1. The criteria are:

a. Malar rash

b. Discoid rash

c. Photosensitivity

d. Oral ulcers

e. Arthritis (nonerosive arthritis)

f. Serositis (pleuritis or pericarditis)

g. Renal disorder (proteinuria or cellular casts)

h. Neurologic disorder (headache, seizures, or psychosis without other cause)

i. Hematologic disorder (hemolytic anemia or any cytopenia)

Table 19–8. Clinical manifestations of SLE at onset and during disease.

Signs and Symptoms	Prevalence at Onset	Prevalence at Any Time
Arthralgia	77%	85%
Rashes	53%	78%
Constitutional	53%	77%
Renal involvement	38%	74%
Arthritis	44%	63%
Raynaud phenomenon	33%	60%
CNS involvement (most commonly headache)	24%	54%
GI (most commonly abdominal pain)	18%	45%
Lymphadenopathy	16%	32%
Pleurisy	16%	30%
Pericarditis	13%	23%

SLE, systemic lupus erythematosis.
Modified from Buyon, JP. Systemic Lupus Erythematosus, Clinical and Laboratory Features in *Primer on the Rheumatic Diseases,* 12th ed. Atlanta, GA: Arthritis Foundation, 2001:336 © 2001. Reprinted with permission of the Arthritis Foundation, 1330 Peachtree St. Atlanta, GA 30309. To order the 12th edition of the *Primer on the Rheumatic Diseases* call 1(800)268-6942 or visit www.arthritis.org.

    j. Immunologic disorder (anti-DNA, anti-SM, or antiphospholipid antibodies)

    k. ANA

  2. The diagnosis of SLE requires the presence of 4 or more of these criteria.

  3. Although the same reservations about using diagnostic criteria clinically that were discussed above in the section of RA apply here, the SLE criteria are frequently used.

  4. The test characteristics of these criteria are given in Table 19–9. Also included in this table are the test characteristics for the various individual criteria.

C. Autoantibodies

  1. Measuring autoantibodies is very important in SLE because they provide important diagnostic information.

  2. ANA and anti-DsDNA

    a. ANA is the most sensitive test for SLE. It is very nonspecific.

    b. Anti-DsDNA is highly specific.

    c. The test characteristics of these tests are given in Table 19–10.

 A negative ANA essentially rules out SLE. A positive anti-DsDNA essentially rules in SLE.

    d. Staining patterns are often reported with the ANA.

      (1) These patterns correlate, to some extent, with the other specific antibodies discussed below and their use has, to a great extent, been supplanted by these tests.

      (2) In general, the meaning of the staining patterns are as follows:

        (a) Homogeneous: Seen in SLE, RA, and drug-induced lupus

        (b) Peripheral: Most specific pattern for SLE

        (c) Speckled: Least specific pattern. Commonly seen with low titer ANAs in people without rheumatic disease

        (d) Nucleolar: Common in patients with scleroderma and Raynaud phenomenon.

  3. Other serologies are helpful; they tend to be closely associated with various subsets of disease.

    a. Anti-RNP: High specificity, common in people with SLE and Raynaud phenomenon.

    b. Anti-Ro: High specificity, common in people with sicca syndrome (dry eyes and dry mouth). Also seen in the rare patient with ANA-negative SLE.

Table 19–9. Test characteristics for the ACR criteria and individual findings in the diagnosis of SLE.

Finding	Sensitivity	Specificity	LR+	LR−
ACR criteria	80%	98%	40	0.2
Malar rash	57%	96%	14	0.45
Discoid rash	18%	99%	18	0.83
Photosensitivity	43%	96%	11	0.59
Oral ulcers	27%	96%	6.8	0.76
Arthritis	86%	37%	1.4	0.38
Serositis	56%	86%	4.0	0.51
Renal disorder	51%	94%	8.5	0.52
Hematologic disorder	20%	98%	10	0.80
Neurologic disorder	59%	89%	5.4	0.46

ACR, American College of Rheumatology; SLE, systemic lupus erythematosis.
Adapted from Black ER. *Diagnostic strategies for common medical problems.* Philadelphia: American College of Physicians, 1999:421.

  c. Anti-histone: High sensitivity and specificity for drug-induced SLE

D. Complement

  1. Complement levels are helpful in tracking the activity of SLE.

  2. C3, C4 and CH50 levels tend to decline during episodes of lupus activity.

Treatment

A. The treatment of SLE is complicated and to a great extent the purview of the rheumatologist.

B. In general, NSAIDs, corticosteroids, and immuno-suppressants are the mainstay of therapy.

C. NSAIDs are generally used for symptomatic relief of inflammatory symptoms with careful monitoring because of their potential nephrotoxic effects.

D. Corticosteroids are commonly used at low levels in long-term therapy and in high levels for disease exacerbations.

E. Cyclophosphamide and azathioprine are the most commonly used immunosuppressants in SLE. They are used most widely for the treatment of lupus nephritis.

CASE RESOLUTION

Mrs. C's laboratory and radiology test results are as follows: Hgb, 10.5 g/dL; Hct, 31.0%; serum ferritin, 95 ng/mL (nl > 45 ng/mL); serum iron, 36 mcg/dL (nl 40–160 mcg/dL);

Table 19–10. Test characteristics for ANA and DsDNA in the diagnosis of SLE.

Test	Sensitivity	Specificity	LR+	LR−
ANA	99%	80%	4.95	0.01
DsDNA	73%	98%	36.5	0.28

ANA, antinuclear antibodies; SLE, systemic lupus erythematosis.
Adapted from Black ER. *Diagnostic strategies for common medical problems.* Philadelphia: American College of Physicians, 1999:423.

TIBC, 400 mcg/dL (nl 230–430); RF, 253 international units/mL (nl < 10 international units/mL); ANA, 2560 titer (nl < 80); Anti-DsDNA, < 10 titer (nl < 10); x-ray films of hand, periarticular erosions of the 3 clinically involved MCP joints.

The diagnosis of RA is now fairly certain. The clinical picture, as well as the laboratory test showing an anemia of chronic inflammation, elevated RF, and positive ANA all support the diagnosis. (About 40% of patients with RA have positive ANAs.) The first step in management is to control Mrs. C's symptoms. NSAIDs and prednisone are likely to accomplish this. There are already signs of joint destruction on the x-ray films, so aggressive therapy with disease-modifying drugs is indicated.

Treatment of RA

A. The treatment for RA has changed rapidly in recent years and is now, like the treatment of SLE, the purview of the rheumatologist.

B. The drugs used to treat the disease are:
1. NSAIDs
2. Corticosteroids

3. Disease-modifying antirheumatic drugs (DMARDs)
   a. Sulfasalazine
   b. Hydroxychloroquine
   c. Gold
   d. Methotrexate
   e. Cyclosporine
   f. Etanercept
   g. Infliximab
   h. Leflunomide

C. NSAIDs
1. Generally used early in the course of the disease for symptom relief while a diagnosis is being made.
2. Rarely, patients with very mild disease can remain on these medications alone.

D. Corticosteroids provide excellent symptom control and can retard progression of RA.

E. DMARDs
1. Provide symptom control and inhibit the chronic joint destruction of RA.
2. Methotrexate is the most commonly used drug in this class.

F. Patients with more severe disease also commonly receive the TNF-α inhibitors etanercept or infliximab or leflunomide, a drug that impairs T-cell function.

CHIEF COMPLAINT

PATIENT 3

Ms. T is a 21-year-old woman who comes to see you complaining of rash and joint pain for the past 2 days. She reports being well until 2 days ago when she awoke with severe pain in both knees and mild pain in both wrists. No other joints were involved. She also noted a nonpruritic rash on her distal arms and legs. She describes the rash as "splotchy." The joint pain has worsened over the last 2 days, and she reports that both her knees are swollen.

At this point, what is the leading hypothesis, and what are the active alternatives? What other tests should be ordered?

ORGANIZING THE DIFFERENTIAL DIAGNOSIS

Ms. T has acute onset polyarticular joint symptoms. From her history of knee swelling, it is likely that she has arthritis rather than arthralgias. The differential diagnosis of acute polyarthritis is extensive; the patient's demographics and associated symptoms help narrow the list.

In a young woman with arthritis and a rash, SLE needs to be considered. As discussed above, rash, arthralgias, and arthritis are among the most common presenting symptoms in patients with SLE. The acuity of the onset and lack of other organ system involvement would be a little unusual for patients with SLE. RA would be less likely given the patient's age; however, Still disease, may present acutely in young patients.

Various infectious arthritides need to be considered. Many viral illnesses can cause arthritis. Parvovirus is probably the most common. Bacterial illnesses can cause polyarthritis in many different ways. Septic arthritides, discussed above, can be polyarticular as can disseminated gonorrhea. Bacterial endocarditis can cause aseptic polyarthritis and often causes arthralgia of multiple joints. Acute rheumatic fever classically causes a migratory polyarthritis and rash and clearly needs to be considered. Lyme disease, discussed above, is most commonly monoarticular. Reactive arthritis, occurring after enteric or urogenital infections, is also a possibility.

Given that the viral arthritides are more common than bacterial ones and, as far as we know, the patient has been previously well, viral arthritis is probably more likely than bacterial disease. Table 19–11 lists the differential diagnosis.

⌄3

On further history, Ms. T reports that 10 days before she came to see you she experienced 2 days of fatigue, myalgias, and fever to 39.4 °C. There were no other symptoms. These symptoms resolved uneventfully.

She reports no travel outside Chicago, where she is in school, for the last year. She has not had a dental cleaning recently and does not use recreational drugs. She is not sexually active.

On physical exam, she appears healthy. Her vital signs are temperature, 36.9 °C; BP, 106/68 mm Hg; pulse, 84 bpm; RR, 14 breaths per minute. On extremity exam, her wrists have normal range of motion. There is pain with extremes of flexion and extension in the wrists and MCPs. There is mildly decreased range of motion and warmth in the knees as well as small effusions.

Skin exam reveals a diffuse erythematous rash with macules on the hands, feet, and distal extremities. Palms and soles are spared. The remainder of the exam was normal. There is no heart murmur.

The patient's history forces us to reorder our differential. The history of a recent febrile illness has to make a viral arthritis or postinfectious arthritis most likely. Lyme disease and bacterial endocarditis remain must not miss diagnoses but are very unlikely given her lack of suspicious exposure and the fact that she is presently well. SLE remains on the differential but is less likely.

Table 19–11. Diagnostic hypotheses for Ms. T.

Diagnostic Hypotheses	Clinical Clues	Important Tests
Leading Hypothesis		
Systemic lupus erythematosus	Multisystem disease Most common in young, African American women	Clinical diagnosis aided by serologies and diagnostic criteria
Active Alternative		
Viral arthritis, parvovirus most common	Usually a history of preceding illness	Antibody titers and serology
Active Alternative—Must Not Miss		
Rheumatic fever	Migratory polyarthritis Carditis Erythema marginatum	Jones criteria
Bacterial arthritis (gonococcal or nongonococcal)	Fever with monoarticular or polyarticular arthritis	Positive synovial (or other body) fluid cultures
Other Alternative		
Reactive arthritis	History of recent colonic or urogenital infection Presence of arthritis, urethritis, and iritis	Clinical diagnosis

In a patient with acute polyarthritis, a detailed history of recent illnesses must be taken.

Is the clinical information sufficient to make a diagnosis? If not, what other information do you need?

Leading Hypothesis: Parvovirus

Textbook Presentation

Parvovirus is commonly seen in young people who are in contact with children (mothers, teachers, daycare workers, and pediatricians). Parvovirus often presents with a macular rash 10 days after a flu-like illness with moderately severe arthralgias of the joints of the upper extremities. There is no fever and symptoms improve over the course of weeks.

Disease Highlights

A. There are 5 major manifestations of the parvovirus infection in humans.

   1. Erythema infectiosum (fifth disease) in children

   2. Acute arthropathy in adults

   3. Transient aplastic crises in patients with chronic hemolytic diseases

   4. Chronic anemia in immunocompromised persons

   5. Fetal death complicating maternal infection prior to 20 weeks gestation.

B. In adults, the acute disease often proceeds in 2 phases with the arthritis following a systemic febrile infection.

1. Initial phase

   a. Nonspecific symptoms such as fever, malaise, headache, myalgia, diarrhea, and pruritus

   b. Generally resembles a nonspecific viral infection.

2. Second phase

   a. Follows initial phase by 10 days

   b. Joint symptoms usually dominate the clinical picture.

      (1) Arthropathy accompanies about 50% of adult infections.

      (2) The arthritis is a symmetric polyarthritis commonly involving the following joints:

         (a) Elbows

         (b) Wrists

         (c) Hands

         (d) Knees

         (e) Ankles

         (f) Feet

   c. Rash

      (1) Usually lasts 2–3 days

      (2) Usually a peripheral macular rash that occasionally spreads to the trunk

      (3) Many different rashes have been described

C. Illness usually occurs between January and June

D. Attack rates of 50–60%

E. Contact with children is common among patients.

F. Other viruses cause arthritis less commonly. These are listed in Table 19–12.

Table 19–12. Common viral causes of arthritis.

Virus	Disease Characteristics
Rubella	Seen in about 50% of infection Occurs occasionally with vaccination Associated with rash
Hepatitis B	Arthritis usually precedes jaundice but is associated with transaminitis Rash may be present
HIV	May be symptoms of seroconversion or occur at other times during illness
Mumps, arboviruses, adenoviruses, coxsackieviruses, and echoviruses all associated with arthritis	

Evidence-Based Diagnosis

A. The diagnosis of parvovirus can be difficult because it can mimic other diseases.

B. Distinguishing the disease from SLE can be challenging.

    1. Both may present with arthritis, arthralgias, and rash

    2. Both are far more common in women

    3. ANA can be transiently elevated in patients with parvovirus.

C. Diagnosis is made by identifying IgM to parvovirus in the serum of patients with a suspicious symptom complex.

MAKING A DIAGNOSIS

Ms. T was treated with NSAIDs and returned in 1 week for follow-up. Laboratory tests were sent. Data returning on the day of the visit were: Chem-7, normal; liver function tests, normal; WBC, 6,800/mcL; Hgb, 12.9 g/dL; Hct, 37.9%; platelet, 182,000/mcL; ESR, 68 mm/h; rapid strep test, negative. Results that were still pending were: ANA, streptococcal antibody titers, blood cultures, stool cultures, and parvovirus titer.

Have you crossed a diagnostic threshold for the leading hypothesis, parvovirus? Have you ruled out the active alternatives? Do other tests need to be done to exclude the alternative diagnoses?

Parvovirus, or another viral arthritis, is high on the differential. Laboratory testing to rule in the most likely disease and rule out other possible diseases is reasonable. The normal liver function tests rule out hepatitis B. Negative blood cultures will make endocarditis even less likely than it is based on the history alone. Lyme disease was thought so unlikely that serologies were not even sent. Stool cultures were sent to evaluate the possibility of a reactive arthritis.

Alternative Diagnosis: Reactive Arthritis

Textbook Presentation

Reactive arthritis classically presents as a subacute arthritis, often involving the knees, ankles, and back. Physical exam reveals arthritis. There may be a history of an antecedent infection and symptoms of urethritis and conjunctivitis.

Disease Highlights

A. Reactive arthritis is an acute arthritis complicating enteric and urogenital infections. This was formerly called Reiter syndrome.

B. Reactive arthritis is often accompanied by other extra-articular manifestations such as urethritis or conjunctivitis.

C. Reactive arthritis is 1 of the seronegative spondyloarthropathies.

D. The bacteria implicated in reactive arthritis are:

    1. *Shigella*

    2. *Salmonella*

    3. *Yersinia*

    4. *Campylobacter*

    5. *Chlamydia*

E. GI infections are equally likely to be the inciting event in men and women, while arthritis complicating chlamydial infection is rare in women.

F. The mean age at diagnosis is 26 years.

G. More often than not, the inciting infection is asymptomatic.

Reactive arthritis often presents without an apparent antecedent infection.

H. Manifestations of the disease begin 2–4 weeks after the inciting infection.

    1. Urethritis is frequently the first finding followed by eye findings and then arthritis.

    2. The asymmetric arthritis has a predilection for the lower extremities.

        a. Knees, ankles, and joints in the feet are the most common locations.

        b. Dactylitis, heel pain, and back pain also occur in 50–60% of patients.

    3. Other associated findings include rash, nail changes, and oral ulcers.

    4. Table 19–13 shows the prevalence of various findings.

Evidence-Based Diagnosis

A. The diagnosis is a clinical one.

B. A high clinical suspicion is warranted in a young patient with an asymmetric oligoarthritis.

Table 19–13. Features of reactive arthritis.

Feature	Prevalence
History of diarrhea	6%
Urethritis	46%
Conjunctivitis	31%
Location of arthritis	
Knees	68%
Ankles	49%
Feet	64%
Fever > 38.3 °C	32%
HLA-B27	81%

From Arnett FC. Incomplete Reiter's syndrome: Clinical comparisons with classical triad. *Ann Rheum Dis* 1979;38(Suppl 1):suppl 73–78. Adapted and reproduced with permission from the BMJ Publishing Group.

Treatment

A. In most patients, symptoms resolve within 1 year.

B. NSAIDs are useful in treating the acute symptoms.

C. Culture positive enteric or chlamydial infections should be treated.

D. A subset of patients experience relapse, development of a chronic arthritis, or development of ankylosing spondylitis.

Alternative Diagnosis: Rheumatic Fever

Textbook Presentation

Rheumatic fever classically presents in a child in the weeks following streptococcal pharyngitis. Five cardinal manifestations are arthritis, carditis, rash, subcutaneous nodules, and chorea. The arthritis is typically migratory, involving the knees, ankles, and hands.

Disease Highlights

A. Rheumatic fever is an inflammatory disease that follows streptococcal pharyngitis by 2–4 weeks.

B. Unlike in children, clinical documentation of a previous streptococcal infection is rare in adults and the most pronounced symptoms are joint pain and stiffness.

C. The arthritis is generally described as a migratory polyarthritis.

1. Individual joints are usually affected for less than a week.

2. The joints in the legs are usually affected first.

3. Subjective complaints are often more prominent than objective findings.

D. Carditis

1. May involve any, or all, parts of the heart—pericarditis, myocarditis, endocarditis, or pancarditis.

2. Endocarditis commonly causes valvular lesions that may progress over years to symptomatic valve disease, especially mitral stenosis.

Evidence-Based Diagnosis

A. The diagnosis of rheumatic fever is based on the Jones Criteria.

B. The criteria require evidence of an antecedent group A streptococcal infection (culture, antibody titer) with either 2 major criteria or 1 major and minor criteria given in Table 19–14.

Treatment

A. Anti-inflammatories

1. Aspirin is the mainstay of therapy.

2. Corticosteroids are given to patients with severe carditis.

B. Antibiotics

1. Penicillin for treatment of pharyngitis

2. Lifelong prophylactic therapy with penicillin is usually recommended after the acute therapy.

CASE RESOLUTION

Parvovirus clearly fits this patient's presentation. Reactive arthritis is possible although the patient's recent illness was not gastrointestinal. Rheumatic fever seems less likely. Although she does have multiple Jones criteria (polyarthritis, arthralgia, elevated erythrocyte sedimentation rate [ESR]) and although the lack of a sore throat during the recent illness is not terribly helpful, the patient does not have a migratory arthritis or evidence of present streptococcal carriage.

Ms. T's blood work came back negative except for a positive ANA (titer 1:80) and a positive parvovirus IgM. She was treated with NSAIDs with good relief of her symptoms. Her rash resolved over 3–4 days, and joint pain was gone at a follow-up visit 2 weeks later.

Table 19–14. Jones criteria for the rheumatic fever.

Major Criteria	Minor Criteria
Polyarthritis	Fever
Carditis (pericarditis, myocarditis, endocarditis)	Arthralgia
Chorea	Inflammatory markers (eg, CRP, ESR)
Rash—Erythema marginatum	PR segment prolongation
Subcutaneous nodules	

CRP, C-reactive protein; ESR, erythrocyte sedimentation rate.

Treatment of Parvovirus

A. The treatment of parvovirus is symptomatic.

B. NSAIDs generally provide good relief of symptoms.

C. Symptoms usually resolve within a couple of weeks, but as many as 10% of patients have symptoms that last longer.

CHIEF COMPLAINT

PATIENT 4

Mr. L is a 55-year-old man who comes to see you complaining of right hip pain. He reports suffering with the pain for about 2 years. The pain is worst in the morning and evening. In the morning, it is associated with stiffness of his hip. The stiffness lasts about 5 minutes and then improves. At the end of the day he routinely feels a dull ache that is worse if he has had a very active day. He recently noticed that he is unable to cross his legs (right over left) without significant discomfort.

At this point, what is the leading hypothesis, and what are the active alternatives? What other tests should be ordered?

ORGANIZING THE DIFFERENTIAL DIAGNOSIS

Mr. L is a middle-aged man with chronic, monoarticular symptoms. The symptoms do not sound inflamma-tory; we have not heard about warmth, erythema, or prolonged morning stiffness.

Reviewing the initial differential diagnosis, the artic-ular process that best fits the history is OA, a chronic, noninflammatory, often monoarticular, arthritis. OA is so common in older adults that it becomes the diagno-sis to disprove in all patients presenting with pain con-sistent with OA. The disease most commonly affects the fingers, knee, hip, and spine. CPPDD is another chronic degenerative arthritis that could produce similar symptoms and should be considered.

In patients with noninflammatory monoarticular symptoms, consider the specific periarticular symptoms that can affect the particular joint.

When considering the periarticular syndromes that cause hip pain it is important to identify where exactly the patient feels the pain. Lumbar spine disease with radicular symptoms can cause pain in the buttocks or lateral hip. Trochanteric bursitis is a common cause of lateral hip pain. Inguinal hernias may cause groin pain. Femoral stress fractures may cause groin or lateral hip pain. Although such stress fractures are rare and are most commonly seen in young women, they should not be missed. Table 19–15 lists the differential diagnosis.

"Hip pain" is a nonspecific complaint. It is important to identify the exact location of the pain.

Leading Hypothesis: OA

Textbook Presentation

OA most commonly presents in older patients with chronic development of joint symptoms. Pain is usually worst with activity and improves with rest. Knees, hips, and hands are most commonly affected. On exam of joints, there is bony enlargement without significant effusions but with mild tenderness along the joint lines and limited range of motion. X-ray films are diagnostic.

Disease Highlights

A. OA is a disease of aging, with peak prevalence in the eighth decade.

B. More common in women than men.

C. Although often referred to as "wear and tear" arthritis, the pathophysiology is actually quite complicated.

D. Joint destruction manifests as loss of cartilage with damage to the underlying bone involving bony sclerosis and osteophyte formation.

E. Joint distribution
1. OA is most common in the knees, hips, hands, and spine.
2. Nearly any joint can be affected.

④

When asked to pinpoint the location of his pain, Mr. L reports that he primarily feels it in the groin. Rest, acetaminophen, and heat all seem to help the pain. He comes in today because he is in more constant pain, and he has begun to limp on bad days. His past history is remarkable only for mild asthma. He denies any previous injury to the hip. He has never been hospitalized or taken corticosteroids. His only medication is albuterol.

Vital signs are temperature, 37.0 °C; RR, 12 breaths per minute; BP, 132/70 mm Hg; pulse, 72 bpm. On physical exam, there is no warmth, erythema, or tenderness around the hip or over the trochanteric bursa. Testicular exam and hernia exam are normal. Flexion and extension of the right hip are nearly normal. There is decreased range of motion in hip rotation with about 20 degrees in internal rotation and 10 degrees in external rotation.

Is the clinical information sufficient to make a diagnosis? If not, what other information do you need?

Table 19–15. Diagnostic hypotheses for Mr. L.

Diagnostic Hypotheses	Clinical Clues	Important Tests
Leading Hypothesis		
Osteoarthritis	Chronic pain in weight-bearing joints	X-ray film of affected joints
Active Alternative		
CPPDD	May present as chronic or acute arthritis	Demonstration of crystals in synovial fluid or classic X-ray findings
Active Alternatives—Nonarticular		
Inguinal hernia	Pain worse with straining	Physical exam
Trochanteric bursitis	Lateral hip pain Tenderness over the bursa	Physical exam X-ray film Response to injection therapy
Lumbar nerve root compression	Positive straight leg raise MRI	Physical exam
Active Alternative—Must Not Miss		
Femoral stress fractures	Most common in young women involved in weight-bearing exercise	MRI Bone scan

3. Non–weight-bearing joints other than the hand, such as the elbow, wrist, and shoulder, are rarely affected by primary OA. The ankle is also not a common location.

F. Classic symptoms include:

1. Pain with activity

2. Relief with rest

3. Periarticular tenderness

4. Occasional mildly inflammatory flares

5. Gelling: Joint stiffness brought on by rest and rapidly resolving with activity.

6. Late in the disease, constant pain with joint deformation and severe disability is common.

G. Physical exam findings

1. Generally there is bony enlargement, crepitus, and decreased range of motion without signs of inflammation or synovial thickening.

2. Knee

a. Crepitus

b. Tenderness on joint line

c. Varus or Valgus displacement of the lower leg related to asymmetric loss of the articular cartilage.

3. Hip

a. Marked decrease in internal and external rotation

b. Groin pain with rotation of the hip

4. Hand

a. Tenderness and bony enlargement of the first carpometacarpal joint

b. Joint involvement in decreasing order of prevalence is DIP, PIP, MCP.

c. Heberden nodes (prominent osteophytes of the DIP joints)

d. Bouchard nodes (prominent osteophytes of the PIP joints)

5. Spine

a. Signs of spinal OA vary depending on location.

b. Pain and limited range of motion are common.

c. Radicular symptoms resulting from osteophyte impingement on nerve roots is seen.

d. Spinal stenosis with associated symptoms can result from bony hypertrophy.

Evidence-Based Diagnosis

A. The diagnosis of OA is clinical, based on a combination of compatible history, physical exam, and radiologic findings.

B. Because of the high prevalence of OA, the diagnosis should lead the differential in any patient with suspicious symptoms.

C. Diagnostic criteria have been established.

1. Hand

a. Pain, aching, or stiffness

b. 3 of the following

(1) Hard tissue enlargement of 2 or more of the following joints:

(a) Second and third DIP joints

(b) Second and third PIP joints

(c) First MCP joint

(2) Hard tissue enlargement of 2 or more DIP joints

(3) Fewer than 3 swollen MCP joints

(4) Deformity of at least 1 of the joints listed in above entries a through c.

2. Hip

a. Hip pain

b. 2 of the following:

(1) ESR < 20 mm/h

(2) Osteophytes on x-ray film

(3) Joint space narrowing on x-ray film

3. Knee: There are multiple criteria, the easiest to remember is:

a. Knee pain

b. Osteophytes on x-ray film, and

c. 1 of the following

(1) Age older than 50 years

(2) Stiffness < 30 minutes

(3) Crepitus

D. The test characteristics for these criteria are shown in Table 19–16.

MAKING A DIAGNOSIS

Mr. L's history and physical exam are very suggestive of OA, but CPPDD remains a possibility. Most of the periarticular syndromes that were considered initially have been made unlikely by the exam. Lumbar spine disease with radicular symptoms would not cause the limited range of motion that is seen on the patient's exam. Patients with trochanteric bursitis usually have more acute symptoms than did this patient, and there is tenderness over the bursa. Mr. L does not have a hernia on exam. Femoral stress fractures may cause groin pain but should not really cause limited range of motion. That said, this

Table 19–16. Test characteristics for the diagnostic criteria for OA.

Joint	Sensitivity	Specificity	LR+	LR–
Hand	94%	87%	7.2	0.07
Hip	89%	91%	9.9	0.12
Knee	91%	86%	6.5	0.10

OA, osteoarthritis.

is a diagnosis that must not be missed, so further consideration should be given.

The working diagnosis of OA was made and the patient was given 1000 mg of acetaminophen twice daily. An x-ray film was ordered.

Have you crossed a diagnostic threshold for the leading hypothesis, OA? Have you ruled out the active alternatives? Do other tests need to be done to exclude the alternative diagnoses?

Alternative Diagnosis: Femoral Stress Fractures

Textbook Presentation

Femoral stress fractures are most commonly seen in young female athletes. Symptoms begin acutely with persistent groin pain that worsens as the day progresses. On physical exam, there is often mild tenderness over the proximal one-third of the femur. Range of motion of the hip is normal. X-ray films are usually normal.

Disease Highlights

A. Like other types of stress fractures, femoral stress fractures are most common

   1. In athletes who have recently increased their level of training

   2. In women

   3. In persons with decreased bone density

B. The most common stress fractures are tibial and metatarsal.

C. Femoral stress fractures usually present with hip or groin pain with preserved range of motion of the hip.

Evidence-Based Diagnosis

A. Stress fractures in general and femoral stress fractures in particular are often not apparent on initial x-ray films.

B. MRI and bone scans are considered the diagnostic test of choice.

Treatment

A. Many stress fractures heal with reduced physical activity and short-term immobilization.

B. Femoral stress fractures may resolve with decreased weight bearing (crutches) or may require casting or internal fixation.

CASE RESOLUTION

The patient's hip x-ray film showed changes consistent with OA.

The combination of a high clinical suspicion, pain, and consistent findings on an x-ray film confirms the diagnosis.

Treatment of OA

A. Nonpharmacologic

   1. Patient education and improved social support have been shown to improve pain and improve the efficacy of pharmacologic interventions.

   2. Physical and occupational therapy can help patients with functional impairment due to OA.

B. Pharmacologic

1. Acetaminophen

    a. Standard initial therapy given its effectiveness and low side-effect profile.

    b. Equally effective to NSAIDs for mild to moderate OA.

2. NSAIDS are probably more effective than acetaminophen for severe OA.

3. Oral combinations of glucosamine and chondroitan sulfate probably are modestly effective in some patients and have a very favorable side-effect profile.

4. Intra-articular medications

    a. Hyaluronic acid given by intra-articular injection may provide a small benefit to some patients.

    b. Intra-articular corticosteroids are very effective for acute flares of OA.

5. Tramadol and opioid analgesics are reasonable choices for patients with severe symptoms.

C. Surgical

1. Arthroscopic surgery for OA is probably ineffective.

2. Hip and knee replacement can have remarkable effects on decreasing pain and improving function in patients in whom conservative therapy has failed.

REVIEW OF OTHER IMPORTANT DISEASES

Periarticular Syndromes

There are textbooks written about the numerous periarticular syndromes that commonly present to primary care physicians, orthopedists, and rheumatologists. Table 19–17 briefly outlines some of the most common.

Table 19–17. Some common periarticular pain syndromes.

Area of Pain	Diagnosis	History	Physical and Diagnostic Evaluation
Neck and shoulder	Acute cervical sprain	Pain and stiffness over neck and upper thoracic vertebrae Often first noticed when rising in the morning	Pain with tilting head Muscle spasm often palpable
	Cervical radiculopathy	Pain and stiffness of cervical spine, usually with radiation to upper back and arm Occasionally manifests solely as pain between spine and scapula	Radicular symptoms can be reproduced with manipulation of cervical spine MRI diagnostic
	Impingement syndrome	Pain inferior to acromioclavicular joint	Tenderness inferior to acromioclavicular joint Pain with passively raising shoulder while preventing "shrugging"
	Rotator cuff tear	Pain similar to above Occurs after injury in younger patients Often spontaneous in older patients	Weakness in abduction Positive Job test (patient resists downward force to an internally rotated, anteriorly stretched arm)
Elbow	Lateral and medial epicondylitis	Pain over tendon insertion on medial and lateral epicondyl	Tenderness at site of pain Exacerbated with wrist flexion (medial) or extension (lateral)
	Olecranon bursitis	Pain over olecranon bursa	Tenderness and swelling over the olecrenon bursa

Table 19–17. Some common periarticular pain syndromes.

Area of Pain	Diagnosis	History	Physical and Diagnostic Evaluation
Hand	DeQuervain tenosynovitis	Pain at the lateral base of the thumb	Worse with pincer grasp Positive Finkelstein maneuver (ulnar deviation of wrist with fingers curled over thumb)
Hip	Trochanteric bursitis	Pain over bursa Patient often notes pain when lying on area at night	Tenderness over bursa Sometimes visualized on x-ray film
	Meralgia paresthetica	Pain or numbness over lateral thigh Often after weight gain or loss	Neuropathic-type pain Abnormal sensation over lateral femoral cutaneous nerve distribution
Knee	Patellofemoral syndrome	Anterior knee pain, often worse climbing or descending stairs	Crepitus beneath patella
	Meniscal and ligamentous injuries	Ligament injuries tend to be traumatic Classically associated with the knee giving way Meniscal injuries may be traumatic or degenerative Knee locking is classic	Ligament injuries will manifest as laxity on exam Meniscal injuries as a click MRI is diagnostic
Foot and ankle	Achilles tendinitis	Pain over distal tendon Pain and stiffness worse after inactivity	Tenderness over insertion of tendon
	Plantar fasciitis	Pain anterior to heel Worse with first standing	History usually diagnostic X-ray film may show heel spur
	Morton neuroma	Pain between the second and third or third and fourth metatarsal heads	Tenderness at the area of pain
Polyperiarticular	Fibromyalgia	Diffuse pain syndrome Often nonrestorative sleep	Diagnosis depends on tenderness at 11 or more specific locations
	Polymyalgia rheumatica	Pain and disability of large muscles of shoulder and hips	Disease is often associated with signs of inflammatory disease (anemia, elevated CRP and ESR)

CRP, C-reactive protein; ESR, erythrocyte sedimentation rate.

Diagnostic Approach: Joint Pain

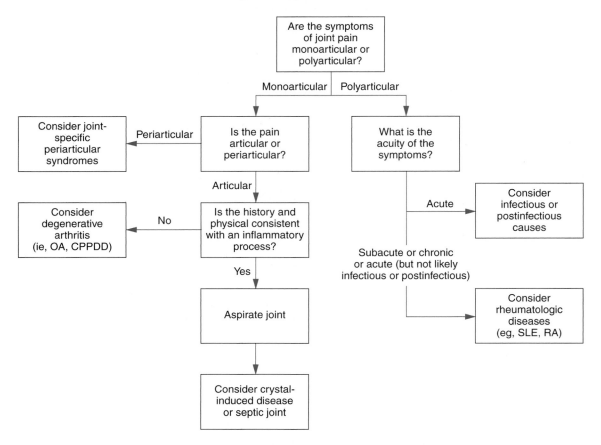

SLE, systemic lupus erythematosus; RA, rheumatoid arthritis; OA, osteoarthritis; CPPDD, calcium pyrophosphate dihydrate deposition disease.

Figure 19–A.

I have a patient with acute renal failure. How do I determine the cause?

CHIEF COMPLAINT

PATIENT 1

Mr. T is 77-year-old man with acute renal failure (ARF).

What is the differential diagnosis of ARF? How would you frame the differential?

CONSTRUCTING A DIFFERENTIAL DIAGNOSIS

ARF is defined as an abrupt decrease in glomerular filtration rate (GFR), with a concomitant increase in serum creatinine, resulting in an inability to maintain fluid and electrolyte balance. It occurs over hours or days and can occur in the presence of previously normal renal function or in patients with chronic renal failure. There is no 1 standard definition, and criteria commonly used include an increase in serum creatinine of > 0.5 mg/dL, an increase of more than 20% above baseline, or a decrease in GFR of at least 50%.

The framework for the differential diagnosis is a combination of anatomic and pathophysiologic:

A. Prerenal (due to renal hypoperfusion)
   1. Hypovolemia
      a. GI fluid loss
      b. Renal loss
      c. Hemorrhage
      d. Third spacing
      e. Decreased effective circulating volume

      (1) Congestive heart failure (CHF)
      (2) Cirrhosis
   2. Hypotension
      a. Sepsis
      b. Cardiogenic shock
      c. Anaphylaxis
      d. Anesthesia- and medication-induced
      e. Relative hypotension below patient's autoregulatory level
   3. Pharmacologic
      a. Nonselective nonsteroidal anti-inflammatory drugs (NSAIDs)
      b. Cyclooxygenase (COX)-2 inhibitors
      c. ACE inhibitors
   4. Large vessel (renal artery or vein)
      a. Thrombosis or embolism
      b. Dissection
B. Intrarenal
   1. Small vessel
      a. Atheroembolism
      b. Malignant hypertension
      c. Scleroderma
      d. Thrombotic thrombocytopenic purpura, hemolytic uremic syndrome, disseminated intravascular coagulopathy
   2. Glomeruli
      a. Rapidly progressive glomerulonephritis (RPGN)
      b. Vasculitis
   3. Tubules
      a. Acute tubular necrosis (ATN)
      b. Tubular obstruction due to uric acid crystals, light chains

4. Interstitium
   a. Acute interstitial nephritis
   b. Bilateral pyelonephritis
   c. Infiltration (lymphoma, sarcoidosis)
C. Postrenal
   1. Mechanical
      a. Ureteral (must be bilateral obstruction to cause ARF)
         (1) Stones
         (2) Tumors
         (3) Hematoma
         (4) Retroperitoneal adenopathy or fibrosis
      b. Bladder neck
         (1) Benign prostatic hyperplasia (BPH) or prostate cancer
         (2) Tumors
         (3) Stones
      c. Urethral
         (1) Strictures
         (2) Tumors
         (3) Obstructed indwelling catheters
   2. Neurogenic bladder

At this point, what is the leading hypothesis, and what are the active alternatives? What other tests should be ordered?

ORGANIZING THE DIFFERENTIAL DIAGNOSIS

Although one etiology may be more likely than the others based on the presentation, the initial testing is generally the same for every patient with ARF.

Mr. T has a classic history for pneumococcal pneumonia, and his hypotension is probably due to pneumococcal sepsis. It is likely he has been hypotensive long enough to have had renal ischemia and consequent ATN. Nevertheless, it is necessary to make sure he does not also have a component of prerenal ARF due to volume depletion. In addition, obstruction due to BPH or prostate cancer is common in his age group and must be ruled out. Post-streptococcal glomerulonephritis is not a consideration since that occurs after group A hemolytic streptococcal infections, not after pneumococcal infections. Table 20–1 lists the differential diagnosis.

Because hypovolemia and obstruction are such treatable causes of ARF, they are always "must not miss" diagnoses.

The evaluation of ARF always begins with urine electrolytes and a urinalysis.

Mr. T felt well until last night, when he had a shaking chill followed by a fever and the onset of a cough productive of rusty colored sputum. His fever has persisted, his cough has worsened, and he feels lethargic. His past medical history is notable only for well-controlled hypertension, treated with lisinopril. He smokes a few cigarettes a day and has 1 drink per week. His physical exam shows temperature, 38.6 °C; BP, 80/60 mm Hg; pulse, 110 bpm; RR, 24 breaths per minute. His mucous membranes appear dry. Lung exam is notable for decreased breath sounds and crackles at the right lung base.

One month ago, his creatinine was 1.4 mg/dL. Laboratory test results now include WBC, 16,000/mcL (70% PMNs, 20% bands, 10% lymphocytes); Hgb, 10.2 g/dL; Hct, 32%; MCV, 88 mcm³; Na, 140 mEq/L; K, 5.4 mEq/L; Cl, 100 mEq/L; HCO₃ mEq/L, 19; BUN, 40 mg/dL; creatinine, 3.8 mg/dL; glucose, 102 mg/dL.

Mr. T receives 1 L of normal saline, with no change in his BP. Urine is obtained prior to the fluid bolus and results include urine sodium, 40 mEq/24 h; urine chloride, 57 mEq/24 h; urine creatinine, 45 mg/kg/24 h; urinalysis showed specific gravity, 1.010; leukocyte esterase, negative; glucose, negative; blood, negative; protein, trace; RBC, 1–2/hpf; WBC, 1–2/hpf; positive granular casts.

Is the clinical information sufficient to make a diagnosis? If not, what other information do you need?

Table 20–1. Diagnostic hypotheses for Mr. T.

Diagnostic Hypotheses	Clinical Clues	Important Tests
Leading Hypothesis		
Acute tubular necrosis	Hypotension from any cause Exposure to toxins (especially IV contrast, aminoglycosides)	FENa Urinalysis
Active Alternative—Must Not Miss		
Hypovolemia	Orthostatic hypotension Sunken eyes Dry axilla History of vomiting or diarrhea Elderly	BUN/creatinine ratio FENa
Obstruction	Incontinence Dribbling Pelvic discomfort	Ultrasound

Leading Hypothesis: ATN

 ATN is not synonymous with ARF; it is 1 etiology of ARF.

Textbook Presentation

The presentation ranges from asymptomatic (with discovery of an increased creatinine on routine laboratory testing) to symptoms of uremia (eg, lethargy, nausea, delirium, seizures, edema, and dyspnea).

Disease Highlights

A. Etiology

  1. Ischemia (due to renal hypoperfusion prolonged enough to cause cell death)

  2. Toxin exposure (IV contrast, aminoglycosides, amphotericin B, cisplatin, Hgb, myoglobin)

B. Epidemiology and prognosis

  1. ATN accounts for 55–60% of ARF in hospitalized patients and for 11% in outpatients

 In-hospital ARF is most commonly caused by ATN due to multiple insults such as hypotension, sepsis, and nephrotoxic drugs.

  2. Can be oliguric (urinary output < 400 mL/d) or nonoliguric

  3. 80% of oliguric patients will need dialysis, compared with 30–40% of nonoliguric patients

  4. Mortality from ATN in hospitalized patients is about 37%; in ICU patients, mortality is about 78%

  5. Risk factors for increased mortality include male sex, advanced age, comorbid illness, malignancy, oliguria, sepsis, mechanical ventilation, multiorgan failure, and severity of illness.

  6. Full renal recovery generally occurs over 1–2 weeks in about 60% of survivors; a "post ATN diuresis," during which urinary output transiently increases, may be seen.

  7. Overall, 5–10% of patients require dialysis; 33% of patients who develop and survive ATN in the ICU require dialysis.

Evidence-Based Diagnosis

 Urine electrolytes, urinalysis, and serum BUN and creatinine are used to distinguish ATN from prerenal states; ultrasound is used to distinguish ATN from obstruction.

A. Urine sodium

  1. Classically, urine sodium is < 20 mEq/L in prerenal states and > 40 mEq/L in ATN.

    a. The sensitivity of urine sodium < 20 mEq/L for distinguishing prerenal states from ATN is 90%, and the specificity is 82%.

b. The LRs for urine sodium < 20 mEq/L distinguishing prerenal states from ATN are LR+ = 5 and LR− = 0.12.

2. When is the urine sodium misleading?

a. Can be increased in prerenal states if the patient has taken a diuretic, or received IV fluids prior to collection of the urine sample

b. Can be low in ATN due to rhabdomyolysis, myoglobinuria, hemolysis, sepsis, cirrhosis, CHF, and radiocontrast nephropathy

c. Is low early in obstruction, and high in obstruction lasting > 4 days

B. Fractional excretion of sodium (FENa)

1.
$$FENa = \frac{urine\ Na/urine\ creatine}{plasma\ Na/plasma\ creatinine} \times 100\%$$

2. Classically, FENa is < 1% in prerenal states and > 2% in ATN.

a. The sensitivity of FENa < 1% for distinguishing prerenal states from ATN is 96%, and the specificity is 95%.

b. The LRs for FENa < 1% distinguishing prerenal states from ATN are LR+ = 19 and LR− = 0.04.

3. Can be low (< 1%) in early ATN and ATN due to rhabdomyolysis, myoglobinuria, hemolysis, sepsis, cirrhosis, CHF, and radiocontrast nephropathy

 FENa is a better test than the urine sodium for distinguishing prerenal states from ATN; however, it is occasionally misleading.

C. Other urine tests

1. Classically, muddy brown granular casts and renal tubular cells are seen; the sensitivity and specificity of these findings are unknown.

2. Specific gravity > 1.015 and urine osmolality > 400 mOsm/kg water are associated with prerenal states.

a. Osmolality can be falsely low in prerenal states because of impairment of concentrating ability from underlying chronic renal disease, an osmotic diuresis, use of diuretics, or diabetes insipidus.

b. Sensitivity and specificity of these findings are unknown.

D. BUN/creatinine ratio

1. Classically, > 20:1 in prerenal states due to reabsorption of urea with sodium

2. Can also be elevated with GI bleeding, use of corticosteroids, intake of a high-protein diet, or increased catabolism (postoperative or infection)

3. Can be low with ARF secondary to rhabdomyolysis, or with decreased production due to malnutrition or liver disease

E. Physical exam

1. See Chapter 21, Syncope, for a discussion of measuring orthostatic vital signs and their usefulness in assessing acute blood loss.

2. The ability of the physical exam to diagnosis hypovolemia is not well studied. Available data show:

a. Orthostatic vital signs: pulse increment > 30 bpm and systolic BP decline > 20 mm Hg have moderate specificity (75% for pulse, 81% for BP) but poor sensitivity (43% for pulse, 29% for BP); LR+ and LR− are both ~1.

b. Sunken eyes (LR+ = 3.4) and dry axilla (LR+ = 2.8) are the best predictors of hypovolemia, but absence of these findings does not rule out hypovolemia.

c. Dry mucous membranes of mouth is not that helpful in ruling in hypovolemia (LR+ = 2) but has the best LR− (LR− = 0.3).

d. One study suggests that a combination of findings (eg, confusion, nonfluent speech, dry mucous membranes, dry/furrowed tongue, extremity weakness, and sunken eyes) is highly predictive of hypovolemia.

MAKING A DIAGNOSIS

Mr. T's FENa is 2.41%. He is treated with IV antibiotics and fluids, with normalization of his BP. A repeat creatinine, done several hours later, is again 3.8 mg/dL.

 Have you crossed a diagnostic threshold for the leading hypothesis, ATN? Have you ruled out the active alternatives? Do other tests need to be done to exclude the alternative diagnoses?

The combination of sepsis, a FENa > 2%, a bland urinalysis, and a lack of exposure to other toxins makes hypotension-induced ATN the most likely diagnosis. You would not expect his creatinine to improve after just a few hours of normotension, so the repeat creatinine of 3.8 mg/dL is not necessarily alarming. However, it is not possible to rule out obstruction based on the information available so far, so it is necessary to do a renal ultrasound. (ARF due to obstruction will be discussed later in the chapter.)

 Exclude urinary tract obstruction in all patients with ARF.

CASE RESOLUTION

The ultrasound shows normal kidneys, with no hydronephrosis. Mr. T's BP remains stable, and at discharge 1 week later, his creatinine is 2.0 mg/dL. He returns to see you 2 weeks later, reporting that his osteoarthritis "flared" after so much time in bed, and he has been using celecoxib for relief. His creatinine is 2.5 mg/dL. You advise him to stop the celecoxib, and a repeat creatinine 2 weeks later is 1.5 mg/dL.

NSAIDs, even selective COX-2 inhibitors, can decrease renal perfusion due to prostaglandin inhibition, leading to a prerenal ARF. Patients with abnormal renal function are at the highest risk for this complication, and such medications should be avoided. Renal function usually returns to baseline after stopping the drug.

Prevention & Treatment of ATN

A. Prevention
1. Identify high-risk patients; established risk factors include
    a. Advanced age
    b. Preexisting renal insufficiency
        (1) Remember that older patients and those with low muscle mass have a decreased creatinine clearance despite a "normal" serum creatinine
        (2) Use the Cockcroft-Gault equation to estimate creatinine clearance
            (a) Accurate only in presence of stable renal function
            (b) Estimated creatinine clearance =
            $$\frac{(140 - \text{age}) \times \text{ideal weight (kg)}}{72 \times \text{serum creatinine (mg/dL)}}$$
            $$(\times 0.85 \text{ for women})$$

 An initial small rise in serum creatinine reflects a marked decrease in GFR: an increase from 0.9 to 1.5 mg/dL represents a loss of 50% of the GFR.

    c. Diabetes
    d. Obesity
    e. Jaundice
2. Optimize intravascular volume
3. Avoid nephrotoxic drugs
    a. IV contrast accounts for 10% of hospital-acquired ARF
        (1) Generally nonoliguric and reversible, with increase in creatinine 24–48 hours after exposure, peak at 3–5 days, and recovery at 7–10 days
        (2) High-risk patients are those with creatinine clearance < 25 mL/min or between 25 mL/min and 50 mL/min *plus* 1 other risk factor (diabetes, recent administration of contrast agent, anticipated large volume of contrast, or CHF).
        (3) Moderate-risk patients are those with creatinine clearance 25–50 mL/min or between 50 mL/min and 75 mL/min *plus* 1 other risk factor.
        (4) Incidence can be reduced with the combination of oral acetylcysteine 600 mg twice daily the day before and the day of the procedure, with infusion of 0.45% saline at 1 mL/kg 6–12 hours before and after the procedure.
            (a) Number needed to treat (NNT) to prevent 1 episode of increase in creatinine = 5
            (b) Recommended for all high-risk patients; optional in moderate-risk patients
        (5) NaHCO$_3$ infusion has also been studied to prevent contrast-induced nephropathy.
            (a) 3 mL/kg/h for 1 hour before the procedure, and then 1 mL/kg/h during the procedure, and for 6 hours after procedure
            (b) Compared with similar infusion with normal saline, NNT to prevent 1 episode of increase in creatinine = 8
    b. Nonselective NSAIDs and COX-2 inhibitors
    c. Aminoglycoside antibiotics (elevated trough level is associated with ATN)
    d. Cis-platinum

B. Treatment

1. Normalize intravascular volume

2. Ensure mean arterial pressure (MAP) is > 70 mm Hg

   a. MAP = ⅓ systolic BP + ⅔ diastolic BP

   b. Elderly patients may need MAP > 80–90 mm Hg

3. Obtain renal consultation within 48 hours

4. Avoid nephrotoxic drugs, especially NSAIDs and IV contrast

5. Adjust doses of drugs for renal impairment as necessary

6. No evidence to support the use of loop diuretics, such as furosemide or low-dose dopamine; both may actually be harmful

7. Indications for acute dialysis

   a. Hyperkalemia

   b. Volume overload

   c. Metabolic acidosis refractory to medical therapy

   d. Uremic pericarditis or encephalopathy

CHIEF COMPLAINT

PATIENT 2

Mr. K is an 80-year-old man brought in by his family with the chief complaint of malaise, anorexia, and confusion for the past 3 days. He is generally healthy and independent, and he had been feeling fine, except for a cold several days ago. Over the last 3 days, his family noticed that he has seemed tired and a little confused. He has been drinking liquids but not eating much. They also report that he has had a couple of episodes of urinary incontinence, something he has never experienced before. His past medical history is notable only for osteoarthritis, for which he takes either acetaminophen or ibuprofen. On physical exam, he is alert and cooperative. His BP is 160/80 mm Hg, pulse is 88 bpm, RR is 16 breaths per minute, and he afebrile. There is no adenopathy, lungs are clear, and cardiac exam is normal. Abdominal exam shows no masses or tenderness. His prostate is mildly enlarged, without nodules. There is no peripheral edema.

Initial laboratory test results include Na, 138 mEq/24 h; K 4.8, mEq/24 h; Cl, 100 mEq/24 h; HCO₃, 20 mEq/L; BUN, 90 mg/dL; creatinine, 7.2 mg/dL.

At this point, what is the leading hypothesis, and what are the active alternatives? What other tests should be ordered?

ORGANIZING THE DIFFERENTIAL DIAGNOSIS

All 3 etiologies of ARF need to be considered. His age, prostatic enlargement, and urinary incontinence all point toward urinary tract obstruction. However, he also could have prerenal ARF from either NSAID use or intravascular volume depletion. He has no history suggesting a specific intrarenal cause, so intrarenal causes would be considered only if no postrenal or prerenal cause could be identified. Table 20–2 lists the differential diagnosis.

Mr. K's urine sodium is 20 mEq/24 h, with a FENa of 1%. He is given 500 mL of 0.9% saline intravenously. A couple of hours later, his creatinine is 7.0 mg/dL, and he reports lower abdominal pain. He has had several episodes of dribbling urine since receiving the IV fluids.

Catheterization can be a diagnostic test in ARF.

After he urinates, a Foley catheter is placed and 500 mL of urine quickly fill the bag.

Is the clinical information sufficient to make a diagnosis? If not, what other information do you need?

Table 20–2. Diagnostic hypotheses for Mr. K.

Diagnostic Hypotheses	Clinical Clues	Important Tests
Leading Hypothesis		
Urinary tract obstruction	Nocturia Incontinence Dribbling Slow stream Abdominal/pelvic discomfort Palpable bladder	Catheterization Postvoid residual Ultrasound
Active Alternative—Most Common		
NSAID use	Medication history, including over-the-counter medications	FENa Stopping medication
Active Alternative—Must Not Miss		
Hypovolemia	Orthostatic hypotension Sunken eyes Dry axilla History of vomiting or diarrhea Elderly	FENa BUN/creatinine ratio Fluid challenge

Leading Hypothesis: Urinary Tract Obstruction

Textbook Presentation

Symptoms vary with site, degree, and rapidity of onset of the obstruction, ranging from severe pain with acute obstruction to mild or no pain. Incontinence and dribbling are common.

Disease Highlights

A. Clinical manifestations

1. Upper ureteral or renal pelvic lesions cause flank pain; lower obstruction causes pelvic pain that can radiate to the ipsilateral testicle or labium.

2. Urinary output

   a. Anuria, if obstruction is complete

      (1) Anuria is defined as < 100 mL of urine per day.

      (2) Also seen in shock, vascular lesions, severe ATN, or severe glomerulonephritis.

   b. Output can be normal or increased with partial obstruction.

   c. Increased output is due to tubular injury that impairs concentrating ability and sodium reabsorption.

   d. Incontinence, dribbling, decreased output, and hematuria may be present.

B. Obstruction accounts for 17% of cases of outpatient ARF, and for 2–5% of cases of inpatient ARF.

C. Patients can have type 1 renal tubular acidosis with hyperkalemia due to tubular injury.

D. Prognosis

1. Complete recovery of renal function occurs if total ureteral obstruction is relieved within 7 days; little or no recovery occurs if the total obstruction is present for 12 weeks.

   a. Complete or prolonged partial obstruction can lead to tubular atrophy and irreversible loss of renal function.

   b. Obstruction is a rare cause of end-stage renal disease.

2. Prognosis of partial obstruction is unpredictable.

Evidence-Based Diagnosis

A. Urine electrolytes are not very helpful.

B. Postvoid residual is normally < 100 mL; it will be increased only if obstruction is distal to the ureters.

C. Renal ultrasound

1. Has a sensitivity of 80–85% for detecting postrenal ARF, defined as finding dilatation of the collecting system *and* the site of the obstruction

2. There are 3 settings in which obstruction can occur without dilatation of collecting system.

    a. Within the first 1–3 days, due to relative lack of compliance of collecting system

    b. Can have hydronephrosis without ureteral dilatation in retroperitoneal fibrosis, which is better seen on CT scan

    c. With obstruction so mild that there is no impairment in renal function

3. Duplex ultrasound can identify unilateral obstruction early by detecting an increased resistive index compared with the other kidney; however, it cannot be used to diagnose bilateral obstruction.

D. CT scan can detect sites of obstruction missed on ultrasound.

E. Intravenous pyelography

    1. Used if site of obstruction cannot be seen on ultrasound or CT

    2. Especially useful for identifying papillary necrosis or caliceal blunting from previous infection

MAKING A DIAGNOSIS

A renal ultrasound shows bilateral ureteral dilatation and hydronephrosis, confirming the diagnosis of urinary tract obstruction. He is admitted to the hospital, and over several days, his creatinine returns to baseline of 1.5 mg/dL. The catheter is removed, and he urinates with his usual mild difficulty starting the stream. Several days after discharge, he arrives in the emergency department, reporting that he cannot urinate at all. As instructed, he has avoided all NSAID use but has been taking pseudoephedrine for cold symptoms.

Have you crossed a diagnostic threshold for the leading hypothesis, urinary tract obstruction? Have you ruled out the active alternatives? Do other tests need to be done to exclude the alternative diagnoses?

No further tests are necessary to diagnose the cause of his ARF; however, it is important to determine the cause of the urinary tract obstruction, and that of his new, related problem, acute urinary retention.

Related Diagnosis: Acute Urinary Retention

Acute urinary retention is most commonly seen in older men with prostatic hypertrophy causing bladder neck obstruction (seen in 10% of men in their 70s and up to 33% of men in their 80s). The risk is increased for older men, for those with moderate to severe lower urinary tract symptoms, for those with a flow rate < 12 mL/sec, and for those with a prostate volume > 30 mL by transrectal ultrasound.

In women, acute urinary retention is usually due to neurogenic bladder, and in younger patients, it is usually due to neurologic disease. Medications that commonly induce urinary retention in susceptible patients include antihistamines, anticholinergics, antispasmodics, tricyclic antidepressants, narcotics, and α-adrenergic agonists.

1. BPH

Textbook Presentation

The classic presentation is urinary frequency, nocturia, reduced stream, and dribbling at the end of urination in an older man.

Disease Highlights

A. Defined as microscopic (histologic evidence of cellular proliferation), macroscopic (actual enlargement of the prostate), or clinical (symptoms resulting from macroscopic BPH)

B. Symptoms include lower urinary tract symptoms, bladder outlet obstruction, hematuria, urinary tract infections

C. Prostate size does not correlate with symptom severity.

    1. Prostate growth is 0.4 mL/year in younger men; 1.2 mL/year in older men.

    2. However, men with prostates > 30 mL, and especially > 40 mL, are more likely to have symptoms.

    3. Can use International Prostate Symptom Score to assess severity of symptoms and assess response to therapy.

        a. There are 7 questions to be answered on a 0 to 5 scale, yielding a potential total of 35 points (Table 20–3).

        b. 0–7 = mild BPH, 8–19 = moderate BPH, 20–35 = severe BPH

Table 20–3. International Prostate Symptom Score.

Over the past month, how often ...	Not at All	< 1 Time in 5	< Half the Time	About Half the Time	> Half the Time	Almost Always
have you had a sensation of not emptying your bladder completely after you finished urinating?	0	1	2	3	4	5
have you had to urinate again less than 2 hours after you finished urinating?	0	1	2	3	4	5
have you found you stopped and started again several times when you urinated?	0	1	2	3	4	5
have you found it difficult to postpone urination?	0	1	2	3	4	5
have you had a weak urinary stream?	0	1	2	3	4	5
have you had to push or strain to begin urination?	0	1	2	3	4	5
did you most typically get up to urinate from the time you went to bed at night until the time you got up in the morning?	0	1	2	3	4	5

Scoring key: 0–7, mild; 8–19, moderate; 20–35, severe.

Modified, with permission, from Barry MJ et al. The American Urological Association symptoms index for benign prostatic hyperplasia. *J Urol.* 1992;148:1549.

Evidence-Based Diagnosis

A. Guidelines recommend all patients have a digital rectal exam, urinalysis, and serum creatinine; other testing (urodynamics, imaging) is optional.

B. A prostate specific antigen should be checked in those men who would consider treatment for prostate cancer.

C. Urinary flow rates, urodynamic measurements, and amount of postvoid residual do not correlate well with symptoms.

D. Digital rectal exam

   1. Cannot ascertain anterior or posterior extension or feel entire posterior surface.

   2. Therefore, prostate size is underestimated by 25–55% on digital rectal exam, compared with transrectal ultrasound; the underestimation increases the larger the prostate volume.

 The prostate is even bigger than you think it is on digital rectal exam.

Treatment

A. Indications for surgical intervention include moderate to severe symptoms not responsive to medical therapy, acute urinary retention, recurrent infections or hematuria, and azotemia.

B. The α-blockers terazosin and tamsulosin have been shown to be superior to placebo in reducing lower urinary tract symptoms and increasing flow rates.

C. 5-α-reductase inhibitors

   1. Finasteride reduces symptoms when the prostate is > 40 mL.

   2. Slow onset of action: weeks to months

   3. Might also reduce risk of acute urinary retention and need for surgery.

CASE RESOLUTION

He is catheterized, and 500 mL of urine is obtained. Because the urinary retention was precipitated by the use of an α-adrenergic agent (pseudoephedrine), he is given tamsulosin and the catheter is removed on a trial basis. He is again unable to urinate. He then undergoes transurethral resection of the prostate (TURP) with resolution of his urinary symptoms. His creatinine stays at 1.5 mg/dL throughout these events.

Treatment of Urinary Tract Obstruction

A. Relieve the obstruction immediately.

   1. Modalities

      a. Foley catheter for bladder neck obstruction

      b. Suprapubic catheter if Foley is not possible

      c. Percutaneous nephrostomy tubes for ureteral obstruction

   2. Consequences

      a. Rapid decompression of the bladder can theoretically lead to hematuria and even hypotension; not generally seen clinically

      b. Will often see a postobstructive diuresis; ie, an initial urinary output of 500–1000 mL/h

         (1) Represents an attempt to excrete fluid retained during the period of obstruction

         (2) Not necessary to replace entire urinary output; doing so will increase the diuresis

         (3) Should treat with normal replacement fluids

B. Correct the underlying cause of the obstruction.

CHIEF COMPLAINT

Mrs. F is a 63-year-old woman with a history of diastolic dysfunction, hypertension, and osteoarthritis. Her usual medications are atenolol, lisinopril, and acetaminophen, and her usual serum creatinine is 1.5 mg/dL. Three weeks ago, she came to see you reporting severe pain, erythema, and swelling of her right first metatarsophalangeal joint. You diagnosed gout, and prescribed indomethacin 25 mg 3 times daily to use until the gout resolved. She returned for follow-up yesterday, reporting that the gout had resolved in a few days, but that she kept taking the indomethacin because it helped her arthritis so much. Despite your reservations, you agree to refill the prescription because she clearly feels so much better than usual. Today you receive the results of the blood tests you ordered during the visit: Na, 141 mEq/24 h; K, 5.0 mEq/24 h; Cl, 100 mEq/24 h; HCO_3, 20 mEq/L; BUN, 32 mg/dL; creatinine, 2.5 mg/dL.

At this point, what is the leading hypothesis, and what are the active alternatives? What other tests should be ordered?

ORGANIZING THE DIFFERENTIAL DIAGNOSIS

At this point, the differential for her new renal insufficiency is quite broad, but it is logical to focus on the 1 new intervention since her last visit, the use of indomethacin. Through prostaglandin inhibition, NSAIDs can cause decreased renal blood flow, leading to a prerenal state. NSAIDs are also 1 of the classes of drugs most commonly associated with an intrarenal disease, interstitial nephritis. Although obstruction must always be considered, she is having no urinary symptoms and has no risk factors. Table 20–4 lists the differential diagnosis.

Table 20–4. Diagnostic hypotheses for Mrs. F.

Diagnostic Hypotheses	Clinical Clues	Important Tests
Leading Hypothesis		
NSAID-induced renal hypoperfusion	Use of NSAIDs History of renal disease CHF	FENa Stopping the medication
Active Alternative		
Interstitial nephritis	Flank pain Hematuria	Stopping the medication Urine eosinophils Renal biopsy

Mrs. F's urine sodium is 35 mEq/24 h, and the FENa is 1.5%. Urinalysis shows 2+ protein, 3 RBCs/hpf, 5–10 WBCs/hpf, and no casts.

Is the clinical information sufficient to make a diagnosis? If not, what other information do you need?

Leading Diagnosis: NSAID-Induced Renal Hypoperfusion

Textbook Presentation
ARF caused by NSAIDs is usually asymptomatic and is most commonly detected by finding an increased serum creatinine.

Disease Highlights
A. Can occur with nonselective NSAIDs and COX-2 inhibitors.

B. Seen within 3–7 days of starting therapy

C. Renal prostaglandins are not important regulators of blood flow in normal kidneys.

D. Release of prostanglandins is increased by underlying glomerular disease, renal insufficiency, hypercalcemia, and vasoconstrictors such as angiotensin II and norepinephrine, which are released in volume depletion, CHF, and cirrhosis.

E. Prostaglandin inhibition in such patients can lead to significant decreases in renal blood flow, consequent reversible renal ischemia, and ARF.

Evidence-Based Diagnosis
A. FENa should be < 1%. (Sensitivity and specificity are unknown.)

B. Should reverse when the drug is stopped.

Treatment
Stop the exposure.

MAKING A DIAGNOSIS

You call Mrs. F and tell her to stop taking the indomethacin. One week later, her creatinine is still 2.5 mg/dL. Urine eosinophils are negative.

Have you crossed a diagnostic threshold for the leading hypothesis, NSAID-induced renal hypoperfusion? Have you ruled out the active alternatives? Do other tests need to be done to exclude the alternative diagnoses?

Mrs. F's FENa is higher than expected for NSAID-induced renal hypoperfusion. She has not used diuretics or received IV fluids, both of which can cause a falsely elevated urine sodium and FENa. In addition, her creatinine has not improved. Therefore, it is unlikely that prostaglandin inhibition is the reason for her renal insufficiency.

Alternative Diagnosis: Interstitial Nephritis

Textbook Presentation

Classic symptoms include renal insufficiency, hematuria, pyuria with WBC casts, fever, and eosinophilia. The full syndrome is rarely seen today since it occurs primarily with methicillin-induced acute interstitial nephritis.

Disease Highlights

A. Interstitial nephritis is found in 2–3% of all renal biopsies, and in up to 15% of patients who had a biopsy done for ARF.

B. Etiology

   1. In 1 case series, 10% of cases were caused by infection, 85% of cases were caused by medications, and 4% of cases were idiopathic.

   2. Can be caused by many medications

     a. Antibiotics—most commonly ampicillin, ciprofloxacin, penicillin G, rifampin, sulfonamides

     b. NSAIDs—most commonly fenoprofen, ibuprofen, indomethacin, naproxen, aspirin, phenylbutazone, piroxicam

     c. COX-2 inhibitors

     d. Diuretics—most commonly furosemide

     e. Anticonvulsants—most commonly phenytoin

     f. Cimetidine, omeprazole, allopurinol

   3. Can be caused by sarcoidosis, and streptococcal and viral infections

C. Clinical manifestations

   1. Renal manifestations develop within 3 weeks in 80% of patients, with an average delay of 10 days (range 1 day to 18 months; longer delays often seen with NSAIDs).

   2. Symptoms develop more rapidly if patient is rechallenged with the offending drug.

   3. Clinical presentation is often incomplete.

     a. The most suggestive presentation, a combination of renal insufficiency, mild proteinuria, abnormal urinalysis, normal BP, no edema, and flank pain, is seen in less than 25% of cases.

     b. Hematuria (usually microscopic), pyuria, and flank pain are each seen in about 50% of cases.

     c. Extrarenal symptoms (fever, rash) are seen in < 50% of cases (< 10% of cases of NSAID-induced interstitial nephritis)

     d. Proteinuria is more prominent in NSAID-induced interstitial nephritis (often nephrotic range with NSAIDs; otherwise, usually < 1 g/d)

     e. Less than 20% of patients are oliguric.

The absence of fever, rash, eosinophilia, or eosinophiluria does *not* rule out interstitial nephritis.

D. Prognosis

   1. Most patients improve within 6–8 weeks and return to baseline renal function.

   2. Diffuse infiltrates and frequent granulomas on biopsy, intake of the offending drug for longer than 1 month, delayed response to prednisone, and persistent renal failure after 3 weeks are predictors of irreversible injury.

Evidence-Based Diagnosis

A. Sensitivity of urine eosinophils is 67% and specificity is 83% (LR+ = 3.9; LR− = 0.39).

B. FENa usually > 1%

C. Gallium scan

   1. Substantial renal uptake in acute interstitial nephritis, but also see uptake in glomerulonephritis, pyelonephritis, and other conditions

   2. Sensitivity and specificity are not well defined.

   3. No uptake with ATN, so possibly useful in distinguishing ATN from acute interstitial nephritis

D. Renal biopsy is gold standard.

CASE RESOLUTION

Her urinalysis is consistent with interstitial nephritis, and the lack of urine eosinophils does not rule out the diagnosis. Renal biopsy is performed, which shows inflammatory infiltrates in the interstitium. Her renal function returns to baseline after several weeks without any exposure to NSAIDs.

Treatment of Acute Interstitial Nephritis

A. Stop exposure, if possible.

B. Corticosteroids are sometimes used, but there are no prospective randomized clinical trials.

1. Consider in patients whose renal function does not improve within 1 week of stopping exposure, after biopsy confirms diagnosis.

2. Consider empiric trial in patients who have worsening renal function and suspected acute interstitial nephritis, and who are poor candidates for biopsy.

3. NSAID-induced acute interstitial nephritis is less responsive to corticosteroid therapy.

4. Should see improvement in 2–3 weeks.

Summary Table

	Prerenal	Intrarenal	Postrenal
History	History of hemorrhage, vomiting or diarrhea, burns, pancreatitis, CHF, or cirrhosis Elderly	Hypotension from any cause Exposure to toxins (especially IV contrast, aminoglycosides) Infections	Nocturia Incontinence Dribbling Slow stream Flank pain Anuria Abdominal or pelvic discomfort
Physical exam	Orthostatic hypotension Sunken eyes Dry axilla	Edema Livedo reticularis Rash Petechiae	Palpable bladder Enlarged prostate
Urine sediment	Bland	Granular casts (ATN) or WBCs + casts (AIN) or RBCs + casts (GN)	Bland or RBCs
Protein	None or low	None or low, EXCEPT GN, when there is proteinuria	Low
FENa (%)	< 1	> 1	< 1 (acute); > 1 chronic

CHF, congestive heart failure; ATN, acute tubular necrosis; AIN, acute interstitial nephritis; GN, glomerulonephritis.

I have a patient with syncope.
How do I determine the cause?

CHIEF COMPLAINT

PATIENT 1

Mr. M is a 23-year-old medical student who had an episode of syncope this morning after entering his anatomy lab for the first time. He is quite alarmed (and embarrassed).

What is the differential diagnosis of syncope? How would you frame the differential?

CONSTRUCTING A DIFFERENTIAL DIAGNOSIS

Syncope is the transient complete loss of consciousness. The differential diagnosis is easily remembered by considering the brain's requirements to maintain consciousness. Derangement of any of these requirements may result in syncope. Consciousness requires the following:

1. Organized electrical activity

2. Glucose

3. Oxygen

4. A functional delivery system to deliver oxygen and glucose. This in turn requires open vascular conduits and adequate BP.

By far, most causes of syncope result from inadequate BP. Therefore, it is useful to look at the determinants of BP.

BP = cardiac output (CO) × total peripheral resistance (TPR)

CO = stroke volume (SV) × heart rate (HR)

Simple substitution: BP = SV × HR × TPR

SV = end-diastolic volume (EDV) − end-systolic volume (ESV)

Simple substitution: BP = (EDV − ESV) × HR × TPR

In summary, the differential diagnosis of syncope can be remembered by considering the requirements for consciousness (ie, BP [determined by EDV, ESV, HR, TPR], organized electrical activity, glucose, oxygen, and open vascular conduits).

Differential Diagnosis of Syncope

A. BP = (EDV − ESV) × HR × TPR
  1. Inadequate EDV (poor filling)
     a. Dehydration
     b. Hemorrhage
     c. Pulmonary embolism (PE)
  2. Elevated ESV (inadequate emptying)
     a. Aortic stenosis
     b. Asymmetric septal hypertrophy
  3. Heart rate disorders
     a. Tachycardias
        (1) Ventricular tachycardia (VT)
        (2) Supraventricular tachycardia associated with accessory pathway (Wolff-Parkinson-White syndrome [WPW])
     b. Bradycardias
        (1) Neurocardiogenic syncope
        (2) Sinus node disorders
           (a) Sinus bradycardia (< 35 beats per minute)
           (b) Sinus pauses (> 3 seconds or > 2 seconds with symptoms)
        (3) Atrioventricular (AV) block (second- or third-degree)

    (4) Hypersensitive carotid syndrome (cardio-inhibitory type)

4. Decreased TPR (vasodilatation)

    a. Drugs (α-blockers, vasodilators, nitrates, tricyclic antidepressants, and phenothiazines)

    b. Hypersensitive carotid (vasodepressor type)

    c. Sepsis (usually causes protracted hypotension rather than syncope)

    d. Addison disease (usually causes protracted hypotension rather than syncope)

B. Disorganized electrical activity: Generalized seizures

C. Hypoglycemia

    1. Iatrogenic (eg, insulin and sulfonylureas)

    2. Insulinomas (exceedingly rare)

D. Hypoxemia (usually results in impaired consciousness or coma rather than syncope)

E. Obstructed vascular conduits

    1. Vertebral obstruction

        a. Vertebrobasilar insufficiency

        b. Subclavian steal

    2. Bilateral carotid obstruction

Mr. M reports that he was in his usual state of health and felt perfectly well prior to entering the anatomy dissection room. Upon viewing the cadaver, he felt queasy and warm. He became diaphoretic and collapsed to the floor. When he regained consciousness, he was not confused. The instructor told him that he was unconscious for only a few seconds.

> **At this point, what is the leading hypothesis and what are the active alternatives? What tests should be ordered?**

ORGANIZING THE DIFFERENTIAL DIAGNOSIS

Mr. M's history is classic for neurocardiogenic syncope. Neurocardiogenic syncope is often precipitated by a highly emotional event or painful stimulus. Patients may experience nausea, diaphoresis, and then brief syncope with a rapid return to normal consciousness. It is also important to consider other common causes of syncope such as dehydration or medications. "Must not miss" diagnoses include cardiac syncope and seizures. Clues that might suggest a cardiac cause include any history of structural heart disease, congestive heart failure (CHF), ischemic heart disease, significant murmurs, advanced age, or syncope that occurs with exercise. Lastly, seizures should be considered. They are usually accompanied by a prolonged postictal period characterized by lethargy and confusion. Table 21–1 lists the differential diagnosis.

Mr. M reports no diarrhea or vomiting, and he is not taking any medications. He has no known heart disease and exercises vigorously without symptoms. There is no history of confusion following the syncope, tonic-clonic activity, or incontinence. On physical exam, his BP and pulse are normal and do not change with standing. Cardiac exam reveals a regular rate and rhythm without a significant murmur, JVD, or S_3 gallop.

> **Is the clinical information sufficient to make a diagnosis? If not what other information do you need?**

Leading Hypothesis: Neurocardiogenic (Vasovagal) Syncope

Textbook Presentation

Neurocardiogenic syncope typically develops in young patients following prolonged standing or in association with pain or anxiety (ie, phlebotomy). Lightheadedness, nausea, and diaphoresis may precede syncope, which is brief.

Disease Highlights

A. Most common cause of syncope (approximately 33% of cases)

B. Pathophysiology (Figure 21–1)

C. Situational syncope is a variant of neurocardiogenic syncope, which follows micturation particularly while upright after excessive alcohol ingestion.

Evidence-Based Diagnosis

A. History

    1. Abdominal discomfort prior to syncope increases the likelihood of neurocardiogenic syncope; LR+ 8, LR− 0.93

Table 21–1. Diagnostic hypotheses for Mr. M.

Diagnostic Hypotheses	Clinical Clues	Important Tests
Leading Hypothesis		
Neurocardiogenic syncope (faint)	Preceding pain, anxiety, fear or prolonged standing Rapid normalization of consciousness Absence of heart disease	Tilt table if recurrent
Active Alternatives—Most Common		
Dehydration	History of vomiting, diarrhea, poor oral intake	Orthostatic measurement of BP and pulse
Medications	History of α-blockers, other antihypertensive medication	Orthostatic measurement of BP and pulse
Active Alternatives—Must Not Miss		
Cardiac syncope	History of prior heart disease (CHF, CAD) Unprovoked syncope Syncope with exercise Significant murmur Irregular pulse JVD or S_3	ECG Echocardiogram Stress test Electrophysiologic study
Seizure	Prolonged period of lethargy, confusion, or amnesia following syncope suggesting postictal period Tonic-clonic activity Incontinence Tongue biting	EEG

2. Nausea after syncope also increases the likelihood of neurocardiogenic syncope; LR+ 3.5, LR– 0.9

B. Laboratory and radiologic tests

1. Patients with a typical history and no evidence of heart disease do not require further testing.

2. Patients with an atypical history (ie, without a clear precipitant) require an ECG, echocardiogram, and occasionally tilt-table testing.

3. Tilt-table testing is particularly useful in patients with recurrent events in whom the diagnosis is unclear. The patient is initially supine for 20–45 minutes. The table is then tilted to 60–80 degrees and the patient kept upright for 30–45 minutes during which time the pulse and BP are continuously monitored.

   a. Criteria for a positive test include the reproduction of the presyncopal or syncopal symptoms with hypotension, bradycardia, or both.

   b. Sensitivity is 32–85% and specificity ≅ 90%, but they cannot be precisely determined due to the lack of a gold standard. Furthermore, estimates vary depending on tilt table angle, duration, and medications used. A variety of medications can increase sensitivity but decrease specificity (eg, isoproterenol and nitrates).

C. Carotid hypersensitivity is another variant of neurally mediated syncope.

1. Precipitated by pressure on carotid body (eg, buttoning collar, shaving, or cervical motion).

2. Hypotension or syncope may develop secondary to bradycardia, vasodilatation, or both (mixed).

3. Diagnosis

   a. Carotid sinus massage (CSM) for 5–10 seconds during continuous electrocardiographic monitoring producing symptoms and > 3 second pause or > 50 mm Hg drop in BP

Pathophysiology of Neurocardiogenic Syncope

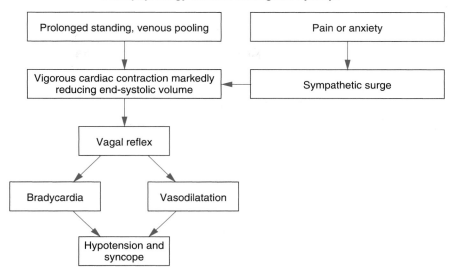

Figure 21–1.

   b. CSM is contraindicated in patients with carotid bruits, recent cerebrovascular accident, myocardial infarction (MI) (within 6 months), or severe dysrrhythmias.

4. Pacemakers can be useful in patients with syncope secondary to cardio-inhibitory carotid hypersensitivity.

MAKING A DIAGNOSIS

Mr. M's well-defined precipitant for neurocardiogenic syncope and typical premonitory symptoms combined with the absence of red flags for serious cardiac syncope (such as CHF, ischemic heart disease, advanced age, or abnormal physical exam) makes neurocardiogenic syncope the most likely diagnosis. Tilt-table testing is not indicated in patients with isolated episodes of well-defined neurocardiogenic syncope. Other diagnostic testing is not warranted.

CASE RESOLUTION

> 1
>
> Mr. M is reassured, and although embarrassed, he feels much better. After explaining the pathophysiology of his disorder, you initiate standard recommendations for the prevention of further episodes.

Treatment of Neurocardiogenic Syncope

A. Patients should be reassured, instructed to avoid triggers, and become supine if they notice the premonitory signs of an impending faint.

B. β-Blockers slow HR and improve ventricular filling. While successful in short-term trials, long-term placebo controlled trials have not demonstrated a benefit. The use of β-blockers is therefore controversial. Other therapies have included fludrocortisone and selective serotonin reuptake inhibitors.

C. "Rate drop" dual chamber pacemakers (triggered by a sudden drop in HR) may be effective in some patients with recurrent severe neurocardiogenic syncope associated with profound bradycardia or asystole. This should only be considered in severe drug refractory cases.

CHIEF COMPLAINT

PATIENT 2

Mr. C is a 65-year-old man who comes to see you with a chief complaint of syncope. He reports that he was sitting at home watching television when he suddenly lost consciousness without any warning. His wife reports that he was unresponsive for approximately 30 seconds. There was no tonic-clonic activity or incontinence, and the patient was not confused after regaining consciousness.

At this point, what is your leading hypothesis and what are the active alternatives? What other tests should be ordered?

ORGANIZING THE DIFFERENTIAL DIAGNOSIS

Mr. C's sudden loss of consciousness without warning or precipitant and his age raise the possibility of some form of cardiac syncope. Active alternatives include orthostatic syncope (secondary to dehydration, hemorrhage, or drugs) and hypoglycemia-induced syncope. Hypoglycemia-induced syncope is usually preceded by either confusion or sympathetic stimulation producing tremulousness, nervousness, or diaphoresis and occurs almost exclusively in diabetic patients taking insulin, sulfonylureas, or thiazolidinediones. "Must not miss" alternatives include PE, which is an uncommon cause of syncope. Neurocardiogenic syncope is unlikely because syncope occurred while Mr. C was sitting and was not preceded by any pain or anxiety. The absence of any postsyncopal confusion makes seizure unlikely. Table 21–2 lists the differential diagnosis.

Table 21–2. Diagnostic hypotheses for Mr. C.

Diagnostic Hypotheses	Clinical Clues	Important Tests
Leading Hypothesis		
Cardiac syncope	History of CAD, CHF, or valvular heart disease Syncope while supine or with exercise Palpitations S_3, JVD, or significant murmur	ECG Echocardiogram Stress test Event monitor EP study
Active Alternatives—Most Common		
Dehydration or hemorrhage	History of vomiting, diarrhea, poor oral intake History of melena or rectal bleeding Positive fecal occult blood test	Orthostatic measurement of BP and pulse
Medications	History of α-blockers, other antihypertensive medication	Orthostatic measurement of BP and pulse
Hypoglycemia	Insulin, sulfonylureas, or thiazolidinediones therapy	Glucose measurement at time of event
Active Alternatives—Must Not Miss		
PE	Risk factors for PE Pleuritic chest pain or dyspnea Loud S_2 Unexplained persistent hypotension Right heart strain on ECG (right bundle-branch block, right axis deviation) or right ventricular dilatation on echocardiogram	Ventilation-perfusion scan Helical CT scan Leg dopplers Angiogram

Past medical history reveals that Mr. C has suffered from 2 MIs. Subsequently, he has dyspnea upon walking more than 20 yards. Mr. C also has diabetes mellitus. His medications include atenolol, aspirin, atorvastatin, insulin, and lisinopril. On physical exam his BP is 128/70 mm Hg with a pulse of 72 bpm, which is regular. There is no significant change upon standing. His lung exam is clear, and cardiac exam reveals prominent JVD and a loud S_3 gallop. There is no significant murmur. He has 2+ pretibial edema, and his rectal exam reveals guaiac-negative stool. Finally, Mrs. C reports that she took Mr. C's blood glucose when he passed out and that the reading was 120 mg/dL.

Is the clinical information sufficient to make a diagnosis? If not, what other information do you need?

Mr. C's history of MI dramatically increases the likelihood of some form of cardiac syncope. Furthermore, his history of dyspnea on minimal exertion, jugular venous distention (JVD), and S_3 gallop all suggest CHF. CHF in turn markedly increases the likelihood of VT. His lack of postural BP change argues against orthostatic syncope from dehydration, hemorrhage, or medications. His normal blood glucose at the time of the event effectively rules out hypoglycemia. PE is possible but less likely.

Leading Hypothesis: Cardiac Syncope

Textbook Presentation

Cardiac syncope refers to syncope secondary to a disorder arising within the heart. Arrhythmias (either tachyarrhythmias or bradyarrhythmias) are the most common disorders, although occasionally syncope may be secondary to severe valvular heart disease (eg, aortic stenosis). Classically, patients with cardiac syncope are elderly patients with known heart disease (ie, CHF or coronary artery disease [CAD]) who experience sudden syncope, which may occur without warning. Patients may have palpitations.

Disease Highlights

A. The presence of heart disease is the single most important prognostic factor in patients with syncope.

B. Cardiac syncope is associated with increased mortality.

1. The 1-year mortality rate in patients with cardiac syncope is 18–33%, compared with 6% in patients with syncope of unknown cause.

2. Sudden cardiac death (presumably arrhythmogenic) occurs in 50% of patients with CHF.

3. Subsequent mortality in patients experiencing syncope increases with the severity of heart disease.

   a. Class 1–2 CHF, OR 7.7

   b. Class 3–4 CHF, OR 13.5

C. Although there are a large number of cardiac dysrhythmias, only a relative few produce syncope. Most supraventricular tachyarrhythmias will not cause syncope because the AV node limits the ventricular response rate. The most common arrhythmias associated with syncope include

1. Tachycardias

   a. VT

      (1) 21% of patients with heart disease have inducible VTs

      (2) Long QT syndrome: Consider if there is a family history of sudden death

   b. Supraventricular tachycardias associated with an accessory pathway (eg, atrial fibrillation with WPW)

2. Bradycardias: 34% of patients with heart disease have significant bradycardias

   a. Sinus node dysfunction

      (1) Sinus bradycardia (< 35 bpm)

      (2) Sinus pauses > 3 seconds (or > 2 seconds with symptoms)

   b. AV heart block (second- or third-degree)

   c. Atrial fibrillation with a *slow* ventricular response

Evidence-Based Diagnosis

A. History

1. Syncope in patients with suspected or certain heart disease

   a. Preexistent cardiac disease increases the risk of cardiac syncope, and the absence of cardiac disease markedly decreases the risk of cardiac syncope.

   b. Syncope during exertion or while supine increases the likelihood of cardiac syncope. However, since neither of these features is sensitive for cardiac syncope, their absence does not diminish the likelihood of cardiac syncope.

2. Syncope in patients without known or suspected heart disease: Palpitations increased the likelihood of cardiac syncope (Table 21–3).

Table 21–3. Sensitivity, specificity, and LRs for cardiac syncope.

Clinical Feature	Sensitivity	Specificity	LR+	LR–
Patients with suspected or certain heart disease				
Prior history of cardiac disease	95%	55%	2.1	0.09
Syncope while supine	12%	98%	6	0.90
Syncope with effort	14%	96%	3.5	0.90
Patients without suspected or certain heart disease				
Palpitations	75%	87%	5.8	0.29

B. Laboratory tests

1. An abnormal ECG increases the OR of cardiac arrhythmias in patients without neurocardiogenic syncope (OR, 23.5 [CI, 7–87]).

2. Certain ECG findings may suggest particular cardiac etiologies.
   a. ECG evidence of prior MI or a long QT interval increases the likelihood of VT.
   b. ECG findings of significant bradycardia, second- or third-degree AV block increase the likelihood of a significant bradycardia.
   c. Bundle branch block (BBB) suggests intermittent AV block even if the patient has a negative electrophysiologic study. Consider long-term loop recording in such patients.
   d. RV strain (S1Q3T3) or right BBB suggests PE.
   e. Ischemic changes suggests MI.
   f. Delta wave or short PR interval suggests an accessory pathway.

3. Echocardiograms
   a. Used to assess left ventricular function
   b. Used to assess valve function (eg, aortic stenosis, although this is rare in the absence of a significant murmur)
   c. VT is much more common in presence of left ventricular dysfunction.

4. Exercise testing
   a. Particularly useful in patients with syncope induced by exertion
   b. Also obtained in patients with cardiac disease

5. Holter monitoring: External cardiac leads are applied to the patient and a 24- to 48-hour recording of the cardiac rhythm is made
   a. Diagnostic yield is only 7–21%

   b. Usually nondiagnostic due to
      (1) Absence of arrhythmia during study
      (2) Absence of symptoms during arrhythmia
   c. Diagnostic only if
      (1) Arrhythmia captured **and** patient symptomatic during arrhythmia
      (2) Rhythm normal during symptoms (excludes an arrhythmia)

6. External loop recorders
   a. External devices that can be worn for up to 1 month. A continuous recording is made.
   b. If symptoms occur, most recent 2–5 minutes can be frozen in memory and transmitted by telephone.
   c. Relative short duration of monitoring (1 month) still limits sensitivity.
   d. Sensitivity is 14% compared with long-term implantable loop recorder

7. Electrophysiologic (EP) studies are invasive procedures that use a right heart catheterization. During EP studies, stimuli are delivered to the heart in order to detect bradyarrhythmias and accessory pathways and to elicit tachyarrhythmias.
   a. Sensitivity is 90% for VT.
   b. Patients with inducible VT are often treated with an automatic implantable cardiac defibrillator (AICD).
   c. To detect intermittent bradyarrhythmias, several measurements are made.
      (1) The atria are paced at rapid rates and then the pacing is terminated. Prolonged sinus node recovery time (SNRT) predicts sinus node dysfunction and some patients benefit from pacemaker insertion.

(2) Prolonged conduction through the bundle of His (HV interval) predicts AV block.

(3) Sensitivity for bradyarrhythmias is low (33%).

d. Overall diagnostic yield of EP studies

(1) 36% in patients with heart disease

(2) 22% in patients with abnormal ECGs

(3) 14% in select patients with normal ECGs and without heart disease

e. Indications for EP studies in patients with syncope include

(1) Unexplained syncope in patients with structural heart disease.

(2) Prior MI associated with ejection fraction < 40%

(3) Bifascicular block

(4) Prior MI associated with late potentials on signal averaged ECG

(5) Monitoring suggests sinus node dysfunction or AV block

f. Risk of EP studies include cardiac perforation, MI, AV fistulae (< 3%), deep venous thrombosis, and PE.

8. Implantable loop recorders have been used successfully in some patients with recurrent unexplained syncope. This may be particularly useful at detecting bradycardias missed by EP studies.

> 2
>
> Mr. C's serum troponin levels are undetectable (thus excluding acute MI). The ECG shows Q waves in leads V1–V4 and II, III and aVF consistent with prior anterior and inferior MI. The PR interval is normal. There is no evidence of sinus bradycardia, sinus pause, or AV block. The QRS width is normal excluding BBB. An echocardiogram reveals severe left ventricular dysfunction with hypokinesis of the anterior and inferior walls. The ejection fraction is estimated to be 25%. The aortic valve is normal without evidence of aortic stenosis.

Mr. C's ECG and echocardiogram confirm severe left ventricular dysfunction, markedly increasing the likelihood of some form of cardiac syncope. In particular, patients with left ventricular dysfunction are at high risk for VT. There are no ECG findings to suggest bradycardia (ie, heart block, BBB, sinus bradycardia). The leading hypothesis is revised to VT.

Revised Leading Hypothesis: VT

Textbook Presentation

Patients with VT may be asymptomatic or have symptoms that range from palpitations to lightheadedness, near syncope, syncope, or sudden cardiac death. VT occurs most commonly in patients with CAD and CHF and should be seriously considered when patients with preexisting CAD or CHF present with syncope.

Disease Highlights

A. ECG criteria

1. ≥ 3 consecutive wide complex (QRS ≥ .12 seconds) beats (Figure 21–2)

2. Supraventricular tachycardias can also occasionally manifest wide QRS complexes.

3. ECG criteria that increase the likelihood that the wide complex tachycardia is VT include fusion beats, capture beats, AV dissociation or a QRS width > .14 seconds.

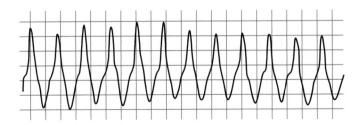

Figure 21–2. Ventricular tachycardia.

4. A history of CAD or CHF increases the likelihood that the wide complex tachycardia is ventricular.

5. Sustained VT is defined as VT lasting longer than 30 seconds.

B. Etiology

1. Ischemic heart disease

2. CHF

3. Hypertrophic cardiomyopathy

4. Valvular heart disease

5. Drugs (antiarrhythmic drugs and drugs that prolong the QT interval)

6. Electrolyte disorders (hypokalemia, hypocalcemia, hypomagnesemia)

7. Congenital disorders

   a. Congenital heart disease

   b. Long QT syndrome

      (1) The ECG of affected families demonstrates long refractory periods (long QT intervals)

      (2) Affected patients are at risk for sudden cardiac death from a form of VT called torsades de pointes.

      (3) Associated with congenital neural deafness

8. Miscellaneous other causes

C. Prognosis: VT is a potentially life-threatening arrhythmia. In patients with VT the following are predictors of mortality:

1. Prior cardiac arrest: 1-year mortality is 20%

2. Left ventricular dysfunction and VT: 2-year mortality is > 30%

3. VT post MI: 2-year mortality is 30%

4. Inducible VT on EP study: 2-year mortality is 50%

The 4 factors that predict sudden death or important cardiac arrhythmias are (1) history of CHF, (2) history of ventricular arrhythmias, (3) abnormal ECG, and (4) age ≥ 45. Patients in whom cardiac syncope is suspected should be admitted for evaluation.

MAKING A DIAGNOSIS

The pretest probability of ventricular tachycardia is very high. If routine inpatient monitoring fails to document a significant symptomatic arrhythmia, an EP study is

appropriate. You still wonder if a significant bradyarrhythmia or a PE might be responsible for Mr. C's syncope.

Have you crossed a diagnostic threshold for the leading hypothesis, VT? Do other tests need to be done to exclude the alternative diagnoses?

Alternative Diagnosis: Bradycardia from Sick Sinus Syndrome (SSS)

Textbook Presentation

The presentation of SSS depends on the duration and severity of the bradyarrhythmia. When the bradyarrhythmia is severe and prolonged patients may experience sudden syncope. With less severe bradycardia, patients may experience weakness, dyspnea on exertion, angina, transient ischemic attacks, or near syncope. Since the bradyarrhythmia may be short lived, patients may recover without intervention.

Disease Highlights

A. Episodic failure of sinus node

B. Most common indication for pacemaker placement

C. Often seen in the elderly due to fibrosis and degeneration of sinus node

D. Underlying CAD is common and contributes to the pathogenesis of SSS in some patients.

E. Electrical manifestations may include

1. Sinus bradycardia < 40 bpm

2. Sinus pauses > 2 seconds

3. Sinus arrest (with an escape junctional rhythm)

4. Sinoatrial exit block (inability of the sinus impulse to exit the sinus node)

F. Concomitant AV conduction disturbances are common.

G. Associated in some patients with supraventricular tachyarrhythmias, particularly atrial fibrillation (tachy-brady syndrome). Such patients may complain of palpitations. The bradycardia often follows termination of the tachycardia.

SSS should be suspected in patients with atrial fibrillation and a slow ventricular response who are not taking digoxin or AV nodal–blocking drugs (eg, β-blockers, verapamil).

Evidence-Based Diagnosis

A. Simultaneous symptoms and ECG findings (sinus bradycardia, significant pauses or sinus exit block) establishes the diagnosis.

B. Holter monitoring may be used but is often nondiagnostic due to the intermittent nature of the disorder.

C. External cardiac event monitors allow for a longer period of monitoring and correlation with symptoms.

D. Carotid sinus massage may cause prolonged pauses in patients with SSS (> 3 seconds).

E. Internal loop recorders have also been used.

F. Pharmacologic studies: Adenosine slows sinus node activity. Small studies suggest patients with SSS have delayed sinus node recovery following adenosine administration. The diagnostic accuracy is similar to EP studies.

G. EP studies:

    1. Useful in patients with severe symptoms when simultaneous rhythm abnormalities and symptoms are unavailable.

    2. SNRT and sinoatrial conduction time (SACT) can be measured.

    3. SNRT (see above) is 70% sensitive, 90% specific). Normal results do not rule out SSS.

    4. SACT: Measures the conduction from the sinus node to the atria.

Treatment

A. Discontinue any medications that may adversely affect sinus function, such as digoxin, β-blockers, sympatholytic agents, verapamil, diltiazem, certain antiarrhythmics, methyldopa, lithium, and cimetidine. (If β-blockers or other drugs cannot be discontinued, patients may require pacemaker.)

B. Pacemakers

    1. Atrial pacing is associated with a lower incidence of complications (eg, CHF, embolization, total morbidity and mortality) than isolated ventricular pacing.

    2. Pacemaker indications

      a. Documented **symptomatic** sinus node dysfunction

      b. Chronotropic incompetence: In this condition, the sinus rate does not increase appropriately with physical activity, leading to a relative bradycardia and symptoms.

      c. Pacemakers are often used when SSS is suspected but cannot be confirmed.

      (1) Patients with HR < 40 bpm and prior symptoms

      (2) EP study shows long SNRT in patients with prior symptoms

Alternative Diagnosis: Bradycardia due to AV Heart Block

Textbook Presentation

Depending on the duration and severity of the heart block, patients with AV block may be asymptomatic or complain of palpitations, angina, transient ischemic attacks, near syncope, or syncope.

Disease Highlights

A. Secondary to conduction abnormalities in the AV node, bundle of His, or bundle branches.

B. Etiology

    1. Fibrosis and CAD are most common.

    2. Drugs (eg, β-blockers, verapamil, digoxin, amiodarone).

 The combination of verapamil and β-blockers should always be avoided. There is a high incidence of subsequent AV block and CHF.

    3. Hyperkalemia

    4. Valvular heart disease

    5. Increased vagal tone

C. Classification (Table 21–4, Figure 21–3)

Treatment

A. Withdraw drugs that impair AV conduction.

B. Correct electrolyte abnormalities

C. Pacemakers: Precise indications are complex. In general, pacing is recommended for patients with Mobitz II second-degree AV block and third-degree AV block. Pacing is usually not indicated in first-degree AV block or Mobitz I second-degree AV block.

Alternative Diagnosis: PE

Textbook Presentation

PE is covered extensively in Chapter 11, Dyspnea and will only be discussed here briefly. While there is wide variation in the presentation of PE, only 5% of patients with PE experience syncope. Furthermore, PE is an un-

Table 21–4. Classification of heart block.

Type	Atrial Ventricular Conduction	ECG Findings	Clinical Findings	Treatment
First degree	1:1	PR interval > .2 s QRS width usually WNL	None	None
Second degree Mobitz I	Intermittent	Progressive lengthening of PR interval until p wave is not conducted and QRS absent. Next PR interval shorter than PR prior to dropped beat QRS width usually WNL	Associated with inferior MI Rarely progresses to third-degree AV block	Observation or atropine
Second degree Mobitz II	Intermittent	Intermittent nonconduction of p waves More severe infranodal damage, QRS may be widened	Associated with anterior MI Often progresses to third-degree AV block	Pacemaker
Third degree	None	P waves not conducted Complete AV disassociation Ventricular rate depends on escape pacemakers	Associated with CAD, drugs, degeneration, abnormal electrolytes, bradycardia, hypotension	Pacemaker

WNL, within normal limits; MI, myocardial infarction; AV, atrioventricular; CAD, coronary artery disease.

usual cause of syncope. Surprisingly, the subset of patients with PE in whom syncope develops and yet survive to arrive at the hospital may be hemodynamically stable, relatively asymptomatic, and have normal or near normal oxygen saturation. Consider PE as a cause of syncope in patients with a history of risk factors for PE, dyspnea, or pleuritic chest pain, physical exam findings of unexplained hypotension, tachycardia, JVD, a loud S_2, cor pulmonale, or ECG or echocardiographic findings that suggest right heart strain (S1Q3T3, right BBB). An unexplained pulmonary infiltrate may be a sign of infarction from pulmonary embolus.

CASE RESOLUTION

After 24 hours, Mr. C is feeling well. He is anxious to go home. The telemetry reveals normal sinus rhythm without evidence of intermittent AV block or VT. Stress testing is performed and shows evidence of prior MI but no acute ischemia.

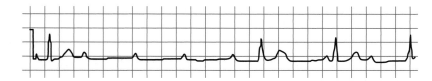

Figure 21–3. Third-degree atrioventricular block.

The sensitivity of telemetry is inadequate to exclude life-threatening arrhythmias such as VT. Furthermore, none of the alternative diagnoses are suggested by the history, physical exams, or laboratory test results (such as hypoglycemia, dehydration, orthostatic hypotension, SSS, or AV heart block). After careful discussion with Mr. C, you order an EP study.

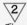

The EP study demonstrates inducible sustained VT, placing the patient at high risk for spontaneous lethal ventricular arrhythmias. An AICD is placed. At follow-up 12 months later, Mr. C is doing well and has no subsequent syncopal events. His AICD has delivered 5 shocks.

Treatment of VT

A. The management of acute VT evolves rapidly and is beyond the scope of this text. Please see appropriate ACLS guidelines.

B. Prevention of recurrent VT and sudden cardiac death
   1. Optimize electrolytes
   2. Treat CHF (ACE inhibitors, β blockade, and spironolactone have all been shown to decrease mortality.)
   3. Evaluate and treat ischemic heart disease
   4. Treatment options include AICD, antiarrhythmic drugs (especially class III agents), catheter ablation, and combinations of the above. AICDs have been used with increasing frequency in combination with antiarrhythmic therapy to minimize the number of delivered shocks. Consultation is advised.

CHIEF COMPLAINT

PATIENT

Mrs. S is a 60-year-old woman who arrives at the emergency department via ambulance after an episode of syncope. The patient reports that she was eating dinner, and the next thing she knew she was in the emergency department. Mr. S reports that he found his wife lying on the floor next to the dining room table when he came home. At that time, Mrs. S was conscious but lethargic. The food and plate were scattered on the floor. There was no evidence of incontinence. On physical exam, her vital signs are normal. HEENT exam reveals a contusion over the right eye and bruising along the right half of her tongue. Cardiac and pulmonary exams are normal. Abdominal exam is unremarkable. Stool is guaiac negative. Neurologic exam is nonfocal.

 At this point, what is your leading hypothesis and what are the active alternatives? What other tests should be ordered?

ORGANIZING THE DIFFERENTIAL DIAGNOSIS

The remarkable feature of Mrs. S's history is the prolonged period of lethargy and confusion that persisted until she reached the emergency department. This is highly suggestive of a postictal period following a seizure. The patient's bruised tongue increases the suspicion that she suffered a seizure. Another consideration is hypoglycemia, which can also cause a prolonged period of lethargy or confusion. Patients with cardiac or neurocardiogenic syncope tend to regain consciousness almost immediately and do not usually suffer from prolonged confusion, lethargy, or memory loss. Therefore, despite the absence of witnessed tonic-clonic activity, the prolonged period of confusion and amnesia is highly suggestive of seizures. Table 21–5 lists the differential diagnosis.

Patients with syncope should be asked, "What was the next thing you remember?" Patients who do not remember the ambulance ride or suffer a period of amnesia **following the event** (> 5 minutes) should be evaluated for seizures.

Table 21–5. Diagnostic hypotheses for Mrs. S.

Diagnostic Hypotheses	Clinical Clues	Important Tests
Leading Hypothesis		
Seizure	Prolonged period of lethargy, confusion, amnesia suggesting postictal period Tonic-clonic activity Incontinence Prior stroke, CNS tumor, or neurologic disease Abnormal neurologic exam	EEG Contrast-enhanced CT or MRI scan
Active Alternatives—Most Common		
Hypoglycemia	Diabetes mellitus treated with either insulin, thiazolidinediones, or sulfonylureas	Glucose measurement at time of event

The patient reports no prior history of epilepsy, CNS tumor or stroke. She has no history of cerebrovascular disease or head trauma. She has no history of diabetes and is not taking any medications. She does not remember any antecedent event. She has no cardiac history and walks 2 miles every day without dyspnea or chest pain. She reports no history of melena or hematochezia.

Is the clinical information sufficient to make a diagnosis? If not, what other information do you need?

Leading Hypothesis: Seizures

Textbook Presentation

Generalized seizures classically present with tonic-clonic activity, loss of postural tone, incontinence, and a prolonged postictal period of lethargy. The purpose of this review is to focus on features that help distinguish seizures from syncope.

Disease Highlights

A. 3% of US population suffers a seizure in their lifetime

B. Seizures account for 1–7% of patients with syncope

C. Etiology of seizure and prevalence in patients over age 60

1. Idiopathic, ≅ 35%
2. Ischemic, 49%
3. CNS tumor, 11%
   a. Primary CNS tumor, 35%
   b. Metastatic, 59%
4. CNS trauma, 3%
5. CNS infection, 2%
6. Withdrawal states (ie, alcohol)

Evidence-Based Diagnosis

A. Postictal confusion is the most sensitive clinical feature (Table 21–6). The absence of a postictal period makes seizures unlikely (sensitivity 94%, LR– 0.09).

B. Tongue laceration, unusual posturing, and limb jerking are the most specific clinical features and substantially increase the likelihood of seizure (specificity 97–88%, LR+ 16–5.6).

C. Certain symptoms are unusual in patients with seizures and reduce the likelihood of seizure.
   1. Diaphoresis preceding spell, LR 0.17
   2. Chest pain preceding spell, LR 0.15
   3. Palpitations, LR 0.12
   4. Dyspnea prior to spell, LR 0.08
   5. CAD, LR 0.08
   6. Syncope with prolonged standing, LR 0.05

D. Convulsive syncope
   1. Tonic-clonic activity is not specific for seizures.
   2. 15% of patients with other causes of syncope experience limb jerking, a phenomenon referred to as **convulsive syncope.**

Table 21–6. Sensitivity, specificity, and LRs for seizures.

Clinical Feature	Sensitivity (%)	Specificity (%)	LR+	LR−
Cut tongue	45	97	16	0.56
Head turning	43	97	13	0.59
Unusual posturing	35	97	13	0.67
Bedwetting	24	96	6.4	0.79
Limb jerking noted by others	69	88	5.6	0.35
Prodromal trembling	29	94	4.9	0.76
Prodromal preoccupation	8	98	4.3	0.94
Prodromal hallucinations	8	98	4.3	0.94
Postictal confusion	94	69	3.0	0.09

Modified from *Journal of the American College of Cardiology*. Sheldon Robert, et al. Historical criteria that distinguish syncope from seizures, 40:142–148. Copyright © 2002. With permission from American College of Cardiology Foundation.

3. Patients with convulsive syncope have short-lived tonic-clonic activity (< 10 seconds) and either no postictal period or short postictal periods (< 1 minute).

4. Patients who appear to have refractory "seizure disorders" and nonspecific abnormalities on EEG should undergo tilt-table testing to rule out neurocardiogenic syncope with secondary tonic-clonic activity.

E. Sheldon developed a point score to distinguish seizures from syncope (Table 21–7). Point scores of ≥ 1 suggest seizures (sensitivity, 94%; specificity, 94%; LR+, 16; LR−, 0.06).

F. An EEG is indicated in the evaluation of patient with possible seizures. The finding of spike and wave patterns increases the likelihood of a seizure disorder.

1. Sensitivity (between episodes) EEG, 35–50%

2. Sensitivity increases with sleep deprivation

3. Specificity, 98%

G. Neuroimaging (either contrast-enhanced CT or MRI) should be performed in adults with new-onset seizures.

1. 37% have structural lesions

2. 15% of adults with new-onset seizures and nonfocal neurologic exams have structural lesions on neuroimaging

MAKING A DIAGNOSIS

The patient's EEG revealed intermittent right temporal spike and wave pattern.

The patient's history of a postictal period and tongue biting are highly suggestive of seizures, which was confirmed on the EEG. Since structural lesions and ischemia are common in adults with new-onset seizures, neuroimaging is required.

CASE RESOLUTION

An MRI scan revealed a solitary right temporal lobe mass. Subsequent biopsy demonstrated a glioblastoma multiforme. The patient underwent surgical resection and was treated with anticonvulsive therapy. She died approximately 6 months later.

Table 21–7. A point score to distinguish seizures from syncope.[a]

Criteria	Points
Waking with cut tongue	2
Abnormal behavior (eg, limb jerking, prodromal trembling, preoccupation, hallucinations)	1
Lost consciousness with emotional stress	1
Postictal confusion	1
Head turning to 1 side	1
Prodromal deja vu	1
Any presyncope	−2
Lost consciousness with prolonged standing	−2
Diaphoresis before a spell	−2

[a]Point scores of ≥ I suggest seizures.
Modified from *Journal of the American College of Cardiology*. Sheldon Robert, et al. Historical criteria that distinguish syncope from seizures, 40:142–148. Copyright © 2002. With permission from American College of Cardiology Foundation.

CHIEF COMPLAINT

PATIENT 4

Mrs. P is a 39-year-old woman who arrives at the emergency department via ambulance with abdominal pain and syncope. She was in her usual state of health until the morning of admission when increasing left lower quadrant abdominal pain developed. The pain increased in intensity and became quite severe. Upon standing, she lost consciousness and collapsed to the floor. She recovered quickly and was helped to a chair by her husband. When she stood several minutes later, she briefly lost consciousness again. The patient reports that her abdominal pain is much better. Her vital signs are BP, 105/60 mm Hg; pulse, 85 bpm; temperature, 37.0 °C; and RR, 18 breaths per minute. Her cardiac and pulmonary exams are normal, and abdominal exam reveals mild left lower quadrant tenderness. Her ECG is normal and her Hct is normal at 36.0%.

 At this point, what is your leading hypothesis and what are the active alternatives? What other tests should be ordered?

ORGANIZING THE DIFFERENTIAL DIAGNOSIS

Several features of Mrs. P's syncope are noteworthy. First, her syncope occurred in association with abdominal pain raising the possibility of neurocardiogenic syncope. Second, she had 2 episodes of syncope upon standing. This raises the possibility of orthostatic syncope from either dehydration or hemorrhage. Reviewing the remaining differential diagnoses at the beginning of the chapter, her young age and absence of preexistent cardiovascular disease argue against cardiac syncope. Aortic stenosis is unlikely in patients without a significant systolic murmur. Medications and PE are possibilities. Her rapid restoration of consciousness argues against a seizure. Table 21–8 lists the differential diagnosis.

Table 21–8. Diagnostic hypotheses for Mrs. P.

Diagnostic Hypotheses	Clinical Clues	Important Tests
Leading Hypothesis		
Neurocardiogenic syncope (faint)	Preceding pain, anxiety, fear or prolonged standing Rapid normalization of consciousness Absence of heart disease	Tilt table if recurrent
Active Alternatives—Most Common		
Orthostatic syncope	History of vomiting, diarrhea, decreased oral intake, melena, bright red blood per rectum or other blood loss	Orthostatic measurement of BP and pulse
Medications	History of α-blockers, other antihypertensive medication	Orthostatic measurement of BP and pulse
Active Alternatives—Must Not Miss		
PE	Risk factors for PE Pleuritic chest pain or dyspnea Loud S_2 Unexplained persistent hypotension Right heart strain on ECG (right bundle-branch block, right axis deviation) or right ventricular dilatation on echocardiogram	Ventilation-perfusion scan Helical CT scan Leg dopplers Angiogram

Further history reveals that Mrs. P is not taking any medications and did not have any chest pain or dyspnea. She has no risk factors for PE (eg, oral birth control pills, prolonged immobilization, recent surgery or postpartum period, cancer, or known hypercoagulable state). Your initial assessment is neurocardiogenic syncope secondary to transient abdominal pain.

As discussed in the first case presentation, neurocardiogenic syncope is often precipitated by pain, is brief, and is followed by a rapid restoration of consciousness. Many of Mrs. P's features are consistent with this diagnosis. However, both episodes of syncope occurred immediately after standing providing a clue that her syncope was in fact orthostatic. In addition, although her abdominal pain is improved, it is still unexplained. You elect to check her BP and pulse for orthostatic change.

Mrs. P's BP while supine was 105/60 mm Hg with a pulse of 85 bpm, which changed when sitting to BP of 95/50 mm Hg with a pulse of 90 bpm. Upon standing her BP fell to 60/0, her pulse was 140 bpm, and she lost consciousness. She was quickly laid down and again rapidly regained consciousness.

The patient's volume status is always assessed based on the clinical, **not laboratory** exam. Orthostatic measurement of BP and pulse are critical. Life-threatening hypovolemia may be overlooked if the BP and pulse are not measured while the patient is standing.

Mrs. P's profound drop in BP upon standing, reflex tachycardia, and recurrent syncope clearly indicate that she is syncopal due to orthostatic hypotension. This is not consistent with neurocardiogenic syncope. You revise the leading hypothesis to orthostatic syncope.

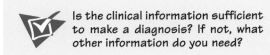

Is the clinical information sufficient to make a diagnosis? If not, what other information do you need?

Leading Hypothesis: Orthostatic Hypotension

Textbook Presentation

Patients with orthostatic hypotension often have obvious sources of fluid or blood loss. Common causes include vomiting, diarrhea, inadequate fluid intake, or GI bleeding (hematemesis, melena, or bright red blood per rectum). Occasionally, orthostatic hypotension may develop secondary to massive but occult internal bleeding (rupture of abdominal aortic aneurysm, splenic rupture, retroperitoneal hemorrhage, or ruptured ectopic pregnancy). Finally, orthostatic hypotension may occur without volume loss, particularly in the elderly.

Disease Highlights

A. Symptoms may include lightheadedness, visual blurring, near syncope, or syncope. Some patients are asymptomatic.

B. Accounts for 20–30% of patients with syncope

C. The distinguishing feature is the occurrence of syncope when arising

D. Definition

   1. > 20 mm decrease in systolic BP upon standing

   2. > 10 mm decrease in diastolic BP upon standing

   3. Or > 30 bpm increase in pulse upon standing

E. Etiology

   1. Dehydration

      a. Decreased oral intake

      b. GI losses (vomiting, diarrhea)

      c. Urinary losses

         (1) Uncontrolled diabetes mellitus

         (2) Salt losing nephropathy

         (3) Adrenal insufficiency

      d. Over-dialysis

   2. Hemorrhage

3. Medications

   a. α-Blockers (Syncope occurs in 1% of patients taking their first dose.)

   b. Diuretics

   c. Vasodilators

   d. Tricyclic antidepressants

   e. Phenothiazines

   f. Alcohol and opiates

4. Prolonged bed rest

5. Autonomic insufficiency (characterized by a fall in BP upon standing *without* a concomitant increase in pulse)

   a. Diabetes mellitus

   b. Other neurologic disorders (ie, Parkinson disease, multiple sclerosis, and numerous others)

6. Elderly (20–30% patients > 65 years old)

7. Postprandial hypotension, particularly common in the elderly

Evidence-Based Diagnosis

Several studies assessed the impact of phlebotomy on volunteers. Phlebotomy removed a moderate (450–630 mL) to large (630–1150 mL) volume of blood.

A. The most sensitive measure for large blood loss was postural increase in pulse > 30 bpm (sensitivity 97%, LR– .03) (Table 21–9). The sensitivity falls dramatically if the patient sits instead of stands (39–78%)

B. Supine measurements of BP and pulse were not sensitive for even large blood loss (sensitivity 12–33%).

C. Any abnormal finding on orthostatic maneuvers strongly suggested volume loss (specificity 94–98%; LR+, 3.0–48).

D. The sensitivity of orthostatic measurements is greatest if the supine and standing BPs are compared. If the supine BP is not measured, 67% of orthostatic patients may not be identified.

E. Patients should stand for 1 minute before the measurement of the upright BP.

F. No measure was very sensitive for moderate blood loss (0–27%).

G. Profound blood loss may occasionally paradoxically produce bradycardia. (The reduction in ESV may trigger the neurocardiogenic reflex.)

H. The admission Hct does not accurately reflect the severity of acute hemorrhage. A fall in Hct may take 24–72 hours.

Table 21–9. Accuracy of physical exam for large blood loss (630–1150 mL).

Clinical Finding	Sensitivity (%)	Specificity (%)	LR+	LR–
Supine heart rate > 100 bpm	12	96	3.0	0.9
Supine hypotension < 95 mm Hg	33	97	11.0	0.7
Postural increase in pulse > 30 bpm	97	98	48.0	0.03

Modified with permission from *Journal American Medical Association*. McGee Steven, et al. Is This patient hypovolemic? 1999;281:1022–1029.

MAKING A DIAGNOSIS

Mrs. P reports that she has not suffered from any diarrhea or vomiting and has taken in normal amounts of fluid. She denies any hematemesis, melena, or bright red blood per rectum.

It is important to remember that Mrs. P presented with syncope *and* abdominal pain. Although the pain has improved, it has not resolved; it may provide an important clue to the underlying etiology. Given the profound orthostatic hypotension and the lack of external blood or volume loss, internal bleeding must be considered as a source of her abdominal pain and syncope. In the differential diagnosis you consider ruptured spleen, ruptured abdominal aortic aneurysm, and ruptured ectopic pregnancy. The lack of trauma argues against splenic rupture and the patient's age and gender are atypical for abdominal aortic aneurysm.

It is important to remember the patient's chief complaint because it usually holds the most important clues to the diagnosis.

CASE RESOLUTION

Mrs. P reports that she missed her last menstrual period. An abdominal ultrasound is performed and reveals 750 mL of fluid (presumed to be blood) in the pelvis. A urine pregnancy test is positive.

Although the final diagnosis of ectopic pregnancy was not considered initially, a careful clinical exam confirmed orthostatic syncope. Once that diagnosis was made, the differential diagnosis could be narrowed and the underlying cause determined. It is instructive to note that her initial Hct was normal because the remaining intravascular blood had not yet been diluted by any oral or IV fluids.

Initial Hgb measurements will not accurately reflect the magnitude of blood loss in a patient with recent hemorrhage.

Treatment of Orthostatic Hypotension

A. Acute blood loss: Blood transfusion is appropriate in the orthostatic patient with acute blood loss.

B. Acute plasma loss (diarrhea, vomiting, or decreased oral intake)

1. Patients able to tolerate oral intake: oral rehydration

2. Patients unable to tolerate oral intake: IV hydration

   a. Normal saline is preferred.

   b. Usually 500 mL to 1 L boluses are given over 1 hour

   c. Smaller boluses may be given to fragile patients (ie, those with a history of renal failure or CHF).

   d. Repeat orthostatic BP measurements are made following each bolus as well as a lung and cardiac exam to ensure the patient has not received excessive fluid.

   e. Bolus therapy should be continued until orthostatic hypotension resolves.

C. Chronic orthostatic hypotension

1. Hydration (soup or sports drinks containing sodium)

2. Remove offending agents (diuretics, α-blockers, nitrates, tricyclic antidepressants, phenothiazines)

3. Patients are advised to arise slowly (sitting on the side of the bed, prior to standing), avoid large meals and excessive heat and use waist high support hose.

4. Fludrocortisone is initial drug of choice. Monitor patients for hypokalemia and hypertension.

5. α-Agonists have also been used successfully.

    a. Ephedrine, pseudoephedrine, phenylephrine, and midodrine have been used.

    b. Side effects include urinary retention, hypertension, and worsening CHF

6. Caffeine can be useful.

7. Erythropoietin is helpful in anemic patients.

Mrs. P had 2 large bore IVs placed and was typed and crossed for RBC transfusions. CBC, PT, PTT, and platelet counts were measured and a 1 L bolus of normal saline was given while waiting for the packed RBCs. After volume and blood resuscitation, she underwent surgical exploration and removal of her ruptured fallopian tube.

REVIEW OF OTHER IMPORTANT DISEASES

Aortic Stenosis

Textbook Presentation

Aortic stenosis is usually diagnosed incidentally during routine exam rather than due to symptoms. Typically, aortic stenosis produces a loud crescendo-decrescendo systolic murmur at the right second intercostal space, which may radiate to the neck and apex. When aortic stenosis becomes very severe, patients may have any of the 3 cardinal symptoms: CHF (dyspnea), syncope, or angina.

Disease Highlights

A. Thickening and calcification of valve leaflets results in **progressive** obstruction to blood flow.

B. Severe aortic stenosis is characterized by valve area < 1 cm or mean aortic valve gradient > 50 mm Hg.

C. Left ventricular hypertrophy develops to compensate for the obstruction.

D. Etiology

    1. Degeneration of a previously normal valve

2. Congenital bicuspid valve

    a. 1–2% of population is born with congenital bicuspid valve

    b. Severe aortic stenosis develops at an earlier age in patients with congenital bicuspid valves.

3. Rheumatic heart disease

Evidence-Based Diagnosis

A. Physical exam findings modestly increase the likelihood of severe aortic stenosis: a late peaking systolic murmur (LR+ 4.4), palpable delay in the carotid upstroke (LR+ 2.6), an absent A2 (LR+ 4.5).

B. The likelihood of severe aortic stenosis is markedly reduced in patients without a systolic murmur LR− 0.1. A systolic murmur ≥ grade 2 is found in approximately 75% of patients.

C. Doppler echocardiogram is the initial test of choice to assess for aortic stenosis.

Treatment

A. Mechanical correction

    1. Valve replacement is the treatment of choice. Subsequent survival approaches the age-matched normal population.

    2. Definite indications for valve replacement

        a. Severe aortic stenosis in **symptomatic** patients

            (1) Mortality is markedly increased in symptomatic patients unless they undergo valve replacement. The mortality for patients not undergoing valve replacement follows:

                (a) Aortic stenosis and angina: 50% 5-year mortality

                (b) Aortic stenosis and syncope: 50% 3-year mortality

                (c) Aortic stenosis and dyspnea: 50% 2-year mortality

        b. Severe aortic stenosis in **asymptomatic** patients undergoing coronary artery bypass grafting (CABG) or other valve surgery

    3. Possible indications

        a. Moderate aortic stenosis in asymptomatic patients undergoing CABG or other valve surgery

        b. Severe aortic stenosis in asymptomatic patients with ejection fraction < 50%, hypotension during exercise, or VT

    4. Standard preoperative evaluation includes angiography in patients with risk factors or symptoms of CAD to determine whether the patient needs concomitant CABG.

5. Mechanical and bioprosthetic valves have been used.

  a. Mechanical valves have greater durability and a significantly lower rate of failure and need for replacement. They are associated with a lower all-cause mortality than bioprosthetic valves.

  b. Mechanical valves are associated with an increased risk of thromboembolism and infection. Patients with mechanical valves require lifelong anticoagulation therapy.

  c. Bioprosthetic valves are reserved for patients who have a contraindication to warfarin therapy or are believed to be noncompliant. They may also be used in elderly patients (whose life expectancy makes replacement unlikely).

  d. Another alternative is the Ross procedure in which the pulmonary valve is removed and used as the aortic valve. The pulmonary artery is reconstructed to create the pulmonary valve. The survival of these grafts is good and patients do not require anticoagulation therapy.

6. Balloon valvotomy is a poor option. It provides only temporary relief (6–12 months) and does not improve survival. Complications occur in 10–20%. Reserved for palliation in patients with other serious (or lethal) comorbidities.

B. Other treatment

  1. Standard endocarditis prophylaxis

  2. Vigorous exercise should be discouraged in patients with moderate to severe aortic stenosis.

Cerebrovascular Disease & Syncope

Although physicians commonly consider carotid artery obstruction in the differential diagnosis of patients with syncope, unilateral obstruction of the carotid will not result in syncope. Therefore, evaluation of the anterior circulation is not indicated in the patient with syncope. On the other hand, impairment of the posterior circulation may cause syncope due to interruption of blood flow to the reticular activating system. This may occur in the subclavian steal syndrome, vertebrobasilar insufficiency, and basilar artery occlusion. These disorders should be considered whenever patients have syncope and other symptoms referable to the brainstem (ie, diplopia, vertigo, ataxia, weakness).

1. Subclavian Steal

Textbook presentation

Classically, patients have symptoms referable to the brainstem and cerebellum that occur with arm exercise. Vertigo, ataxia, visual blurring, diplopia, weakness, and syncope may occur. Due to the subclavian obstruction, the brachial BP is significantly lower on the involved side than on the uninvolved side.

Disease Highlights

A. Secondary to stenosis in the subclavian artery. This lowers BP in the subclavian artery distal to the obstruction and causes blood to flow retrograde down the vertebral artery into the subclavian artery (distal to the obstruction). This "steals" blood from the basilar artery.

B. Usually secondary to atherosclerosis, often associated with atherosclerotic disease in the circle of Willis impairing collateral circulation

C. Due to concomitant carotid artery atherosclerosis, hemispheric ischemia is more likely to develop

D. Posterior ischemic events are rare.

Evidence-Based Diagnosis

A. Upper extremity claudication occurs in 33% of patients.

B. Systolic BP gradient > 20 mm between the 2 arms seen in 94% of patients.

C. Most patients have a diminished radial pulse and subclavian bruit on the involved side.

D. Duplex exam, magnetic resonance angiography, and conventional angiography can demonstrate subclavian artery stenosis and flow reversal in the vertebral artery.

E. The finding of significant subclavian artery stenosis does not confirm that the patient's symptoms are secondary to subclavian steal.

  1. Only a subset of patients with subclavian stenosis have reversal of flow (steal) from the ipsilateral vertebral artery.

  2. Even with reversal of flow (steal), many patients with subclavian steal are asymptomatic due to collateral flow to the brainstem through the circle of Willis and the uninvolved vertebral artery.

Treatment

A. The optimal therapy for patients with symptomatic subclavian steal is uncertain.

B. Many patients improve with time without treatment.

C. Surgical bypass, angioplasty, and stents have all been used successfully.

D. In patients with concomitant carotid artery obstruction, carotid endarterectomy may improve subclavian steal by improving flow through the circle of Willis.

Diagnostic Approach: Syncope

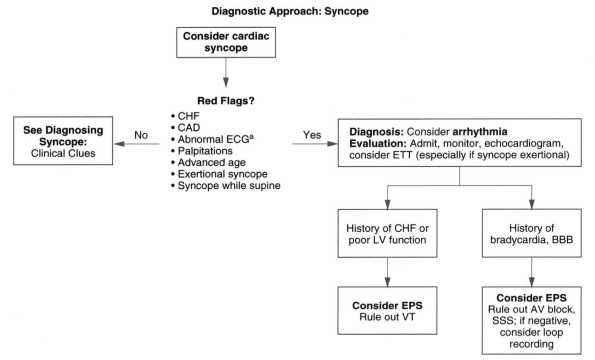

^aAn ECG is probably unnecessary in young patients who present with classic neurocardiogenic syncope without heart disease. All other patients should have an ECG.

CHF, congestive heart failure; CAD, coronary artery disease; ETT, exercise tolerance test; LV, left ventricular; BBB, bundle branch block; EPS, electrophysiologic study; AV, atrioventricular; SSS, sick sinus syndrome.

Figure 21–A.

Diagnosing Syncope: Clinical Clues

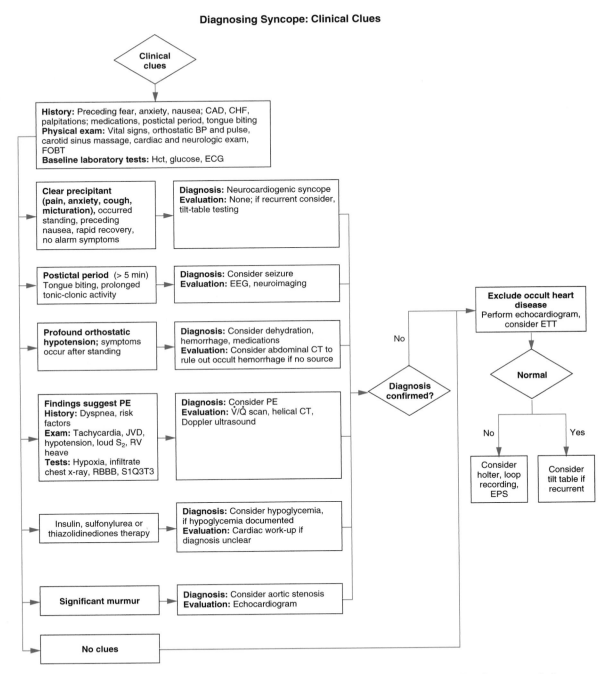

CAD, coronary artery disease; CHF, congestive heart failure; EEG, electroencephalogram; PE, pulmonary embolism; JVD, jugular venous distention; RV, right ventricular; RBBB, right bundle-branch block; V̇/Q̇, ventilation-perfusion; ETT, exercise tolerance test; EPS, electrophysiologic study.

Figure 21–B.

I have a patient with unintentional weight loss. How do I determine the cause?

CHIEF COMPLAINT

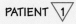

Mrs. M is an 85-year-old woman who comes to the office complaining of weight loss. She is quite concerned that she has something dreadful.

What is the differential diagnosis of unintentional weight loss? How would you frame the differential?

CONSTRUCTING A DIFFERENTIAL DIAGNOSIS

Significant unintentional weight loss is defined as > 5% loss of usual body weight in the last 6–12 months. The causes of unintentional weight loss can be organized into disorders that increase energy demands (eg, hyperthyroidism), cause nutrient loss (eg, diarrhea or diabetes), or decrease energy intake (eg, anorexia).

Decreased energy intake is the most common mechanism of unintentional weight loss and can be organized into disorders involving 1 of 4 systems: the psychosocial system (required to ensure access to food and an appetite), the neurologic system, the GI system (organized from diseases of the mouth to rectum), and systemic diseases.

Differential Diagnosis of Unintentional Weight Loss

A. Increased energy demands
 1. Hyperthyroidism
 2. Chronic obstructive pulmonary disease
 3. Cardiac cachexia
 4. Fever
 5. Malignancy
 6. Emotional states (eg, mania, schizophrenia)

B. Nutrient loss
 1. Diarrhea syndromes
  a. Inflammatory bowel disease (IBD) (eg, Crohn disease, ulcerative colitis)
  b. Celiac sprue
  c. Bacterial overgrowth syndromes
  d. Pancreatic insufficiency
  e. Chronic infection (*Giardia lamblia*, *Clostridium difficile*, *Entamoeba histolytica*)
  f. Lactose intolerance
 2. Urinary: Uncontrolled diabetes mellitus

C. Decreased energy intake
 1. Psychosocial
  a. Poverty (15% of patients over 65 live below the poverty line)
  b. Isolation
  c. Immobility or inadequate transportation
  d. Depression
  e. Anxiety
  f. Alcoholism
 2. Neurologic
  a. Dementia
  b. Stroke
  c. Parkinson disease
 3. GI (organized from mouth to rectum)
  a. Poor dentition (50% of patients edentulous by age 65)
  b. Anosmia

   c. Esophageal disorders

     (1) Esophageal stricture or web

     (2) Dysmotility

     (3) Esophageal cancer

   d. Gastric disorders

     (1) Peptic ulcer disease (PUD)

     (2) Gastric cancer

     (3) Gastroparesis

     (4) Gastric outlet obstruction

   e. Small bowel diseases

     (1) Mesenteric ischemia

     (2) Crohn disease

     (3) Celiac sprue

   f. Pancreatic disease

     (1) Acute pancreatitis

     (2) Chronic pancreatitis

     (3) Pancreatic cancer

   g. Hepatic disease

     (1) Hepatitis

     (2) Cholelithiasis

     (3) Cirrhosis

     (4) Hepatocellular carcinoma

   h. Colonic diseases

     (1) Chronic constipation

     (2) Colon cancer

     (3) IBD

4. Systemic diseases

   a. Iatrogenic

     (1) Drugs (eg, digoxin, loop diuretics, diltiazem, levodopa)

     (2) Medical diets

     (3) Radiation

   b. Inflammatory

     (1) Polymyalgia rheumatica, temporal arteritis

     (2) Rheumatoid arthritis

     (3) Systemic lupus erythematosus

   c. Infectious

     (1) HIV

     (2) Subacute bacterial endocarditis (SBE)

     (3) Tuberculosis

   d. Metabolic: uremia, hypercalcemia

   e. Cancer: Carcinoma of the pancreas, lung, GI tract

The 4 most common causes of unintentional weight loss are cancer (GI, lung, and lymphoma), 27%; nonmalignant GI diseases, 17%; depression and alcoholism, 14%; and unknown, 22%. Endocrine disorders account for 7% of unintentional weight loss. Although cancer is the most common cause, it is not the cause in the majority of patients. The yield of various diagnostic tests in the evaluation of patients with unintentional weight loss is shown in Table 22–1.

Mrs. M reports that she has lost weight over the last 6 months. She denies any diarrhea, loose, or difficult to flush stools. She reports that her appetite is poor and she feels fatigued.

At this point, what is the leading hypothesis and what are the active alternatives? What tests should be ordered?

ORGANIZING THE DIFFERENTIAL DIAGNOSIS

The patient's history is typical of many patients complaining of weight loss. Patients report an unspecified amount of

Table 22–1. Yield of diagnostic tests in the evaluation of patients with unintentional weight loss.

Test	Yield
Chest x-ray	41%
Serum chemistry	2%
FOBT	18%
CBC	14%
Thyroid function tests	24%
Urinalysis	3%
UGI/EGD	12–44%
BE/FS/colonoscopy	15%

FOBT, fecal occult blood test; UGI, upper GI series; EGD, esophagogastroduodenoscopy; BE, barium enema; FS, flexible sigmoidoscopy.

Modified with permission Blackwell Publishing. Thompson MP, Morris LK. Unexplained weight loss in the ambulatory elderly. *J Am Geriatr Soc.* 1991;39:497–500.

weight loss, associated with anorexia. The first step in the evaluation is to verify that weight loss did in fact occur.

Approximately 50% of patients who complain of weight loss have not lost weight. Clinicians should verify the weight loss or document significant changes in the patient's clothing or belt size.

Mrs. M does not remember her prior weight but reports that her clothes are much too loose. Indeed, she has gone out to buy clothes 2 sizes smaller.

Mrs. M's change in clothing size suggests true and significant weight loss. Since the history does not suggest diarrhea or malabsorption, the leading hypothesis should include diseases associated with decreased energy intake, focusing on the most common causes of cancer, digestive diseases, and psychosocial problems. Active alternatives are diseases associated with increased energy expenditure (eg, hyperthyroidism). Must not miss alternatives include systemic diseases associated with decreased intake (eg, HIV, SBE, temporal arteritis). Finally, malabsorption should be reconsidered if the evaluation is negative, since patients with malabsorption may not have diarrhea or foul stools. Table 22–2 lists the differential diagnosis.

The second step in evaluating patients with documented weight loss determines whether the patient has symptoms suggestive of diarrhea or malabsorption. If not, consider diseases associated with decreased intake or increased demand.

Table 22–2. Diagnostic hypotheses for Mrs. M.

Diagnostic Hypotheses	Clinical Clues	Important Tests
Leading Hypothesis		
Cancer		
Stomach	Early satiety	EGD or upper GI
Colon	Change in stools Hematochezia Positive FOBT	Colonoscopy
Lung	Cough, hemoptysis Tobacco use	Chest x-ray
Pancreas	Abdominal pain Jaundice, dark urine (bilirubinuria)	Abdominal ultrasound or CT scan
Active Alternatives—Most Common		
Nonmalignant GI disease		
Dental	New ill-fitting dentures	
Esophageal disease	Dysphagia	Upper GI series/EGD
PUD	Early satiety Nausea Melena NSAID use	Upper GI series/EGD
Pancreatitis	Alcohol use Jaundice	Lipase Abdominal ultrasound or CT scan
Hepatitis	Alcohol use Jaundice	AST, ALT, bilirubin

Table 22–2. Diagnostic hypotheses for Mrs. M. (continued)

Diagnostic Hypotheses	Clinical Clues	Important Tests
IBD	Diarrhea Hematochezia	Colonoscopy
Depression	History of loss Prior depression Postpartum state Family history Multiple somatic symptoms (> 6) Positive depression screen	Complaints of feeling down or anhedonia
Alcoholism	Quantity of alcohol use Family- or work-related problems Family history of alcoholism Elevated AST and MCV	CAGE or TWEAK questionnaire
Hyperthyroidism	Increased sweating Nervousness Goiter Tachycardia Atrial fibrillation Lid lag or retraction Fine tremor Hyperactive reflexes	TSH
Active Alternatives—Must Not Miss		
HIV	Fevers, lymphadenopathy, recurrent pneumonias History of high-risk sexual contacts or injection drug use	HIV
Subacute bacterial endocarditis	History of valvular heart disease, murmur	Blood cultures ESR
Temporal arteritis	Proximal muscle soreness Headache Visual loss Temporal artery tenderness	ESR

TSH, thyroid-stimulating hormone.

Finally, a thorough review of systems, physical exam, and basic laboratory exam (CBC, urinalysis, renal panel, liver panel, FOBT, ESR, TSH and chest x-ray) are critical in evaluating patients with unintentional weight loss. The myriad of diseases associated with unintentional weight loss make it vital to search for clues before beginning a more expensive and indiscriminate investigation.

Mrs. M reports no early satiety, nausea, or vomiting. She reports that she never smoked cigarettes, has no unusual cough, and has not experienced any episodes of hemoptysis. She has had no change in her bowel habits or blood in her stool. She has had dentures for many years without change. She has not experienced dysphagia, odynophagia, abdominal pain, jaundice, change in the color of her urine, and has no history of hepatitis. She has not noticed any tremulousness, heat intolerance, or swelling over her thyroid. She denies having any headaches, fevers, or history of known valvular heart disease or injection drug use.

(continued)

On physical exam, Mrs. M looks quite cachectic. She appears apathetic (Figure 22–1). Her vital signs are stable. HEENT exam reveals no oral lesions or adenopathy. Lungs are clear to percussion and auscultation. Cardiac exam reveals a regular rate and rhythm, with a grade I–II flow systolic murmur along the left sternal border. Her abdomen is scaphoid, without hepatosplenomegaly or mass. Rectal exam reveals guaiac-negative stool. Neurologic exam is normal, including a Mini-Mental Status Exam.

Is the clinical information sufficient to make a diagnosis? If not what other information do you need?

Mrs. M's history and physical do not clearly point to a specific disease process. There are no clues to suggest a GI disorder or features of any of the systemic diseases associated with decreased intake (HIV, SBE, temporal arteritis). Given her cachectic appearance, your primary concern is that she has an underlying malignancy. Her apparent apathy also raises the possibility of depression. Hyperthyroidism seems unlikely given her sluggish demeanor.

Leading Hypothesis: Cancer Cachexia

Textbook Presentation

Patients with cancer cachexia often have advanced disease. They suffer from anorexia, fatigue, and other symptoms specific to their particular malignancy. The cancer may have been diagnosed before the weight loss or the weight loss may lead to the diagnosis.

Disease Highlights

A. Cancer diagnoses account for 27% of cases of unexplained weight loss.

B. The most common malignancies associated with weight loss are GI, lung, and lymphoma.

C. Weight loss is one of the most common presenting symptoms in patients with lung cancer (comparable to cough). It is more frequent than dyspnea, hemoptysis, or chest pain.

D. Unintentional weight loss is common in cancer patients.

   1. Incidence: 13–25% over 3–4 years in prospective studies

   2. At the time of diagnosis, 24% of patients with cancer have lost weight.

E. Mortality is increased in all patients who lose weight, especially if the weight loss is secondary to malignancy.

   1. The 2-year mortality rate in all patients with weight loss is 35%.

   2. The 2-year mortality rate in patients with weight loss due to unknown cause is 18%.

   3. The 2-year mortality rate in patients with weight loss secondary to cancer is 62%.

F. Recurrence of breast cancer was more common in women with weight loss than those without (84% vs 10%).

G. Weight loss increases risk of immobility, deconditioning, and adversely affects immunity. The risk of pulmonary embolism, decubitus ulcers, and pneumonia are increased.

H. Mechanisms for weight loss are anorexia (secondary to medication, radiation, chemotherapy, alteration in taste and smell, nausea, depression) and increased resting energy expenditure.

Evidence-Based Diagnosis

Truly *occult malignancy* is unusual. Most malignancies become apparent on thorough history, physical exam, and

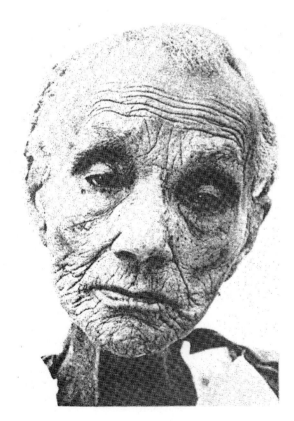

Figure 22–1. Mrs. M. (Reproduced, with permission, from Thomas FB et al. *Ann Intern Med.* 1970;72: 679–685.)

basic laboratory exam (CBC with differential, liver panel, renal panel, urinalysis, erythrocyte sedimentation rate [ESR], fecal occult blood test [FOBT] and chest x-ray), or follow-up of noted abnormalities. In one study of patients with unexplained weight loss, only 1 of 59 patients was found to have occult malignancy after a thorough history, physical, chest x-ray and basic laboratory exam.

Treatment

A. Nutritional support

1. In many patients, artificial nutritional support is not effective.

2. Certain subgroups of patients may benefit from nutritional support.

   a. Head and neck cancer (after radiation therapy)

   b. Bowel obstruction

   c. Surgery patients (particularly upper GI tract cancer)

   d. Patients receiving high-dose chemotherapy

3. Enteral support is appropriate if the bowel is functional.

B. Treat underlying malignancy

C. Medroxyprogesterone and megestrol

1. Decreases nausea and anorexia and increases weight gain

2. Mortality rate is increased due to the risk of thromboembolic events.

3. Other side effects include hyperglycemia, endometrial bleeding, edema, hypertension, adrenal suppression, and insufficiency.

D. Corticosteroids

1. Decrease anorexia and nausea

2. May increase quality of life and feeling of well-being.

3. Because of the side effects, corticosteroids are often reserved for patients with terminal disease.

E. Prokinetic drugs (metoclopramide) can decrease anorexia and nausea and improve early satiety.

MAKING A DIAGNOSIS

Clearly, a diagnosis is not yet apparent. The data suggest that when the cause of unintentional weight loss is malignant, there are usually clues on history, physical, or on laboratory testing. You elect to check a CBC, liver panel, renal panel, urinalysis, chest film, and screening mammogram. Finally, you elect to schedule Mrs. M for a colonoscopy, since she has never undergone colon cancer screening.

Surprisingly, Mrs. M's laboratory evaluation is strikingly normal. Her CBC is normal without evidence of iron deficiency anemia (which could indicate gastric or colon cancer). The chest x-ray is also normal, making lung cancer unlikely, particularly in a patient who never smoked. ALT (SGPT), AST (SGOT), alkaline phosphatase, and bilirubin are normal (an elevation can suggest hepatic metastasis or obstruction due to pancreatic cancer), and her renal panel is normal. There was no hematuria on urinalysis (which could suggest renal cell carcinoma or bladder cancer). Her mammogram and colonoscopy were normal.

Have you crossed a diagnostic threshold for the leading hypothesis, cancer cachexia? Have you ruled out the active alternatives? Do other tests need to be done to exclude the alternative diagnoses?

Alternative Diagnosis: Depression

Textbook Presentation

Depression may follow a recognizable loss or occur without a clear precipitant. Classically, patients complain of profound sadness, lack of interest in activities (anhedonia), sleep and appetite disturbances, impaired concentration, and other symptoms. Patients may lose or gain weight. Patients may experience suicidal or homicidal thoughts.

Disease Highlights

A. Point prevalence of major depressive disorder (MDD) in primary care is 4.8–8.6%. Lifetime prevalence is 16.2%. Minor depression is twice as common.

B. Depression is the second most common condition seen in primary care practices.

C. It is the fourth leading cause of disability: 59% of patients have severe or very severe role impairment.

D. Criteria for MDD requires depressed mood or anhedonia for at least 2 weeks along with ≥ 4 of the following: significant appetite or weight change, sleep disturbance, psychomotor agitation or retardation, fatigue, feelings of worthlessness, impaired concentration, or suicidal ideation. Minor depression requires 2–4 symptoms.

E. Risk factors for major depression

1. Prior episode of depression

2. Postpartum

3. Comorbid medical illness

4. Absence of social support

5. Female sex (2–3 times more common than in males)

6. Family history (first-degree relative)

7. Stressful life events

8. Substance abuse

F. Associated anxiety: 50% of patients have anxiety symptoms

   1. 10–20% of patients with MDD have evidence of panic disorder

   2. 30–40% of depressed patients meet the criteria for generalized anxiety disorder

   3. Conversely, 91% of patients with agoraphobia manifest MDD within 3 years.

   4. Patients with anxiety and MDD are at higher risk for suicide.

G. Minor depression

   1. 10–18% progress to major depression within 1 year.

   2. 20% have moderate to severe disability

Evidenced-Based Diagnosis

A. Depression is often missed on routine evaluation. In patients in whom depression was subsequently diagnosed, only 8.8% were found to be depressed during routine interview.

B. Signs and symptoms are not very sensitive or specific in inpatients admitted for a variety of reasons

   1. "Downhearted or blue," 60% sensitive and 85% specific

   2. "Feel like crying," 45% sensitive and 87% specific

   3. Depressed mood is 100% sensitive but only 33% specific; LR+ 2.1

   4. Suicidal ideations were insensitive for depression (40–50%) but more specific (91–96%); LR+ 5.6–9.7

   5. Somatic GI symptoms were common in depressed inpatients 88–100% (depending on age group).

C. Screening tools increase identification of patients with depression by 2- to 3-fold (an absolute increase of 10–47%).

D. US Preventive Services Task Force concluded that 2 questions perform as well as longer screening instruments (a positive response to either question sensitivity, 96%; specificity, 57%; LR+, 2.2; LR–, 0.07)

   1. "During the past month, have you felt down, depressed or hopeless"

   2. "During the past month, have you often been bothered by little interest or pleasure in doing things?"

E. Many medical illnesses are associated with depression (eg, 20–45% of cancer patients are depressed, and 40% of Parkinson disease patients are depressed). Therefore, care must be taken before ascribing weight loss to depression.

 The diagnosis of depression does not exclude other serious illnesses causing weight loss. Ideally, patients should be monitored to ensure weight gain following treatment of their depression.

F. Clinical clues include

   1. Recent stress or loss

   2. Chronic medical illness, chronic pain syndromes

   3. > 6 physical symptoms: Men with major depression averaged 6.5 symptoms, compared with 3.7 symptoms in men with other diagnoses

   4. Higher patient ratings of symptom severity

   5. Lower patient rating of overall health

   6. Physician perception of encounter as difficult

   7. Substance abuse (23% have MDD)

   8. Overestimation of weight loss

      a. In patients who overestimated their weight loss (by more than .5 kg), no organic cause was found in 73% and cancer was unlikely (6%).

      b. In patients who underestimated their weight loss (by more than 1 kg), cancer was diagnosed in 52%.

Treatment

A. Work-up should include TSH, drug history (alcohol abuse, glucocorticoids, oral contraceptives, H_2-blockers, cocaine) and screening tests (ie, basic metabolic panel, liver function tests, CBC) to rule out other medical conditions.

B. Assess suicide risk: Ideation, intent, or plan

   1. Have you been having thoughts of dying?

   2. Do you have a plan?

   3. Does patient have the means (eg, weapons) to succeed?

   4. Presence of psychotic symptoms

   5. Substance abuse

   6. History of prior attempts

7. Family history of suicide or recent exposure to suicide.

8. Patients at risk for suicide should be referred for emergent psychiatric evaluation.

C. Pharmacotherapy

   1. Based on number of symptoms and functional impairment.

   2. *Not* influenced by whether or not there is understandable explanation (ie, stress). In grief reactions, signs of MDD should be treated if symptoms persist for more than 2 months.

   3. Multiple classes of medications are effective; selective serotonin reuptake inhibitors are first-line due to low frequency of adverse effects.

   4. Treat for 4–5 months *after* clinical recovery (usually takes 3.6 months).

   5. For patients with multiple recurrences, lifetime therapy may be indicated.

D. Other options are cognitive behavioral therapy and interpersonal psychotherapy.

E. Pharmacotherapy *with* psychotherapy more effective than either alone.

F. Indications for referral include psychotic features, substance abuse, panic disorder, agitated depression, severe depression, bipolar depression, suicidality, relapsing depression, dysthymia.

▽
1

Mrs. M reports no unusual stresses or losses. She has been widowed for 15 years and feels that she has come to terms with her husband's death. She lives with her daughter and regularly sees family members and remains actively involved in her church. She denies feeling down, depressed, or hopeless in the last month and denies loss of interest or pleasure in doing things.

Mrs. M's answers to the screening questions make depression highly unlikely (LR− 0.07). Although her appearance seems antithetical to hyperthyroidism, you wonder if that possibility should be pursued.

Alternative Diagnosis: Hyperthyroidism

Textbook Presentation

Classically, patients with hyperthyroidism present with a myriad of symptoms and signs obvious to the experienced observer. Symptoms include palpitations, heat intolerance, increased sweating, insomnia, tremulousness, diarrhea, and *weight loss.* Signs of hyperthyroidism include sinus tachycardia, frightened stare, an enlarged goiter, a fine resting tremor, and exophthalmos (only if the hyperthyroidism is secondary to Graves disease). Other manifestations may include hyperpigmentation, pruritus, and thinning of hair. Complications include osteoporosis, tracheal obstruction (from the goiter), tachyarrhythmias (particularly atrial fibrillation), high output congestive heart failure, anemia, and proximal muscle weakness.

Disease Highlights

A. Prevalence, 0.3%.

B. Hyperthyroidism is actually an endocrine syndrome caused by several distinct pathophysiologic entities (Table 22–3).

Evidence-Based Diagnosis

A. History and physical

   1. Certain findings of hyperthyroidism are quite specific (ie, lid lag and lid retraction) and help rule in the diagnosis (99% specific, LR+, 17–32).

   2. Clinical findings are not highly sensitive. Therefore, absent clinical findings do not allow hyperthyroidism to be ruled out.

      a. Goiter is present in 70–93% of cases.

      b. Lid lag is present in 19% of cases.

      c. Heart rate > 90 bpm is present in 80% of cases.

      d. Tremor is present in 84–96% of cases.

      e. Ophthalmopathy is present in 25–50% of patients with Graves disease.

      f. Hyperreflexia is present in 25% of cases.

B. Elderly patients

   1. Prevalence of hyperthyroidism in elderly is 2–3%.

   2. Cardiovascular findings and weight loss more common in the elderly, whereas goiter and adrenergic overactivity are less common (tachycardia, nervousness, sweating, hyperreflexia and heat intolerance), resulting in the phenomenon *apathetic hyperthyroidism of elderly.*

      a. Weight loss is the most common finding (75–100%).

      b. Atrial fibrillation is seen in 35–54% of cases.

      c. Symptoms suggestive of congestive heart failure are present in 67% of cases.

      d. Heat intolerance is present in 15% of cases.

      e. Hyperreflexia occurs in 28% of cases.

Table 22–3. Distinguishing features of several hyperthyroid states.

Disease	Pathogenesis/Important Features	TSH	T4, FTI or T3	Thyroid Scan and Other Tests
Graves disease	Autoimmune production of thyroid-stimulating antibody binds and stimulates TSH receptor. Exophthalmos parenthysis (unique to Graves—may be unilateral or bilateral)	↓	↑	Diffusely increased Elevated TSI
Toxic multinodular goiter	Most common form in elderly	↓	↑	Heterogeneous Increased uptake
Subacute thyroiditis	Viral or immune inflammatory attack on thyroid resulting in neck pain, tenderness, and release of hormone	↓	↑	Decreased uptake Elevated ESR
Toxic adenoma	Autonomously functioning benign thyroid nodule	↓	↑	Hot nodule, rest of gland is suppressed
Iodine or amiodarone	Amiodarone[a] may cause the release of T4 and T3	↓	↑	Usually decreased
TSH-producing adenoma	Autonomously functioning benign *pituitary* adenoma. May cause bitemporal hemianopsia. Galactorrhea develops in 33% of women	↑	↑	Diffusely increased
Factitious or iatrogenic	Self or physician induced	↓	↑	T4/FTI more elevated than T3

[a]Amiodarone causes hypothyroidism in 20% of patients by impairing conversion of T4 to T3.
TSI, thyroid-stimulating immunoglobin; ESR, erythrocyte sedimentation rate.

   f. Eye manifestations are present in < 50% of cases.

   g. Goiter is present in 50% of cases.

   h. Agitation, confusion, and depression may also be seen.

Consider hyperthyroidism in elderly patients with weight loss (OR 8.7), tachycardia (OR 11.2), atrial fibrillation or apathy (OR 14.8). Hyperthyroidism was not even considered in 54% of admitted patients in whom hyperthyroidism was subsequently diagnosed.

C. Laboratory tests

   1. Thyroid stimulating hormone (TSH) is the test of choice.

      a. Sensitivity > 99%, specificity > 99%

      b. LR+ > 99; LR– < .01

      c. Low TSH, indicates hyperthyroidism

      d. Normal TSH, indicates euthyroidism

      e. High TSH, indicates hypothyroidism

   2. Exception occurs when the pituitary itself is diseased (rare).

      a. Pituitary adenoma producing TSH produces hyperthyroidism with increased TSH and free thyroxine index (FTI).

      b. Pituitary destruction (ie, sarcoidosis) produces hypothyroidism with decreased TSH and FTI.

   3. The total T4 is less accurate than the FTI because the total T4 is affected by alterations in thyroid binding globulin (TBG). [Elevations in TBG leads to increased T4 but the free T4 and FTI remain normal. A normal free T4 level (or FTI) and normal TSH in such patients confirms the patient is euthyroid despite the elevated total T4.]

   4. Occasionally, patients with hyperthyroidism have isolated elevations in T3, or T3 thyrotoxicosis. In such patients, the TSH is still suppressed.

   5. Certain features can help to distinguish the etiology of hyperthyroidism (Table 22–3).

CASE RESOLUTION

A TSH on Mrs. M is completely suppressed (< 0.1 mcU/mL). The T4 is elevated at 20 mcg/dL (nl 5–11.6) and the FTI is 22 (nl 6–10.5). You diagnose hyperthyroidism. A thyroid scan reveals heterogeneous uptake consistent with a toxic multinodular goiter.

Treatment of Hyperthyroidism

A. β-Blockers can be used to decrease the sympathetic simulation.

B. Definitive treatment of hyperthyroidism depends on underlying etiology.

   1. Graves disease
      a. Antithyroid drugs
         (1) May cause agranulocytosis
         (2) 60–70% of patients relapse within 1 year.
      b. Radioactive iodine
         (1) Used successfully for over 60 years.
         (2) Patients usually require subsequent lifelong thyroid hormone replacement.
         (3) Pretreatment with antithyroid drugs is recommended for elderly patients and patients with cardiovascular disease to prevent the transient worsening of thyrotoxicosis.
      c. Surgery is occasionally used, particularly if the goiter is troublesome.

   2. Toxic multinodular goiter
      a. Elderly: Consider radioactive iodine; monitor for hypothyroidism
      b. Large goiter: Consider surgery

   3. Subacute thyroiditis
      a. Aspirin or nonsteroidal anti-inflammatory drugs (NSAIDs) decrease thyroid inflammation.
      b. β-Blockers decrease symptoms of hyperthyroidism until inflammation subsides.
      c. Prednisone and ipodate can be used in severe cases.

   4. TSH-producing pituitary adenoma (rare): Transphenoidal hypophysectomy and radiation therapy (directed at the pituitary) have been used. Octreotide has also been used to suppress TSH secretion.

Due to her advanced age, you elect to have her treated with radioactive iodine. Six months later she returns on replacement levothyroxine. Laboratory exam reveals that she is euthyroid. She complains that her clothes are now too tight.

In short, Mrs. M had unintentional weight loss and no clinical clues. The initial concern about cancer and depression are appropriate, but many patients end up with alternative diagnoses. Despite her apathetic appearance, Mrs. M suffered from hyperthyroidism and, in fact, she presented with symptoms commonly seen in elderly patients.

CHIEF COMPLAINT

PATIENT 2

Mr. O is a 55-year-old man who complains of weight loss. He reports that he has tried for years to lose weight (unsuccessfully) but that recently he has lost more and more weight without effort. He was initially pleased but recently has become concerned. He reports that altogether he has lost 30 pounds in the last 6 months (from 200 lbs to 170 lbs).

At this point, what is the leading hypothesis and what are the active alternatives? What other tests should be ordered?

ORGANIZING THE DIFFERENTIAL DIAGNOSIS

Mr. O has clearly suffered from verifiable significant weight loss (> 5% in 6 months). As noted above, the second step in the evaluation of patients with *documented* weight loss is to determine whether or not the patient is having symptoms that suggest diarrhea or malabsorption.

Mr. O reports no diarrhea, large foul-smelling stools, or difficult to flush stools. He reports that he previously moved his bowels once a day but lately only once every other day. He attributes this to his decreased appetite.

Since Mr. O's weight loss is not clearly secondary to malabsorption or diarrhea, the likely mechanism is either decreased energy intake or increased energy expenditure. Decreased intake may result from cancer, GI, psychosocial disease, or systemic disease. Increased demand may occur in hyperthyroidism. A thorough review of systems, psychosocial history, physical exam, and basic laboratory studies (including TSH) should be performed. Table 22–4 lists the differential diagnosis, which is similar to Mrs. M's.

Mr. O has a decreased appetite and feels full quickly after starting to eat. He has not noticed any melena or hematochezia or any jaundice. He has never been a tobacco smoker. He denies night sweats or swollen lymph nodes. He denies any dysphagia or odynophagia but does admit to NSAID use. He reports that he takes 600 mg of ibuprofen 2–3 times a day for his arthritis. He denies any abdominal pain. He reports that he has not felt down, depressed, or hopeless during the past month nor has he been bothered by a lack of interest in activities. He drinks 2 beers about once a month. Finally, he denies symptoms associated with a variety of systemic diseases including fevers, muscle aches (other than his arthritic knees), or headaches.

Physical exam reveals a thin but otherwise healthy appearing middle-aged man. Vital signs are normal. The remainder of his exam is completely normal.

Laboratory tests, including CBC, differential, hepatic panel, renal panel, urinalysis, ESR, and TSH, are normal. A chest x-ray is normal without mass or adenopathy.

Is the clinical information sufficient to make a diagnosis? If not what other information do you need?

The cause of Mr. O's weight loss is not obvious. However, his early satiety and NSAID use are clues that he might have PUD or other gastric pathology. You revise your leading hypothesis to PUD. The change in bowel habits also raises the possibility of colon cancer.

Colon cancer causing subtotal obstruction may present with hematochezia or change in bowel habits, which can manifest as either constipation *or diarrhea.*

All medications (prescription and over the counter) should be carefully scrutinized in patients complaining of unexplained weight loss. Some medications cause anorexia directly, others through various organ toxicities.

Leading Hypothesis: PUD

Textbook Presentation

The pain of PUD is classically described as a dull or hunger-like pain in the epigastrium that is either exacerbated or improved by food intake. The pain is often worse on waking and may radiate to the back. Nausea and early satiety may be seen.

Disease Highlights

A. 250,000 cases per year in the United States

B. 1.5–2 times more common in males than females

C. Etiology: Most ulcers are secondary to either NSAIDs or *Helicobacter pylori*

    1. *H pylori* infection

        a. Asymptomatic in 70% of patients

        b. Peptic ulcer develops in 15% of infected patients.

        c. May cause duodenal or gastric ulcers

            (1) Duodenal ulcers are associated with increased acid secretion.

Table 22–4. Diagnostic hypotheses for Mr. O.

Diagnostic Hypotheses	Clinical Clues	Important Tests
Leading Hypothesis		
Cancer		
Stomach	Early satiety	EGD or upper GI
Colon	Change in stools Hematochezia Positive FOBT	Colonoscopy
Lung	Cough, hemoptysis Tobacco use	Chest x-ray
Pancreas	Abdominal pain Jaundice, dark urine (bilirubinuria)	Abdominal ultrasound or CT scan
Active Alternatives—Most Common		
Nonmalignant GI disease		
Dental	New ill-fitting dentures	
Esophageal disease	Dysphagia	Upper GI series/EGD
PUD	Early satiety Nausea Melena NSAID use	Upper GI series/EGD
Pancreatitis	Alcohol use Jaundice	Lipase Abdominal ultrasound or CT scan
Hepatitis	Alcohol use Jaundice	AST, ALT, bilirubin
IBD	Diarrhea Hematochezia	Colonoscopy
Depression	History of loss Prior depression Postpartum state Family history Multiple somatic symptoms (> 6) Positive depression screen	Complaints of feeling down or anhedonia
Alcoholism	Quantity of alcohol use Family- or work-related problems Family history of alcoholism Elevated AST and MCV	CAGE or TWEAK questionnaire
Hyperthyroidism	Increased sweating Nervousness Goiter Tachycardia Atrial fibrillation Lid lag or retraction Fine tremor Hyperactive reflexes	TSH

Table 22–4. Diagnostic hypotheses for Mr. O. (continued)

Diagnostic Hypotheses	Clinical Clues	Important Tests
Active Alternatives—Must Not Miss		
HIV	Fevers, lymphadenopathy, recurrent pneumonias History of high-risk sexual contacts or injection drug use	HIV
Subacute bacterial endocarditis	History of valvular heart disease, murmur	Blood cultures ESR
Temporal arteritis	Proximal muscle soreness Headache Visual loss Temporal artery tenderness	ESR

(2) Gastric ulcers are associated with diffuse gastritis, decreased acid secretion, and an increased risk of gastric cancer.

   d. *H pylori* is a major risk factor for gastric cancer (but rarely causes it).

2. NSAIDs

   a. 25% of all adverse drug reactions involve NSAIDs

   b. 16,500 deaths/y from NSAID-associated GI bleeding

   c. Gastric ulcers are 5 times more common than duodenal ulcers.

   d. Prevalence of symptoms or complications

      (1) Endoscopic lesions, 80%

      (2) Endoscopic ulcers, 20%

      (3) Dyspepsia, 10%

      (4) Hospitalizations, 2.2%/y

      (5) Death, 0.15%/y

      (6) Death in patients who hemorrhage, 10%

   e. Ulcers are most likely in the first 1–3 months of NSAID use.

   f. There is an increased risk of ulcer if any of the following are present:

      (1) Concurrent warfarin use; relative risk increases 10–15 times

      (2) High dose NSAIDs; relative risk increases 10 times

      (3) Age > 60; relative risk increases 5–6 times

      (4) Concurrent glucocorticoid use; relative risk increases 4–5 times

      (5) Prior ulcer or hemorrhage; relative risk increases 4–5 times

      (6) Concomitant *H pylori* infection; relative risk increases 3.53 times compared to NSAIDs alone

      (7) Female sex

      (8) Nonselective NSAIDs (with cyclooxygenase (COX)-1 activity)

3. Zollinger-Ellison syndrome is a rare cause of PUD.

D. Complications: Bleeding can vary from massive hemorrhage (with hematemesis and melena or hematochezia) to iron deficiency anemia and guaiac-positive stools (see Chapter 14, GI Bleeding).

Evidence-Based Diagnosis

A. History and physical

   1. 60% of NSAID-associated ulcers are asymptomatic

   2. 25% of non-NSAID ulcers are asymptomatic

   3. First sign of ulcer may be life-threatening complication (hemorrhage or perforation): > 50% of patients with serious to life-threatening complication had no prior symptom.

   4. 31–55% of patients with benign gastric ulcer noted weight loss.

      a. ≅ 50% lost 10–20 lbs

      b. 21% lost > 20 lbs

      c. PUD is found more often in patients undergoing esophagogastroduodenoscopy (EGD) for weight loss than for dyspepsia.

A significant number of patients with NSAID-induced ulcers do not experience pain. Anemia, GI bleeding, early satiety, and weight loss can be the only symptom of PUD.

5. < 33% of patients with dyspepsia have PUD

6. Best predictors of PUD are a history of NSAID use and *H pylori* infection (Table 22–5).

7. Poor clinical predictors for discriminating ulcer from nonulcer dyspepsia include

  a. Response to antisecretory therapy

  b. Epigastric tenderness

  c. The quality of the pain

B. Laboratory

  1. *H pylori* testing

    a. Options include invasive and noninvasive testing

      (1) Invasive: histology, culture, urease test

      (2) Noninvasive: serology, stool antigen, urea breath test

    b. All options share a > 90% sensitivity and specificity.

    c. Serology useful for diagnosis but remains positive long after therapy, so it cannot be used to assess eradication.

    d. Stool antigen, breath test, or urease can assess eradication.

    e. Sensitivity of urease test or breath test fall significantly with acid blockade.

  2. Ulcer diagnosis

    a. EGD is more sensitive than upper GI series (92% vs 54%) and is useful to rule out other serious pathology.

    b. Indications for EGD (Figure 22–2)

      (1) Hemorrhage

      (2) Anemia

      (3) Weight loss

      (4) Early satiety

      (5) New onset of symptoms in persons older than 45 years

      (6) Suspicion very high

      (7) Patients who do not respond to initial therapy

MAKING A DIAGNOSIS

Despite the absence of pain, the early satiety, weight loss, and history of NSAID use convinces you to order an EGD.

 The EGD reveals 2 gastric ulcers 1.5 cm in size. Pathology reveals organisms consistent with *H pylori*.

 Have you crossed a diagnostic threshold for the leading hypothesis, gastric ulcer? Have you ruled out the active alternatives? Do other tests need to be done to exclude the alternative diagnoses?

You conclude that the likely cause of Mr. O's weight loss is gastric ulcer. You elect to initiate therapy without further testing.

 Altogether, malignant and nonmalignant GI disease is responsible for weight loss in 28% of patients and the yield of EGD 12–44%. EGD should be considered in the evaluation of patients with unexplained weight loss.

Table 22–5. Pretest probability of PUD in patients with dyspepsia.

Age	Neither *H pylori* or NSAIDs	Current NSAID use	*H pylori* infection
40 years	1%	5%	20%
75 years	3%	20%	30%

PUD, peptic ulcer disease; NSAID, nonsteroidal anti-inflammatory drug.

Diagnostic Approach: Peptic Ulcer Disease

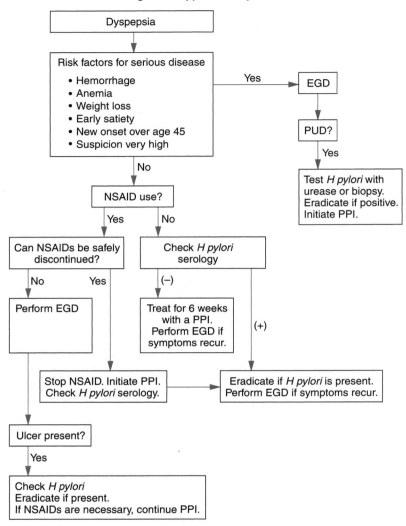

EGD, esophagogastroduodenoscopy; PUD, peptic ulcer disease; NSAIDs, nonsteroidal anti-inflammatory drugs; PPI, proton pump inhibitors.

Figure 22–2.

CASE RESOLUTION

Mr. O received eradication therapy, a proton pump inhibitor (PPI), and stopped his ibuprofen. Three months later, his appetite is excellent. He is advised to use acetaminophen for his arthritis pain and to perform nonimpact physical activities.

Treatment of PUD

A. *H pylori* and ulcer

   1. Eradication markedly decreases recurrence from 60–100% to 15%.

   2. Regimens require multiple simultaneous medications using a PPI and usually 2 distinct antibiotics.

   3. Increased incidence of *H pylori* resistance has led to the recommendation for posttreatment testing.

4. Patients requiring continued NSAIDs
   a. Most experts recommend *H pylori* eradication
   b. Continued PPI therapy prevents rebleeding more effectively than eradication *alone.*
B. Prevention of PUD
   1. Minimize dose and duration of NSAIDs
   2. Avoid certain high-risk nonselective NSAIDS, such as ketorolac, piroxicam and indomethacin, which increased the relative risk of PUD
   3. COX-2 inhibitors have been shown to decrease the incidence of PUD and bleeding compared with nonselective NSAIDs. However, recent studies have suggested an increase risk of myocardial infarction associated with the use of COX-2 inhibitors. Their current role is uncertain.
   4. High-dose misoprostol is effective at preventing NSAID-induced ulcers but poorly tolerated.
   5. High-dose PPI is slightly less effective than misoprostol but better tolerated (net prevention similar): Consider in high-risk patients taking nonselective NSAIDs or aspirin.
   6. H_2-receptor blockers do not prevent NSAID-induced ulcers.

CHIEF COMPLAINT

PATIENT 3

Mr. A is a 62-year-old man who complains of recent weight loss. He reports that he has lost 15 pounds over the last 6–9 months, and that his clothes no longer fit. He denies diarrhea but admits to abdominal bloating and having several large stools a day that are difficult to flush. He reports that his appetite is not what it used to be but attributes that to his recent separation from his wife.

The cause of Mr. A's weight loss is not immediately clear. The recent separation from his wife suggests that social issues may be important. You ask him if he will elaborate on what happened with his wife and how he feels about the separation.

Mr. A reports that they have not gotten along for years. She seemed to blame everything on his drinking, but he assures you that alcohol was definitely not a problem. Further, he reports that he is glad she is out of his life.

> **At this point, what is the leading hypothesis, and what are the active alternatives? What other tests should be ordered?**

ORGANIZING THE DIFFERENTIAL DIAGNOSIS

Mr. A's social history raises several possibilities. First, you suspect that his drinking is a problem and might be contributing to his weight loss. Alternatively, he may be more depressed than he acknowledges or simply adjusting to lifestyle changes precipitated by his separation. Finally, although he denies diarrhea, his large frequent stools raise the possibility of some form of malabsorption. Table 22–6 lists the differential diagnosis.

On further questioning, Mr. A reports that he drinks 2 or so alcoholic beverages a night. He proudly states that he has never missed work due to a hangover and never drinks before noon. When you ask him how much alcohol he uses in each drink and whether anyone else has commented on his drinking, he gets defensive and reminds you he is here because he is losing weight.

 Is the clinical information sufficient to make a diagnosis? If not, what other information do you need?

Mr. A's defensiveness increases your suspicion of alcoholism. You wonder how much alcohol consumption is normal and how to screen him more thoroughly for alcoholism.

Table 22–6. Diagnostic hypotheses for Mr. A.

Diagnostic Hypotheses	Clinical Clues	Important Tests
Leading Hypothesis		
Alcoholism	Quantity of alcohol use Family- or work-related problems Family history of alcoholism Elevated AST and MCV Difficult to control hypertension	CAGE or TWEAK questionnaire
Active Alternatives—Most Common		
Depression	History of loss Prior depression Family history Multiple somatic symptoms (> 6) Positive depression screen	Admission of feeling down or anhedonia
GI diseases that cause malabsorption	Diarrhea Foul, oily, or difficult to flush stools Iron deficiency anemia Hematochezia Vitamin B_{12} deficiency Edema (hypoalbuminemia) Calcium oxalate stones (secondary to fat malabsorption)	CBC with differential Albumin ESR Vitamin B_{12} Ferritin
IBD	Family history History of uveitis Erythema nodosum Rectal abscess	Colonoscopy P-ANCA, ASCA antibodies Consider enteroclysis for Crohn disease
Bacterial overgrowth	Prior bowel surgery Small bowel diverticula	Quantitative jejunal aspirates D-xylose breath test
Chronic pancreatitis	History of heavy alcohol use	Calcifications on plain film and CT scan ERCP
Celiac disease	Family history Neurologic disorders	IgA endomysial Ab Anti-tGT Ab

Leading Hypothesis: Alcoholism

Textbook Presentation

Patients with alcoholism present along a continuum, from the functioning executive to the homeless alcoholic. Psychosocial complications include job loss, marital difficulties, loss of driving license, and violent behavior. Medical complications may include pancreatitis, gastritis, cirrhosis, vitamin deficiency, cardiomyopathy, hypertension, malnutrition, weight loss, and death. Weight loss may be multifactorial secondary to decreased caloric intake during intoxication or due to alcohol-related illnesses (gastritis, pancreatitis, cirrhosis). Alcoholism is difficult to recognize early, when intervention may prevent progression.

Disease Highlights

A. Categories and definitions of patterns of alcohol use (1 drink is defined as 1.5 oz of liquor, 5 oz of wine, or 12 oz of beer)

1. Moderate drinking
   a. Men: ≤ 2 drinks/d
   b. Women: ≤ 1 drink/d
   c. Persons older than 65 years: ≤ 1 drink/d

2. At-risk drinking
   a. Men: > 14 drinks/wk or > 4 drinks per occasion
   b. Women: > 7 drinks/wk or > 3 drinks per occasion

3. Hazardous drinking: At risk for consequences from alcohol

4. Harmful drinking: Alcohol causing physical or psychological harm

5. Alcohol abuse: ≥ 1 of the following events in 1 year:

    a. Recurrent use resulting in failure to fulfill major role or obligations

    b. Recurrent use in hazardous situations

    c. Recurrent alcohol-related legal problems (eg, driving while intoxicated)

    d. Continued use despite social or interpersonal problems caused or exacerbated by alcohol

6. Alcohol dependence: ≥ 3 of the following events in 1 year:

    a. Tolerance (increased amounts to achieve effect)

    b. Withdrawal

    c. A great deal of time spent obtaining, using, or recovering from alcohol; important activities given up or reduced because of alcohol

    d. Drinking more or longer than intended

    e. Persistent desire or unsuccessful efforts to cut down or control alcohol use

    f. Continued use despite knowledge of a psychological problem exacerbated by alcohol

B. Prevalence of hazardous drinking among women is 4–5% and among men is 14–18%.

C. Prevalence of alcohol abuse and dependence is 7–16%.

D. Alcohol is involved in 40% of all traffic fatalities and 20–37% of emergency department trauma. Alcoholism is estimated to cause 100,000 deaths annually.

E. Women are more likely to deny alcohol-related problems and to have associated eating disorders, depression, and panic disorders than men.

Evidence-Based Diagnosis

A. Clinical clues

    1. Family, work or legal problems

    2. Accidents

    3. Violence

    4. Depression

    5. Substance abuse (7 times higher in alcoholics)

    6. Hypertension

    7. Abnormal liver enzymes

    8. Macrocytosis

    9. Anemia

    10. Thrombocytopenia

    11. Family history of alcoholism

B. Self reporting of alcohol ingestion may be inaccurate, particularly in patients who have recently ingested alcohol.

    1. Sensitivity of self report of ≥ 4 drinks per day, 47%

    2. Sensitivity of self report of ≥ 20 drinks per week, 20%

C. Laboratory studies may increase the suspicion of alcoholism but are insensitive and should not be used to rule out the diagnosis.

    1. GGT elevation: Sensitivity, 42–52%; specificity, 76%; LR+, 1.7; LR−, 0.8

    2. Increased MCV: Sensitivity, 24%; specificity, 96%; LR+, 6; LR−, 0.8

D. **CAGE** questionnaire

    1. Highly accurate for lifetime history of alcohol abuse and dependence

    2. Sensitivity is 77–94% and specificity is 79–97%.

    3. Less sensitive for heavy alcohol use (without abuse).

    4. Questions (positive is defined as ≥ 2 affirmative answers)

        a. Have you ever felt you should **Cut** down on your drinking?

        b. Have people **Annoyed** you by criticizing your drinking?

        c. Have you ever felt bad or **Guilty** about your drinking?

        d. Have you ever taken a drink first thing in the morning (**Eye** opener) to steady your nerves or get rid of a hangover?

E. **TWEAK** questionnaire is the optimal screening tool for heavy alcohol use or dependence in women and racially mixed groups (positive is defined as ≥ 2 affirmative answers)

    1. **Tolerance:** Can you hold more than 6 drinks (total), or ≥ 3 drinks before you feel the effects?

    2. **Worried:** Are friends or relatives worried or have they complained about your drinking?

    3. **Eye opener:** Do you sometimes take a drink first thing in the morning?

    4. **Amnesia:** Have you forgotten things that occurred while you were drinking?

    5. **Kut down:** Have you felt the need to cut down on your drinking?

MAKING A DIAGNOSIS

Mr. A's history of "2 or so" drinks per night suggest at-risk drinking. Furthermore, his marital separation, while possibly multifactorial, raises the real possibility of alcohol abuse. You elect to administer the CAGE and TWEAK questionnaires.

Mr. A reports that of course he tried to **cut** down while he was married. Fortunately, since his separation he no longer feels that restraint. He admits to feeling **annoyed** with other family members who have suggested he cut down. (He is certain that his wife turned them against him.) He denies feeling **guilty** about his drinking and has never taken an **eye** opener. Mr. A reports that he has always been able to "hold his liquor" and that 6 drinks in an evening is not uncommon if he is having fun (**tolerance**). He acknowledges that occasionally he hears funny stories about himself from these parties that he cannot recollect (**amnesia**).

Mr. A reluctantly reports that he received 2 tickets for driving while intoxicated within the past year. He feels mildly guilty about this but assures you he knows better than to make that mistake again. He reiterates that he has never missed work due to his drinking but did miss several family events because he was "partying."

Mr. A has 2 positive responses to the CAGE questionnaire and 4 positive responses to the TWEAK questions. Both suggest abuse or dependence. His failure to fulfill family obligations and his continued drinking despite legal problems clearly classifies his drinking pattern as alcohol abuse. His tolerance, time spent using alcohol, and missing of important activities also suggest dependence. You elect to check a CBC and a liver panel. The CBC shows macrocytosis (enlarged RBCs) and the liver panel shows a mildly elevated AST and ALT. The elevation in AST is more marked than the elevation in ALT, a pattern commonly seen in alcoholic hepatitis.

Clearly, Mr. A suffers from alcohol abuse and dependence. This may be the sole cause or a contributing cause of his weight loss. You elect to initiate a treatment plan and reevaluate him once he is abstinent.

CASE RESOLUTION

You have a frank discussion of the issues with Mr. A. You acknowledge that his marital difficulties are complex, but that many features of his alcohol use suggest dependence and abuse. The missed family gatherings, alcoholic blackouts, tolerance, tickets for driving while intoxicated, and abnormal blood test results all suggest this is a serious medical problem. Mr. A confides that he is frightened to go "cold turkey." He feels shaky and agitated whenever he stops drinking. You suggest admission to a detoxification unit. Mr. A listens carefully and agrees to be admitted.

Treatment of Alcohol Abuse & Dependence

A. Components of effective interventions for hazardous drinkers include:
   1. Feedback on clinical assessment
   2. Comparison to drinking norms
   3. Discussion of the adverse effects of alcohol
   4. Statement of the recommended drinking limits
   5. Prescription to "Cut down on your drinking"
   6. Patient educational material (www.niaaa.nih.gov)
   7. Drinking diary
   8. Follow-up office sessions and phone contact

B. Physician feedback, discussion, and prescription to cut down have been demonstrated to reduce drinking (OR 1.95). Hospitalizations were also decreased by the intervention.

C. Alcohol withdrawal (see Chapter 8, Delirium & Dementia)

D. Relapse prevention: Several options
   1. Alcoholics Anonymous (AA), a 12-step program
   2. Motivational enhancement therapy
   3. Therapy to develop cognitive behavioral coping skills.
   4. Naltrexone, disulfiram, and topiramate may help decrease the relapse rate.
   5. Treatment of depression, if present.

FOLLOW-UP OF MR. A

Two months later, Mr. A returns to your office. His mood is clearly better. He proudly reports that he is "on the wagon" and feeling better. He attends AA meetings 5–7 nights per week. However, he remains concerned about his weight. He reports that his appetite is better and he is eating well but has not regained any weight.

At this point, what is the leading hypothesis, and what are the active alternatives? What other tests should be ordered?

Mr. A's response to your intervention is rewarding. It is surprising that his weight is not improving particularly in light of his improved appetite. During his previous visit, he mentioned difficult to flush, large stools and you wonder if part of his weight loss is secondary to malabsorption. You revisit the common causes of malabsorption and diarrhea. (See Figure 22–3; Table 22–7 for a complete differential diagnosis of chronic diarrhea.)

ORGANIZING THE DIFFERENTIAL DIAGNOSIS

Mr. A denies ever being diagnosed with acute pancreatitis. He does remember multiple episodes of abdominal pain over the years following a night of binging. He did not seek medical care but remained at home drinking only clear fluid for several days until the pain subsided. He denies any history of bowel surgery, family history of IBD, hematochezia, recent antibiotic use, or travel. Table 22–8 lists the differential diagnosis.

Mr. A's history of alcohol abuse and recurrent pain leads you to suspect that he may have chronic pancreatitis.

Is the clinical information sufficient to make a diagnosis? If not, what other information do you need?

Leading Hypothesis: Chronic Pancreatitis

Textbook Presentation

Patients typically seek medical attention for longstanding postprandial abdominal pain. Frequent, loose, malodorous bowel movements are common, and weight loss occurs. Patients may note that several flushes are required to clear the toilet. A prior history of alcoholism and acute pancreatitis are clues to the diagnosis.

Disease Highlights

A. Usually secondary to recurrent acute pancreatitis, primarily from alcohol abuse

B. Pancreatic *insufficiency* is a common late finding. Manifestations include

    1. Weight loss secondary to anorexia and steatorrhea

    2. Steatorrhea:

        a. Floating stools not specific for steatorrhea (bacterial gas may also result in floating stools)

        b. Difficult to flush stools, weight loss, oil in the bowl suggests steatorrhea

    3. Despite malabsorption, elderly patients may not have diarrhea.

    4. Diabetes develops secondary to destruction of islet cells.

        a. Ketoacidosis is rare.

        b. Hypoglycemia is common due to loss of glucagon production.

C. Pseudocysts develop in 10–25% of patients with chronic pancreatitis.

D. Pancreatic cancer develops in 4% of patients within 20 years.

Evidence-Based Diagnosis

A. Amylase and lipase elevations are not reliably seen in chronic pancreatitis.

B. Pancreatic calcifications on plain films has a sensitivity of 30%.

C. CT scan has a sensitivity of 74–90% and a specificity of 85%.

D. Endoscopic retrograde cholangiopancreatography (ERCP) is the gold standard (reveals strictures and obstructions).

E. Specialized tests of pancreatic function (secretin stimulation test sensitivity and specificity 80–90%) can document pancreatic insufficiency in the occasional patient with normal ERCP yet chronic pancreatitis.

F. Tests for steatorrhea

Diagnostic Approach: Chronic Diarrhea

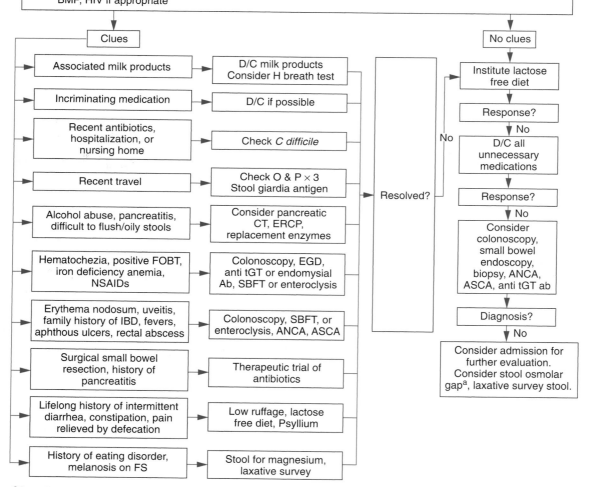

History:

Dietary: Association with milk products, mints, gums, caffeine, ruffage
Medications: Including over-the-counter medications, antacids, recent antibiotics, metformin
Social: Recent travel, alcohol use, risk factors for HIV
Family: Jewish descent, family history of IBD or celiac sprue
Clinical clues: History of pancreatitis, alcohol use; manifestations of IBD (erythema nodosum, uveitis, aphthous ulcers, rectal abscess, fever, hematochezia)
Surgical: Prior small bowel or gastric resection, cholecystectomy

Physical exam: Include comprehensive exam, weight, FOBT. Look for signs of malabsorption, pallor, edema, easy bruisability

Labs: CBC with differential, stool cultures, O & P (or stool giardia antigen), stool *C difficile* toxin, TSH, LFTs, BMP, HIV if appropriate

Clues — No clues

Clues	
Associated milk products	D/C milk products Consider H breath test
Incriminating medication	D/C if possible
Recent antibiotics, hospitalization, or nursing home	Check *C difficile*
Recent travel	Check O & P × 3 Stool giardia antigen
Alcohol abuse, pancreatitis, difficult to flush/oily stools	Consider pancreatic CT, ERCP, replacement enzymes
Hematochezia, positive FOBT, iron deficiency anemia, NSAIDs	Colonoscopy, EGD, anti tGT or endomysial Ab, SBFT or enteroclysis
Erythema nodosum, uveitis, family history of IBD, fevers, aphthous ulcers, rectal abscess	Colonoscopy, SBFT, or enteroclysis, ANCA, ASCA
Surgical small bowel resection, history of pancreatitis	Therapeutic trial of antibiotics
Lifelong history of intermittent diarrhea, constipation, pain relieved by defecation	Low ruffage, lactose free diet, Psyllium
History of eating disorder, melanosis on FS	Stool for magnesium, laxative survey

Resolved?

No clues:
Institute lactose free diet
Response? → No
D/C all unnecessary medications
Response? → No
Consider colonoscopy, small bowel endoscopy, biopsy, ANCA, ASCA, anti tGT ab
Diagnosis? → No
Consider admission for further evaluation. Consider stool osmolar gap[a], laxative survey stool.

[a]Osmolar gap = Measured fecal osmolarity-calculated fecal osmolarity
Calculated fecal osmolarity = $2 \times (Na^+ + K^+)$; osmolar gap < 50 mOsm in secretory diarrhea; osmolar gap is increased in malabsorptive diarrheas.
IBD, inflammatory bowel disease; FOBT, fecal occult blood test; O & P, ova and parasites; LFTs, liver function tests; BMP, basic metabolic panel; NSAIDs, nonsteroidal anti-inflammatory drugs; FS, flexible simoidoscopy; D/C, discontinue; ERCP, endoscopic retrograde cholangiopancreatography; EGD, esophagogastroduodenoscopy; SBFT, small bowel follow through.

Figure 22–3.

Table 22–7. Differential diagnosis of chronic (> 4 weeks) diarrhea.

Most common in developed countries

   a. Irritable bowel syndrome
   b. Lactose intolerance
   c. Inflammatory bowel disease
   d. Chronic infection
   e. Idiopathic

Organized by mnemonic **VITAMIN—V**ascular, **I**atrogenic, **I**nfectious, **T**oxic, **T**raumatic, **A**llergic, **M**etabolic/endocrine, **M**iscellaneous, **I**nflammatory, **N**eoplastic

  1. **Vascular:** Ischemic colitis
  2. **Iatrogenic**
    a. Medications and additives
      i. Antibiotics, metformin, antiarrhythmics, chemotherapy, antacids, laxatives (usually denied by patients)
      ii. Nonabsorbed sweeteners (ie, sorbitol in mints), caffeine
    b. Radiation
    c. Bowel surgery
      i. Ileal resection leads to nonabsorbed bile acids causing colonic diarrhea
      ii. Larger bowel resection lead to short bowel syndrome
      iii. Gastrectomy causes dumping syndrome
  3. **Infectious**
    a. *Clostridium difficile, Giardia lamblia, Entamoeba histolytica*
    b. Bacterial overgrowth
    c. HIV-related infections
  4. **Toxin**
    a. Celiac sprue
    b. Chronic pancreatitis (alcohol)
  5. **Allergic:** Food allergy
  6. **Metabolic/Endocrine**
    a. Lactose intolerance
    b. Hyperthyroidism
    c. Adrenal insufficiency
  7. **Miscellaneous:** Irritable bowel syndrome
  8. **Inflammatory**
    a. Crohn disease
    b. Ulcerative colitis
    c. Collagenous colitis
  9. **Neoplastic**
    a. Colon cancer
    b. VIPoma
    c. Carcinoid tumor

---

1. Normal fecal fat is ≤ 7 g/d on 75–100 g fat diet.
2. Patients with primarily watery diarrhea may excrete up to 13 g of fecal fat per day.
3. ≥ 14 g/d defines steatorrhea
4. Stool Sudan III stain (qualitative) is 90% sensitive for fecal fat ≥ 10 g/d.
5. Acid steatocrit (performed on spot stool specimen) is 100% sensitive and 95% specific.

MAKING A DIAGNOSIS

A CT scan of the abdomen reveals multiple areas of pancreatic calcifications consistent with chronic pancreatitis. A Sudan stain for fecal fat is positive consistent with fat malabsorption.

(continued)

Table 22–8. Diagnostic hypotheses for Mr. A on follow-up.

Diagnostic Hypotheses	Clinical Clues	Important Tests
Leading Hypothesis		
Chronic pancreatitis	History of acute pancreatitis Alcohol abuse	Calcifications on plain film and CT scan ERCP
Active Alternatives—Most Common		
Lactose intolerance	Symptoms of gas and diarrhea following ingestion of milk or ice cream Onset after gastroenteritis	Improvement with lactose free diet Hydrogen breath test
Bacterial overgrowth	History of bowel surgery Blind loop Small bowel diverticula Chronic pancreatitis	Quantitative jejunal aspirates Abnormal D-xylose breath test
Crohn disease	Family history Jewish descent Uveitis, erythema nodosum Sclerosing cholangitis Hematochezia Rectal abscess Apthous ulcers Polymicrobial urinary tract infection	Colonoscopy P-ANCA and ASCA antibodies Enteroclysis
Ulcerative colitis	Family history Jewish descent Uveitis, erythema nodosum Sclerosing cholangitis Hematochezia	Colonoscopy P-ANCA and ASCA antibodies
Celiac disease	Family history Neurologic disorders (ataxia, headaches) Dermatitis herpetiformis	IaA endomysial Ab Anti-tGT Ab
Active Alternatives—Must Not Miss		
Chronic infection (eg, *C difficile, Giardia lamblia, Entamoeba histolytica*)	Recent antibiotic use Hospitalization, long-term facility Fresh water intake Travel	Stool *C difficile* toxin Stool *Giardia* antigen Stool O & P

 Have you crossed a diagnostic threshold for the leading hypothesis, chronic pancreatitis? Have you ruled out the active alternatives? Do other tests need to be done to exclude the alternative diagnoses?

Alternative Diagnosis: Bacterial Overgrowth

Textbook Presentation

Classically, patients often had some type of surgical blind loop that allowed for bacterial multiplication. Patients may experience longstanding diarrhea and weight loss.

Disease Highlights

A. Mechanism: Bacteria digest carbohydrates producing gas and osmotically active byproducts and fatty acids. Fatty acids injure mucosa and contribute to diarrhea. Lactase deficiency may also occur.

B. Etiologies

1. Chronic pancreatitis

   a. Occurs in 40% of chronic pancreatitis cases

   b. Secondary to decreased motility from obstruction, narcotics, or surgery

2. Intestinal dysmotility

3. Achlorhydria (autoimmune or secondary to PPI)

4. Small intestinal diverticula

5. Blind loops

6. Strictures (Crohn disease, radiation, surgery)

7. Resection of ileocecal valve (allows retrograde colonization from heavily colonized colon into ileum)

8. Immunodeficiency states

9. Cirrhosis (occurs in up to 60% of patients with cirrhosis)

10. Alcoholism

11. End-stage renal disease

C. Bacteria may utilize B_{12}, leading to B_{12} deficiency.

Evidence-Based Diagnosis

A. Healthy older patients may also have bacterial overgrowth without any symptoms, making diagnosis difficult.

B. Gold standard is quantitative jejunal aspirates demonstrating $> 10^5$ bacteria.

C. D-xylose breath test is usually abnormal secondary to bacterial digestion of xylose releasing radiolabeled C14. Sensitivity and specificity approximately 90%. (Avoid in pregnant women.)

D. Consider bacterial overgrowth if upper GI series demonstrates hypomotility or obstruction or diverticula.

E. Weight loss may occur without diarrhea (17% of children).

F. Therapeutic trials of antibiotics may be necessary.

Treatment

A. Eliminate drugs that reduce intestinal motility or reduce gastric acidity.

B. A variety of oral antibiotics have been used for 7–10 days (amoxicillin and clavulanate, cephalexin, TMP-SMX and metronidazole, norfloxacin, oral gentamicin, and metronidazole). Rotating course of antibiotics has been used in some patients.

C. Correct vitamin K and B_{12} deficiency.

Alternative Diagnosis: IBD

Crohn disease and ulcerative colitis are idiopathic conditions with a genetic component. They are found most commonly in patients of Jewish descent or among patients with a family history of IBD. In addition to intestinal manifestations, extraintestinal manifestations that may be seen include the following: uveitis, erythema nodosum, large joint peripheral arthritis and ankylosing spondylitis, sclerosing cholangitis, secondary amyloidosis, and venous thromboembolism. The risk of colon cancer is proportional to the amount of the colon involved and the duration of disease.

1. Crohn Disease

Textbook Presentation

Crohn disease may present in a variety of ways, including chronic abdominal pain, diarrhea, weight loss, enterocutaneous fistulas, and acute abdominal pain, even mimicking acute appendicitis.

Disease Highlights

A. Transmural inflammation leads to fistula formation, strictures, and obstruction. Complications of fistulas include abscess formation, peritonitis, enterocutaneous fistulas (most commonly perianal), and enterovesicular fistulas (resulting in polymicrobial urinary tract infection).

B. Manifestations

1. Can involve any part of GI tract with normal "skip areas" between involved areas

   a. 80% of patients have small bowel involvement (most often in terminal ileum)

   b. 50% of patients have ileocolitis

2. Nonspecific symptoms may precede diagnosis by many years.

3. Diarrhea may occur due to

   a. Small bowel disease impairing absorption

   b. Ileal disease may lead to bile malabsorption resulting in bile deficiency and finally causing steatorrhea.

   c. Bacterial overgrowth secondary to strictures

4. Abdominal pain, weight loss, and fever

5. B_{12} deficiency (secondary to ileal disease)

6. Calcium oxalate renal stones (Fat malabsorption binds intestinal calcium leading to increased ox-

alate absorption. This in turn causes hyperoxaluria and predisposes patients to kidney stones.)

7. Hypocalcemia and osteomalacia; fat malabsorption leads to vitamin D deficiency.

8. Gross bleeding less frequent than in ulcerative colitis

9. Aphthous ulcers

Evidence-Based Diagnosis

A. Colonoscopy is often useful with biopsy.

B. Enteroclysis is superior to small bowel follow through (SBFT) for evaluation of small bowel and ileum, although AGA guidelines recommend SBFT over enteroclysis for patients with chronic diarrhea. Some centers are utilizing capsule endoscopy. (A swallowed pill transmits radioimages to a receiver.)

C. Serologies are still being evaluated. Patients with Crohn disease tend to be P-ANCA negative and ASCA positive. The reverse is true in ulcerative colitis. Sensitivities range from 40% to 60%; specificities, 90%.

Treatment

A. Primary: Several initial options

  1. 5 Aminosalicylic acid (5-ASA)

  2. Antibiotics

B. Several options for nonresponders or patients with severe disease

  1. Corticosteroids can be added to 5-ASA, antibiotics

  2. Azathioprine or its active metabolite 6 mercaptopurine (6MP)

  3. Methotrexate

  4. TNF antagonists (eg, infliximab)

C. Adjunctive therapy

  1. Treat lactose intolerance if present

  2. Antibiotics, CT-guided drainage of abscesses

  3. Multivitamins

  4. Total parenteral nutrition

    a. Necessary if patient is unable to maintain adequate nutrition.

    b. May also produce remission in refractory cases.

  5. Surgery

    a. May be required for the management of massive hemorrhage, fulminant colitis, abscesses, peritonitis, obstruction, or disease refractory to medical therapy.

    b. High rate of recurrence following surgery (10–15%/y clinical recurrence, 80% endoscopic recurrence).

    c. 5-ASA, metronidazole, and 6MP have been demonstrated to reduce postoperative recurrences.

  6. Bile acid resins for patients with watery diarrhea and ileal disease

  7. Monitor for colon cancer if colonic involvement.

2. Ulcerative Colitis

Textbook Presentation

Typically, diarrhea and hematochezia are presenting symptoms.

Disease Highlights

A. Primarily mucosal disease. (Occasionally, severe inflammation may extend deeper, involving muscular layers resulting in dysmotility and toxic megacolon.)

B. Strictly limited to colon

C. Starts at rectum and proceeds proximally in a *continuous fashion;* may be limited to rectum or involve rectosigmoid or entire colon

D. Decreased risk among smokers (opposite of Crohn disease)

E. Common symptoms include rectal bleeding and diarrhea.

F. Anemia, fever, and increasing diarrhea are seen with more extensive disease.

G. Complications

  1. Massive hemorrhage (rare)

  2. Toxic megacolon

  3. Stricture

  4. Cancer risk is increased unless the disease is limited to proctitis or very distal colitis. Increased risk begins 7–8 years after onset of disease.

Evidence-Based Diagnosis

A. Sigmoidoscopy or colonoscopy demonstrates loss of vascular markings, erythema, friability, and exudates in a continuous fashion extending from the rectum proximally.

B. Biopsy specimen reveals crypt abscesses, branching crypts, and glandular atrophy.

C. Serologies are still being evaluated. Patients are likely to be P-ANCA positive and ASCA negative; sensitivities range from 40% to 60%; specificities, 90%.

Treatment

A. Exclude acute infectious processes (*Salmonella, Shigella, Campylobacter, Escherichia coli 0157:H7, C difficile, E histolytica*).

B. Topical 5-ASA preparations (suppositories and enemas) for those with disease limited to rectum and distal colon. Enemas can be used for disease that extends to 30–40 cm.

C. Corticosteroid foams and enemas
  1. Not superior to 5 ASA compounds
  2. Budesonide may be preferred corticosteroid. Significant first-pass hepatic metabolism leads to lower systemic toxicity.

D. Oral 5-ASA can also be used.

E. Oral or systemic corticosteroids can be added to 5-ASA for more severe disease or nonresponders.

F. Antibiotics may be useful in select ill patients, particularly those with toxic megacolon or peritonitis.

G. Cyclosporine, 6MP, and infliximab have been effective in some patients with severe, corticosteroid refractory disease.

H. Adjuvant therapy
  1. Persistent diarrhea
    a. Test for lactose intolerance
    b. Avoid fresh fruits, vegetables, and caffeine
  2. Surveillance colonoscopy: AGA recommendations (for ulcerative colitis and Crohn disease):
    a. Pancolitis: first colonoscopy after 8 years. Repeat every 1–2 years.
    b. Left-sided colitis: first colonoscopy after 15 years. Repeat every 1–2 years
  3. Supplemental iron
  4. Fish oils and nicotine (transdermal) have been demonstrated to induce remission in some patients.
  5. Total parenteral nutrition when patients are unable to maintain adequate nutrition
  6. Antidiarrheals must be used with caution (if at all) due to the increased risk of toxic megacolon
  7. Surgery (colectomy) curative. Indications include:
    a. Patients with high-grade dysplasia, carcinoma in situ or cancer on surveillance colonoscopy
    b. Massive hemorrhage
    c. Toxic megacolon
    d. Intractable disease

CASE RESOLUTION

Mr. A's history and CT scan point strongly toward chronic pancreatitis. It would be reasonable to exclude chronic infection (*C difficile, Giardia,* and *E histolytica*) with a single stool for ova and parasites and stool for *C difficile* toxin. IBD is possible but unlikely. Since bacterial overgrowth can complicate chronic pancreatitis, an empiric trial of antibiotics could be given if therapy for chronic pancreatitis is unsuccessful.

Treatment of Chronic Pancreatitis

A. Abstinence from drinking is vital (but not universally effective at halting progression).

B. Analgesia is necessary; opioid dependence is a common problem.

C. Pancreatic enzymes given with meals can decrease pain and improve nutritional status.

D. Diabetes should be treated, but care must be taken to avoid hypoglycemia. Metformin should be avoided due to concomitant alcoholism.

E. ERCP, stenting, and surgery are useful in selected patients.

F. Pseudocysts require surgical or endoscopic drainage.

Mr. A is given pancreatic enzymes. He reports that his diarrhea and bloating are greatly improved. Six months later he is back to his baseline weight.

REVIEW OF OTHER IMPORTANT DISEASES

Celiac Disease

Textbook Presentation

Classically, chronic diarrhea, steatorrhea, and weight loss are present. Iron and vitamin deficiencies may be seen.

Disease Highlights

A. Prevalence of 1:300–1:500 in Northern Europeans

B. Secondary to immune reaction to gliadin a component of the wheat protein. Antibodies develop to gliadin, transglutaminase (tTG), and endomysin.

C. Clinical manifestations

1. Usually presents between ages 10 and 40 years, although may be recognized in patients aged 60–80 years

2. Symptoms precipitated by exposure to wheat protein (gluten) and resolve within weeks to months on gluten-free diet.

3. Disease may be asymptomatic or mild causing only iron deficiency or elevated liver function tests.

4. Vitamin deficiencies may cause ataxia and headaches.

5. Osteopenia (secondary to vitamin D deficiency)

6. Associated with dermatitis herpetiformis

7. Far more common in patients with Down syndrome

Evidence-Based Diagnosis

A. Small bowel biopsies traditionally used to confirm the diagnosis. The necessity of biopsy in patients with positive IgA endomysial antibody (IgA EMA) or IgA tGT antibody is unclear.

B. Many antibodies available for testing (Table 22–9)

1. IgA tGT and IgA EMA are tests of choice.

2. Sensitivity is lower with gluten-free diet or low levels of disease activity.

Treatment

A. Gluten-free diet (no wheat, rye, and barley)

B. Some patients also require oats-free diet

C. Lactose avoidance may be necessary due to concomitant lactase deficiency.

D. Correct iron, folic acid, vitamin B_{12}, and vitamin D deficiencies.

E. IgA gluten antibodies should fall with gluten-free diet. Increasing titers suggest dietary noncompliance.

F. Pneumococcal vaccine is recommended by some experts.

G. Rarely corticosteroids or other immunosuppressives have been necessary in patients with refractory celiac sprue.

Table 22–9. Test characteristics for celiac sprue.

Test	Sensitivity (%)	Specificity (%)	LR+	LR–
Anti tGT	95–98	94–98	47	0.04
IgA endomysial antibody	85–95	97–100	60	0.1
Antigliadin IgA antibody	80–90	85–95	8.5	0.17
Antigliadin IgG antibodies	75–85	75–90	4.4	0.24

Diagnostic Approach: Unintentional Weight Loss

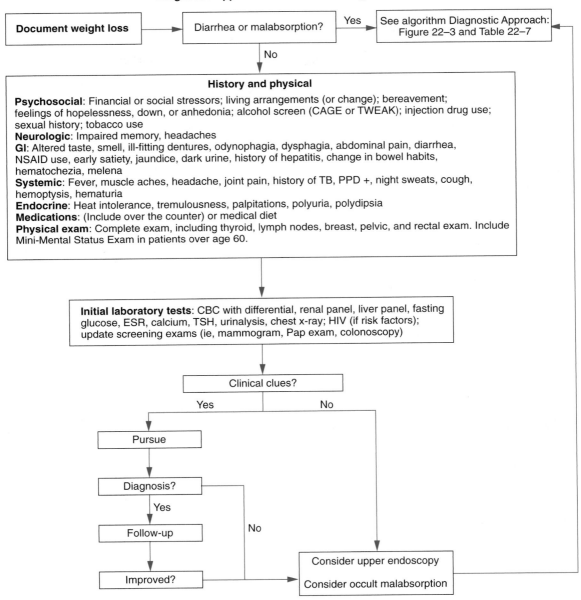

TB, tuberculosis; ESR, erythrocyte sedimentation rate.

Figure 22–A.

I have a patient with wheezing or stridor. How do I determine the cause?

CHIEF COMPLAINT

PATIENT 1

Mr. C is a 32-year-old man with occasional wheezing.

What is the differential diagnosis of wheezing? How would you frame the differential?

CONSTRUCTING A DIFFERENTIAL DIAGNOSIS

Wheezing and stridor are symptoms of airflow obstruction. These sounds are caused by the vibration of the walls of pathologically narrow airways. **Wheezing** is a musical sound produced primarily during expiration by airways of any size. **Stridor** is a single pitch, inspiratory sound that is produced by large airways with severe narrowing.

Stridor is often a sign of impending airway obstruction and should be considered an emergency.

The differential diagnosis for airway obstruction is large. It is best remembered by an anatomic approach. Stridor may be caused by severe obstruction of any airway proximal to the distal airways (see A through D in the differential diagnosis outline below). A more clinical approach to the differential appears in the algorithm at the end of the chapter.

A. Nasopharynx and oropharynx
   1. Tonsillar hypertrophy
   2. Pharyngitis
   3. Peritonsillar abscess
   4. Retropharyngeal abscess
B. Laryngopharynx and larynx
   1. Epiglottitis
   2. Paradoxical vocal cord movement (PVCM)
   3. Anaphylaxis and laryngeal edema
   4. Postnasal drip
   5. Benign and malignant tumors of the larynx and upper airway
   6. Vocal cord paralysis
C. Trachea
   1. Tracheal stenosis
   2. Tracheal malacia
   3. Goiter
D. Proximal airways
   1. Foreign-body aspiration
   2. Bronchitis
E. Distal airways
   1. Asthma
   2. Chronic obstructive pulmonary disease (COPD)
   3. Pulmonary edema
   4. Pulmonary embolism
   5. Bronchiectasis

1

Mr. C has been having symptoms for 1–2 years. His symptoms have always been so mild that he has never sought care. Over the last month, he has been more symptomatic with wheezing, chest tightness, and shortness of breath. His symptoms are worse with exercise and worse at night. He notes that he often goes days without any symptoms.

 At this point, what is the leading hypothesis, and what are the active alternatives? What other tests should be ordered?

ORGANIZING THE DIFFERENTIAL DIAGNOSIS

The presence of wheezing, chest tightness, and shortness of breath places asthma at the top of the differential diagnosis. Although asthma is by far the most likely diagnosis, other diseases that could account for recurrent symptoms of airway obstruction should be kept in mind. Allergic rhinitis can cause cough and wheezing, although shortness of breath is unlikely. Vocal cord dysfunction, such as PVCM, is frequently confused with asthma. COPD can also cause intermittent pulmonary symptoms. Table 23–1 lists the differential diagnosis.

On further history, Mr. C reports that he had asthma as a child and was treated for years with theophylline. He was without symptoms until he moved 2 years ago.

He reports that his symptoms are worst when he has a cold, when he jogs, and when he is around dogs or cats. His symptoms are usually only chest tightness and dyspnea. Only when his symptoms are at their worst does he hear wheezing. He does not smoke cigarettes.

On physical exam he appears well. His vital signs are BP, 120/76 mm Hg; RR, 14 breaths per minute; pulse, 72 bpm; temperature, 36.9 °C. His lung exam is normal without wheezes or prolonged expiratory phase. His peak flow is 550 L/min or 87% of predicted.

 Is the clinical information sufficient to make a diagnosis? If not, what other information do you need?

Leading Hypothesis: Asthma

Textbook Presentation

Asthma commonly presents as recurrent episodes of dyspnea, often with chest tightness, cough, and wheezing. Patients usually report stereotypical triggers (eg, allergens, cold weather, exercise) and rapid response to β-agonist inhalers. Asthma is so common that most patients have diagnosed themselves prior to presentation.

Disease Highlights

A. Definition: The NIH/NHLBI definition of asthma is "A chronic inflammatory disease of the airways in

Table 23–1. Diagnostic hypotheses for Mr. C.

Diagnostic Hypotheses	Clinical Clues	Important Tests
Leading Hypothesis		
Asthma	Episodic and reversible airflow obstruction	Peak flow PFTs Methacholine challenge Response to treatment
Active Alternative		
Allergic rhinitis	Rhinitis with seasonal variation	Response to treatment
Vocal cord dysfunction	Voice pathology accompanies airflow obstruction	Abnormal vocal cord movement visualized
Active Alternative—Must Not Miss		
COPD	Presence of smoking history	PFTs

which many cells and cellular elements play a role." "In susceptible individuals, this inflammation causes recurrent episodes of wheezing, breathlessness, chest tightness, and cough, particularly at night and/or in the early morning. These episodes are usually associated with widespread but variable airflow limitation that is often reversible either spontaneously or with treatment."

B. Clinical manifestations

1. Asthma is recurrent and intermittent. Patients will have periods with no or only mild symptoms.

2. Asthma usually presents during childhood but presentation as an adult is not uncommon.

3. People with asthma have fluctuation of airway function.

    a. Airway function is most commonly measured with peak expiratory flows (PEFs).

    b. Values are generally lowest in the morning and highest at mid-day.

    c. PEF will vary by more than 20% in asthmatic patients over the course of the day.

4. Identifying exacerbating factors and timing of symptoms is important. It aids in the diagnosis of asthma (exacerbating factors are stereotypical) and in treatment (if the factors are reversible).

    a. Asthma frequently worsens at night (probably related to decreased mucociliary clearance, airway cooling, and low levels of endogenous catecholamines).

    b. Asthma frequently worsens with exercise (probably related to airway cooling and drying).

    c. Viral infections are a common cause of asthma exacerbation.

    d. Occupational agents may cause or exacerbate asthma by a number of mechanisms:

        (1) Corrosive agents (ammonia)

        (2) Pharmacologic agents (organophosphates)

        (3) Reflex bronchoconstriction (ozone)

        (4) IgE-mediated (latex)

 Asthma should be in the differential diagnosis of any patient with intermittent respiratory symptoms.

C. Classification: The present classification scheme for asthma helps focus attention on the severity of the asthma and dovetails nicely with treatment considerations (Table 23–2).

Table 23–2. Classification of asthma severity.

Classification	Symptoms	Lung Function
Mild intermittent	Symptoms less than twice a week Asymptomatic between exacerbations and brief exacerbations Nighttime symptoms < twice monthly	PEF > 80% of predicted
Mild persistent	Symptoms between once a day and twice a week Asymptomatic between exacerbations but exacerbations may limit activity Nighttime symptoms > twice monthly	PEF > 80% of predicted
Moderate persistent	Daily symptoms Exacerbations limit activity Nighttime symptoms > weekly.	PEF 60–80% of predicted
Severe persistent	Continual symptoms Symptoms chronically limit physical activity Frequent nighttime symptoms	PEF < 60% of predicted

PEF, peak expiratory flow.

D. Exacerbations or "flares"

1. Asthma exacerbations are periods of increased disease activity identified by increased airflow obstruction (and therefore increased symptoms) and increased medication use.

2. Exacerbations may or may not be caused by an identifiable trigger.

3. Management of an exacerbation depends on an accurate assessment of the cause of the exacerbation and the risk to the patient.

Evidence-Based Diagnosis

A. There is no 1 specific test to diagnose asthma; the diagnosis is a clinical one, based on multiple findings in the history, physical, and a few simple tests.

B. Most asthma cases are easy to diagnose and are usually made by the patient.

C. Asthma is common and is easily recognized when it presents with intermittent wheezing.

D. Diagnosing asthma is challenging when it presents in atypical ways. Asthma should be high in the differential diagnosis when a patient has any of the following intermittent symptoms:

1. Wheezing
2. Dyspnea
3. Cough
4. Chest tightness

E. The key points in establishing the diagnosis of asthma are:

1. Episodic symptoms of airflow obstruction
2. Reversibility of the airflow obstruction
3. Exclusion of other likely diseases

F. There are not great data on the test characteristics of various symptoms of asthma.

1. One large study interviewed nearly 10,000 patients regarding symptoms of asthma in the preceding 12 months.

   a. 225 of these people had asthma, defined as reporting that they had asthma and that a medical professional had confirmed the diagnosis.

   b. The test characteristics are shown in Table 23–3.

   c. As expected, the presence of wheezing or wheezing and dyspnea were the most predictive findings.

Table 23–3. Test characteristics of symptoms for the diagnosis of asthma.

Criteria	Sensitivity	Specificity	LR+	LR−
Wheezing	74.7%	87.3%	5.77	0.29
Wheezing and dyspnea	65.2%	95.1%	13	0.37
Wheezing without URI symptoms	59.8%	93.6%	12	0.42
Nocturnal chest tightness	49.3%	86.4%	3.5	0.59
Dyspnea at rest	47.1%	94.9%	9.4	0.56
Exertional dyspnea	69.3%	75.7%	2.88	0.41
Nocturnal dyspnea	46.2%	96%	11.5	0.56
Nocturnal cough	49.3%	72.3%	1.75	0.71
Chronic cough	21.5%	95.2%	4.4	0.82
Chronic phlegm	22.7%	93.3%	3.29	0.83
Chronic bronchitis	12.5%	98.2%	6.5	0.89

URI, upper respiratory infection.

Adapted from Sistek D et al. Clinical diagnosis of current asthma: predictive value of respiratory symptoms in the SAPALDIA study. Swiss Study on Air Pollution and Lung Diseases in Adults. *Eur Respir J.* 2001;17:214–219.

(1) Notice that patient symptoms are much more helpful for ruling in rather than ruling out the diagnosis of asthma.

(2) In the 25% of patients in the study who had asthma but no symptoms of wheezing, the most common symptom was exercise-related dyspnea, present in 57% of the patients.

2. In another study, which used a methacholine challenge test to diagnose asthma, 90% specificity was achieved for making the diagnosis of asthma with the question, "Do you cough during or after exercise?"

G. Other clues that make the diagnosis more likely are outlined in the NIH/NHLBI guidelines:

1. Diurnal variability in PEF (> 20% variability between best and worst)

2. Symptoms occur or worsen in the presence of:

a. Exercise

b. Viral infections

c. Animals with fur or feathers

d. House dust mites

e. Mold

f. Smoke

g. Pollen

h. Weather changes

i. Laughing or hard crying

j. Airborne chemicals or dust

3. Symptoms occur or worsen at night.

H. There is some evidence that persons with asthma describe their dyspnea differently from people with other cardiorespiratory disease. They are more likely to refer to symptoms of chest tightness or constriction.

I. Most guidelines recommend spirometry to help make the diagnosis of asthma. The following all support the diagnosis of asthma:

1. Decreased forced expiratory volume in 1 second (FEV_1)

2. Decreased FEV_1/forced vital capacity (FVC) ratio

3. Reversibility (defined as > 12% improvement with bronchodilators)

J. Other tests

1. Pulmonary function tests and chest film are useful mainly in excluding other diseases.

2. Methacholine challenge

a. Can be very helpful in diagnosing asthma in patients who have a suspicious history but normal pulmonary function tests (PFTs)

b. < 20% decrease in FEV_1 has a 95% negative predictive value

MAKING A DIAGNOSIS

Mr. C's clinical history is consistent with asthma. He has intermittent pulmonary symptoms of wheezing, dyspnea, and chest tightness. Multiple points in his history raise the probability of asthma as the diagnosis. These include the childhood history of asthma and the exacerbating factors. His normal peak flow does not exclude the diagnosis because he is not experiencing an exacerbation. At this point, a diagnostic and therapeutic trial of asthma medication would be reasonable.

Mr. C was given an albuterol inhaler. He was told to use 2 puffs about 30 minutes before exercise or expected animal exposure. On follow-up 6 weeks later, Mr. C reported marked improvement in his symptoms. He was able to exercise without difficulty as long as he was using his inhalers and could spend short amounts of time around friends' pets. He suffered one upper respiratory tract infection during the last 6 weeks. He found his symptoms worse during this time. He used his inhaler about 4 times daily with good relief of symptoms.

Have you crossed a diagnostic threshold for the leading hypothesis, asthma? Have you ruled out the active alternatives? Do other tests need to be done to exclude the alternative diagnoses?

Because asthma is very common and the initial treatment is benign, the treatment threshold is low. A therapeutic and diagnostic trial of medication is nearly always appropriate.

CASE RESOLUTION

The patient's history and response to therapy confirms the diagnosis of asthma. The patient has no nasal symptoms that would suggest allergic rhinitis. COPD is unlikely without a smoking history. Vocal cord dysfunction will be discussed below and is also unlikely. Congestive heart failure (CHF) is unlikely given the patient's age, the absence of a history of heart disease, and his response to bronchodilators.

The patient continued taking albuterol as needed. The following year, Mr. C's symptoms worsened after a move into a new house. His asthma was maintained with inhaled corticosteroid therapy for 6 months. He was able to wean these medications after he had carpets in his house replaced with hardwood floors.

Treatment of Asthma

A. The goals of asthma therapy are to:

1. Prevent chronic symptoms such as nighttime wakening

2. Maintain normal pulmonary function (assessed by PEF and spirometry)

3. Maintain normal levels of physical activity; this can be a challenge. Because many patients become accustomed to the limitation by their breathing, they may not be able to objectively report whether their breathing is limited.

4. Prevent exacerbations

B. Therapy includes treatment of asthma itself and treatment of exacerbating factors.

1. Exacerbating factors are treated with pharmacologic and nonpharmacologic interventions.

   a. Smoking cessation and removal of second-hand smoke

   b. Air pollution (Ozone, SO_2, NO_2)

   c. Gastroesophageal reflux disease (GERD)

   d. Common allergens

   e. Dander, dust, mold, insects

2. Asthma therapy is aimed at treating the factors that cause asthma and its symptoms. The drugs are summarized in Table 23–4.

3. A usual course of therapy follows:

   a. Short-acting β_2-agonists are used as-needed for mild intermittent asthma and exercise-induced asthma.

   b. In patients with mild persistent asthma (or once a patient is using short-acting β_2-agonists more than twice weekly) inhaled corticosteroids are added. The dose of inhaled corticosteroids is escalated for control of symptoms.

   c. Long-acting β_2-agonists should be considered for nocturnal symptoms and for maintenance after short-acting β_2-agonists and inhaled corticosteroids are used.

   d. Leukotriene antagonists and theophylline can also be used for maintenance after short-acting β_2-agonists and inhaled corticosteroids are used.

Table 23–4. Pharmacotherapy of asthma.

Medication	Purpose	Common Adverse Effects
Short acting β_2-agonists	Immediate relief of symptoms	Tachycardia, jitteriness
Inhaled corticosteroids	Mainstay of chronic therapy	Thrush, dysphonia, potentially osteopenia at high doses
Long-acting β_2-agonists	Long-term therapy when inhaled corticosteroids have not adequately controlled symptoms. Useful for nocturnal symptoms	Tachycardia, jitteriness
Leukotriene antagonists	Long-term therapy when inhaled corticosteroids have not adequately controlled symptoms	No significant adverse effects
Systemic corticosteroids	Immediate therapy for exacerbations or long-term therapy in patients with refractory asthma	Traditional corticosteroid side effects (weight gain, hyperglycemia, bone loss)
Theophylline	Similar to long-acting β_2-agonists but used less frequently	Dose-related tachycardia, nausea, jitteriness

e. Systemic corticosteroids are reserved for the treatment of exacerbations and refractory cases.

 At each visit, review a patient's medications and carefully review symptoms. Focus on any limitations of activity related to asthma.

C. Refractory cases

1. Most cases of asthma can be well controlled. There are a number of considerations if asthma is refractory to treatment.

2. Is the patient compliant?

3. Are there unaccounted for or untreated precipitants? (Consider GERD, sinusitis, and allergies.)

4. Is the diagnosis correct? (Consider other causes of chronic intermittent airway obstruction.)

5. Are there rare diseases present that can cause or worsen asthma? (Consider Churg-Strauss disease, allergic bronchopulmonary aspergillosis.)

D. Exacerbations

1. Appropriate treatment for exacerbations of asthma is based on a detailed history and physical exam focused on determining the cause, duration, and severity of the exacerbation.

2. History

  a. Duration of exacerbation

    (1) Very brief exacerbations (hours) may improve with β-agonists alone while longer exacerbations will likely need corticosteroids.

    (2) Because early treatment leads to better outcomes, it is important that patients monitor their own disease and know how to initiate appropriate treatment and contact their physician when necessary.

  b. Precipitants

    (1) Is there a clear precipitant of the exacerbation that needs to be treated or removed (eg, sinusitis, allergen exposure)?

    (2) Is there an exacerbating factor that hospital admission might avoid (eg, house painting, recent insect extermination)?

  c. Severity of disease. The following are risk factors of asthma-related death. Hospital admission is nearly always indicated for patients with an exacerbation and 1 of these factors:

    (1) History of sudden severe exacerbations

    (2) Prior admission to an ICU

    (3) Recent emergency department visits or hospitalizations

    (4) Use of more than 2 canisters of β-agonist in the past month

    (5) Current use or recent discontinuation of systemic corticosteroids

    (6) Difficulty perceiving airflow obstruction

    (7) Comorbid medical or psychiatric disease

3. Physical exam

  a. The lung exam is generally a poor marker of the severity of disease.

  b. Lack of wheezing can either reflect improved or worsening airflow.

 Patients whose decreased wheezing is accompanied by worsening distress likely have worsening airflow obstruction. Conversely, a patient whose decreased wheezing is accompanied by lessened respiratory distress likely has improved airflow obstruction.

4. Other tests

  a. Chest x-ray is only helpful for identifying the uncommon concomitant infection or complication (eg, pneumothorax).

  b. Spirometry is most helpful in determining severity of exacerbation.

    (1) A moderate exacerbation will have an FEV_1 or PEF 50–80% of predicted and moderate symptoms.

    (2) A severe exacerbation will have an FEV_1 or PEF 50–80% of predicted with severe symptoms, physical findings, or concerning history.

 Spirometry and the history of the patient's prior exacerbations are the most important pieces of information for making admission decisions.

E. Treatment

1. Figure 23–1 is adapted from the NIH/NHLBI Guidelines for the Diagnosis and Management of Asthma and is a guide to the management of asthma exacerbations.

2. Recognize that the differentiation of mild, moderate and severe exacerbations is based not only on spirometry but on history and physical as well.

Initial Evaluation and Treatment of an Asthma Exacerbation

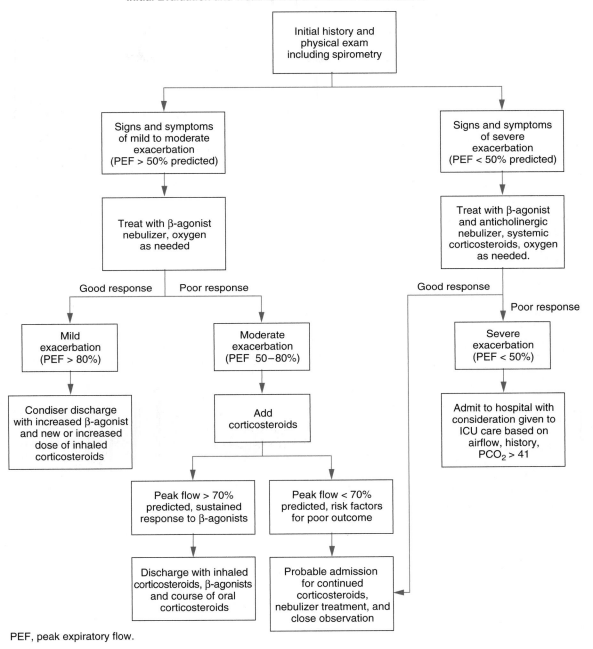

PEF, peak expiratory flow.

Figure 23–1.

CHIEF COMPLAINT

PATIENT 2

Mrs. P is a 62-year-old woman who arrives at the emergency department with shortness of breath and wheezing. She says that the symptoms have been present for 3 days. The symptoms are present both at rest and with exertion and have not improved with an albuterol inhaler.

She reports that she has had these symptoms on and off for 6 years. When the symptoms occur, they generally last for hours to a few days. She had been diagnosed with asthma and taken both long- and short-acting β-agonists, inhaled corticosteroids, and prednisone before coming off all medications 1 year ago. She stopped her medications herself out of frustration with side effects and perceived lack of efficacy. She decided instead to treat herself with yoga and meditation. She reports no episodes since this decision.

Presently she denies cough, chest pain, fever, or rhinitis. She does report hoarseness that occurs when her breathing is bad.

Past medical history is remarkable only for depression and hypertension. Her only medication is enalapril. She has no known drug allergies. She does not smoke cigarettes.

At this point, what is the leading hypothesis, and what are the active alternatives? What other tests should be ordered?

ORGANIZING THE DIFFERENTIAL DIAGNOSIS

As discussed above, asthma is very common and should be considered in anyone with intermittent pulmonary symptoms. There are some points in Mrs. P's history that argue against asthma. Her symptoms have not improved with a β-agonist, and it seems that she came off an aggressive asthma regimen without ill effects. PVCM is a syndrome of episodic adduction of the vocal cords producing wheezing and stridor. The lack of response to bronchodilators and associated hoarseness are clues to this diagnosis. GERD is a very common diagnosis (see

Chapter 6, Chest Pain). It can cause and worsen asthma and can cause hoarseness via irritation of the vocal cords. Angioedema occurs when vascular permeability increases leading to swelling of subcutaneous tissues. Airway compromise can occur. It is usually associated with other signs of disease such as facial swelling, tongue swelling, or hives. Table 23–5 lists the differential diagnosis.

Hoarseness and dysphonia are nonspecific findings that can be associated with any anatomic or functional abnormality of the vocal cords, asthma, or GERD.

2

On further history, she reports that her symptoms are moderate for her. She had been intubated once in the past during a flare.

On physical exam, the patient is in moderate to severe respiratory distress. Her voice is hoarse and "squeaky." Her vital signs are temperature, 37.1 °C; pulse, 110 bpm; BP, 140/90 mm Hg; RR, 32 breaths per minute. There is a harsh wheeze heard throughout the lungs that is loudest in the anterior neck. The remainder of the physical exam was normal.

PEF is 300 L/min, 70% of predicted.

Is the clinical information sufficient to make a diagnosis? If not, what other information do you need?

Leading Hypothesis: PVCM

Textbook Presentation

PVCM typically presents as episodic attacks of respiratory distress accompanied by wheezing or stridor or both. The respiratory distress is often accompanied by voice pathology and a lack of response to traditional asthma therapy.

Disease Highlights

A. PVCM has gone by many names including vocal cord dysfunction, episodic laryngeal dyskinesia, Munchausen stridor, psychogenic stridor, and factitious asthma.

Table 23–5. Diagnostic hypotheses for Mrs. P.

Diagnostic Hypotheses	Clinical Clues	Important Tests
Leading Hypothesis		
Paradoxical vocal cord movement	Episodic airflow obstruction associated with stridor	Laryngoscopy demonstrating abnormal vocal cord movement
Active Alternative—Most Common		
Asthma	Episodic and reversible airflow obstruction	Peak flow PFTs Methacholine challenge Response to treatment
Active Alternative		
Gastroesophageal reflux disease	May cause or worsen asthma and cause voice pathology	Identification of esophageal and laryngeal abnormalities on endoscopy
Active Alternative—Must Not Miss		
Angioedema	Often associated with hives and causative exposure	Clinical presentation with or without risk factors

B. Most commonly occurs in younger patients (< 35 years) but can be seen in any age.

C. Female predominance

D. Disease often occurs in patients with psychiatric diagnoses.

E. The symptoms are not produced consciously.

F. During asymptomatic disease, there are no abnormalities of lung function:

1. Spirometry is normal.

2. There is none of the increased variability in airway function seen with asthma.

3. Bronchoprovocation tests are normal.

Evidence-Based Diagnosis

A. Given the prevalence of asthma and the similarity of the presentation, asthma needs to be excluded in any patient with PVCM.

B. Clues to the differentiation of the diseases are:

1. The lack of exacerbating factors (eg, exercise, allergens, sleeping) common in asthma.

2. The lack of response to asthma medications.

3. The occasional disappearance of symptoms during sleep.

4. The striking voice pathology during attacks.

5. The preponderance of auscultatory findings in the neck.

6. Flow-volume loop abnormalities in the inspiratory phase suggesting a fixed extrathoracic airway obstruction.

C. The definitive diagnosis is made on laryngoscopy.

1. There is adduction of the vocal cords often leaving only a diamond-shaped opening between the cords during flares.

2. There is generally normal vocal cord function between flares.

MAKING A DIAGNOSIS

Given Mrs. P's history and physical findings, PVCM was suspected, but the history of asthma and the severity of the dyspnea were concerning. An albuterol nebulizer was started and an otolaryngologist was called to evaluate the patient.

Have you crossed a diagnostic threshold for the leading hypothesis, PVCM? Have you ruled out the active alternatives? Do other tests need to be done to exclude the alternative diagnoses?

The diagnosis of PVCM is certainly likely given the patient's history and physical exam findings. Asthma still needs to be ruled out with spirometry and, if necessary, bronchoprovocation. The other important diagnosis to consider is angioedema.

 Asthma is significantly more prevalent that PVCM. Any patient in whom the diagnosis of PVCM is considered should have asthma ruled out.

Alternative Diagnosis: Angioedema

Textbook Presentation

The presentation of angioedema is usually an acute swelling of the face, lips, tongue, and larynx. Patients nearly always have a history of angioedema or a risk factor for it.

Disease Highlights

A. The onset of angioedema is usually rapid, over minutes to, at most, hours.

B. Angioedema may be caused by.

1. ACE inhibitors

2. Allergic reactions

3. Hereditary and acquired forms of C1-inhibitor deficiency

C. The presentation can range from mild, only sensed by the patient; to disfiguring, obvious to the casual observer; to life-threatening laryngeal involvement.

D. The diverse causes of angioedema produce symptoms by different mechanisms, have different presentations, and different treatments.

1. Histamine-related angioedema

   a. Almost always accompanied by pruritus and urticaria (hives).

   b. Usually related to an allergic exposure such as an insect bite or a food.

   c. Urticaria can also be chronic, caused by allergy, drug effect, autoimmune phenomena, or malignancy.

2. Nonhistamine-related angioedema (caused by elevated levels of bradykinin)

   a. Most commonly the result of ACE inhibitor therapy

   b. Deficiency of C1-inhibitor also causes elevated bradykinin levels as well as elevated C2b levels, another cause of angioedema.

Evidence-Based Diagnosis

A. A diagnosis of angioedema is clinical, based on the recognition of angioedema and associated symptoms.

B. Angioedema most commonly presents as swelling of the lips, tongue, or both.

C. Figure 23–2 presents a useful algorithm for considering the differential diagnosis and treatment of angioedema.

Treatment

A. The most critical aspect of the management of angioedema is airway stabilization.

B. All patients receive H_1- and H_2-blockers as well as corticosteroids.

C. Patients with airway compromise or any intraoral swelling should also receive epinephrine.

D. Patients need to be closely monitored because intubation is sometimes necessary.

E. Patients with C1-inhibitor deficiency can be treated with androgens or C1-inhibitor concentrate. Androgens increase the production of C1-inhibitor.

CASE RESOLUTION

2 A helium oxygen mixture was given to the patient briefly before laryngoscopy was performed. The findings on laryngoscopy were consistent with PVCM. The patient was counseled in the emergency department on ways to improve her airflow and symptoms subsided over the next hour. The patient spent 2 days in the hospital, experiencing only 1 mild episode of dyspnea during the period of observation.

The findings on laryngoscopy are diagnostic of PVCM. Except for ACE inhibitor therapy, there is little evidence or history supporting angioedema; the patient has no facial swelling, and there are no findings on laryngoscopy.

Treatment of PVCM

A. There are no controlled trials of treatments for PVCM.

B. Speech therapy, concentrating on laryngeal relaxation seems to be the most effective therapy.

C. Psychiatric intervention is suggested for patients with psychiatric illness.

D. Acute attacks may be quite hard to manage.

1. Helium oxygen mixtures have been suggested to obtain better flow through the narrowed larynx.

2. Instructing the patient to lay his tongue on the floor of the mouth and breath through pursed lips may also help.

Differential Diagnosis and Treatment of Angioedema

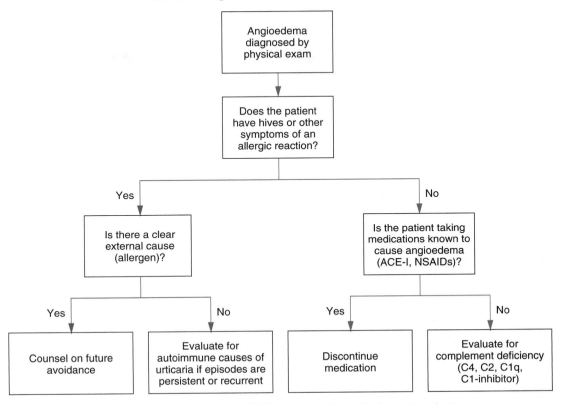

ACE-I, angiotensin-converting enzyme inhibitors; NSAIDs, nonsteroidal anti-inflammatory drugs.

Figure 23–2.

CHIEF COMPLAINT

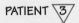

Mr. S is a 50-year-old man who arrives at the emergency department with sore throat, fever, and wheezing. He reports being well until 2 days ago when his sore throat started. Over the next 2 days, the sore throat became progressively more severe and he lost his voice. On the morning of admission he measured a fever of 38.0 °C and wheezing. He was also unable to eat because of the pain. He has never had similar symptoms before.

At this point, what is the leading hypothesis, and what are the active alternatives? What other tests should be ordered?

ORGANIZING THE DIFFERENTIAL DIAGNOSIS

Mr. S has an acute illness that is most likely infectious in nature. The symptoms are not recurrent making asthma, the most common cause of airway obstruction, unlikely. Acute infectious causes need to be considered first. These include common conditions such as pharyngitis and rare but serious causes such as epiglottitis and retropharyngeal abscess. Angioedema is a possibility, but the infectious symptoms (fever and pain) and the lack of visible swelling make this less likely. Aspiration of a foreign body could cause either a pneumonia or infection of the soft tissues of the neck resulting in fever. However, the history would be more suspicious. Table 23–6 lists the differential diagnosis.

On physical exam, Mr. S is in obvious distress. He is uncomfortable, is sitting upright, and speaks in a muffled voice. His vitals signs are temperature, 38.3 °C; pulse, 110 bpm; BP, 128/88 mm Hg; RR, 18 breaths per minute. Exam of the oropharynx is notable only for mild tonsillar edema without exudates. There is diffuse cervical lymphadenopathy and significant tenderness over the anterior neck. The neck is supple. Lungs are clear, but there is stridor transmitted from the neck.

Is the clinical information sufficient to make a diagnosis? If not, what other information do you need?

The patient's physical exam makes pharyngitis a less likely cause of his symptoms. His pharynx is patent, and there is more distal stridor.

Leading Hypothesis: Epiglottitis

Textbook Presentation

Fever and sore throat are usually the presenting symptoms. There can be evidence of varying degrees of airway obstruction including wheezing, stridor, and drooling. The disease has become significantly less common in children since the use of the *Haemophilus* vaccine.

Disease Highlights

A. Epiglottitis is an infectious disease, classically caused by *Haemophilus influenzae* that causes swelling of the epiglottis and supraglottic structures.

B. Can rapidly cause airway compromise so the diagnosis is always considered an airway emergency.

C. Classic presentation is a patient with sore throat, muffled "hot potato" voice, drooling, and stridor.

D. *H influenzae* is cultured in only a minority of adult patients; respiratory viruses are the likely cause of most cases of epiglottitis.

E. Epiglottitis is a difficult diagnosis because initial presentation is often identical to pharyngitis.

Evidence-Based Diagnosis

A. The gold standard for diagnosis is visual identification of swelling of the epiglottis.

   1. Can be done with direct or indirect laryngoscopy.

Table 23–6. Diagnostic hypotheses for Mr. S.

Diagnostic Hypotheses	Clinical Clues	Important Tests
Leading Hypothesis		
Pharyngitis	Sore throat often with fever, exudates and lymphadenopathy	Clinical exam Throat culture
Active Alternative—Must Not Miss		
Epiglottitis	Sore throat with muffled voice, stridor, and anterior neck tenderness	Direct visualization with laryngoscopy
Retropharyngeal abscess	Similar to epiglottitis with more prominent neck symptoms (stiff, painful)	Lateral neck x-ray or CT scan of the neck
Other Alternative		
Foreign body aspiration	Usually history of acute-onset pain or airway obstruction	Documentation of foreign body directly or radiographically

2. In patients with signs of severe disease (eg, muffled voice, drooling, and stridor), an experienced physician should perform direct laryngoscopy and be prepared to insert an endotracheal tube or perform a tracheostomy (if airway control cannot be obtained).

B. The classic symptoms of muffled voice, drooling, and stridor are seen very rarely and signify imminent airway obstruction.

1. Sitting erect and stridor are independent predictors of subsequent airway intervention (RRs of 4.8 and 6.2 respectively).

2. In 1 study, patients requiring intubation were sitting erect at presentation 47% of the time and stridor was present 42% of the time. In patients not requiring intubation, 10% were sitting erect and stridor was present in only 6%.

C. Common symptoms and signs of patients with epiglottitis are as shown in Table 23–7.

D. Lateral neck films, a commonly used diagnostic tool, have a sensitivity of about 90%. The classic finding is the "thumb sign" of a swollen epiglottis.

 A normal lateral neck film does not rule out epiglottitis. Laryngoscopy should be performed in a patient with a high clinical suspicion of epiglottitis, even if the neck film is normal.

Table 23–7. Prevalence of the signs and symptoms of epiglottitis.

Symptoms and Signs	Frequency
Sore throat	95%
Odynophagia	94%
Muffled voice	54%
Pharyngitis	44%
Fever	42%
Cervical adenopathy	41%
Dyspnea	37%
Drooling	30%
Sitting erect	16%
Stridor	12%

Reproduced from Frantz TD, Rasgon BM, Quesenberry CP Jr. Acute epiglottitis in adults. Analysis of 129 cases. *JAMA.* 1994;272:1358–1360. Copyright © 1994. American Medical Association. All rights reserved.

MAKING A DIAGNOSIS

Mr. S's history is very concerning. His upright posture, voice changes, and stridor are not only indicative of epiglottitis but also for imminent airway closure. None of these findings would be seen with pharyngitis, and a foreign-body aspiration does not fit the history. Retropharyngeal abscess remains a possibility.

 Given the concern for epiglottitis, lateral neck films were obtained, and an otolaryngologist was called to examine the patient's upper airway.

 Have you crossed a diagnostic threshold for the leading hypothesis, epiglottitis? Have you ruled out the active alternatives? Do other tests need to be done to exclude the alternative diagnoses?

Alternative Diagnosis: Retropharyngeal Abscess

Textbook Presentation

Retropharyngeal abscess can be seen in either children or adults. Patients usually have symptoms similar to those seen in epiglottitis but commonly have a history of a recent upper respiratory infection or trauma from recently ingested materials (bones), or procedures (pulmonary or GI endoscopy).

Disease Highlights

A. Symptoms can sometimes help differentiate retropharyngeal abscess from epiglottitis.

B. Patients with retropharyngeal abscesses often will sense a lump in their throat.

C. Patients are often most comfortable supine with neck extended (very different from epiglottitis).

Evidence-Based Diagnosis

A. The diagnosis of retropharyngeal abscess is made when a thickening of the retropharyngeal tissues is seen on lateral neck films.

B. Plain films are probably not 100% sensitive, so when films are normal and clinical suspicion is high, CT scanning should be done to verify the diagnosis.

Treatment

A. Retropharyngeal abscesses are usually polymicrobial.

B. Treatment is both medical and surgical.

1. Surgical drainage should be accomplished as soon as possible.

2. Many antibiotics have been suggested. Coverage of gram-positive organisms and anaerobes make clindamycin a common choice.

CASE RESOLUTION

The patient's lateral neck film showed probable acute epiglottitis with a thumb sign. An otolaryngologist visualized the epiglottis and, given the patient's symptoms and severity of the visualized airway obstruction, placed an endotracheal tube. Mr. S was admitted to the ICU and treated with a second-generation cephalosporin. Blood and epiglottis cultures were negative.

The patient's infection was diagnosed on the lateral neck films. Evaluation by an otolaryngologist and intubation were necessary because of the patient's signs and symptoms of airway obstruction and the actual obstruction visualized on laryngoscopy.

Treatment of Epiglottitis

A. Airway control

1. All patients should be admitted to the ICU for close monitoring.

2. Patients with signs or symptoms of airway obstruction should be intubated electively.

3. Elective intubation is preferred because intubation in a patient with epiglottitis can be very difficult.

4. Some advocate prophylactic intubation of all patients.

 Epiglottitis is an airway emergency. Patients need to monitored extremely closely and not left alone until the airway is stable.

B. Antibiotics

1. Necessary to cover *H influenzae*.

2. Second- and third-generation cephalosporins are usually recommended.

CHIEF COMPLAINT

Mrs. A is 52-year-old woman who comes to your office with shortness of breath and wheezing. She reports that her symptoms have been present for about 2 years. She reports almost constant, mild dyspnea that is worst with exercise or when she has a cold. Only rarely does she feel "nearly normal." She also complains of a mild cough productive of clear sputum. She does not feel that her cough is much of a problem as it is significantly better since she stopped smoking 2 years ago.

 At this point, what is the leading hypothesis, and what are the active alternatives? What other tests should be ordered?

ORGANIZING THE DIFFERENTIAL DIAGNOSIS

Because of the patient's chronic dyspnea and wheezing, as well as her smoking history, COPD and asthma should be high in the differential diagnosis. CHF is also a possibility. The patient's smoking history is a risk factor for coronary disease, the most common cause of CHF, and she suffers from nearly constant dyspnea that is worse with exertion. Bronchiectasis could cause symptoms of dyspnea, cough, and sputum production, but the patient's sputum production seems to be a minor symptom, unlike what is usually seen in bronchiectasis. Tuberculosis should probably be considered in the differential. Tuberculosis can cause chronic cough and dyspnea. Given the chronic nature of the symptoms, if tuberculosis were the cause, we would expect to hear about weight loss and other constitutional signs. Table 23–8 lists the differential diagnosis.

Mrs. A. reports a 60 pack-year history of smoking. She stopped 2 years ago, after smoking 2 packs a day for 30 years, when her chronic cough began to worry her. She reports that she still coughs but only rarely brings up sputum.

She has not experienced fever, chills, weight loss, or peripheral edema. She does say that when her breathing is bad it is worse when lying down. She has never had symptoms consistent with paroxysmal nocturnal dyspnea.

Orthopnea is a very nonspecific symptom. It is found in many types of cardiopulmonary disease.

Is the clinical information sufficient to make a diagnosis? If not, what other information do you need?

Leading Hypothesis: COPD

Textbook Presentation

Presenting symptoms of COPD include progressive dyspnea, decreased exercise tolerance, cough, and sputum production. The onset is usually slow and progressive with occasional acute exacerbations. A long smoking history is present in almost all patients with COPD who live in industrialized countries.

Disease Highlights

A. COPD is defined in the WHO/NHLBI Global Strategy for the Diagnosis, Management, and Prevention of Chronic Obstructive Pulmonary Disease as a "disease state characterized by airflow limitation that is not fully reversible. The airflow limitation is usually both progressive and associated with an abnormal inflammatory response of the lungs to noxious particles or gases."

Table 23–8. Diagnostic hypotheses for Mrs. A.

Diagnostic Hypotheses	Clinical Clues	Important Tests
Leading Hypothesis		
COPD	Chronic irreversible airway obstruction with a smoking history	Spirometry and sometimes imaging
Active Alternative—Most Common		
Asthma	Episodic and reversible airflow obstruction	Peak flow PFTs Methacholine challenge Response to treatment
Active Alternative—Must Not Miss		
CHF	Presence of risk factors and consistent physical exam findings	Echocardiography
Other Alternative		
Bronchiectasis	Chronic, heavy, purulent sputum production	CT scan of the chest

B. COPD should be considered in any patient with a smoking history who has pulmonary complaints. These complaints can be:

1. Mild (smokers' cough or lingering colds)

2. Moderate (chronic cough, sputum production, and dyspnea)

3. Severe (activity-limiting dyspnea with life-threatening exacerbations)

C. COPD can also be seen in patients without a smoking history but with significant exposure to second-hand smoke, occupational dust and chemicals and, especially in less developed countries, indoor air pollution from cooking stoves.

D. Because of the wide variation in disease course, it is impossible to give an average amount of exposure necessary to cause disease.

1. Pulmonary symptoms usually develop after about 10 years of exposure.

2. Airflow obstruction may develop later.

E. Diagnosis of early, minimally symptomatic COPD is important because it may allow for more appropriate treatment of mild symptoms (cough) and may provide extra incentive for smoking cessation.

F. Emphysema and chronic bronchitis are currently being used less as descriptors of types of COPD.

1. Emphysema is a pathologic term not accurately correlating with its general clinical usage.

2. Chronic bronchitis is the presence of mucus production for most days of the month, 3 months of a year, for 2 successive years. This symptom does not relate to the airflow obstruction that causes the morbidity in COPD.

3. Due to the overlap and lack of specificity of these 2 terms, COPD should be used as the diagnostic term.

G. Two staging systems provide a way of categorizing patients by symptoms and prognosis.

1. The WHO/NHLBI outlines stages of COPD (Table 23–9) that are useful for both diagnosis and management of patients. They are based mainly on spirometry and are thus very easy to use.

2. Other indices, such as the recently published BODE index, take into account other patient features, such as body mass index, degree of dyspnea, and exercise tolerance, and are very useful prognostically.

Evidence-Based Diagnosis

A. The diagnosis of COPD is based on history, physical exam, and ancillary tests (primarily spirometry). The diagnosis is clinical, based on a history of pulmonary complaints, exposure to a causative agent (usually cigarette smoke) and, at least in the later stages of disease, airflow obstruction.

B. History

1. History is important in all patients but is crucial in patients with mild disease in whom spirometry is unlikely to be helpful.

2. Important symptoms are:

Table 23–9. WHO/NHLBI stages of COPD.

Stage	Spirometry	Symptoms
0 At Risk	Normal	Chronic cough and sputum production
1 Mild COPD	$FEV_1/FVC < 70\%$ $FEV_1 > 80\%$	Chronic cough and sputum production often without dyspnea
2A Moderate COPD	$FEV_1 = 50\text{-}80\%$	Chronic dyspnea possibly with intermittent exacerbations
2B Moderate COPD	$FEV_1 = 30\text{-}50\%$	Chronic dyspnea probably with intermittent exacerbations
3 Severe COPD	$FEV_1 < 30\%$	Also may be diagnosed with $PaO_2 < 60$ mm Hg, $PaCO_2 > 50$ mm Hg or cor pulmonale

COPD, chronic obstructive pulmonary disease; FEV_1/FVC, forced expiratory volume in 1 second/forced vital capacity.
Pauwels RA, Buist AS, Calverley PM, Jenkins CR, Hurd SS. Global strategy for the diagnosis, management, and prevention of chronic obstructive pulmonary disease. NHLBI/WHO Global Initiative for Chronic Obstructive Lung Disease (GOLD) Workshop summary. *Am J Respir Crit Care Med.* 2001;163:1256–1276.

a. Smoker's cough

b. Lingering colds

c. Chronic cough

d. Sputum production

e. Dyspnea

f. Decreased exercise tolerance

C. Physical exam

1. The physical exam is useful mainly in patients with more advanced disease.

2. No findings are sensitive enough to exclude a diagnosis of COPD.

3. The test characteristics for some of the physical exam findings are listed in Table 23–10.

 The absence of wheezing does not rule out, or significantly decrease the likelihood of, COPD.

D. Spirometry

1. Because the results of spirometry are part of the information required to make a diagnosis of COPD, there is no good data on their test characteristics.

2. For the diagnosis of COPD, the most important spirometric values are postbronchodilator, since COPD is defined by irreversible airway obstruction.

3. In general, spirometry is significantly more useful in patients with more advanced disease and is most helpful when used with other clinical findings.

4. Typically spirometry in COPD reveals:

a. Increased total lung capacity secondary to air trapping

b. Decreased FEV_1 and FVC due to airflow obstruction

5. The test characteristics for spirometry, alone and in combination with clinical findings, in a middle-aged smoker are listed in Table 23–11.

E. Other tests

1. Spirometry with bronchodilator response

a. Recommended to rule out asthma. Patients with completely reversible airflow obstruction likely have asthma.

b. Also helpful in gauging the response to treatment and the prognosis. Patients with greater airflow reversibility have a better prognosis.

2. Chest x-ray is generally not useful in diagnosing COPD.

a. Some findings are suggestive

(1) Upper lobe bullous disease (least common but almost diagnostic)

(2) Flattened diaphragm on the lateral chest film

(3) Large retrosternal air space

(4) Hyperlucency of the lungs

(5) Diminished distal vascular markings

b. Chest film is always recommended to rule out other causes of symptoms.

3. ABG measurement is recommended in patients with $FEV_1 < 40\%$ predicted or with right heart failure.

4. Testing for α_1-antitrypsin deficiency (a rare cause of COPD) is recommended in patients:

a. In whom COPD develops before age 45 years

Table 23–10. Test characteristics for physical exam findings in COPD.

Criteria	Sensitivity	Specificity	LR+	LR−
Subxiphoid cardiac impulse	4–27%	97–99%	≈ 8	≈ 1
Absent cardiac dull LLSB	15	99	15	≈ 1
Diaphragmatic excursion < 2 cm	13	98	6.5	≈ 1
Early inspiratory crackles	25–77	97–98	8–38.5	≈ 1
Any unforced wheeze	13–56	86–99	1–56	≈ 1

COPD, chronic obstructive pulmonary disease; LLSB, left lower sternal border.

Modified from McGee SR. Evidence-based Physical Diagnosis. Philadelphia, PA: Saunders, 2001:382. With permission from Elsevier.

Table 23–11. Test characteristics for spirometry in a middle-aged smoker.

Criteria	Sensitivity	Specificity	LR+	LR−
FEV$_1$	10–40%	90%	1–4	0.7–1.0
FEV$_1$/FVC	20–50	90	2–5	0.6–0.9
History of bronchitis or emphysema, > 70 pack-year history, decreased breath sounds	67	98	33.5	0.34

FEV$_1$/FVC, forced expiratory volume in 1 second/forced vital capacity.
Adapted from Black ER. Diagnostic strategies for common medical problems. Philadelphia: American College of Physicians, 1999:362.

b. Who do not have a smoking history or suspicious exposure

In general, any patient with a smoking history who complains of chronic cough, sputum production, or dyspnea should be considered to have COPD if no other diagnosis can be made. Additional testing can help establish the diagnosis and assess severity.

MAKING A DIAGNOSIS

On the physical exam, Mrs. A appears well. Her vital signs are normal. The only findings on lung exam are decreased breath sounds and a slightly prolonged expiratory phase. Her chest x-ray is normal. Some of the results of her PFTs are shown in Table 23–12.

Have you crossed a diagnostic threshold for the leading hypothesis, COPD? Have you ruled out the active alternatives? Do other tests need to be done to exclude the alternative diagnoses?

The patient's history and physical exam is certainly consistent with the diagnosis of COPD. She has a smoking history, persistent cough, and dyspnea. Her physical exam reveals findings of decreased breath sounds. The chest film does not argue for another diagnosis.

Her PFTs are also supportive of the diagnosis. Most importantly there is an irreversible decrease in airflow. The severity of disease is surprising given the patient's mild symptoms. The low DLCO (carbon monoxide diffusing capacity), suggesting loss of a portion of the Hgb/air interface, and lack of response to bronchodilators portend a poor prognosis.

Asthma and CHF, the alternative diagnoses, are very unlikely. The irreversibility of the airway disease excludes asthma as a potential cause. The lack of purulent sputum excludes bronchiectasis. CHF remains a much less likely possibility because it often causes an elevated DLCO. The PFTs also do not support a diagnosis of CHF.

Alternative Diagnosis: Bronchiectasis

Textbook Presentation

Dyspnea and chronic, purulent sputum production are usually present in patients with bronchiectasis. There is usually a history of a chronic infection that has led to airway destruction.

Disease Highlights

A. Chronic sputum production is the hallmark of the clinical presentation of bronchiectasis.

B. The disease is caused by the combination of an airway infection and an inability to clear this infection because of impaired immunity or anatomic abnormality (congenital or acquired). Bronchiectasis can be the result of common (viral infection) or rare (Kartagener syndrome) underlying diseases.

  1. Pertussis and tuberculosis were the classic causes of bronchiectasis.

  2. Some of the common causes now are:

    a. Postviral, often with lymphadenopathy causing airway obstruction

    b. *Aspergillus fumigatus,* mainly in association with allergic bronchopulmonary aspergillosis

    c. *Mycobacterium avium* complex infection, usually causing middle lobe disease

Table 23–12. Pulmonary function test results for Mrs. A.

| Test | Prebronchodilator | | Postbronchodilator | |
	Result	% of Predicted	Result	% Change
Total lung capacity (L)	6.92	128		
Forced vital capacity (L)	3.03	91	2.90	−4.0
FEV$_1$ (L)	1.03	43	1.00	−4.0
FEV$_1$/FVC (%)	34	NA	34	0
DLCO (mL/min/mm Hg)	50			

FEV$_1$/FVC, forced expiratory volume in 1 second/forced vital capacity; DLCO, carbon monoxide diffusing capacity of the lungs.

    d. Cystic fibrosis

    e. HIV

C. The most common bacteria isolated from the sputum of people with bronchiectasis are *H influenzae, Pseudomonas aeruginosa,* and *Streptococcus pneumoniae.*

D. Complications of the disease include hemoptysis and rarely amyloidosis, given the chronic levels of inflammation.

Evidence-Based Diagnosis

A. The diagnosis of bronchiectasis depends on recognizing the clinical symptoms (chronic sputum production) and demonstrating airway destruction, usually by high-resolution CT scanning.

B. Symptoms and their prevalence

    1. Dyspnea and wheezing, 75%

    2. Pleuritic chest pain, 50%

C. Signs and their prevalence

    1. Crackles, 70%

    2. Wheezing, 34%

D. Differentiation of bronchiectasis from COPD can sometimes be difficult as both may present with cough, sputum production, dyspnea, and airflow limitation. Important points in the differentiation are as follows:

    1. Sputum production is heavy and chronic in bronchiectasis, while it is only truly purulent in COPD during exacerbations.

    2. There is usually a smoking history associated with COPD.

    3. Spirometry is not helpful since bronchiectasis can cause both airflow limitation and airway hyperreactivity.

    4. Imaging (CT scan) will show diagnostic airway changes in bronchiectasis. In COPD, imaging may or may not demonstrate parenchymal destruction.

Treatment

A. Antibiotics are used both to treat flares of disease and to suppress chronic infection.

B. Pulmonary hygiene

    1. Chest physiotherapy

    2. There may be a role for bronchodilators, mucolytics, and anti-inflammatory medication.

C. Surgery is mainly used to treat airway obstruction, to remove destroyed and chronically infected lung tissue, and to treat life-threatening hemoptysis.

CASE RESOLUTION

Given the minor role that sputum production plays in Mrs. A's disease, the diagnosis of COPD is nearly definite.

Mrs. A is given an ipratropium bromide inhaler, and she reports mild improvement in her symptoms. A month later, the medication was changed to an albuterol and ipratropium combination inhaler, which controlled her symptoms better. Four months later, she arrives at the emergency department with acute worsening of her symptoms at the time of an upper respiratory tract infection. She is admitted with an exacerbation of COPD.

Treatment of COPD

A. Management of stable disease

1. Nonpharmacologic and preventive therapy

   a. Smoking cessation or removal of other inhaled toxic agents

   b. Exercise programs if allowable from a cardiovascular standpoint

   c. Vaccination against influenza and pneumococcal pneumonia

2. Pharmacologic

   a. Ipratropium bromide

      (1) Mainstay of therapy

      (2) Initial therapy for symptomatic patients

      (3) Also recommended for patients with $FEV_1 < 50\%$ of predicted regardless of symptoms

   b. β-Agonists

      (1) Short-acting medications are useful if the patient's response to ipratropium is insufficient.

         (a) Can be used as-needed or on a scheduled basis

         (b) Combinations with ipratropium are useful

      (2) Long-acting medications are useful for treatment of nocturnal symptoms.

   c. Theophylline

      (1) May be used in patients with inadequate response to β-agonists and ipratropium

      (2) Narrow therapeutic window limits usefulness

   d. Inhaled corticosteroids

      (1) Use remains somewhat controversial

      (2) There is some evidence that inhaled corticosteroids decrease symptoms but do not effect rate of decline in pulmonary function.

   e. Home oxygen is recommended for persons with chronic hypoxia or cor pulmonale.

B. Management of exacerbations

1. Evaluation

   a. Patients who are likely to have the worst outcomes have low baseline FEV_1, PaO_2, pH, and high PCO_2. Discharge of such patients from an emergency department should be done with great care.

   b. All patients should have a chest x-ray to look for complicating illnesses, such as pneumonia.

   c. Unlike in the assessment of asthma exacerbations, spirometry is of little value in making admission decisions.

2. Therapy

   a. Ipratropium bromide should be given to all patients with addition of β-agonists if necessary.

   b. Systemic corticosteroids are effective when given for up to 2 weeks. There is no evidence that inhaled corticosteroids are effective.

3. Antibiotics are effective for more severe exacerbations. It is unclear which is the most effective antibiotic.

4. Oxygen therapy is beneficial.

   a. Oxygen does carry a risk of hypercapnea and respiratory failure.

   b. The development of respiratory failure is somewhat predictable.

   c. The following equation identifies patients who are at high risk for CO_2 retention and for requiring mechanical ventilation: $pH = 7.66 - 0.00919 \times PaO_2$. If the calculated pH is greater than the patients true pH, he is at high risk for being intubated. Sensitivity is $\cong 80\%$.

 If a patient with a COPD exacerbation requires oxygen, it should be provided and not withheld for fear of causing CO_2 retention. If respiratory failure does ensue, it is the fault of the COPD and not of the physician who administered the oxygen.

5. Noninvasive positive pressure ventilation (eg, bilevel positive airway pressure) decreases rates of intubation, length of stay, and in-hospital mortality in patients with severe exacerbation.

6. Mucolytics, theophylline, and chest physiotherapy have no role in the treatment of COPD exacerbations.

Diagnostic Approach: Wheezing and Stridor

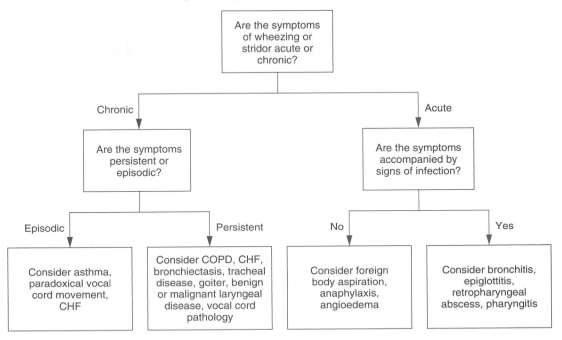

COPD, chronic obstructive pulmonary disease; CHF, congestive heart failure.

Figure 23–A.

Index

Page numbers followed by italic *f* or *t* denote figures or tables, respectively. Entries followed by *W* indicate topics that can be found on the Web at: www.symptomtodiagnosis.com.